Phlebotomy
Essentials

DISCARD

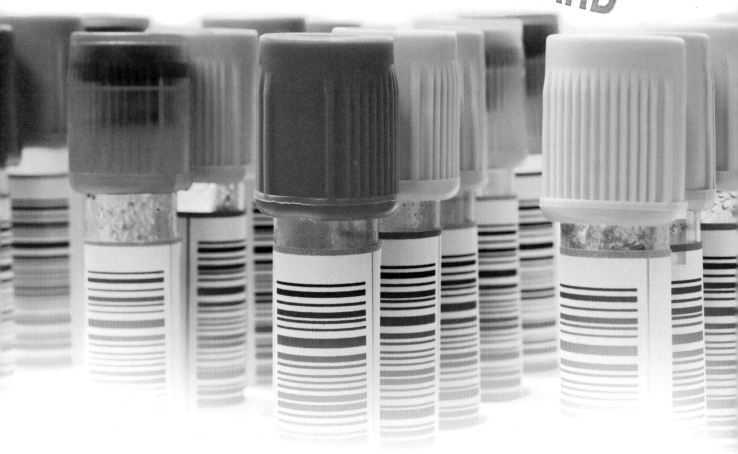

Ruth E. McCall, BS, MT (ASCP)
Retired Director of Phlebotomy and Clinical
    Laboratory Assistant Programs
Central New Mexico (CNM) Community College
Albuquerque, New Mexico

Cathee M. Tankersley, BS, MT (ASCP)
President, NuHealth Educators, LLC
Faculty Emeritus
Phoenix College
Phoenix, Arizona

Wolters Kluwer

Philadelphia • Baltimore • New York • London
Buenos Aires • Hong Kong • Sydney • Tokyo

Acquisitions Editor: Jonathan Joyce
Product Development Editor: Paula Williams
Editorial Assistant: Tish Rogers
Marketing Manager: Shauna Kelley
Production Project Manager: Marian Bellus
Design Coordinator: Terry Mallon
Artist/Illustrator: Jen Clements
Manufacturing Coordinator: Margie Orzech
Prepress Vendor: Aptara, Inc.

6th edition

© 2016 Wolters Kluwer

9 8 7 6 5 4 3 2

Printed in the United States of America

978-1-4511-9452-4
Library of Congress Cataloging-in-Publication Data
available upon request

LWW.com

To my husband John, for his love and patience; my sons Chris and Scott, and daughter-in-law Tracy, for their encouragement; my grandchildren Katie and Ryan for the joy they bring me; and to the memory of my parents Charles and Marie Ruppert, who taught me the value of perseverance.

Ruth E. McCall

To the memory of my wonderful husband, Earl Lynn Tankersley, whose unconditional love was the wind beneath my wings for 50 years.

Cathee M. Tankersley

Reviewers

The following reviewers provided valuable information and feedback during the updating of this edition of *Phlebotomy Essentials*. We thank all these professionals for their time, talent, and expertise.

Justin Abeyta, AS
Sr Clinical Laboratory Science Instructor
Lab Sciences
Arizona Medical Training Institute
Mesa, Arizona

Diana Alagna, RN
Medical Assistant Program Director
Medical Assisting
Stone Academy
Waterbury, Connecticut

Rhonda Anderson, PBT(ASCP)ᶜᵐ
Program Manager/Phlebotomy Instructor
Corporate and Career Development, Direct Care
Phlebotomy Program
Greenville Technical College
Greenville, South Carolina

Judy C. Arbique, MLT, ART(CSMLS), BHSc
Capital District Health Authority
Member CLSI G41 Document
Development Committee
Halifax, Nova Scotia, Canada

Belinda Beeman, CMA (AAMA), PBT(ASCP), MEd
Professor and Curriculum Coordinator
Medical Assisting
Goodwin College
East Hartford, Connecticut

Judith Blaney, MCLS
Phlebotomy Internship Coordinator
Allied Health
Manchester Community College
Manchester, New Hampshire

Kathy Bode, RN, BS, MS
Professor of Nursing Program
Allied Health Program Coordinator
Nursing and Allied Health
Flint Hills Technical College
Emporia, Kansas

Diane Butera, ASCP
CPT Instructor
Phlebotomy
Fortis Institute
Wayne, New Jersey

Marie Chouest, LPN
LPN Instructor
Health Sciences
Northshore Technical Community College
Bogalusa, Louisiana

Becky M. Clark, MEd, MT(ASCP)
Professor
Medical Laboratory Technology
J. Sargeant Reynolds Community College
Richmond, Virginia

Kelly Collins, MA, CPT1
Teacher
Allied Health
Tulare Adult School
Tulare, California

Silvia de la Fuente, MA, AHI
Phlebotomy Instructor
Allied Health Institute
Medical Programs and Phlebotomy
Estrella Mountain Community College
Avondale, Arizona

Desiree DeLeon, ASCP(PBT)ᶜᵐ, RN
RN Phlebotomy Instructor
Medical Lab Sciences
Central New Mexico Community College
Albuquerque, New Mexico

Mary Doshi, MA, MLS(ASCP)
Associate Professor/MLT Program Director
Medical Technology
San Juan College
Farmington, New Mexico

Amy Eady, MT(ASCP), MS(CTE), RMA
Director of Allied Health
Allied Health
Montcalm Community College
Sidney, Michigan

Kathleen Fowle, CPT
Certified Phlebotomist and Instructor
Pinellas Technical College
St. Joseph's Hospital
Clearwater, Florida

Tammy Gallagher, MT(ASCP)
Lead Phlebotomy Instructor
Emergency Medical Services
Butler County Community College
Butler, Pennsylvania

Faye Hamrac, MT, MS, BS
Phlebotomy Instructor
Health Sciences/Phlebotomy
Reid State Technical College
Evergreen, Alabama

Jacqueline Harris, CMA (AAMA), AHI (AMT)
Allied Health Program Chair
Medical Assisting, HCA, Medical Lab Tech
Wright Career College
Wichita, Kansas

Ronald Hedger, DO
Associate Professor of Primary Care
Clinical Education
Touro University Nevada
Henderson, Nevada

Angela Hernandez, LPN II
Adjunct Professor
Phlebotomy/Medical Assisting/Health Science Careers
University of New Mexico Continuing Education
Albuquerque, New Mexico

Eleanor Hooley, MT (ASCP)
Educator
Allied Health Department
Vancouver Community College
Vancouver, BC, Canada

Jamie Horn, RMA, RPT, AHI
Medical Instructor
Medical Programs
Warren County Career Center
Warren, Pennsylvania

Bob Kaplanis, PBT, MT(ASCP)
Systems Technical Director - POCT
Laboratory Sciences of Arizona/Banner Health
Laboratory Sciences of Arizona/Sonora Quest
  Laboratories
Tempe, Arizona

Konnie King Briggs, CCT, CCI; PBT(ASCP); CPCI, ACA
Healthcare Instructor
Healthcare Continuing Education
Houston Community College
Houston, Texas

Theresa Kittle, CPT
Adjunct Instructor
Healthcare
Rockford Career College
Rockford, Illinois

Judy Kline, NCMA, RMA
Medical Assistant Instructor
Health Science Medical Assisting
Miami Lakes Technical Education Center
Miami Lakes, Florida

Anne-Marie Martel, MT
Vice-chairholder
CLSI G41 Document Development Committee
  Scientific Affairs
Ordre Professionnel Des Technologistes
  Medicaux Du Quebec
Montreal, Quebec, Canada

Peggy Mayo, MEd
Associate Professor
Multi-Competency Health Technology
Columbus State Community College
Columbus, Ohio

Andrea Minaya, MA, CPT
MA/CPT Lab Assistant and CPT Administrator
Medical Assistant and Certified Phlebotomy
  Technician
Fortis Institute
Wayne, New Jersey

Linda Pace, CMA, CPC-A
Director, Medical Assisting/Phlebotomy
Medical Assisting and Phlebotomy
Red Rocks Community College
Lakewood, Colorado

Nicole Palmieri, BSN, RN; CCMA, CPT, CET, CPCT
Instructor
Medical Assistant, Phlebotomy, Cardiac/EKG
Patient Care Technician
Advantage Career Institute
Eatontown, New Jersey

Paula Phelps, RMA
Online Education Coordinator
Allied Health
Cowley County Community College
Arkansas City, Kansas

Deyal Riley, CPT, CHI(NHA)
Instructor
Healthcare
Washtenaw Community College
Ann Arbor, Michigan

Ann Robinson, BS, MA, RPBT, LPN
Laboratory Coordinator
Phlebotomy, CNA, RMA, Surg Tech, LPN
Sports Medication
Tulsa Technology Center
Tulsa, Oklahoma

Kristie Rose, MA, PBT(ASCP), CMP
Program Manager/Instructor
Phlebotomy-Health Sciences
Eastern Florida State College
Cocoa, Florida

Diana Ross, RPT(AMT)
Career Services Coordinator
Pima Medical Institute
Mesa, Arizona

Suzanne Rouleau, MSN, RN, HHS
Educator
Allied Health
Manchester Community College
Manchester, Connecticut

Michael Simpson, BA, MS, MT(ASCP)
Clinical Laboratory Instructor
Clinical Laboratory Science
College of Southern Nevada
Clark County, Nevada

Maria V. Suto, BA, CPT
Faculty
Medical Assisting/Certified Phlebotomy Technician
Fortis Institute
Wayne, New Jersey

Phillip Tate, DA
Author, Anatomy & Physiology
Lubbock, TX

Joseph Tharrington, CPT1, CPT2, CPT (AMT) RPT, MA
Northern & Central Coast Regional
Director/Instructor
Phlebotomy, Medical Assisting
Academy Education Services (DBA) Clinical
  Training Institute
Santa Maria, California

Tina Veith, MA
Phlebotomy Instructor
Phlebotomy
Allied Health Careers Institute
Murfreesboro, Tennessee

Janet Vittori, BS, MT(ASCP)
POC Specialist
HonorHealth John C Lincoln Medical Center
Phoenix, Arizona

Amy Vogel, MHA
Program Director, Phlebotomy Technician
Allied Health
Harrisburg Area Community College
Harrisburg, Pennsylvania

Sharon F. Whetten, MEd, BS, MT(ASCP)
Education Coordinator
TriCore Reference Laboratories
Albuquerque, New Mexico

Kari Williams, BS, DC
Director, Medical Office Technology Program
Medical Office Technology
Front Range Community College
Westminster, Colorado

Rebecca C. Wilkins, MS, MT(ASCP), SM(ASCP)
Part-time Faculty Instructor
Health Science—MLT/Phlebotomy Program
San Juan College
Farmington, New Mexico

About the Authors

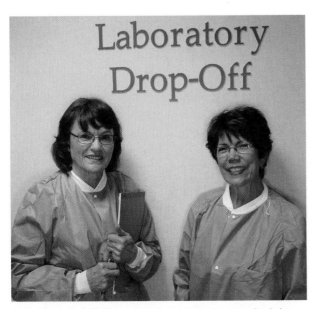

Ruth E. McCall (left) and Cathee M. Tankersley (right).

Ruth McCall received her bachelor's degree from the University of Iowa and her medical technology certificate from Saint Joseph's School of Medical Technology in Phoenix, Arizona, and has worked or taught in the area of Clinical Laboratory Sciences and Health Care Education since 1969. Ruth retired from her position as Director of the Phlebotomy and Clinical Laboratory Assistant Programs after 18 years of teaching in the Health, Wellness and Public Safety Department at Central New Mexico (CNM) Community College. While at CNM Ruth was instrumental in the creation and development of the Clinical Laboratory Assistant Program, and helped it become one of the first programs at CNM offered entirely through distance education. Ruth participated with science instructors from a local high school in a program that introduced the students to health careers and was the first CNM phlebotomy instructor to teach phlebotomy to high school students through concurrent enrollment. She has lectured on phlebotomy topics at conferences throughout the United States, served as an expert witness in phlebotomy injury cases, and especially enjoyed participating in a medical technology exchange trip to China. Most recently Ruth had the privilege of being a member of the CLSI Working Group

charged with the sixth revision of the H3 (now GP41) Venipuncture Standard, and the working group that updated the sixth revision of the H4 (now GP42) Capillary Puncture Standard. She was most recently a contributor to the committee working on the seventh edition of the GP41 Venipuncture Standard.

Ruth loves the outdoors. She enjoys hiking in the beautiful southwest, downhill skiing in the mountains of Colorado, and walks along the ocean in Cocoa Beach, Florida. She has been married for over 48 years to her husband, John, and has two sons, Christopher and Scott. Christopher and his wife Tracy are parents of her fantastic grandchildren, Katie and Ryan.

Cathee Tankersley recently retired as Faculty Emeritus after 27 years of teaching at Phoenix College in the Health Enhancement Department. She has worked or taught in the area of Clinical Laboratory Sciences and Health Care Education since graduating from New Mexico State University in Medical Technology in 1964. Cathee has been active in many professional organizations since she became a medical technologist. She has served on many committees at the state and national level. While at St. Joseph's Hospital and Medical Center, she was the Director of the Medical Technology Program during her last 2 years at that facility. Her tenure at Phoenix College has been as Clinical Coordinator for the MLT Program, Director of the EKG and EEG Programs, and as the Phlebotomy Program Director from 1982 until 2006. While at PC, she established one of the first accredited phlebotomy programs in the United States. In 2000, she developed and directed the first and at present, the only college-based Law Enforcement Phlebotomy Program in the United States. In 2010, she worked with the Arizona Governor's Office of Highway Safety to maintain current curricular materials for law enforcement phlebotomy and helped to prepare it for dissemination to other states.

Cathee served on the initial National Credentialing Agency for Laboratory Personnel (NCA) Phlebotomy Certification Committee as chair from 1983 to 1985. She was one of the original six members of the National Accrediting Agency for Clinical Laboratory Sciences (NAACLS) Approval Committee for Phlebotomy Programs in 1985. She went on to serve as the chair of that committee from 1993 to 1995. Since 1997 when she established her company, NuHealth Educators, LLC, she has been a healthcare educator and consultant for several organizations. She has served as an expert witness in the area of phlebotomy techniques and has lectured at numerous conferences across the United States.

Ruth and Cathee have collaborated for over 25 years on textbook writing and as presenters at national and state conferences.

Family is very important to Cathee and she feels very fortunate to have her two children, Todd and Jaime, and daughter-in-law, Chris and two wonderful grandsons, Trevor and Connor in Phoenix where they help her keep her life in balance and in joy.

Preface

Phlebotomy Essentials, sixth edition, was written for all who want to correctly and safely practice phlebotomy. The authors have over 70 years of combined experience in laboratory sciences, phlebotomy program direction, and teaching many different levels and diverse populations of phlebotomy students. As with previous editions, the goal of *Phlebotomy Essentials*, sixth edition, is to provide accurate, up-to-date, and practical information and instruction in phlebotomy procedures and techniques, along with a comprehensive background in phlebotomy theory and principles. It is appropriate for use as an instructional text or as a reference for those who wish to update skills or study for national certification.

Organization

Much care has been taken to present the material in a clear and concise manner that encourages learning and promotes comprehension. A good deal of time was spent organizing and formatting the information into a logical and student-friendly reading style in an order that allows the reader to build on information from previous chapters.

The book is divided into four units. Unit I, The Healthcare Setting, presents a basic description of the healthcare system and the role of the phlebotomist within it. Major topics include communication skills, healthcare financing, and delivery with an emphasis on clinical laboratory services, quality assurance, and legal issues and their relationship to the standard of care, and comprehensive instruction in infection control and safety.

Unit II, Overview of the Human Body, provides a foundation in medical terminology and a basic understanding of each of the body systems, including associated disorders and diagnostic tests. An entire chapter is devoted to the circulatory system, with special emphasis on the vascular system, including blood vessel structure, vascular anatomy of the arm, and blood composition.

Unit III, Blood Collection Procedures, describes phlebotomy equipment (including the latest safety equipment and order of draw) and proper procedures and techniques for collecting venipuncture and capillary specimens based upon the latest CLSI standards. Also included is an extensive explanation of preanalytical variables, complications, and procedural errors associated with blood collection.

Unit IV, Special Procedures, offers information and instruction on how to handle special blood and nonblood specimen collections and the latest in point-of-care instruments and testing. Routine and special handling and processing of specimens, with an emphasis on the latest rules of safety are described in this section. Included in this unit is an overview of the Laboratory Information System (LIS); how it supports the laboratory process and is an essential part of the network of healthcare communication. Also included is nonblood specimens and testing information, which can be an important part of phlebotomist's responsibilities, as well as arterial puncture for those phlebotomists who currently draw ABGs or who anticipate advancing beyond venous collection.

Features

The sixth edition includes various features meant to help the reader learn and retain the information in *Phlebotomy Essentials*.

- Brand new to this edition are the applicable **NAACLS competencies** listed at the beginning of each chapter to serve as an aid to the instructors of approved programs or programs seeking approval, and an assurance to students that they are learning material expected of a graduate of a phlebotomy program.

- **Key Terms** and **Objectives** head each chapter and help students recognize important terms and concepts they will come across while reading the chapter.

- Consistently organized step-by-step **Procedures** with an explanation or rationale for each step assist the student in learning and understanding phlebotomy techniques.

- More **Key Points** emphasize important concepts to enhance student learning and reinforce the significance of the stated information.

- **Cautions** highlight critical information to help students identify and avoid dangerous practices.

- **FYIs** add interesting notes and fun facts that will enhance practical application of the information.
- **Memory Joggers** offer a proven way to aid some students in remembering important information.
- More **Study and Review Questions** at the conclusion of each chapter provide a review of content covered in the chapter.
- New additional **Case studies** bring concepts to life and enhance critical thinking skills at the end of each chapter.
- A **Media Menu** at the end of each chapter points out online student resources available for that chapter.
- **Book icons** throughout the text refer readers *to Student Workbook for Phlebotomy Essentials* and *Phlebotomy Exam Review*, available for separate purchase, for further opportunities to enrich their learning.
- **Online icons** throughout the text refer readers to corresponding videos and animations on the book's companion website that bring the content to life (see "Additional Resources," below, for more information on these resources).

The content in this new edition of *Phlebotomy Essentials* was designed in accordance with applicable National Accrediting Agency for Clinical Laboratory Science (NAACLS) competencies. Procedures have been written to conform to the latest OSHA safety regulations and, wherever applicable, standards developed by the Clinical and Laboratory Standards Institute (CLSI).

Additional Resources

Phlebotomy Essentials, sixth edition, includes additional resources for both instructors and students that are available on the book's companion website at http://thepoint. lww.com/McCallPE6e.

INSTRUCTORS
Approved adopting instructors will be given access to the following additional resources:

- Lesson Plans
- Critical Thinking Questions
- Wimba Test Generator
- Image Collection
- Appendix D (from text)
- PowerPoint Slides with Images and Tables

- LMS Cartridges
- Signature Papers (i.e., HIPAA/confidentiality forms, bloodborne pathogen statements, assumption of risk form, health declaration form)
- Log Examples
- Lab Skills Evaluation Checklists (i.e., venipuncture, skin puncture, special test procedures)

STUDENTS
Students who have purchased *Phlebotomy Essentials*, sixth edition, have access to the following additional resources:

- Interactive games and exercises that offer a fun way to study and review. Exercise types include Look and Label, Word Building, Body Building, Roboterms, Interactive Crossword Puzzles, Quiz Show, and Concentration.
- 25 procedure videos
- Animations of key concepts
- Audio flash cards and a flash card generator
- An audio glossary

See the inside front cover of this text for more details, including the passcode you will need to gain access to the website.

Related Titles

The authors of this textbook have created the following two titles, available for separate purchase, that correspond to *Phlebotomy Essentials*, sixth edition, to create an ideal study package for phlebotomy training programs. Each corresponds to this main textbook in chapter sequence.

- Companion Workbook (available for separate purchase) provides students with chapter-by-chapter exercises to reinforce text material, assessment tools to evaluate their skills, realistic scenarios to gauge their grasp of key concepts, and skills logs to chart their progress. The Workbook includes key terms matching exercises, chapter review questions, crossword puzzles, skill and knowledge drills, requisition activities, case studies, and procedure evaluation forms.
- Companion Exam Review book (available for separate purchase) prepares students for all of the national certification exams in phlebotomy.

Acknowledgments

The authors sincerely wish to express their gratitude to the many individuals who gave of their time, talent, and expertise to make this edition of *Phlebotomy Essentials* current and accurate.

- Judy Arbique
- Katy Babcock
- David Berg
- Daven J. Byrd
- Theresa McGillvray-Dodd
- Irene Hales
- Joyce Hall
- Judy Herrig
- Angela Hernandez
- Glenda Hiddessen
- Tammy Jackson
- Scott Leece
- Anne-Marie Martel
- Charez Norris
- Phil Tate
- Jaime Tankersley
- Chris and Connor Tankersley
- Sharon Whetten

A special thanks to all the people at **Mayo Clinic and TriCore Laboratories**, especially Mary Gannon, Matt Jones, and Sharon Whetten.

And, sincere appreciation to our two contributing POCT experts,

- **Bob Kaplanis,** PBT, MT (ASCP) | System Technical Specialist—POCT | Banner Hospitals | Laboratory Sciences of Arizona/Sonora Quest Laboratories
- **Janet Vittori,** MT (ASCP), Point of Care Coordinator, Laboratory Supervisor, John C Lincoln Hospital, Phoenix, Arizona.

In addition, we would like to thank our illustrator Jonathan Dimes, and our photographers Bruce Knapus and John McCall.

Finally, we would like to thank *Acquisitions Editor* **Jonathan Joyce** and the production and editorial staff at Wolters Kluwer, especially those with whom we worked most closely, with a special thank you to *Product Development Editor* **Paula Williams**, *Creative Services Art Director* **Jennifer Clements** and *Supervisor of Product Development* **Eve Malakoff-Klein** for their patience, support, and dedication to this endeavor and an extra special thank you to Eve for stepping in and taking the lead when it was really needed. We also extend a special thank you to our compositor **Indu Jawwad** and her team at Aptara for their patience and professionalism as they brought together the many components of our texts.

Ruth E. McCall
Cathee M. Tankersley

Brief Contents

Detailed Contents

2   Quality Assurance and Legal Issues in Healthcare   35

UNIT II   OVERVIEW OF THE HUMAN BODY   101

4 Medical Terminology 103

UNIT III   BLOOD COLLECTION PROCEDURES   177

7   Blood Collection Equipment, Additives, and Order of Draw   179

8   Venipuncture Procedures   209

9 Preanalytical Considerations 263

10 Capillary Puncture Equipment and Procedures 293

UNIT IV   SPECIAL PROCEDURES   327

12 Computers and Specimen Handling and Processing   373

List of Procedures

User's Guide

Connecting Learning to Practice

Phlebotomists have a critical role within the healthcare system. At Wolters Kluwer, we believe your text should not only help you understand the critical tasks associated with your chosen profession, but also prepare you to step into the role of a practicing phlebotomist. This User's Guide provides a tour of the elements of *Phlebotomy Essentials* to help you do just that.

Laying the Foundation

To practice effectively, you need strong content understanding. Consistent chapter opening elements let you preview what each chapter has to offer.

NACCLS Competencies show you what you'll need to know on Day 1 of your first job.

Key Terms, listed at the beginning of each chapter and defined in the glossary, help you "talk the talk" of your profession.

Objectives provide a quick overview of the content covered within the chapter and what you're going to learn.

Chapter 14

Arterial Puncture Procedures

NAACLS Entry Level Competencies

3.6 Discuss the properties of arterial blood, venous blood, and capillary blood.

4.2 Describe the types of patient specimens that are analyzed in the clinical laboratory.

4.3 Define the phlebotomist's role in collecting and/or transporting these specimens to the laboratory.

6.00 Follow standard operating procedures to collect specimens.

Key Terms
Do Matching Exercise 14-1 in the WORKBOOK to gain familiarity with these terms.

abducted	brachial artery	FiO_2	steady state
ABGs	collateral	L/M	ulnar artery
Allen test	circulation	radial	
arteriospasm	femoral artery	artery	

Objectives

Upon successful completion of this chapter, the reader should be able to:

1 Demonstrate knowledge of practices, terminology, hazards, and complications related to arterial blood collection, and identify and analyze arterial puncture sites according to site-selection criteria and the advantages and disadvantages of each site.

2 Describe arterial blood gas (ABG) procedure including patient assessment and preparation, equipment and supplies, and commonly measured ABG parameters.

3 Perform the modified Allen test; explain how to interpret results and describe what to do based upon the results.

Enhancing Your Learning

Did you know that free, online resources can help you be more successful? Or that boxes within the text can make your studying easier? Don't overlook the tools we've built into this book to help you graduate with high marks, and a high level of confidence in your abilities!

Key Points highlight important concepts to help you study and ensure you carry your knowledge into the clinical setting.

 Key Point Adequate circulation via the ulnar artery must be verified before puncturing the radial artery. If ulnar blood flow is weak or absent, the radial artery should not be punctured.

Caution Boxes provide a heads-up about potential mistakes to help you avoid them.

CAUTION *Never* select a site in a limb with an AV shunt or fistula. It is a patient's lifeline for dialysis and should not be disturbed; also, venous and arterial blood mix together at the site.

Icons throughout the text let you know where related material in the workbook or exam review can help you practice putting what you've learned to work.

See the arm labeling exercise in WORKBOOK Labeling Exercise 14-1.

Memory Joggers help you to learn and provide for easy recall of key tips and facts long after you've entered the workplace.

 Memory Jogger The median nerve lies medial to the brachial artery, which lies medial to the biceps tendon. The order from lateral to medial can be remembered by the mnemonic TAN, where T stands for tendon, A for artery, and N for nerve.

FYI Boxes provide interesting, relevant information and add context to the materials you're learning.

 The radial pulse can be felt on the thumb side of the wrist approximately 1 in above the wrist crease.

Study and Review Questions

See the EXAM REVIEW for more study questions.

1. **The primary reason for performing arterial puncture is to**
   a. determine hemoglobin levels.
   b. evaluate blood gases.
   c. measure potassium levels.
   d. obtain calcium values.

2. **The first-choice location for performing arterial puncture is the**
   a. brachial artery.
   b. ulnar artery.
   c. femoral artery.
   d. radial artery.

3. **ABG supplies include**
   a. 18-gauge needles.
   b. heparinized syringes.
   c. tourniquets.
   d. all of the above.

4. **Commonly measured ABG parameters include**
   a. pH.
   b. $PaCO_2$.
   c. O_2 saturation.
   d. All of the above.

5. **A phlebotomist has a request to collect an ABG** ... **patient is breathing room** ... **tomist arrives to collect** ... **tient is still on a ventilator.** ... **ebotomist do?**
   a. ... ly supervisor and ask how to
   b. ... atient's nurse to determine
   c. Draw the ABG and note the oxygen setting on the request.
   d. Take the patient off the ventilator and draw the specimen.

6. **The purpose of the modified Allen test is to determine**
   a. blood pressure in the ulnar artery.
   b. if collateral circulation is present.
   c. if the patient is absorbing oxygen.
   d. the clotting time of both arteries.

7. **Which of the following is an acceptable angle of needle insertion for radial ABGs?**
   a. 10 degrees
   b. 20 degrees
   c. 45 degrees
   d. 90 degrees

8. **Which of the following complications are associated with arterial puncture?**
   a. Arteriospasm
   b. Hematoma
   c. Infection
   d. All of the above

9. **Which of the following can cause erroneous ABG values?**
   a. The presence of air bubbles in the specimen
   b. Delay in analysis exceeding 30 minutes
   c. Inadequate mixing results in microclots
   d. All of the above

10. **Which of the following would cause you to suspect that a thrombus had formed in the artery while you were collecting an ABG?**
    a. A hematoma quickly forms at the site.
    b. The patient complains of extreme pain.
    c. The pulse distal to the site is very weak.
    d. All of the above.

Study and Review Questions test how well you understand each chapter's major concepts.

thePoint. *View the Introductory and Identification Processes Required Prior to Blood Specimen Collection video at http://thepoint.lww.com/McCall6e.*

Online Icons point you to free resources available on thePoint.lww.com that provide supplemental information and help you to better understand the topics presented.

Media Menus recap and highlight all of the resources available for each chapter.

MEDIA MENU

Online Ancillaries (at http://thepoint.lww.com/McCall6e)
- Videos:
  - Rapid Detection of Strep
  - Routine Urinalysis
  - Throat Swab Collection
- Interactive exercises and games, including Look and Label, Word Building, Body Building, Roboterms, Crossword Puzzles, Quiz Show, and Concentration
- Audio flash cards and flash card generator
- Audio glossary

Internet Resources
- **Center for Phlebotomy Education:** http://www.phlebotomy.com/
- **Centers for Disease Control and Prevention (CDC): NP swab collection video.** http://www.cdc.gov/pertussis/clinical/diagnostic-testing/specimen-collection.html
- **Clinical Laboratory Science Internet Resources Website:** http://www.clinlabnavigator.com/Links/new-review/clinical-laboratory-science-internet-resources.html
- **LabCorp (Laboratory Corporation of America):** https://www.labcorp.com/wps/portal/provider/testmenu/
- **Mayo Medical Laboratories:** http://mayomedicallaboratories.com/it-mmlfiles/Urine_Preservatives10.pdf

Other Resources
- McCall R, Tankersley C. *Student Workbook for Phlebotomy Essentials.* 6th ed. (Available for separate purchase.)

Stepping into Success

Do you feel like you learn better when you understand not only the what, but also the why of what you're learning? We think you do. *Phlebotomy Essentials* provides many opportunities for you to step into the shoes of practicing phlebotomists and understand what wearing those shoes feels like!

Case Studies help you see exactly how the concept you're learning might present itself in the real world. You'll start to think like you're already in practice so you're fully ready for the workforce when you graduate.

Case Studies

See the WORKBOOK for more case studies.

Case Study 4-1: Lab Orders

A physician orders ASAP blood cultures on an ER patient with a diagnosis of FUO.

QUESTIONS
1. When should the blood cultures be collected?
2. Where is the patient located?
3. What does the diagnosis abbreviation FUO mean?

Case Study 4-2: Misinterpreted Instructions

A phlebotomy student is doing a clinical rotation with a laboratory in a medical clinic. A patient comes in for a TB test. The phlebotomist in charge thinks that it would be a good learning experience for the student to administer the test. The student is a little reluctant. The phlebotomist tells her not to worry, writes out the instructions shown below, and goes about processing specimens that are ready to be centrifuged. Phlebotomist's instructions:

Choose a clean site on the inside of the arm below the elbow.

Procedure 14-1: Modified Allen Test

PURPOSE: To assess collateral circulation through the ulnar artery
EQUIPMENT: None

Step	Rationale/Explanation
1. Have the patient make a tight fist.	A tight fist partially blocks blood flow, causing temporary blanching until the hand is opened.
2. Use the middle and index fingers of both hands to apply pressure to the patient's wrist, compressing both the radial and ulnar arteries at the same time.	Pressure over both arteries is needed to obstruct blood flow, which is required to be able to assess blood return when pressure is released. Note: If the patient is unable to make a fist, the hand can be held above heart level for 30–60 seconds during steps 2 and 3.

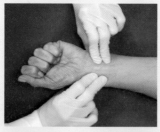

Practicing phlebotomy means successfully performing a variety of **procedures**. Our visual, step-by-step instructions can help you get ready to do just that!

3. While maintaining pressure, have the patient open the hand slowly. It should appear blanched or drained of color.	Blanched appearance of the hand verifies temporary blockage of both arteries. Note: The patient must not hyperextend the fingers when opening the hand, as this can cause decreased blood flow and misinterpretation of results.

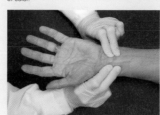

Strengthening Your Learning

Ever feel like you're struggling to keep up in class? Make sure you're taking advantage of all of the tools available to help you own your success!

Student Workbook for Phlebotomy Essentials provides new tools and resources to help you supplement your text and build on your learning. Activities include:

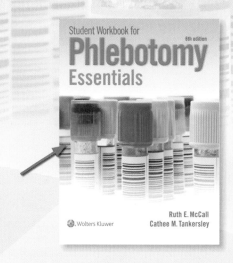

- **Matching activities** to help you learn the terms and concepts that professional phlebotomists need to know.
- **Labeling exercises** to help you recognize important equipment, tools, and procedures.
- **Knowledge drills** to reinforce core concepts and principles discussed in the text.
- **Skills drills** to help you make the transition from the classroom to clinical practice.
- **Chapter and unit crossword puzzles** that offer a fun way to reinforce and assess your knowledge.
- **Chapter review questions** to test your comprehension as you progress through the text and build your knowledge.
- **Case studies** that let you see how your newfound knowledge and skills can be put into practice.

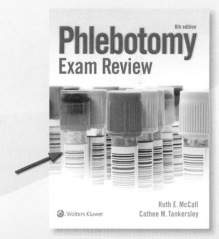

Want to sit for certification? Do you know that, on average, certified phlebotomists earn more money than those who opt not to obtain certification? If you're considering certification, then consider *Phlebotomy Exam Review*, which can help you prepare for several national exams.

In addition to the tools outlined in this user's guide, you have access to a variety of free resources at **http://thePoint.lww.com/McCall6e**. These items can help make learning exciting and effective, and include:

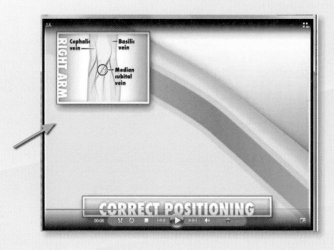

- Interactive games and activities offer that a fun way to study and review.
- Videos and animations that illustrate important procedures and concepts
- Study tools, like audio flash cards, a flash card generator, and an audio glossary, that can help you check your learning

Get Your Customized Success Play

Ever had a study plan that was completely customized for you? Now you can by purchasing prepU for Phlebotomy Essentials Exam Review. prepU is an adaptive quizzing engine that is simple to use and extraordinary in what it can do to help you learn!

- **Personalized Quiz Builder:** PrepU uses data gathered from student performance to create personalized quizzes that focus on exactly what each student needs to understand! After each quiz, PrepU adapts to continue helping students progress on their next quiz!

- **Personalized Reports:** PrepU gives students feedback about their performance—broken down by topic—so students know exactly where to focus their study efforts.

- **Quick and Meaningful Remediation:** PrepU offers an Answer Key for each completed quiz including rationales for each answer with specific textbook pages to help students quickly remediate.

Take a look at these solutions at **thePoint. lww.com/McCall6e**

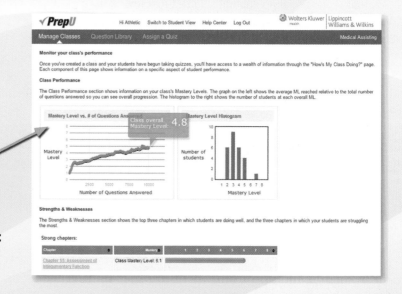

Unit I

The Healthcare Setting

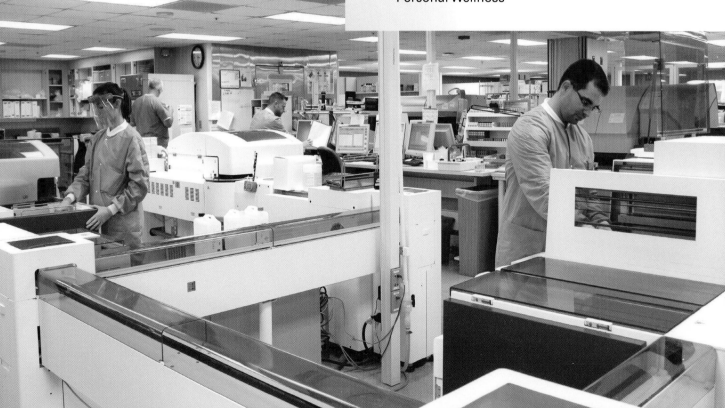

Chapter 1

Phlebotomy: Past and Present and the Healthcare Setting

NAACLS Entry Level Competencies

1.00 Demonstrate knowledge of the healthcare delivery system and medical terminology.

4.2 Describe the types of patient specimens that are analyzed in the clinical laboratory.

4.3 Define the phlebotomist's role in collecting and/or transporting these specimens to the laboratory.

9.00 Communicate (verbally and nonverbally) effectively and appropriately in the workplace.

9.1 Maintain confidentiality of privileged information on individuals according to federal regulations (e.g., HIPAA).

9.2 Demonstrate respect for diversity in the workplace.

9.3 Interact appropriately and professionally.

9.5 Comply with the American Hospital Associations' Patient's Bill of Rights and the Patient's Bill of Rights from the workplace.

9.6 Model professional appearance and appropriate behavior.

Key Terms

Do Matching Exercise 1-1 in the WORKBOOK to gain familiarity with these terms.

ACA	CPT	Medicaid	primary care
ACO	exsanguinate	Medicare	proxemics
AHCCCS	HIPAA	MLS	reference
case manager	HMOs	PCP	laboratories
certification	ICD-10-PCS	PHI	secondary care
CLIA '88	IDNs	PHS	tertiary care
CMS	kinesic slip	phlebotomy	third-party
communication	kinesics	PM	payer
barriers	MCOs	polycythemia	

Objectives

Upon successful completion of this chapter, the reader should be able to:

1 Demonstrate basic knowledge of terminology for healthcare settings including the national healthcare organizations that contributed to the evolution of phlebotomy and the role of the phlebotomist today.

2 Describe the basic concepts of verbal and nonverbal communication as they relate to the professional image and proper telephone protocol in the health care.

3 Compare types of healthcare institutions and the methods used by providers for coverage.

4 List the personnel levels in the clinical analysis areas of the laboratory and the types of laboratory procedures performed in each of the areas.

Overview

Health care today has evolved into an integrated delivery system (IDS) offering a full range of services intended to ensure that the patient gets what is needed at the right time and in the right way. In addition to physicians, nurses, and patient support personnel, allied health professionals such as clinical laboratory personnel play an important role in the delivery of patient care. The clinical laboratory provides physicians with some of medicine's most powerful diagnostic tests. The value of laboratory service has become even more important with the passage of new healthcare legislation. It is predicted that in the very near future the clinical laboratory's crucial diagnostic data will greatly influence physicians' decisions and positively affect those who manage patient outcomes and costs. Before patient test results can be reported to the physician, specimens must be collected and analyzed. Phlebotomists have been **key players** in this process for some time and their role increases in value each year. In addition to blood collection skills, successful specimen collection requires the phlebotomist to demonstrate professionalism, good communication and public relations skills, and a working knowledge of the healthcare delivery system. An understanding of phlebotomy from a historical perspective helps phlebotomists appreciate the significance of their role in health care today.

Phlebotomy: The Past

Since very early times, people have been fascinated by blood and have believed in some connection between the blood racing through their veins and their well-being. From this belief, certain medical principles and procedures dealing with blood evolved, some surviving to the present day.

An early medical theory developed by Hippocrates (460 to 377 BC) stated that disease was the result of excess substance—such as blood, phlegm, black bile, and yellow bile—within the body. It was thought that removal of the excess would restore balance. The process of removal and extraction became the treatment and could be done either by expelling disease materials through the use of drugs or by direct removal during surgery. One important surgical technique was venesection (cutting a vein), used in the process of bloodletting. Venesection—which comes from the Latin words *vena,* "vein," and *sectio,* "cutting"—was the most common method of general bloodletting. It involved cutting into a vein with a sharp instrument and releasing blood in an effort to rid the body of evil spirits, cleanse the body of impurities, or, as in Hippocrates' time, bring the body into proper balance. It often meant withdrawing large quantities of blood from a patient to cure or prevent illness and disease. *Venesection* is another word for **phlebotomy**, which comes from the Greek words *phlebos,* "vein," and *tome,* "incision."

Some authorities believe phlebotomy dates back to the last period of the Stone Age, when crude tools were used to puncture vessels and allow excess blood to drain out of the body. A painting in a tomb showing the application of a leech to a patient evidences bloodletting in Egypt in about 1400 BC. Early in the Middle Ages, barber–surgeons flourished. By 1210, the Guild of Barber–Surgeons had been formed in Paris; it divided the surgeons into Surgeons of the Long Robe and Surgeons of the Short Robe. Soon the Short Robe surgeons were forbidden by law to do any surgery except bloodletting, wound surgery, cupping, leeching, shaving, tooth extraction, and enema administration.

To distinguish their profession from that of the Long Robe surgeon, barber–surgeons placed a striped pole, from which a bleeding bowl was suspended, outside their doors. The pole represented the rod squeezed by the patient to promote bleeding and the white stripe on the pole corresponded to the bandages, which were also used as tourniquets. Soon, handsomely decorated ceramic bleeding bowls (Fig. 1-1) came into fashion and were passed down from one generation to the next. These bowls, which often doubled as shaving bowls, usually had a semicircular area cut out on one side to facilitate placement of the bowl under the chin.

During the 17th and early 18th centuries, phlebotomy was considered a major therapeutic (treatment) process, and anyone willing to claim medical training could perform phlebotomy. The lancet, a tool used for cutting the vein during venesection, was perhaps the most prevalent medical instrument of the times. The

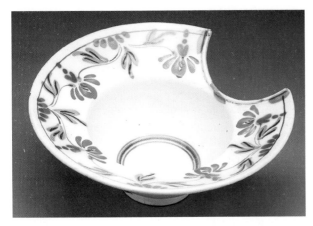

Figure 1-1 A bleeding bowl. (Courtesy of Robert Kravetz, MD, Chairman, Archives Committee, American College of Gastroenterology.)

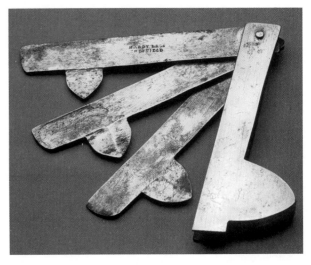

Figure 1-2 Typical fleams. (Courtesy of Robert Kravetz, MD, Chairman, Archives Committee, American College of Gastroenterology.)

usual amount of blood withdrawn was approximately 10 mL, but excessive phlebotomy was common.

(i) Excessive phlebotomy is thought to have contributed to George Washington's death in 1799, when he was diagnosed with a throat infection and the physician bled him four times in 2 days. It was because of Washington's request to be allowed to die without further medical intervention that the physician did not completely **exsanguinate** him, or remove all his blood.

During this same period, phlebotomy was also accomplished by cupping and leeching. The art of cupping required a great deal of practice to maintain the high degree of dexterity necessary to avoid appearing clumsy and thus frighten the patient away. Cupping involved the application of a heated suction apparatus, called the "cup," to the skin to draw the blood to the surface. Then the capillaries in that area were severed by making a series of parallel incisions with a lancet or fleam. The typical fleam was a wide double-edged blade at right angles to the handle. Eventually, multiple fleams (Fig. 1-2) were attached and folded into a brass case for easy carrying. The blades were wiped clean with only a rag; therefore, they readily transmitted a host of blood-borne infections from patient to patient.

(i) Dry cupping (cupping without superficial incisions) is still used today by many alternative medical practitioners. It is believed the suction penetrates deep into the tissues mobilizing blood flow and causing the tissues to release harmful toxins that can be removed from the body.

Fleams were used for general phlebotomy to open an artery or, more commonly, a vein to remove large amounts of blood. For more localized bloodletting, leeches were used. This procedure involved enticing the *Hirudo medicinalis*, a European medicinal leech, to the spot needing bloodletting with a drop of milk or blood on the patient's skin. After the leech engorged itself with blood, which took about an hour, it was allowed to drop off. By the mid-18th century, leeching was widely practiced in Europe, especially in France. Leeches were kept in special vessels that were filled with water and had perforated tops, so that the leeches could breathe. Early leech jars were glass and later ones ceramic (Fig. 1-3).

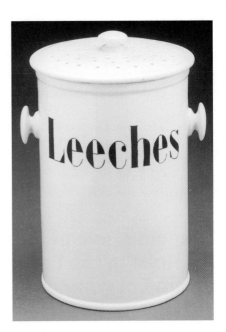

Figure 1-3 A leech jar. (Courtesy of Robert Kravetz, MD, Chairman, Archives Committee, American College of Gastroenterology.)

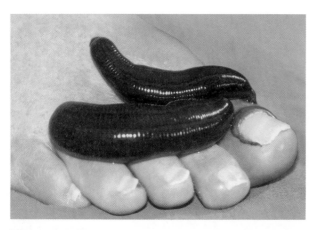

Figure 1-4 A toe with leech. (Courtesy of Robert Kravetz, MD, Chairman, Archives Committee, American College of Gastroenterology.)

Within the last decade, leeches have made a comeback as defenders from the complications of microsurgical replantation. The value of leech therapy (Fig. 1-4) is found in the worm's saliva, which contains a local vasodilator (substance that increases the diameter of blood vessels), a local anesthetic, and hirudin, an anticoagulant (a substance that prevents clotting).

Phlebotomy: The Present

The practice of phlebotomy continues to this day; however, principles and methods have improved dramatically. Today, phlebotomy is performed to

- obtain blood for diagnostic purposes and to monitor prescribed treatment.
- remove blood for transfusions at a donor center.
- remove blood for therapeutic purposes, such as treatment for **polycythemia**, a disorder involving the overproduction of red blood cells.

Phlebotomy is primarily accomplished by one of two procedures:

- Venipuncture, which involves collecting blood by penetrating a vein with a needle and syringe or other collection apparatus.
- Capillary puncture, which involves collecting blood after puncturing the skin with a lancet.

The Changing Role of the Phlebotomist in the Emerging Healthcare Environment

Healthcare delivery systems are constantly changing. Advances in laboratory technology are making point-of-care testing (POCT) commonplace, and services that were once unique to the laboratory are now being

provided at many other locations. The development of teams and the sharing of tasks have become necessary as healthcare organizations attempt to find the balance between cost-effective treatment and high-quality care. Work responsibilities have been revised, so that many types of healthcare professionals are cross-trained in a number of techniques and skills, including phlebotomy. Consequently the term *phlebotomist* is applied to any individual who has been trained in the various techniques used to obtain blood for laboratory testing or blood donations. A competent clinical phlebotomist must have good manual dexterity, special communication skills, good organizational skills, and a thorough knowledge of laboratory specimen requirements and departmental policies. A selection of duties and responsibilities associated with the role of phlebotomist are listed in Box 1-1.

Regardless of which member of the healthcare team performs phlebotomy techniques, quality assurance demands that the highest standards be maintained and approved procedures followed.

Consequently there is a standardized educational curriculum with a recognized body of knowledge, skills, and standards of practice for the phlebotomy profession that was developed by the **National Accrediting Agency for Clinical Laboratory Sciences (NAACLS)**. Many hospitals, vocational schools, and colleges offer structured phlebotomy programs that include classroom instruction and clinical practice. These programs, can apply for NAACLS approval. Whether approved by NAACLS or not, most programs not only train students in phlebotomy procedures, but also prepare them for national certification or state licensure.

Official Recognition

ⓘ For information about specific state laboratory regulations and licensure, go to that state's DHS or HHS web site, for instance, Michigandhs.gov.

CERTIFICATION

Certification is a voluntary process by which an agency grants recognition to an individual who has met certain prerequisites in a particular technical area. Certification indicates the completion of defined academic and training requirements and the attainment of a satisfactory score on an examination. This is confirmed by the awarding of a title or designation. Phlebotomist certification is signified by initials that the individual is allowed to display after his or her name. Examples of national agencies that certify phlebotomists, along with

Box 1-1

Duties and Responsibilities of a Phlebotomist

Typical Duties

- Prepare patients and site for specimen collection following nationally recognized standards and institution's guidelines.
- Collect venipuncture and capillary specimens for testing following nationally recognized standards and institutional procedures.
- Prepare specimens for proper transport, ensuring the integrity and stability of the sample.
- Adhere to all HIPAA and confidentiality guidelines, including all Code of Conduct and Integrity programs instituted by the employer.
- Transport and dispatch samples efficiently by prioritizing specimens to ensure desired turnaround times.
- Comply with safety rules, policies, and guidelines for the area, department, and institution.
- Provide quality customer service for all internal and external customers.

Additional Duties as Required

- Assist in collecting and documenting monthly workload and record data.
- Perform quality-control protocols as specified in standard operating procedures, and perform and document instrument and equipment maintenance.
- Participate in continuing education programs such as Quality, Safety, Lean/Six Sigma, and Customer Service.
- Collect and perform point-of-care testing (POCT) following all standard operating procedures.
- Prepare drafts of procedures for laboratory tests according to standard format.
- Perform appropriate laboratory computer information operations.
- Provide proper instruction to patients/customers for container specimen collection.
- Perform front-office duties required by institution including scheduling, coding, itinerary updates, and obtaining Advance Beneficiary Notice (ABN).
- Train new technicians and students in duties and responsibilities.

the title and corresponding initials awarded, are listed in Table 1-1.

> ⓘ Certified lab professionals earn more money than those who are not certified according to the ASCP's 2013 Wage Survey. Noncertified staff level phlebotomists (PBT), for example, reported that they make an average of $13.87 per hour, but the average wage for certified PBTs is $15.93, a 13.8% differential.

LICENSURE

Licensure is the act of granting a license. A license in health care is an official document or permit granted by a state agency that gives legal permission for a person to work in a particular health profession. Without a license, it would be against the law for a person to practice that profession in that state. Typically, the individual must meet specific education and experience requirements and pass an examination before the license is granted. The license indicates competency only at the time of examination. As a demonstration of

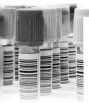

Table 1-1: Phlebotomist Title and Initials Awarded by Certification Agency*

Certification Agency	Certification Title	Certification Initials
American Medical Technologists	Registered Phlebotomy Technician	RPT(AMT)
American Certification Agency	Certified Phlebotomy Technician	CPT(ACA)
American Society for Clinical Pathology	Phlebotomy Technician	PBT(ASCP)
National Center for Competency Testing	National Certified Phlebotomy Technician	NCPT(NCCT)

*Mailing and e-mail addresses and telephone numbers for the phlebotomy certification agencies listed and several others can be found in McCall R. Tankersley, C. *Phlebotomy Exam Review*. 6th ed. Baltimore, MD: Lippincott Williams & Wilkins; 2016.

continued competency, states normally require periodic license renewal, by either reexamination or proof of continuing education.

i Some states have several levels of licensure for certain professions. For example, California offers three levels of phlebotomy licensure: Limited Phlebotomy Technician (LPT), Certified Phlebotomy Technician I (CPT I), and Certified PhlebotomyTechnician II (CPT II).

CONTINUING EDUCATION

Continuing education is designed to update the knowledge or skills of participants and is generally geared to a learning activity or course of study for a specific group of health professionals, such as phlebotomists. Many organizations, such as the American Society for Clinical Pathology (ASCP), the American Society for Clinical Laboratory Sciences (ASCLS), and the American Medical Technologists (AMT), sponsor workshops, seminars, and self-study programs that award **continuing education units (CEUs)** to those who participate. The most widely accepted CEU was created by the **International Association for Continuing Education and Training (IACET)** to provide a standard unit of measurement to determine continuing education and training activities for diverse providers and purposes. One CEU equals 10 contact hours of participation in an organized experience under responsible sponsorship, capable direction, and qualified instruction (International Association for Continuing Education and Training. Retrieved January 21, 2014, from http://www.iacet.org/ceus/about the ceu).

Most certifying and licensing agencies require CEUs or other proof of continuing education for renewal of credentials. These requirements are intended to encourage professionals to expand their knowledge base and stay up to date. It is important for phlebotomists to participate in continuing education to be aware of new developments in specimen collection and processing, personal safety, and patient care.

Patient Interaction

As a member of the clinical laboratory team, the phlebotomist plays an important role in how the laboratory is portrayed to the public. The phlebotomist is often the only real contact the patient has with the laboratory. In many cases, patients equate this encounter with the caliber of care they receive while in the hospital. Positive "customer relations" involves promoting goodwill and a harmonious relationship with fellow employees,

visitors, and especially patients. A competent phlebotomist with a professional manner and a neat appearance helps to put the patient at ease and establish a positive relationship.

RECOGNIZING DIVERSITY

Despite similarities, fundamental differences among people arise from nationality, ethnicity, and culture as well as from family background, life experiences, and individual challenges. These differences affect the personal health beliefs and behaviors of both patients and the providers, for example, the phlebotomist.

Culturally aware healthcare providers enhance their potential for more rewarding interpersonal experiences and greater job satisfaction. A continued awareness and knowledge of cultural differences by all employees can protect an organization from civil rights violations, promote an inviting workplace, and increase innovation and teamwork. More importantly, the healthcare organization benefits greatly in improved patient satisfaction with the services provided.

Critical factors in providing healthcare services that meet the needs of diverse populations include understanding the

- beliefs and values that shape a person's approach to health and illness.
- health-related needs of patients and their families according to the environments in which they live.
- knowledge of customs and traditions related to health and healing.
- attitudes toward seeking help from healthcare providers.

Key Point By recognizing and appreciating diversity, the phlebotomist promotes goodwill and harmonious relationships that directly improve health outcomes, the quality of services, and customer satisfaction.

State how each quality contributes to professional attitude in Knowledge Drill 1-7 in the WORKBOOK.

PROFESSIONALISM

Professionalism is defined as the conduct and qualities that characterize a professional person. As part of a service-oriented industry, persons performing phlebotomy must practice professionalism.

The public's perception of the phlebotomy profession is based on the image created by the phlebotomist's conduct and appearance. In fact, general appearance and grooming directly influence whether the phlebotomist is perceived as a professional. It has been said that people form opinions of a person within the first 3 seconds of meeting, and this judgment on the superficial aspect of a person sets an image in the observer's mind that can affect the interaction.

Conservative clothing, proper personal hygiene, and physical well-being contribute to a professional appearance. It should be noted that healthcare institutional policies for attire are influenced by a federal standard that requires employers to provide protective clothing for laboratory workers, including phlebotomists.

Besides displaying a professional appearance, a person performing phlebotomy is required to display attitudes, personal characteristics, and behaviors consistent with accepted standards of professional conduct. Some of the personal behaviors and characteristics that make up this professional image are as follows:

Self-Confidence

A phlebotomist who displays self-confidence has the ability to trust his or her own personal judgment. A phlebotomist's perception of self has an enormous impact on how others perceive him or her, and "perception is reality." The more self-confidence a phlebotomist has, the more professional he or she appears. Many factors affect being perceived as self-confident, for example, erect posture, professional appearance, courage, and tactfulness in communication.

Integrity

Integrity as a concept has to do with a personal feeling of "wholeness" derived from honesty and consistency of character; this can be seen in the person's actions, values, and beliefs. Professional standards of integrity or honesty require a person to do what is right regardless of the circumstances and in all situations and interactions. For example, a phlebotomist often functions independently and may be tempted to take procedural shortcuts when pressed for time. A phlebotomist with integrity understands that following the rules for collection is essential to the quality of test results; therefore, he or she respects those rules regardless of circumstances.

Compassion

Compassion is a human emotion prompted by others' experiences and concerns; it is considered to be one of the greatest of virtues by major religious traditions. It is differentiated from empathy only by the level of emotion, as it tends to be more intense. Compassion means being sensitive to a person's needs and willing to offer reassurance in a caring and humane way. A phlebotomist may show compassion by appreciating the fear that illness or the unknown generates, by using empathy to sense others' experiences, and by demonstrating a calm and helpful demeanor toward those in need.

Self-Motivation

A person with motivation finds the workplace stimulating no matter what the tasks may entail. Motivation is a direct reflection of a person's attitude toward life. A phlebotomist who exhibits self-motivation takes initiative to follow through on tasks, consistently strives to improve and correct behavior, and takes advantage of every learning opportunity that is offered. A phlebotomist who is motivated makes every effort to provide excellence in all aspects of patient care in which he or she is involved.

Dependability

Dependability and work ethic go hand in hand. An individual who is dependable and takes personal responsibility for his or her actions is extremely refreshing in today's environment. A phlebotomist who works hard and shows constant, reliable effort and perseverance is a valuable asset to a healthcare organization. This set of values makes a person a desirable candidate for new job opportunities and ultimately promotions in the healthcare setting or anywhere.

Ethical Behavior

A phlebotomist should know that there are policies designed to regulate what should or should not be done by those who work in the healthcare setting. This system of policies or principles is called a *code of ethics*. Ethics are centered on an individual's conduct. Ethical behavior means making the right choices to maintain a high level of personal respect, and, respect for one's profession.

In health care, ethical behavior requires conforming to a standard of right and wrong conduct so as to avoid harming patients in any way. A code of ethics, although not enforceable by law, leads to uniformity and defined expectations for the members of that profession. Professional organizations, such as ASCP, have developed a code of ethics for laboratory professionals.

Key Point The Latin phrase *primum non nocere* which means "first do no harm" describes one of the fundamental principles of health care. Although it does not include this exact phrase, the promise "to abstain from doing harm" is part of the Hippocratic oath given to new physicians and other healthcare professionals as they begin their practice.

The primary objective in any healthcare professional's code of ethics must always be to safeguard the patient's welfare. A guide to working with that principle in mind is a document of accepted quality-care principles developed by the American Hospital Association (AHA) and the related patient rights.

PATIENTS' RIGHTS

All patients in a healthcare setting have rights and should be informed of these rights when care is initiated. In a hospital or outpatient surgery center, the patient must sign a statement that these rights have been explained, and the signed statement must be made a part of the patient's medical record. It has been found that patients who are informed about their treatments and prognoses and are considered in the decision-making process are more satisfied with their care.

Almost two decades ago, the federal government recognized the need to strengthen consumer confidence in the fairness and responsiveness of the healthcare system. The result was *The Patient Bill of Rights in Medicare and Medicaid*. Medicare now requires that patients be informed of their rights, including the right to know what treatment they can expect, who will be treating them, the right to refuse treatment, and the right to confidentiality.

To affirm the importance of a strong relationship between patients and their healthcare providers, the AHA publishes and disseminates a statement of patient rights and responsibilities. The AHA brochure or a similar pamphlet should be provided to consumers during inpatient admission procedures as evidence of patient advocacy or support. This easy-to-read brochure is called *The Patient Care Partnership* and is designed to help patients understand their expectations during their hospital stay with regard to their rights and responsibilities. It states that the first priority of all healthcare professionals, including phlebotomists, is to provide high-quality patient care in a clean and safe environment, while also maintaining the patient's personal rights and dignity by being sensitive to differences in culture, race, religion, gender, and age. Expectations listed in the brochure are summarized in Box 1-2.

CONFIDENTIALITY

Patient confidentiality is seen by many as the ethical cornerstone of professional behavior in the healthcare field. It serves to protect both the patient and the practitioner. The healthcare provider must recognize that all patient information is absolutely private and confidential. Healthcare providers are bound by ethical standards and various laws to maintain the confidentiality of each person's health information.

Any questions relating to patient information should be referred to the proper authority. Unauthorized release of information concerning a patient is considered an invasion of privacy. In 1996, a federal law was passed requiring all healthcare providers to obtain a patient's consent in writing before disclosing medical information such as a patient's test results, treatment, or condition to any unauthorized person. That law is the **Health**

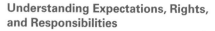

Box 1-2

The Patient Care Partnership

Understanding Expectations, Rights, and Responsibilities

What to Expect during Your Hospital Stay

- High-quality hospital care
- A clean and safe environment
- Involvement in your care
- Protection of your privacy
- Help when leaving the hospital
- Help with your billing claims

Adapted from the American Hospital Association's brochure. *The Patient Care Partnership*. Retrieved February 14, 2014 from http://www.aha.org. See that document for more details.

Insurance Portability and Accountability Act (HIPAA) of 1996.

HIPAA

As a person's health information has become more easily transferable from one facility or entity to the next through electronic exchange, a growing problem with a person's rights and confidentiality has arisen. The HIPAA law was enacted in order to more closely secure this information and regulate patient privacy. HIPAA provisions protect a broad range of health information. Safeguarding the confidentiality of **protected health information (PHI)** is one of the primary aims of the HIPAA privacy rule. The law defines PHI as "individually identifiable health information that is transmitted by electronic media; maintained in any medium described in the definition of electronic media or transmitted or maintained in any other form or medium." The law established national standards for the electronic exchange of PHI and states that patients must be informed of their rights concerning the release of PHI and how it will be used. Penalties for HIPAA violations include disciplinary action, fines, and possible jail time.

The law states that healthcare workers (HCWs) must obtain the patient's written authorization for any use or disclosure of PHI unless the use or disclosure is for treatment, payment, or healthcare operations. To avoid litigation in this area, all HCWs and students must sign a confidentiality and nondisclosure agreement affirming that they understand HIPAA and will keep all patients' information confidential.

Communication Skills

Phlebotomy is both a technical and a people-oriented profession. Many different types of people or customers interact with phlebotomists. Often, the customer's perception of the healthcare facility is based on the employees they deal with on a one-to-one basis, such as a phlebotomist. Customers expect high-quality service. A phlebotomist who lacks a good bedside manner (the ability to communicate with courtesy and compassion toward the patient) increases the chances of becoming part of a legal action should any difficulty arise while a specimen is being obtained. Favorable impressions result when HCWs respond properly to patient needs, and this occurs when there is good communication between the healthcare provider and the patient.

COMMUNICATION DEFINED

Communication is a skill. Defined as the means by which information is exchanged or transmitted, communication is one of the most important processes that takes place in the healthcare system. This dynamic and constantly changing process involves three components: verbal skills, nonverbal skills, and the ability to listen.

Test your knowledge of communication components in Labeling Exercise 1-1 in the WORKBOOK.

COMMUNICATION COMPONENTS

Verbal Communication

Expression through the spoken word is the most obvious form of communication. Effective healthcare communication should be an interaction in which both participants play a role. It involves a *sender* (speaker), a *receiver* (listener), and, when complete, a process called *feedback,* creating what is referred to as the *communication feedback loop* (Fig. 1-5). Accurate verbal exchange depends upon feedback. It is through feedback that the listener or receiver is given the chance to clarify ideas or correct miscommunication, which may be due to preformed biases or barriers.

Normal human behavior sets up many **communication barriers** (prejudices or personalized filters) that become obstructions to hearing and understanding what has been said and are frequent causes of miscommunication. Examples of communication barriers are language limitations, cultural diversity, emotions, age, gender, and physical disabilities such as hearing loss.

To encourage good verbal communication, the phlebotomist should use a vocabulary that is easily understood by his or her clients. To avoid creating suspicion and distrust in individuals from other countries, the phlebotomist should be aware of cultural differences and avoid clichés and nonverbal cues that could be misunderstood. It is important for good communication that the phlebotomist practice active listening to what is being said.

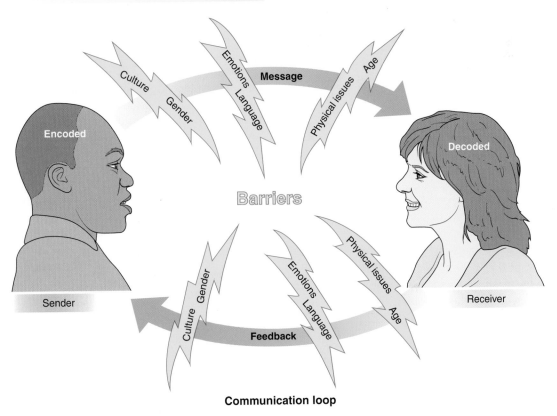

Communication loop

Figure 1-5 The verbal communication feedback loop.

Active Listening

True communication is not just about speaking. It is more difficult to communicate than just to speak, because effective communication requires that the listener participate by focusing on what is being said and giving appropriate feedback. It is always a two-way process. The ordinary person can absorb verbal messages at about 500 to 600 words per minute, and the average speaking rate is only 125 to 150 words per minute. Therefore, to avoid distraction, the listener must use the extra time for active listening. Active listening means taking positive steps through feedback to ensure that the listener is interpreting what the speaker is saying exactly as the speaker intended. Listening is the foundation of good interpersonal communication. The phlebotomist will find that listening carefully to what is being said and watching for nonverbal cues is the way to quickly build mutual trust with patients.

Nonverbal Communication

It has been stated that 80% of language is unspoken. Unlike verbal communication, formed from words that are one-dimensional, nonverbal communication is multidimensional and involves the following elements.

Kinesics

The study of nonverbal communication is also called **kinesics**; it includes characteristics of body motion and language such as facial expression, gestures, and eye contact. Figure 1-6 illustrates an exaggerated and simplified form of the six emotions that are most easily read by nonverbal facial cues. Body language, which most often is conveyed unintentionally, plays a major role in communication because it is continuous and more reliable than verbal communication. In fact, if the verbal and nonverbal messages do not match, it is called a **kinesic slip**. When this happens, people tend to trust what they see rather than what they hear.

As health professionals, phlebotomists can learn much about patients' feelings by observing nonverbal communication, which seldom lies. The patient's face often tells the health professional what the patient will not reveal verbally. For instance, when a patient is anxious, nonverbal signs may include tight eyebrows, an intense frown, narrowed eyes, or a downcast mouth (Fig. 1-6A). Researchers have found that certain facial appearances, such as a smile, are universal expressions of emotion. Worldwide, we all recognize the meaning of a smile; however, strong cultural customs often dictate when it is used.

> **Key Point** To communicate effectively with someone, it is important to establish good eye contact. A patient or client may be made to feel unimportant and more like an object rather than a human being if eye contact is not established.

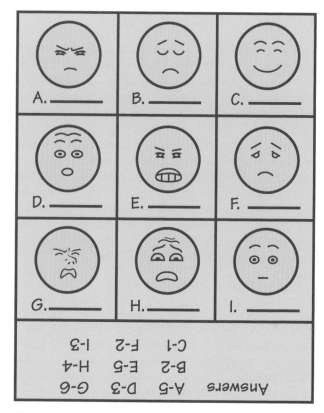

Figure 1-6 Nonverbal facial cues. Can you match the sketches with the correct effects? (1) Happy, (2) sad, (3) surprise, (4) fear, (5) anger, (6) disgust.

Proxemics

Proxemics is the study of an individual's concept and use of space. This subtle but powerful part of nonverbal communication plays a major role in patient relations. Every individual is surrounded by an invisible "bubble" of personal territory in which he or she feels most comfortable. The size of the bubble or territorial "zone of comfort" depends on the individual's needs at the time. Four categories of naturally occurring territorial zones and the radius of each are listed in Table 1-2. These zones are very obvious in human interaction. It is necessary, in the healthcare setting, to enter personal or intimate zones; if this is not carefully handled, the

Table 1-2: Territorial Zones and Corresponding Radii

Territorial Zone	Zone Radius
Intimate	1–18 in
Personal	1½–4 ft
Social	4–12 ft
Public	More than 12 ft

patient may feel threatened, insecure, or out of control. Most phlebotomists' work is in the intimate zone as they search and palpate to find a vein and perform venipuncture. In this close proximity to the patient, many other factors come into play that affect the interaction, such as conduct, hygiene, grooming, and appearance.

Appearance

Most healthcare facilities have dress codes because it is understood that appearance makes a statement. The impression the phlebotomist makes as he or she approaches the patient sets the stage for future interaction. The right image portrays a trustworthy professional. A phlebotomist's physical appearance should communicate cleanliness and confidence as shown in Figure 1-7. Lab coats, when worn, should completely cover the clothing underneath and should be clean and pressed. Shoes should be conservative and polished. Close attention should be paid to personal hygiene. Bathing and deodorant use should be a daily routine. Strong perfumes or colognes should not be worn. Hair

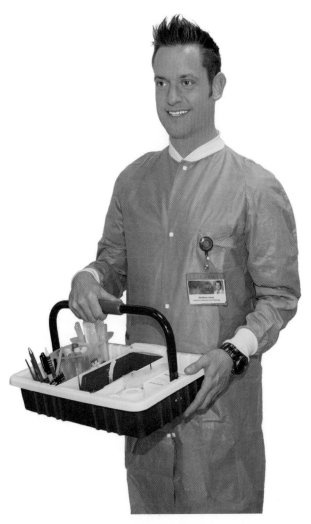

Figure 1-7 A picture of a confident and professional phlebotomist.

and nails should be clean and natural-looking. Long hair must be pulled back and fingernails kept short for safety's sake. In addition, according to current CDC hand hygiene guidelines, HCWs with direct patient contact cannot wear artificial nails or extenders.

Key Point Phlebotomists will find that when dealing with patients who are ill or irritable, a confident and professional appearance will be most helpful to them in doing their job.

Touch

Touching can take a variety of forms and convey many different meanings. For example, accidental touching may happen in a crowded elevator. Social touching takes place when a person grabs the arm of another while giving advice. Today, therapeutic touch that is designed to aid in healing has found a new place in medical practice. This special type of nonverbal communication is very important to the well-being of human beings and even more so to those suffering from disease.

Because medicine is a contact profession, touching privileges are granted to and expected of HCWs under certain circumstances. Whether a patient or healthcare provider is comfortable with touching is based on his or her cultural background. Because touch is a necessary part of the phlebotomy procedure, it is important for the phlebotomist to realize that, patients are often much more aware of your touch than you are of theirs; there may even be a risk of the patient questioning the appropriateness of touching. Generally speaking, patients respond favorably when touch conveys a thoughtful expression of caring.

EFFECTIVE COMMUNICATION IN HEALTH CARE

It is not easy for the patient or the health professional to face disease and suffering every day. For many patients, being ill is a fearful and even terrifying experience; having blood drawn only contributes to their anxiety. Patients reach out for comfort and reassurance through conversation. Consequently, the phlebotomist must understand the unusual aspects of healthcare communication and its importance in comforting the patient.

Communication between the health professional and patient is more complicated than normal interaction. Not only is it often emotionally charged, but it also involves, in many instances, other people who are close to the patient and who may tend to be critical of the way the patient is handled. Recognizing the elements in healthcare communication—such as empathy, control, trust, and confirmation—will help the phlebotomist to interact with the patient successfully.

Elements in Healthcare Communication

Empathy

Defined as identifying with the feelings or thoughts of another person, empathy is an essential factor in interpersonal relations. It involves putting yourself in the place of another and attempting to feel like that person. Thoughtful and sensitive people generally have a high degree of empathy. Empathetic health professionals help patients handle the stress of being in a healthcare institution. A health professional who recognizes the needs of the patient and allows the patient to express his or her emotions helps to validate the patient's feelings and gives the patient a very necessary sense of control.

Control

Feeling in control is essential to an individual's sense of well-being. People like to think that they can influence the way things happen in their lives. An important element relating to communication in the healthcare setting is recognizing fear in patients, which stems from a perceived lack of control. A hospital is one of the few places where individuals give up control over most of the personal tasks they normally perform. Many patients perceive themselves as unable to cope physically or mentally with events in a hospital because they feel fearful and powerless owing to this loss of control. Consequently, the typical response of the patient is to act angry, which characterizes him or her as a "bad patient," or to act extremely dependent and agreeable, which characterizes him or her as a "good patient."

If a patient refuses to have blood drawn, the phlebotomist should allow that statement of control to be expressed and even agree with the patient. Patients who are allowed to assert that right will often change their minds and agree to the procedure because then it is their decision. Sharing control with the patient may be difficult and often time-consuming, but awareness of the patient's need is important.

Respect and Confirmation

Respect is shown in both a positive feeling for a person and in specific action demonstrating that positive feeling. It is an attitude that conveys an understanding of the importance of that person as an individual. Believing that all people are worthy of respect at some level is extremely important in healthcare communication. The effect of honoring and respecting the person as a unique individual is confirmation of the patient's presence and needs.

If a HCW shows disrespect for a patient, it cannot help but be noticed by the patient and may affect the patient's condition in a negative way. Too often, busy HCWs such as phlebotomists, resort to labeling patients when communicating with coworkers and even with patients themselves. They may say, for example, "Oh, you're the one with no veins" or "You're the bleeder, right?" Such communication is dehumanizing and is a subtle way of "disconfirming" patients. A confirming exchange with the patient in the first example could be, "Mrs. Jones, I seem to remember that we had a hard time finding a suitable vein last time we drew your blood." Or, in the second case, "Mr. Smith, wasn't there a problem getting the site to stop bleeding after the draw last time?"

Trust

Another variable in the process of communication is trust. Trust, as defined in the healthcare setting, is the unquestioning belief by the patient that health professionals are performing their job responsibilities as well as they possibly can. As is true with most professionals, healthcare providers tend to emphasize their technical expertise while at times completely ignoring the elements of interpersonal communication that are essential in a trusting relationship with the patient. Having blood drawn is just one of the situations in which the consumer must trust the health professional. Developing trust takes time, and normally, phlebotomists spend very little time with each patient. Consequently, during this limited interaction, the phlebotomist must do everything possible to win the patient's confidence by always appearing knowledgeable, honest, and sincere.

In summary, by recognizing the elements of empathy, control, trust, respect, and confirmation, the phlebotomist can enhance communication with patients and assist in their recovery by making the interaction pleasant even when the blood draw is difficult. Understanding these communication elements will help when they are used with other means of communication, such as using the telephone.

Telephone Communication

At present, the telephone is a fundamental part of communication. It is used 24 hours a day in the laboratory. To phlebotomists or laboratory clerks, it becomes just another source of stress, bringing additional work and uninvited demands on their time. The constant ringing and interruption of the workflow may cause laboratory personnel to overlook the effect their style of telephone communication has on the caller. To maintain a professional image, every person given the responsibility of answering the phone should review proper protocol. Each one should be taught how to answer, put someone on hold, and transfer calls properly. To promote good communication, proper telephone etiquette (Table 1-3) should be followed.

The Healthcare Setting

Virtually everyone in the United States becomes a healthcare consumer at some time. For many, working through the bureaucracy involved in receiving health care can be

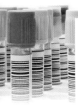

Table 1-3: Proper Telephone Etiquette

Proper Etiquette	Communication Tips	Rationale
Answer promptly.		• If the phone is allowed to ring too many times, the caller may assume that the people working in the laboratory are inefficient or insensitive.
State your name and department.		• The caller has the right to know to whom he or she is speaking.
Be helpful.	Ask how you can be of help to the caller and facilitate the conversation. Keep your statements and answers simple and to the point so as to avoid confusion.	• When a phone rings, it is because someone needs something. Because of the nature of the healthcare business, the caller may be emotional and may benefit from hearing a calm, pleasant voice at the other end.
Prioritize calls.	Inform a caller if he or she is interrupting a call from someone else.	• It takes an organized person to coordinate several calls. Being able to triage is an important skill that takes a knowledgeable and experienced person to handle it well.
	Always ask permission before putting a caller on hold in case it is an emergency that must be handled immediately.	• The caller needs to know where he or she is in the queue. Handling an important call or an emergency immediately will save the laboratory from problems in the future.
Transfer and put on hold properly.	Tell a caller when you are going to transfer the call or put it on hold and learn how to do this properly. Note: Do not leave the line open, and do not keep the caller waiting too long.	• Disconnecting callers while transferring or putting them on hold irritates them. • Leaving the line open so that other conversations can be heard by the person on hold is discourteous and can compromise confidentiality. • Check back with the caller when on hold for longer than expected; this keeps him or her informed of the circumstance. • If a caller is waiting on hold too long, ask if he or she would like to leave a message.
Be prepared to record information.	Have a pencil and paper close to the phone.	• Documentation is necessary when answering the phone at work to ensure that accurate information is transmitted to the necessary person.
	Listen carefully, which means clarifying, restating, and summarizing the information received.	• Reading back the information when complete is one of the best ways to ensure it is correct.
Know the laboratory's policies.	Make answers consistent by learning the laboratory's policies.	• People who answer the telephone must know the laboratory policies to avoid giving the wrong information. Misinformation given to the patient can result in unnecessary worry and additional expense. • Consistent answers help establish the laboratory's credibility, because a caller's perception of the lab involves more than just accurate test results.
Defuse hostile situations.	When a caller is hostile, you might say "I can see why you are upset. Let me see what I can do."	• Some callers become angry because of lost results or errors in billing. • Validating a hostile caller's feelings will often defuse the situation. • After the caller has calmed down, the issue can be addressed.
Try to assist everyone.	If you are uncertain, refer the caller to someone who can address the caller's issue. Remind yourself to keep your attention on one person at a time.	• It is possible to assist callers and show concern even if you are not actually answering their questions. • Validate callers' requests by giving a response that tells them something can be done. • Sincere interest in the caller will enhance communication and contribute to the good reputation of the laboratory.

confusing. Healthcare personnel who understand how health care is organized and financed and their role in the system can help consumers obtain quality care, with minimal repetition of services and consequently at lower cost.

Healthcare Delivery

Two general categories of facilities, inpatient (nonambulatory) and outpatient (ambulatory), support all three (**primary, secondary,** and **tertiary**) levels of health care currently offered in the United States. See Box 1-3 for a listing of services and practitioners associated with the two categories.

AMBULATORY CARE AND OUTPATIENT SERVICES

Changes in healthcare practices that have significantly decreased the amount of time a patient spends in tertiary care or the hospital have led to innovative ways to provide care, including a wide range of ambulatory services defined as medical care delivered on an *outpatient* basis. These services include observation, diagnosis, treatment, and rehabilitation for patients who either do not require an overnight stay in a healthcare facility or after having been discharged from the hospital still require follow-up procedures.

Ambulatory care is generally classified into two types: (a) freestanding medical care settings and hospital-owned clinics and (b) outpatient departments and urgent care facilities. In recent times, outpatient demands have fallen heavily on hospital emergency departments (EDs), which are a very costly way of delivering care and distract the staff from true emergencies.

Today, urgent care centers are seen as a way to decrease the overcrowded emergency rooms and provide significant savings to patients and insurers. These centers were designed to bridge the gap between an injury that is too urgent to wait for the primary care physician and a life-threatening situation that calls for a trip to the emergency room. Over the past several decades, the industry has continued to expand and to gain respect as a viable place to receive care when a person cannot get into a "regular" physician office.

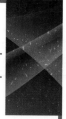 According to the Urgent Care Association of America (UCAOA), the size of the urgent care industry has only been measured in any real way since approximately 2008, and at that time it was estimated that the number of urgent care centers in the United States was approximately 9,000. The suggested growth in the 2008 to 2010 timeframe seemed to be about 300 centers per year, and in 2011 it appeared that growth rate doubled.

Many homebound elderly and those in hospice require ambulatory services where they reside, either in their homes or in assisted living facilities. Usually a home healthcare agency coordinates the services that the physician has ordered. These agencies employ nurses, respiratory therapists, physical therapists, phlebotomists, and other HCWs to provide these services.

PUBLIC HEALTH SERVICE

Another way of delivering health care to the citizens of the United States is through the **Public Health Service (PHS)**. The mission of this primary division under the

Box 1-3

Two Categories of Healthcare Facilities

Outpatient/Ambulatory	Inpatient
Principal source of healthcare services for most people.	The key resource and center of the American healthcare system.
Offer routine care in physician's office to specialized care in a freestanding ambulatory setting.	Offer specialized instrumentation and technology to assist in unusual diagnoses and treatments.
Serve primary care physicians who assume ongoing responsibility for maintaining patients' health.	Serve tertiary care (highly complex services and therapy) practitioners. Usually requires that patients stay overnight or longer.
Serve secondary care physicians (specialists) who perform routine surgery, emergency treatments, therapeutic radiology, and so on in same-day service centers.	Examples are acute care hospitals, nursing homes, extended care facilities, hospices, and rehabilitation centers.

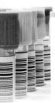

Table 1-4: Examples of Services Provided by Local Health Departments

Vital statistics collection	Tuberculosis screening
Health education	Immunization and vaccination
Cancer, hypertension, and diabetes screening	Operation of health centers
Public health nursing services	Venereal disease clinics

Department of Health and Human Services (HHS) is to promote the protection and advancement of the nation's physical and mental health. It does so by sponsoring and administering programs for the development of health resources, prevention and control of diseases, and dealing with drug abuse. PHS agencies at the local or state level offer defense against infectious diseases that might spread among the populace. These agencies constantly monitor, screen, protect, and educate the public (see Table 1-4 for examples of services provided by local health departments). Public health departments provide their services for little or no charge to the entire population of a region, with no distinction between rich or poor, simple or sophisticated, interested or disinterested. Public health facilities offer ambulatory care services through clinics, much like those in hospital outpatient areas, military bases, and Veterans Administration and Indian Health Service facilities.

As the country moves into reforming health care by controlling costs, streamlining services, and pursuing consolidation, integration between primary prevention and primary/ambulatory care is necessary.

> 🔑 **Key Point** An important component in ensuring that the healthcare system as a whole is sustainable is the **primary care physician (PCP)**. It has been shown that consistent primary care results in better health outcomes and lower spending, including avoidable emergency room visits and hospital care.

Because containment of healthcare costs is the driving force behind managed care and major changes to healthcare coverage, proactive public health programs are increasing as a way to significantly reduce overall healthcare costs.

Healthcare Financing

Health care is expensive, and the cost continues to escalate. Paying for healthcare services involves multiple payers and numerous mechanisms of payment. In an effort to remove barriers to quality and affordable health care, the Patient Protection and Affordable Care Act (PPACA) was passed in March 2013. This recent healthcare legislation, better known as the **Affordable Care Act (ACA)** is primarily about insurance market reform. This new law is to provide the consumer with insurance options and an increased accessibility to *affordable* health care. Insurance reforms are planned to take place over a 4-year period and beyond. As part of the law, everyone in the United States is to have access to health care and no one can be denied coverage or charged more for pre-existing conditions by insurance companies or **third-party payers**.

THIRD-PARTY PAYERS

A third-party payer can be an insurance company, the federal government, a managed care program, or a self-insured company that pays for healthcare services on behalf of its employees. Payment methods used may be either direct or indirect. Payments to the provider by the patient are referred to as direct pay, self-pay, or out-of-pocket pay. Indirect pay involves a third party other than the patient (first party) or the healthcare provider (second party). Some healthcare providers are even beginning to contract directly with the employers to provide health care, thus eliminating insurance carriers. Third-party payers have greatly influenced the direction of medicine.

> ℹ️ The healthcare provider, such as the phlebotomist, in addition to being an employee of an institution that relies on third-party payers for a major portion of its income is also a consumer of health care.

In the past decade, major changes have come about in healthcare payments and third-party reimbursements. Table 1-5 shows methods of payment and coding that have been used to standardize healthcare expenses.

DIAGNOSIS AND BILLING CODES

Healthcare organizations face major challenges in remaining fiscally strong in the coming years due to sweeping reforms in this industry. For that reason, it is imperative that all services be billed correctly and as quickly as possible, but with the advent of new technologies and electronic transfer of data, billing has become even more challenging. The lack of standardization and confusion in the diagnostic and procedural coding led to the passage in 1996 of HIPAA. This bill was designed to improve the efficiency of the healthcare system by establishing

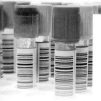

Table 1-5: Methods of Payment and Diagnosis Coding

Method of Payment	Abbreviation	Description
Prospective payment system	PPS	Begun in 1983 to limit and standardize the Medicare/Medicaid payments made to hospitals.
Diagnosis-related groups	DRGs	Originally designed by the American Hospital Association, hospitals are reimbursed a set amount for each patient procedure using established disease categories.
Ambulatory patient classification	APC	A classification system implemented in 2000 for determining payment to healthcare facilities for Medicare and Medicaid patients only.
Fee for service	FFS	Traditional payment model of reimbursement for healthcare services by third-party payers to the healthcare provider after service is rendered.

Diagnosis Codes	Abbreviation	Description
International Classification of Diseases, 9th rev., Clinical Modification	ICD-9-CM	Used in the past by all major payers It grouped together similar diseases and operations for reimbursement.
International Classification of Diseases, 10th rev., Clinical Modification	ICD-10-CM	For coding of diagnoses; contains more codes and covers more content than ICD-9.
International Classification of Diseases, 10th rev., Procedural Coding System	ICD-10-PSC	A procedural classification system for use only in the United States inpatient hospital settings. A clinical modification of ICD-10 that has a much broader range of codes with room for expansion and greater specificity.

standards for electronic data exchange, including coding systems. The goal of HIPAA regulations is to move to one universal procedural coding system (PCS) as the future standard. In 2014, the **Centers for Medicare and Medicaid Services (CMS)** replaced the list of procedure codes found in ICD-9-CM with a new code set called the Procedural Coding System (PCS) or better known as **ICD-10-PCS**, the *International Classification of Diseases–Tenth Revision, Procedural Coding System.* This new ICD must be used by all HIPAA-covered entities. ICD-9 diagnosis and procedure codes can no longer be used.

The **current procedural terminology (CPT)** codes were originally developed in the 1960s by the American Medical Association to provide a terminology and coding system for physician billing. Physicians' offices have continued to use it to report their services. Now all types of healthcare providers use CPT to classify, report, and bill for a variety of healthcare services. In 2014 when the new, ICD-10-PCS procedure codes became available for use in inpatient settings, the CPT procedure codes remained the codes used by physicians for reporting procedures in ambulatory settings and for their professional services in inpatient settings.

REIMBURSEMENT

The history of institutional reimbursement is tied to entitlement programs such as **Medicare** and public welfare in the form of **Medicaid**. Before 1983, hospitals were paid retrospectively and reimbursed for all services performed on Medicare and Medicaid patients. Many changes have been made to federal and state reimbursements since that time. A comparison of Medicare and Medicaid Programs is listed in Box 1-4.

Arizona is the only state that has devised its own system outside of Medicaid, called the **Arizona Health Care Cost Containment System (AHCCCS)**. It differs in that the providers (private physician groups) must bid annually for contracts to serve this population and patients are able to choose their healthcare provider through annual open enrollment.

The Changing Healthcare System

Healthcare systems are currently undergoing major revisions due to an environment that is seen as fragmented and wasteful. The driving force behind these changes is the ever-increasing demands on healthcare services to deliver patient-centered care and improve outcomes at a much lower cost. One of the goals of the ACA is to streamline the delivery of health care by reducing duplication through a new kind of integrated care offered by an **Accountable Care Organization (ACO)**. An ACO is a network of hospitals, physicians, and other healthcare

Box 1-4

Medicare and Medicaid Program Comparison

Medicare	Medicaid
First enacted in 1965.	First enacted in 1965.
Federally funded program for providing health care to persons over the age of 65, regardless of their financial status, and to the disabled.	Federal and state program that provides medical assistance for low-income Americans.
An entitlement program because it is a right earned by individuals through employment.	No entitlement feature; recipients must prove their eligibility.
Financed through Social Security payroll deductions and copayments.	Funds come from federal grants and state and local governments and are administered by the state.
Benefits divided into two categories: Part A, called hospital services, and Part B, called supplementary medical insurance (SMI), which is optional.	Benefits cover inpatient care, outpatient and diagnostic services, skilled nursing facilities, and home health and physician services.

providers who *voluntarily* offer to coordinate care for their Medicare patients. In an ACO, the providers are jointly accountable for the health of their patients, giving them financial incentive to cooperate and seamlessly share information to avoid unnecessary testing and expense.

If the ACO succeeds in offering quality patient care and spending less, they get to share in the savings it achieves for the Medicare program. Today all healthcare organizations and services find they must do more with less and have implemented some form of managed care as a way to survive.

MANAGED CARE

Managed care is a generic term for a payment system that attempts to control cost and access to health care, and strives to meet high-quality standards. Some of the methods used to control costs include

- limiting the providers that the enrollee/patient can use.
- use of primary care physicians as gatekeepers to control referrals.
- use of case managers to monitor and coordinate patients.
- utilization review of all healthcare services.

Most managed care systems do not provide medical care to enrollees; instead, they enter into contracts with healthcare facilities, physicians, and other healthcare providers who supply medical services to the enrollees/clients in the plan.

Benefits or payments paid to the provider are made according to a set fee schedule, and enrollees must comply with managed care policies such as preauthorization for certain medical procedures and approved referral to specialists for claims to be paid. Because the association

of provider, payer, and consumer is the foundation of managed care systems, several concepts have been developed to control this relationship, including gatekeepers and large services networks.

Case Management

One of the most important concepts in managed care is that of the designated **case manager** (primary care provider, gatekeeper), whose responsibility is to coordinate all of a patient's health care. The case manager is an experienced healthcare professional, not necessarily a physician, who knows the patient's condition and needs and where available resources for support and treatment can be found. As the patient's advocate, this person has the responsibility to advise the patient on healthcare needs and coordinate responses to those needs. The case manager's responsibilities also include providing early detection and treatment for disease, which can reduce the total cost of care.

Network Service Systems

Today's large **managed care organizations (MCOs)** evolved from prepaid healthcare plans such as **health maintenance organizations (HMOs)** and **preferred provider organizations (PPOs)**. HMOs are group practices reimbursed on a prepaid, negotiated, and discounted basis of admission. PPOs are independent groups of physicians or hospitals that offer services to employers at discounted rates in exchange for a steady supply of patients. MCOs contract with local providers to establish a complete network of services. The goal of the MCO is to reduce the total cost of care while maintaining patient satisfaction, and this can best be done if the patient can get the right care from the right provider at the right time. To accomplish this, integrated delivery networks (IDNs), also called integrated delivery systems (IDSs), have been developed. An IDN or IDS is a healthcare provider that includes a number of associated medical facilities that can furnish coordinated healthcare services from prebirth to death. Some of the institutions through which the services are offered along this continuum of care are acute care hospitals, ambulatory surgery centers, physician office practices, outpatient clinics, pharmacies, rehabilitation centers, and skilled nursing facilities (SNFs). The focus of an IDN arrangement is holistic, coordinated, cost-effective care rather than fragmented care performed by many medical specialists.

(i) In 2009, according to American Hospital Association, 58% of hospitals were part of integrated delivery networks (IDNs) made up of a group of hospitals, physicians, insurers, other providers, and community agencies that all work together to control costs through coordinated care and often characterized themselves as ACOs.

Medical Specialties

In managed care, the primary physician is most often a family practitioner, pediatrician, or internist. As a manager of a person's care, he or she is expected to refer to the appropriate specialist as needed. Some of the many healthcare areas in which a doctor of medicine (MD) or doctor of osteopathy (DO) can specialize are listed in Table 1-6.

Organization of Hospital Services

Hospitals are often large organizations with a complex internal structure required to provide acute care to patients who need it. Actually the term *hospital* can be applied to any healthcare facility that has these four main characteristics:

- Permanent inpatient beds
- 24-hour nursing service
- Therapeutic and diagnostic services
- Organized medical staff

The healthcare delivery system in hospitals is designed to function 24 hours a day, 7 days a week with high-quality service delivered every hour of the day. This means that the organizational structure has many layers of management arranged by departments or medical specialties. The lines of authority are structured so that functions and services are clustered under similar areas with an executive, such as a vice

president, administering each area. This grouping allows for efficient management of the departments and a clear understanding of the chain of command by the specialized staff in each area. The private practice physicians at the hospital have been granted clinical privileges (i.e., permission to provide patient care at that facility) by a hospital-governing board. These members of the medical team are not actual employees of the facility. However, many hospitals directly employ radiologists, critical care specialists, hospitalists, and a general physician who assumes the care (admission and ongoing treatment) of inpatients in the place of a primary care physician.

(i) Blue Cross and Blue Shield of Kansas City estimates 55% of physicians in the Kansas City area are now employed by hospitals according to an article from The Kansas City Star, December, 2013.

Managed care has led to a reduction in the number of healthcare personnel, whereas the number of services remains the same. This has resulted in cross-trained personnel and the continuous consolidation of services. Such reengineering, as it is called, is designed to make the healthcare delivery system more process-oriented and customer-focused. This shift in design brings significant savings by the efficient use of supplies and space, thereby reducing costs and increasing productivity. Although the lines between former departments are becoming blurred, Table 1-7 shows the services areas that can be considered essential.

Clinical Laboratory Services

Clinical laboratory (lab) services perform tests on patient specimens. Results of testing are used by physicians to confirm health or aid in the diagnosis, evaluation, and monitoring of patient medical conditions. Clinical labs are typically located in hospitals, large reference laboratories, and outpatient clinics.

TRADITIONAL LABORATORIES

There are two major divisions in the clinical laboratory, the clinical analysis area and the anatomical and surgical pathology area. All laboratory testing is associated with one of these two areas (Box 1-5). Large laboratories have organizational arrangements similar to the hospitals based on management structure or hierarchy. People who do similar tasks are grouped into departments (Fig. 1-8), the goal being to perform each task accurately, efficiently, and cost-effectively.

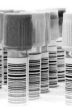

Table 1-6: Medical Specialties

Specialty	Area of Interest	Specialist Title
Allergy and immunology	Disorders of the immune system resulting in hypersensitivity	Allergist–Immunologists
Anesthesiology	Partial or complete loss of sensation, usually by injection or inhalation	Anesthesiologist
Cardiology	Diseases of the heart and blood vessels and cardiovascular surgery, a subspecialty of internal medicine	Cardiologist
Dermatology	Diseases and injuries of the skin; more recently, concerned with skin cancer prevention	Dermatologist
Emergency medicine	Emergent or acute medical care due to trauma, accident, or major medical event	Physician, Medical Specialist
Endocrinology	Disorders of the endocrine glands, such as, sterility, diabetes, and thyroid problems	Endocrinologist
Family medicine	Continuous and comprehensive health care for individuals and family	General or family practitioner
Gastroenterology	Digestive tract and related structural diseases, a subspecialty of internal medicine	Gastroenterologist
Gerontology	Effects of aging and age-related disorders	Gerontologist
Hematology	Disorders of the blood and blood-forming organs	Hematologist
Infectious diseases	Contagious and noncontagious infections caused by pathogenic microorganisms	ID specialist
Internal medicine	Diseases of internal organs and general medical conditions; uses nonsurgical therapy	Internist
Nephrology	Diseases related to the structure and function of the kidney	Nephrologist
Neurology	Disorders of the brain, spinal cord, and nerves	Neurologist
Obstetrics and gynecology	Pregnancy, childbirth, disorders of the reproductive system, and menopause	Gynecologist
Oncology	Tumors, including benign and malignant conditions	Oncologist
Ophthalmology	Eye examinations, eye diseases, and surgery	Ophthalmologist
Orthopedics	Disorders of the musculoskeletal system, including preventing disorders and restoring function	Orthopedist
Otorhinolaryngology	Disorders of the eye, ear, nose, and throat	Otorhinolaryngologist
Pediatrics	Diseases of children from birth to adolescence, including wellness checks and vaccinations	Pediatrician
Primary care physician	Undiagnosed health-related issues and continuous care for varied medical conditions	General practitioner
Psychiatry	Mental illness, clinical depression, and other behavioral and emotional disorders	Psychiatrist
Pulmonary medicine	Function of the lungs; treatment of disorders of the respiratory system	Pulmonologist
Rheumatology	Rheumatic diseases (acute and chronic conditions characterized by inflammation and joint disease)	Rheumatologist
Sports medicine	Injuries or illnesses resulting from participation in athletic activities	Sports medicine specialist
Urology	Urinary tract disease and disorders of the male reproductive system	Urologist

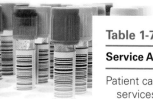

Table 1-7: Essential Service Areas of a Hospital

Service Area	Departments Within Area	Services Performed
Patient care services	Nursing care	Direct patient care. Includes careful observation to assess conditions, administering medications and treatments prescribed by a physician, evaluation of patient care, and documentation in the health record that reflects this. Staffed by many types of nursing personnel including registered nurses (RNs), licensed practical nurses (LPNs), and certified nursing assistants (CNAs).
	Emergency services	Around-the-clock service designed to handle medical emergencies that call for immediate assessment and management of injured or acutely ill patients. Staffed by specialists such as emergency medical technicians (EMTs) and MDs who specialize in emergency medicine.
	Intensive care units (ICUs)	Designed for increased bedside care of patients in fragile condition. Found in many areas of the hospital and named for the type of patient care they provide (e.g., trauma ICU, pediatric ICU, medical ICU).
	Surgery	Concerned with operative procedures to correct deformities and defects, repair injuries, and cure certain diseases. All work is performed by licensed medical practitioners who specialize in surgery.
Support services	Central supply	Prepares and dispenses all the necessary supplies required for patient care, including surgical packs for the operating room, intravenous pumps, bandages, syringes, and other inventory controlled by computer for close accounting.
	Dietary services	Selects foods and supervises food services to coordinate diet with medical treatment.
	Environmental services	Includes housekeeping and groundskeepers whose services maintain a clean, healthy, and attractive facility.
	Health information technology	Maintains accurate and orderly records for inpatient medical history, test results and reports, and treatment plans and notes from doctors and nurses to be used for insurance claims, legal actions, and utilization reviews.
Professional services	Cardiodiagnostics (EKG or ECG)	Performs electrocardiograms (EKGs/ECGs, or actual recordings of the electrical currents detectable from the heart), Holter monitoring, and stress testing for diagnosis and monitoring of therapy in cardiovascular patients.
	Pathology and clinical laboratory	Performs highly automated and often complicated testing on blood and other body fluids to detect and diagnose disease, monitor treatments, and, more recently, assess health. There are several specialized areas of the laboratory called departments or clinical laboratory areas (Box 1-5).
	Electroneurodiagnostic technology (ENT) or electroencephalography (EEG)	Performs electroencephalograms (EEGs), tracings that measure electrical activity of the brain. Uses techniques such as ambulatory EEG monitoring, evoked potentials, polysomnography (sleep studies), and brain-wave mapping to diagnose and monitor neurophysiological disorders.
Professional services	Occupational therapy (OT)	Uses techniques designed to develop or assist mentally, physically, or emotionally disabled patients to maintain daily living skills.
	Pharmacy	Prepares and dispenses drugs ordered by physicians; advises the medical staff on selection and harmful side effects of drugs, therapeutic drug monitoring, and drug use evaluation.
	Physical therapy (PT)	Diagnoses physical impairment to determine the extent of disability and provides therapy to restore mobility through individually designed treatment plans.
	Respiratory therapy (RT)	Diagnoses, treats, and manages patients' lung deficiencies (e.g., analyzes arterial blood gases [ABGs], tests lung capacity, administers oxygen therapy).
	Diagnostic radiology services	Diagnoses medical conditions by taking x-ray films of various parts of the body. Uses latest procedures, including powerful forms of imaging that do not involve radiation hazards, such as ultrasound machines, magnetic resonance (MR) scanners, and positron emission tomography (PET) scanners.

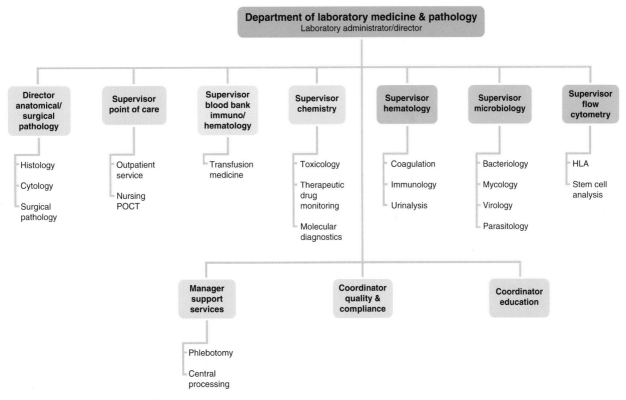

Figure 1-8 An example of a clinical laboratory organizational chart.

📖 **Match laboratory departments with laboratory tests in Matching Exercise 1-4 in the WORKBOOK.**

Clinical Analysis Areas

Hematology

The hematology department performs laboratory tests that identify diseases associated with blood and the blood-forming tissues. The most commonly ordered hematology test is the complete blood count (CBC). The CBC is performed using automated instruments, such as the Beckman Coulter® Counter (Fig. 1-9), that electronically count the cells and calculate results. A CBC is actually a multipart assay reported on a form called a hemogram (Table 1-8).

Coagulation

Coagulation is the study of the ability of blood to form and dissolve clots. Coagulation tests are closely related to hematology tests and are used to discover, identify,

Box 1-5

Two Major Divisions in the Clinical Laboratory

Clinical Analysis Areas	Anatomical and Surgical Pathology
Specimen processing, hematology, chemistry, microbiology, blood bank/immunohematology, immunology/serology, and urinalysis	Tissue analysis, cytologic examination, surgical biopsy, frozen sections, and performance of autopsies

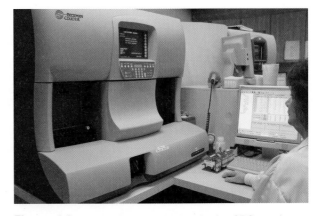

Figure 1-9 A medical technologist checks CBC results on the Beckman Coulter® LH780 Hematology Analyzer.

Table 1-8: Hemogram for Complete Blood Count (CBC) Assay

Name of Test	Abbreviation	Examples of Clinical Significance
Hematocrit	Hct	Values correspond to the red cell count and hemoglobin level; when decreased, indicate anemic conditions.
Hemoglobin	Hgb	Decreased values indicate anemic conditions; values normally differ with age, sex, altitude, and hydration.
Red blood cell count	RBC count	Measure of erythropoietic activity; decreases in numbers are related to anemic conditions.
White blood cell count	WBC count	Abnormal leukocyte response indicative of various conditions, such as infections and malignancies; when accompanied by low WBCs, differential test becomes more specific.
Platelet count	Plt count	Decreased numbers are indicative of hemorrhagic diseases; values may be used to monitor chemotherapy or radiation treatments.
Differential white count	Diff	Changes in the appearance or number of specific cell types signify specific disease conditions; values are also used to monitor chemotherapy or radiation treatments.
Indices		Changes in RBC size, weight, and Hgb content indicate certain types of anemias.
Mean corpuscular hemoglobin	MCH	Reveals the weight of the hemoglobin in the cell, regardless of size. Decreased hemoglobin content is indicative of iron-deficiency anemia, increased hemoglobin content is found in macrocytic anemia.
Mean corpuscular volume	MCV	Reveals the size of the cell. Decreased MCV is associated with thalassemia and iron-deficiency anemia; increased MCV suggests folic acid or vitamin B12 deficiency and chronic emphysema.
Mean corpuscular hemoglobin concentration	MCHC	Reveals the hemoglobin concentration per unit volume of RBCs. Below-normal range means that RBCs are deficient in hemoglobin, as in thalassemia, overhydration, or iron-deficiency anemia; above-normal range is seen in severe burns, prolonged dehydration, and hereditary spherocytosis.
Red blood cell distribution width	RDW	Reveals the size differences of the RBCs. An early predictor of anemia before other signs and symptoms appear.

and monitor defects in the blood-clotting mechanism. They are also used to monitor patients who are taking medications called anticoagulants (chemicals that inhibit blood clotting) or "blood thinners." The two most common coagulation tests are the prothrombin time (PT), used to monitor warfarin therapy, and the activated partial thromboplastin time (aPTT), for evaluating heparin therapy. The **PT** and the calculated standardized unit for the PT called **international normalized ratio (INR)** are measures of the *extrinsic pathway* of coagulation. They are used in conjunction with the activated partial thromboplastin time (aPTT) which measures the *intrinsic pathway* (Table 1-9).

Chemistry

The chemistry department performs most laboratory tests. This department may have subsections such as toxicology, therapeutic drug monitoring, and molecular diagnostics. Highly automated computerized instruments like the cobas® 6000 (Fig. 1-10) used in this area

are capable of performing discrete (individualized) tests or metabolic panels (multiple tests) from a single sample. Physicians are finding with the specificity of new tests, a risk panel for a specific organ is very helpful in diagnosis and prevention.

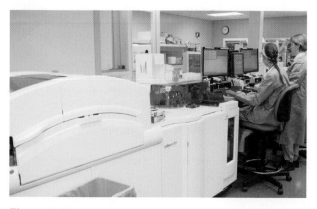

Figure 1-10 Laboratory chemists monitor and review chemistry results from the cobas® 6000 chemistry analyzer.

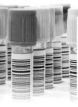

Table 1-9: Common Coagulation Tests

Test	Examples of Clinical Significance
Activated partial thromboplastin time (aPTT)	Prolonged times may indicate stage 1 defects; values reflect adequacy of heparin therapy.
D-dimer	Evaluates thrombin and plasmin activity and is very useful in testing for disseminated intravascular coagulation (DIC); also used in monitoring thrombolytic therapy.
Fibrin split products (FSP)	High levels result in FDP fragments that interfere with platelet function and clotting.
Fibrinogen	Fibrinogen deficiency suggests hemorrhagic disorders and is used most frequently in obstetrics.
Prothrombin time (PT) or international normalized ratio (INR)	Prolonged times may indicate stage 2 and 3 coagulation defects; values are used to monitor warfarin therapy and to evaluate liver disease and vitamin K deficiency.
Thrombin time (TT)	The main use for this test is to detect or exclude the presence of heparin or heparin-like anticoagulants when used in conjunction with other tests for evaluating unexplained prolonged clotting times.

An example of a risk panel being used for cardiovascular assessment includes such tests as follows:

- Apolipoprotein B (ApoB), the primary component of LDL
- 9p21, the strongest genomic marker for coronary artery disease
- N-terminal prohormone of brain natriuretic peptide (NT-proBNP)
- High-sensitivity C-reactive protein (hsCRP)
- Homocysteine, elevated levels increase risk for heart and blood vessel disease
- Fibrinogen, a newly emerging biomarker associated with cardiovascular disease

The use of genetic markers is the new medical model for customized health care or **personalized medicine (PM)**.

 See Appendix A for an expanded list of laboratory tests, sample considerations, and clinical correlation.

Examples of panels that might be ordered to evaluate a single organ or specific body system are given in Table 1-10.

The two most common chemistry specimens are serum and plasma; however, other types of specimens tested include whole blood, urine, and various other body fluids. Examples of tests normally performed in this clinical laboratory section can be found in Appendix A.

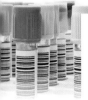

Table 1-10: Disease- and Organ-Specific Chemistry Panels (CMS-Approved)

Panel Grouping	Battery of Selected Diagnostic Tests
Basic metabolic panel (BMP)	Glucose, blood urea nitrogen (BUN), creatinine, sodium, potassium, chloride, carbon dioxide (CO_2), calcium
Comprehensive metabolic panel (CMP)	Albumin, glucose, BUN, creatinine, sodium, potassium, chloride, CO_2, aspartate aminotransferase (AST), alanine aminotransferase (ALT), alkaline phosphatase, total protein, total bilirubin, calcium
Electrolyte panel	Sodium, potassium, chloride, CO_2
Hepatic function panel A	AST, ALT, alkaline phosphatase, total protein, albumin, total bilirubin, direct bilirubin
Lipid panel	Cholesterol, lipoprotein, high-density cholesterol (HDL) triglycerides
Renal function panel	Glucose, BUN, creatinine, sodium, potassium, chloride, CO_2, calcium, albumin, phosphorus

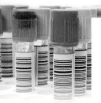

Table 1-11: Common Serology and Immunology Tests

Test	Examples of Clinical Significance
Bacterial Studies	
Antinuclear antibody (ANA)	Positive results indicate autoimmune disorders, specifically systemic lupus erythematosus
FTA-ABS	Fluorescent treponemal antibody absorption test, confirmatory test for syphilis
Rapid plasma reagin (RPR)	Positive screen indicates syphilis; positives must be confirmed
Viral Studies	
Anti-HIV	Screening for human immunodeficiency virus
Cytomegalovirus antibody (CMV)	Screening for evidence of current or past infection
Epstein–Barr virus (EBV)	Presence of this heterophil antibody indicates infectious mononucleosis
Hepatitis B surface antigen (HBsAg)	Demonstrates the presence of hepatitis antigen on the surface of the red cells
HCV	Demonstrates the presence of hepatitis antibodies on the surface of the red cells
General Studies	
Cold agglutinins	Present in cases of atypical pneumonia
High-sensitivity C-reactive protein (hs-CRP)	Increased levels of this protein are present in inflammatory conditions
Human chorionic gonadotropin (HCG)	Present in pregnancy (serum and urine)
Immunoglobulins	Can show presence of five subclasses of antibodies made by immune system to neutralize foreign antigens, such as bacteria or toxins.
Rheumatoid factor (RF)	Presence of antibody indicates rheumatoid arthritis

Serology or Immunology

The term *serology* means the study of serum. Serology tests deal with the body's response to the presence of bacterial, viral, fungal, or parasitic diseases stimulating antigen–antibody reactions that can easily be demonstrated in the laboratory (Table 1-11). Autoimmune reactions, in which autoantibodies produced by B lymphocytes attack normal cells, are becoming more prevalent and can be detected by serologic tests. Testing can be done by polymerase chain reaction (PCR), enzyme-linked immunosorbent assay (ELISA), fluorescent antibodies, agglutination, or precipitation to determine the antibody or antigen present and to assess its concentration or titer.

Urinalysis

The urinalysis (UA) department is often housed in the hematology or chemistry area. Urine specimens may be analyzed manually or using automated instruments like the Iris (Fig. 1-11). UA is a routine urine test that includes physical, chemical, and microscopic evaluations (Table 1-12). The physical examination assesses the color, clarity, and specific gravity of the specimen.

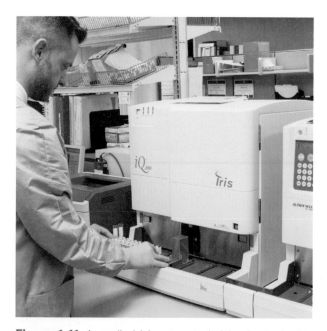

Figure 1-11 A medical laboratory technician loads the Iris automated urine analyzer.

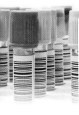

Table 1-12: Common Urinalysis Tests

Test	Examples of Clinical Significance
Physical Evaluation	
Color	Abnormal colors that are clinically significant result from blood melanin, bilirubin, or urobilin in the sample
Clarity	Turbidity may be the result of chyle, fat, bacteria, RBCs, WBCs, or precipitated crystals
Specific gravity	Variation in this indicator of dissolved solids in the urine is normal; inconsistencies suggest renal tubular involvement or ADH deficiency
Chemical Evaluation	
Blood	Hematuria may be the result of hemorrhage, infection, or trauma
Bilirubin	Aids in differentiating obstructive jaundice from hemolytic jaundice, which will not cause increased bilirubin in the urine
Glucose	Glucosuria could be the result of diabetes mellitus, renal impairment, or ingestion of a large amount of carbohydrates
Ketones	Elevated ketones occur in uncontrolled diabetes mellitus and starvation
Leukocyte esterase	Certain white cells (neutrophils) in abundance indicate urinary tract infection
pH	Variations in pH indicate changes in acid–base balance, which is normal; loss of ability to vary pH is indicative of tissue breakdown
Protein	Proteinuria is an indicator of renal disorder, such as injury and renal tube dysfunction
Nitrite	Positive result suggests bacterial infection but is significant only on first-morning specimen or urine incubated in bladder for at least 4 hours
Urobilinogen	Occurs in increased amounts when patient has hepatic problems or hemolytic disorders
Microscopic Evaluation	Analysis of urinary sediment reveals status of the urinary tract, hematuria, or pyuria; the presence of casts and tissue cells is a pathologic indicator.

The chemical evaluation performed using chemical reagent strips screens for substances such as sugar and protein and can be read by hand, visually, or with a urine analyzer. A microscopic examination establishes the presence or absence of blood cells, bacteria, crystals, and other substances.

Microbiology

The microbiology department analyzes body fluids and tissues for the presence of microorganisms, primarily by means of culture and sensitivity (C&S) testing. An automated, computerized identification and susceptibility testing system as shown in Figure 1-12 allows for continuous monitoring, customized antibiotic panels, and the reporting of results more quickly. Results of a C&S tell the physician the type of organisms present and the particular antibiotics that would be most effective for treatment. It is very important to collect, transport, and handle microbiology specimens properly in order to determine the presence of microorganisms and identify them appropriately. An instrument, as shown in Figure 1-13, used only for detection of bloodstream infections makes the observation and identification for microbial growth in the blood culture vials much more efficient.

Subsections of microbiology are bacteriology (the study of bacteria), parasitology (the study of parasites), virology (the study of viruses), and mycology (the study of fungi). Most recently, the mycology section in larger laboratories is using DNA-based testing to identify invasive fungal infections (IFIs) that have

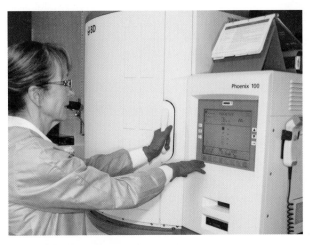

Figure 1-12 A microbiologist checks computer read out for antibiotic sensitivities from the BD Phoenix™ automated microbiology system.

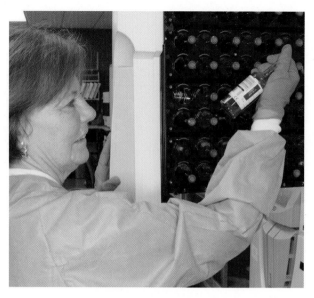

Figure 1-13 A microbiologist reviews blood cultures processed by the BD BACTEC™ FX blood culture instrument.

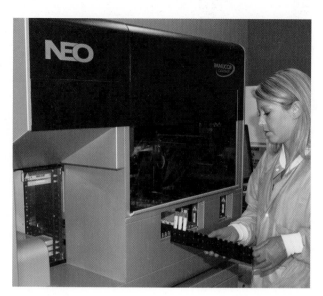

Figure 1-14 NEO Immucor Gamma blood bank automated instrument being loaded with blood samples for type and screen.

become an important issue for patients who are very sick and lack the ability to fight infection (Table 1-13).

(i) Patients who have suppressed immune systems due to aggressive chemotherapy for cancer, organ, and stem cell transplants are susceptible to unusual types of yeast infections that can be deadly unless correctly detected and identified.

Blood Bank or Immunohematology

The blood bank or immunohematology department of the laboratory prepares blood products to be used

for patient transfusions. Blood components dispensed include whole blood, platelets, packed cells, fresh frozen plasma, and cryoprecipitates. Blood samples from all donors and the recipient must be carefully tested before transfusions can be administered so that incompatibility and transfusion reactions can be avoided (Table 1-14). In large clinical laboratories, automation, such as the NEO Immucor Gamma (Fig. 1-14) supports a demanding workload by producing quality-controlled results for type and screen of several hundred tests per hour. Transfusion services offered by the blood bank department collect, prepare, and store units of blood from donors or patients who wish to donate their own units for autologous transfusion should that be needed.

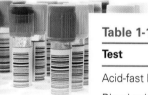

Table 1-13: Common Microbiology Tests

Test	Examples of Clinical Significance
Acid-fast bacilli (AFB)	Positive stain means pulmonary tuberculosis; used to monitor the treatment of TB
Blood culture	Positive culture results (bacterial growth in media) indicate bacteremia or septicemia
CLOtest	Presence of *Helicobacter pylori*
Culture and sensitivity (C&S)	Growth of a pathogenic microorganism indicates infection (culture); in vitro inhibition by an antibiotic (sensitivity) allows the physician to select the correct treatment
Fungus culture and identification	Positive culture detects the presence of fungi and determines the type
Gram stain	Positive stain for specific types of pathogenic microorganisms permits antimicrobial therapy to begin before culture results are known
Occult blood	Positive test indicates blood in the stool, which is associated with gastrointestinal bleeding from carcinoma
Ova and parasites	Microscopic examination of stool sample showing ova and parasites solves many "etiology unknown" intestinal disorders
Viral studies	Tests used to detect or confirm exposure to infection-causing viruses

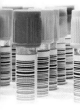

Table 1-14: Common Blood Bank and Immunohematology Tests

Test	Examples of Clinical Significance
Antibody (Ab) screen	Agglutination indicates abnormal antibodies present in patient's blood
Direct antiglobulin test (DAT)	Positive results point to autoimmune hemolytic anemia, hemolytic disease of the newborn (HDN), and transfusion incompatibility
Type and Rh	Determines blood group (ABO) and type (Rh) by identifying agglutinins present or absent
Type and crossmatch	Determines blood group and serves as a general screen for antibodies of recipient's blood; then recipient and donor blood are checked against each other for compatibility
Compatibility testing	Detection of unsuspected antibodies and antigens in recipient's and donor's blood, which could cause a severe reaction if transfused

Cytogenetic and Flow Cytometry

Two areas found in larger labs are cytogenetics and flow cytometry. In cytogenetics, samples are examined microscopically for chromosomal deficiencies that relate to genetic disease. Specimens used for chromosomal studies include fresh blood, solid tissues, prenatal specimens, and bone marrow.

Flow cytometry has many applications in routine clinical diagnosis and is also used for clinical trials and in basic research to analyze and sort cells. The BD FACSCalibur™ as seen in Figure 1-15 is a modular analyzer that can be used for stem cell analysis, T&B leukocyte assay, and human leukocyte antigen (HLA) tissue typing and crossmatching for organ transplants.

Anatomical and Surgical Pathology

Histology

Histology is defined as the study of the microscopic structure of tissues. In this department, pathologists evaluate

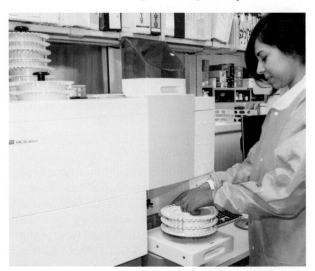

Figure 1-15 Medical Laboratory Scientist loads BD FACSCalibur™ modular analyzer with tissue samples for HLA testing.

samples of tissue from surgeries and autopsies under a microscope to determine if they are normal or pathological (diseased). Histological techniques include two of the most common diagnostic techniques found in the laboratory: (1) biopsy, obtaining samples by removal of a plug (small piece) of tissue from an organ and examining it microscopically, and (2) frozen section, obtaining tissue from surgery and freezing it, then examining it immediately to determine whether more extensive surgery is needed. Before tissues can be evaluated, they must be processed and stained. This is the role of a person called a histologist.

Cytology

Cytology and histology are often confused. Whereas histology tests are concerned with the structure of tissue, cytology tests are concerned with the structure of cells. In this department, cells in body tissues and fluids are identified, counted, and studied to diagnose malignant and premalignant conditions. Histologists often process and prepare the specimens for evaluation by a pathologist or cytotechnologist. The Pap smear, a test for early detection of cancer cells, primarily of the cervix and vagina, is one of the most common examinations performed by this department.

ⓘ The Pap test is named after Dr. George N. Papanicolaou, who developed a staining technique used to detect malignant cells.

SATELLITE LABS

In today's rapidly changing healthcare environment, some laboratory services in large tertiary care facilities have had to set up satellite labs. These specialized labs are located close to the populations they serve in order to facilitate better outcomes for the patients by drastically reducing the **turnaround times (TATs)** for test results. Each satellite lab has a test menu designed for their specific population. Example is a NICU lab in the Newborn ICU area, a critical

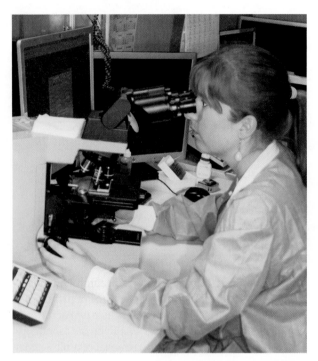

Figure 1-16 A medical technologist checks a differential in the ED Stat lab.

care lab that is close to the operating and recovery room or a STAT lab in the ED. Tests performed in these labs are those needed to respond to medical emergencies, such as the microscopic examination of a newborn's blood in ICU as shown in Figure 1-16.

REFERENCE LABORATORIES

Reference laboratories are large independent laboratories that receive specimens from many different facilities located in the same city, other cities in the same state, or even cities that are out of state. They provide routine and more specialized analysis of blood, urine, tissue, and other patient specimens. One of the benefits of sending specimens to a reference laboratory is the cost per test is reduced due to the high volume of tests that are performed at these sites. Reference laboratories offer "STAT" testing, but since it is off-site the TAT cannot compare to an on-site laboratory. Specimens sent to off-site laboratories must be carefully packaged in special containers designed to protect the specimens and meet federal safety regulations for the transportation of human specimens.

Clinical Laboratory Personnel
LABORATORY DIRECTOR/PATHOLOGIST

The pathologist is a physician who specializes in diagnosing disease, through the use of laboratory

tests results, in tissues removed at operations and from postmortem examinations. It is his or her duty to direct laboratory services so that they benefit both the physician and patient. The laboratory director may be a pathologist or a clinical laboratory scientist with a doctorate. The laboratory director and the laboratory administrator share responsibilities for managing the laboratory.

LABORATORY ADMINISTRATOR/ LABORATORY MANAGER

The lab administrator is usually a technologist with an advanced degree and several years of experience. Duties of the administrator include overseeing all operations involving physician and patient services. Today, the laboratory administrator may supervise several ancillary services, such as radiology and respiratory therapy, or all the laboratory functions in a healthcare system consisting of separate lab facilities across a large geographic area.

TECHNICAL SUPERVISOR

For each laboratory section or subsection, there is a technical supervisor who is responsible for the administration of the area and who reports to the laboratory administrator. This person usually has additional education and experience in one or more of the clinical laboratory areas.

MEDICAL TECHNOLOGIST/MEDICAL LABORATORY SCIENTIST

The medical technologist (MT) or **medical laboratory scientist (MLS)** generally has a bachelor's (BS) degree plus additional studies and experience in the clinical laboratory setting. Some states require licensing for this level of personnel. The responsibilities of the MT/MLS include performing all levels of testing in any area of the laboratory, reporting results, performing quality control, evaluating new procedures, and conducting preventive maintenance and troubleshooting on instruments.

In 2009, the ASCP Board of Registry and the National Certification Agency for Clinical Laboratory Personnel (NCA) were unified into a single certifying agency. All individuals with an active NCA credential were transitioned over to the ASCP Board of Certification (BOC) without further requirements until recertification is due. All CLS (NCA) certificants who had an active credential with NCA were transferred to the BOC as MLS (ASCP).

MEDICAL LABORATORY TECHNICIAN

The medical laboratory technician (MLT) is most often an individual with an associate degree from a 2-year program or certification from a military or proprietary (private) school. As with the MT/MLS, some states may require licensing for MLTs. The technician is responsible for performing routine testing, operating all equipment, performing basic instrument maintenance, recognizing instrument problems, and assisting in problem solving.

> (i) All CLT (NCA) certificants who had an active credential with NCA on October 23, 2009, were transferred to the BOC as MLT (ASCP).

CLINICAL LABORATORY ASSISTANT

Before the arrival of computerized instrumentation in the laboratory, the clinical laboratory assistant (CLA) was a recognized position. Today, because of reductions in laboratory staff, this category of personnel has been revived. A CLA is a person with phlebotomy experience who has skills in specimen processing and basic laboratory testing. CLAs are generalists, responsible for assisting the MLS or MLT with workloads in any area.

PHLEBOTOMIST

The phlebotomist is trained to collect blood for laboratory tests that are necessary for the diagnosis and care of patients. A number of facilities use phlebotomists as laboratory assistants or specimen processors (see Box 1-1 for duties). Formal phlebotomy programs in colleges and private schools usually require a high school diploma or the equivalent to enroll. After completing the program or acquiring 1 year of work experience, a phlebotomist can become certified by passing a national examination. A few states require licensing for this level of personnel.

OTHER LABORATORY PERSONNEL

Other positions in the lab may include the
- laboratory information systems (LIS) manager who ensures proper functioning of the information

processing system, oversees upgrades and maintenance of the software and hardware.
- quality and compliance coordinator who oversees procedures, policies, and processes for continuous quality improvement.
- point-of-care supervisor who works closely with the nursing staff and outpatient services to ensure the quality of POCT results are correct and that the maintenance and QC checks on the POCT instruments are performed correctly by the operators of the instrument at all times.
- education coordinator who oversees all students who are chosen to do their clinical practicum in their laboratory. It is the coordinator's job to verify student credentials, make certain they meet the facility's health and safety requirements, and generally serve as a "gatekeeper" for anyone wishing to intern in that area. He or she also provides educational activities and continuing education for the laboratory personnel.
- supervisor of support services, such as phlebotomy and central processing, makes certain all specimens are correctly collected, received, and prepared for testing. He or she provides phlebotomy and central processing staff with training, technical direction, training support, and resolution of problems that arise in the laboratory on a day-to-day basis.

Clinical Laboratory Improvement Act

The **Clinical Laboratory Improvement Amendments of 1988 (CLIA '88)** is a federal law that allows the CMS in the Department of HHS to regulate all sites performing laboratory testing in the United States. CLIA regulations mandate that all laboratories use the same standards regardless of their location, type, or size. This includes standards for personnel in laboratories performing moderate- and high-complexity testing. Requirements are set for laboratory director, technical consultant, supervisors, and testing personnel. Detailed information may be found at http://www.cdc.gov/clia/regs/subpart_m.aspx.

Study and Review Questions

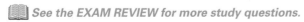 *See the EXAM REVIEW for more study questions.*

1. **Early equipment used for bloodletting included all of the following *except* the**
   a. fleam.
   b. hemostat.
   c. lancet.
   d. leech.

2. **A factor that contributes to the phlebotomist's professional image is**
   a. age.
   b. attitude.
   c. heritage.
   d. religion.

3. The initials for the title granted after successful completion of the American Society for Clinical Pathology phlebotomy examination are

    a. CLPlb.
    b. CLT.
    c. CPT.
    d. PBT.

4. The principles of right and wrong conduct as they apply to professional problems are called

    a. ethics.
    b. kinesics.
    c. proxemics.
    d. rules.

5. The law that established national standards for the electronic exchange of protected health information is

    a. CLIA.
    b. HIPAA.
    c. OSHA.
    d. PHS.

6. Which of the following may be a duty of the phlebotomist?

    a. Analyze specimens
    b. Chart patient results
    c. Perform POCT
    d. Process billing

7. Which of the following is an example of proxemics?

    a. Eye contact
    b. Facial expressions
    c. Personal hygiene
    d. Zone of comfort

8. Which of the following is proper telephone technique?

    a. Being careful of the tone of your voice when answering the phone.
    b. Not identifying yourself to the caller in case there is a problem later.
    c. Listening carefully, but not writing anything down so as to save time.
    d. Waiting for the phone to ring three or four times to appear less anxious.

9. An institution that provides inpatient services is a

    a. clinic.
    b. day surgery.
    c. doctor's office.
    d. hospital.

10. State and federally funded insurance is called

    a. ACO
    b. HIPAA
    c. Medicaid
    d. Medicare

11. The specialty that treats disorders of old age is called

    a. cardiology.
    b. gerontology.
    c. pathology.
    d. psychiatry.

12. The department in the hospital that prepares and dispenses drugs is

    a. central supply.
    b. pharmacy.
    c. physical therapy.
    d. radiology.

13. The microbiology department in the laboratory performs

    a. compatibility testing.
    b. culture and sensitivity testing.
    c. electrolyte monitoring.
    d. enzyme-linked immunoassay.

14. The abbreviation for the routine hematology test that includes hemoglobin, hematocrit, red blood count, and white blood count determinations is

    a. CBC.
    b. CDC.
    c. CPK.
    d. CRP.

15. Which of the following laboratory professionals is specified by CLIA as responsible for the administration of a specific clinical area, such as chemistry?

    a. Laboratory manager
    b. Medical laboratory scientist
    c. Medical laboratory technician
    d. Technical supervisor

Case Studies

 See the WORKBOOK for more case studies.

Case Study 1-1: Telephone Etiquette and the Irate Caller

Sally is a new phlebotomist working for a small hospital in the suburbs of Chicago. As she finds out in a very short time, her coworkers have many different job responsibilities and are required to cover for one another. Today it is Sally's turn to cover the reception area of the lab while the regular person takes a few days off. This is Sally's first time, and she is rather hesitant to answer the first call because she is afraid that she does not know enough to answer all inquiries. Consequently, she lets the phone ring more than 10 times. She finally answers it. The caller, a nurse, sounds irritated. He has been anxious to obtain certain results on a patient. He tells Sally that they were to be faxed 2 days earlier and he has not yet received them. Sally tells him she will transfer him to the technician in the back. Being unfamiliar with this phone, she loses his call in the process. The nurse calls back in a few minutes and wants to speak to "someone who knows what he or she is doing." The other line starts ringing. This time, rather than losing the caller, Sally keeps the line open, puts the phone down on the counter, and calls out "someone please take this call. I have a call on the other line."

QUESTIONS

1. Name three telephone etiquette errors that Sally made.

2. Which error creates the chance for a HIPAA violation to occur? Explain why.

3. What should Sally have done differently that would have prevented all three errors?

4. What responsibility does the laboratory administrator have?

Case Study 1-2: Phlebotomy and PHI

The phlebotomist, Matt, is doing the morning blood collections on the surgery floor of the hospital. As he begins to put the last tube in his cart and head for the clinical lab, the nurse asks him to draw blood from one more patient. She quickly points in the direction of the patient's room and turns to get the requisition. Matt did not see the exact room, so he shouts across the common area, "Do you mean the young, Hispanic man in room 412 who just had an appendectomy?" The nurse put her finger to her mouth and says "shhh" as she hands him the lab requisition.

QUESTIONS

1. Why did the nurse indicate Matt needed to be quiet?

2. What policy had the phlebotomist ignored?

3. What law governs Matt's actions?

4. What should Matt have done?

Bibliography and Suggested Readings

Bishop M, Fody E, Schoeff L. *Clinical Chemistry: Techniques, Principles, Correlations.* 7th ed. Philadelphia, PA: Wolters Kluwer/Lippincott Williams & Wilkins; 2013. www.pbs.org/wgbh/nova/body/leeches.html

Davis A, Appel T. *Bloodletting Instruments in the National Museum of History and Technology.* Washington, DC: Smithsonian Institution Press; 1979.

Fischbach FT, Dunning MB. *Manual of Laboratory and Diagnostic Tests.* 9th ed. Philadelphia, PA: Lippincott Williams & Wilkins; 2014.

Mitchell J, Haroun L. *Introduction to Health Care.* 3rd ed. Albany, NY: Delmar Publishers; 2011.

Sayles N. *Health Information Management Technology: An Applied Approach.* Chicago, IL: AHiMA; 2013.

Williams SJ. *Essentials of Health Services.* 3rd ed. New York, NY: Delmar Publishers; 2013.

 MEDIA MENU

Online Ancillaries (at http://thepoint.lww.com/McCall6e)

- Interactive exercises and games, including Look and Label, Word Building, Body Building, Roboterms, Crossword Puzzles, Quiz Show, and Concentration
- Audio Flash Cards and Flashcard Generator
- Audio Glossary

Internet Resources

- Museum of Quackery. http://museumofquackery.com
- http://www.phlebotomy.com/
- wwwn.cdc.gov/clia/regulatory/
- CMS.gov
- HealthCare.gov
- HHS.gov/HealthCare
- Mghlabtest.partners.org/PhlebotomyInfo.htm

Other Resources

- Ruth McCall and Cathee Tankersley. *Student Workbook for Phlebotomy Essentials.* 6th ed. (Available for separate purchase.)
- Ruth McCall and Cathee Tankersley. *Phlebotomy Exam Review.* 6th ed. (Available for separate purchase.)

Chapter 2

Quality Assurance and Legal Issues in Healthcare

NAACLS Entry Level Competencies

4.1 Describe the legal and ethical importance of proper patient/sample identification.

8.1 Describe quality assurance in the collection of blood specimens.

8.2 Identify policies and procedures used in the clinical laboratory to assure quality in the obtaining of blood specimens.

9.8 Define and use medicolegal terms and discuss policies and protocol designed to avoid medicolegal problems.

Key Terms

Do Matching Exercise 2-1 in the WORKBOOK to gain familiarity with these terms.

- assault
- battery
- breach of confidentiality
- civil actions
- CLSI
- CMS
- CQI
- defendant
- delta check
- deposition
- discovery
- due care
- fraud
- GLPs
- IQCP
- informed consent
- invasion of privacy
- malpractice
- negligence
- NPSGs
- PSC
- plaintiff
- QA
- QC
- quality indicators
- *respondeat superior*
- standard of care
- statute of limitations
- TJC
- threshold values
- tort
- vicarious liability

Objectives

Upon successful completion of this chapter, the reader should be able to:

1. Demonstrate basic knowledge of terminology for national organizations, agencies, and regulations that support quality assurance in health care.

2. Define quality and performance improvement measurements as they relate to phlebotomy, and describe the components of a quality assurance (QA) program and identify areas in phlebotomy subject to quality control (QC).

3. Demonstrate knowledge of the legal aspects associated with phlebotomy procedures by defining legal terminology and describing situations that may have legal ramifications.

Overview

This chapter focuses on quality assurance (QA) and legal issues in health care, including the relationship of both to the practice of phlebotomy. Consumer awareness has increased lawsuits in all areas of society. This is especially true in the healthcare industry. Consequently, it is essential for phlebotomists to recognize the importance of following QA guidelines and understand the legal implications of not doing so.

Quality Assurance in Health Care

As patient care becomes more complex and resources continue to shrink, healthcare institutions search for innovative ways to improve performance and guarantee quality patient care by identifying and minimizing situations that pose risks to patients and employees. Managing risk means the organization must be committed to continuous self-evaluation and process monitoring. Protocols are developed for all processes used and the personnel involved; and when formally adopted, they become the institution's **continuous quality improvement (CQI)** program. Measurement of performance and quality improvement projects are now part of the accreditation requirements for all types of healthcare facilities and are found in every aspect of health care, including phlebotomy. One of the ways to improve quality is through compliance with and use of national standards and regulations.

National Standard and Regulatory Agencies

Do Matching Exercise 2-3 in the WORKBOOK to reinforce your understanding of the services offered by organizations and regulatory agencies in the area of quality assurance.

THE JOINT COMMISSION

One of the key players in bringing quality assessment review techniques to health care is **The Joint Commission (TJC)**. This is an independent, not-for-profit organization charged with, among other things, establishing standards for the operation of hospitals and other health-related facilities and services. Its mission is *to continuously improve health care for the public, in collaboration with other stakeholders, by evaluating healthcare organizations and inspiring them to excel in providing safe and effective care of the highest quality and value.*

TJC is the oldest and largest standards-setting body in health care, presently accrediting and certifying more than 20,000 healthcare organizations (HCOs) and programs in the United States. To receive and maintain TJC's Gold Seal of Approval, an organization must undergo and pass an on-site evaluation by a survey team at least every 3 years (every 2 years for laboratories).

In 2009, TJC implemented key changes that strengthen the focus on quality care and patient safety. The traditional thresholds used in the past for accreditation measurements have been eliminated and, instead, program-specific screening criteria are being used in evaluations and on-site surveys. The revised model for the clinical laboratory incorporates activities intended to reduce total analytical error by improving the pre- and postanalytical processes and more oversight of point-of-care testing. As of 2014, the decision criteria used by an accreditation team have the following four scoring categories:

1. **Direct Impact Standards Requirements.** These are critical care process-related requirements that if not met may pose an immediate risk to patient safety. An example of jeopardizing patient safety is the lack of a quality-control program for each area or specialty in the clinical laboratory services.

2. **Indirect Impact Standards Requirements.** These are planning and evaluation requirements that are less of an immediate threat to patient safety and quality care but, over time, may put patients at risk. An example of an indirect impact on patients would be the lack of documentation for ongoing education of the staff.

3. **Situational Decision Rules.** An example of failure to meet the situational rules would be finding unlicensed personnel working in the facility in a state where licensure is required by law; or practicing outside the scope of license; or misrepresenting information to TJC. Preliminary Denial of Accreditation (PDA) will be recommended if any of the above should be discovered.

4. **Immediate Threat to Health and Safety.** Examples of noncompliance with this requirement would include a blood bank refrigerator temperature out of range, serious problems with specimen labeling, or patient identification (ID). Owing to the severity of this category, the Preliminary Denial of Accreditation (PDA) would be issued until corrective action was validated.

Current Joint Commission standards stress performance improvement by requiring the facility to be directly accountable to the customer. This means that all departments of a healthcare facility should be aware of their customers' expectations and complaints.

To evaluate and track complaints related to HCOs' quality of care, TJC's Office of Quality Monitoring was created. The office has a toll-free line that can help people register their complaints. Information and concerns often come from patients, their families, and healthcare employees. A complaint may be submitted online, by e-mail, fax, or by regular mail. When a report is submitted, TJC reviews any past reports and the organization's most recent accreditation decision. Depending on the nature of the reported concern, TJC will:

- Request a written response to the reported concern from the organization
- Incorporate the concern into a quality-monitoring database that is used to identify trends or patterns in performance
- Conduct an on-site, unannounced assessment of the organization if the report raises serious concerns about a continuing threat to patient safety or a continuing failure to comply with standards
- Review the reported concern and compliance at the organization's next accreditation survey

Patient Safety and Sentinel Events

TJC's commitment to safety for patients and employees in HCOs is a part of their mission for continuous improvement in health care provided to the public. One of the ways this is demonstrated is through its sentinel (early warning) event policy. The intent of this policy is to help HCOs identify significant safety issues and take steps to prevent them from happening again. A sentinel event (SE) is any unfavorable event that is unexpected and results in death or serious physical or psychological injury. Such an event signals the need for immediate investigation and response. An early warning of an undesirable outcome could be any deviation from an acceptable practice that continues to risk a patient or employee's safety. Loss of a limb or any of its function is specifically included as a SE. According to the policy, if a SE occurs, the HCO is required to:

- Perform a thorough and credible analysis of the root cause
- Develop an action plan
- Implement improvements to reduce risk into practice
- Monitor improvements to determine if they are effective

As reported to TJC for the years 1995 through 2005, communication is listed as the leading factor in the root causes of SEs. In 2008, TJC created a new **National Patient Safety Goal (NPSG)**, which states that HCOs must "Implement a standardized approach to 'hand-off' communications, including an opportunity to ask and respond to questions."

National Patient Safety Goals (NPSGs)

TJC's NPSGs program is part of the overall CQI requirements for accreditation. Established in 2002, the review and annual updates are overseen by a safety expert panel as well as physicians, nurses, risk managers, and other healthcare professionals. These safety practices play a significant role in advancing quality care. The goals have specific requirements for protecting patients. The annually updated goals address several critical areas of safety concerns and describe expert-based solutions. Examples of areas addressed are patient ID, communication, healthcare-associated infections, medication safety, and patient involvement.

As of 2014, the NPSGs for the clinical laboratory are as follows:

- **Identify patients correctly.** Use at least two ways to identify patients when providing laboratory services. For example, use the patient's name, an assigned ID number, or other person-specific information, such as date of birth. The patient's room number or physical location cannot be used as an identifier. Label all blood containers and other types of specimens in the patient's presence. Make certain that the correct patient gets the correct blood when they get a blood transfusion.
- **Improve staff communication.** Get important test results to the right staff person on time. Reporting critical results to the responsible caregiver will mean that the patient can be treated more promptly.
- **Prevent infection.** Use the current hand-cleaning guidelines from the Centers for Disease Control and Prevention (CDC) or the current World Health Organization (WHO). Set goals for improving hand cleaning, and use these goals to improve hand cleaning. This will reduce the transmission of infectious agents from staff to patients.

 The exact language of the Goals can be found at www.jointcommission.org.

COLLEGE OF AMERICAN PATHOLOGISTS

Another agency that influences quality care through standards for the laboratory and phlebotomy is the College of American Pathologists (CAP). This national organization is an outgrowth of the American Society for Clinical Pathology (ASCP), a not-for-profit organization for professionals in the field of laboratory medicine. Membership in CAP is exclusively for board-certified pathologists and pathologists in training. CAP offers proficiency testing and a continuous form of laboratory inspection by a team made up of pathologists and laboratory managers. The CAP Inspection and Accreditation Program does not compete with TJC accreditation for healthcare facilities because CAP is designed for pathology/laboratory services only. A CAP-certified laboratory also meets Medicare/Medicaid standards because TJC grants reciprocity (mutual exchange of privileges) to CAP in the area of laboratory inspection.

Key Point The CAP requires documentation in an employee's personnel file to confirm that the employee is qualified to perform the responsibilities for which he or she is assigned.

Do the WORKBOOK Case Study 2-1 exercise to reinforce your understanding of CLIA and CLIAC.

CLINICAL LABORATORY IMPROVEMENT AMENDMENTS OF 1988

The Clinical Laboratory Improvement Amendments of 1988 (CLIA '88) are federal regulations passed by Congress and administered by the **Centers for Medicare and Medicaid Services (CMS)**, an agency that manages federal healthcare programs of Medicare and Medicaid. These regulations establish quality standards that apply to all facilities, including clinics and physicians' office laboratories that test human specimens for the purpose of providing information used to diagnose, prevent, or treat disease and assess health status. The standards address QA, quality control (QC), proficiency testing, laboratory records, and personnel qualifications.

The aim of the standards is to ensure the accuracy, consistency, and reliability of patient test results regardless of the location, type, or size of the laboratory. To assist in administering these regulations, the Clinical Laboratory Improvement Advisory Committee (CLIAC) was formed. Its purpose is to provide technical and scientific advice and guidance to the appropriate people in CMS who are administering the regulations. CLIAC advises on the need for revisions to the standards under which clinical laboratories are regulated and the impact the proposed revisions will have on laboratory practice.

All laboratory facilities subject to CLIA '88 regulations are required to obtain a certificate from the CMS according to the complexity of testing performed there. Three categories of testing are recognized: waived (simple, with a low risk of error), moderate (including provider-performed microscopy), and high complexity. Complexity of testing is based on the difficulty involved in performing the test and the degree of risk of harm to a patient if the test is performed incorrectly. CLIA requirements are more stringent for laboratories that perform moderate- and high-complexity testing than waived testing, and their facilities are subject to routine inspections. Specimen collection is an important part of CLIA inspections, and laboratories that are of moderate- or high-complexity testing are required to have written protocols for patient preparation, specimen collection, labeling, preservation, and transportation.

After discovering significant gaps in the quality of waived testing practices, CMS began on-site visits to approximately 2% of Certificate of Waiver (CoW) laboratories across the country. The on-site visits were known in advance and were intended for education and the gathering of information. CMS has now conducted visits in all 50 states and will continue to visit 2% of the CoW laboratories throughout the United States each year. The CLIAC, in cooperation with CDC, FDA, accrediting agencies and manufacturers, is committed to ensuring that the waived laboratories receive the education needed to produce accurate and reliable test results.

One of the educational tools that CLIAC has developed is the ten QA recommendations for CoW laboratories called **Good Laboratory Practices (GLPs)**. The GLPs emphasize QA in collecting and performing blood work using waived testing kits. They are intended to inform, but are not mandatory. See Box 2-1 for an abbreviated form of the GLPs.

Check out Knowledge Drill 2-4 in the WORKBOOK. This exercise will help you summarize the functions of the national agencies and regulations.

CLINICAL AND LABORATORY STANDARDS INSTITUTE

The **Clinical and Laboratory Standards Institute (CLSI)** is a global, nonprofit, standards-developing organization with representatives from the profession, industry, and government. Its mission is *to develop clinical and laboratory practices and promote their use worldwide.* The organization uses a widespread agreement process to develop voluntary guidelines and standards for all areas of the laboratory. CLSI has grown into a global association of over 2,000 member organizations and more than 1,800 volunteers who are working to improve the quality of medical care through standardization. Phlebotomy program approval, certification examination questions, and the standard of care are based on these important guidelines and standards.

NATIONAL ACCREDITING AGENCY FOR CLINICAL LABORATORY SCIENCES

The **National Accrediting Agency for Clinical Laboratory Sciences (NAACLS)** is recognized by the U.S. Department of Education as an authority on quality clinical laboratory education. Its mission is *to be the premier international agency for accreditation and approval of educational programs in the clinical laboratory sciences and related health professions through the involvement of expert volunteers and its dedication to public service.* NAACLS accreditation process involves an external peer review of the program, including an on-site evaluation, to determine whether the program meets certain established educational standards. The

Box 2-1

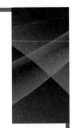

Good Laboratory Practices

1. Keep the manufacturer's current product insert for the laboratory test in use and be sure it is available to the testing personnel. Use the manufacturer's product insert for the kit currently in use; do not use old product inserts.
2. Follow the manufacturer's instructions for specimen collection and handling.
3. Be sure to properly identify the patient.
4. Be sure to label the patient's specimen for testing with an identifier unique to each patient.
5. Inform the patient of any test preparation such as fasting, clean-catch urines, and so forth.
6. Read the product insert prior to performing the test and achieve the optimal result.
7. Follow the storage requirements for the test kit. If the kit can be stored at room temperature but this changes the expiration date, write the new expiration date on the kit.
8. Do not mix components of different kits.
9. Record the patient's test results in the proper place, such as the laboratory test log or the patient's chart, but not on unidentified Post-it notes or pieces of scrap paper that can be misplaced.
10. Perform any instrument maintenance as directed by the manufacturer.

Adapted from U.S. Department of Health and Human Services, Centers for Medicare and Medicaid Services, Clinical Laboratory Improvement Amendments, Good Laboratory Practices. Retrieved on April 14, 2010 from http://www.cms.hhs.gov/clia/downloads/wgoodlab.pdf. See that document for more information. www.clsi.org

NAACLS approval process for phlebotomy programs requires that the program meet educational standards called "competencies" designed to improve student outcomes and maintain quality education.

> **Do Matching 2-3 in the WORKBOOK to reinforce your understanding of regulatory agencies and their purpose.**

Quality Assurance in Phlebotomy

As members of the healthcare team, phlebotomists must understand the significance of their role in providing quality patient care. Due to the advancements in diagnostic techniques and the evolution of personalized medicine, laboratory testing is an even more important part of patient diagnosis and care than ever before. Doctors depend on the test results to be accurate and timely. In today's climate of greater test volume and increased reliance by the physician on the laboratory, all sources of error must be identified and monitored. Preanalytical (before analysis) factors such as patient preparation, specimen collection procedures, and specimen handling can affect the quality of the specimen and in turn affect the validity of test results. Many of these factors fall under the responsibility of the phlebotomist. To ensure consistent quality, specimen collection and handling policies and procedures should be based on

specific guidelines such as those established by TJC, CAP, CLIA, and CLSI. Phlebotomists should strictly adhere to them. Established polices and procedures fall under an overall process called **quality assurance (QA)**.

QA DEFINED

QA and QC are often mistakenly used interchangeably to refer to processes to ensure the quality of a service or product. The terms, however, have different meanings. See Box 2-2. **QA** is defined as a program or process that is designed to prevent problems in the future by evaluating present and past performance. A QA program strives to guarantee quality service through scheduled reviews that look at the appropriateness, applicability, and timeliness of patient care, for instance, the laboratory's response to a comatose patient in the ER. For the past several years as health care has become more complex, there has been an increase in QA processes used by providers as they continually look for better ways to achieve their desired aims and outcomes.

> (i) A study published in Health Affairs in April 2011 revealed that the standard methods hospitals use to detect medical errors fail over 90% of the time.

If errors are caused by processes that fail, it becomes very important to adopt appropriate process improvement (PI) techniques to identify inadequacies, and make

Box 2-2

Quality Assurance Versus Quality Control in the Clinical Laboratory

	Quality Assurance (QA)	Quality Control (QC)
Definition	Refers to processes used to create standardization for quality service or product and prevention of problems	Specific activities and techniques that are performed to fulfill the requirements for a quality service or product
As a tool	QA is a managerial tool for laboratory supervisors	QC is a corrective tool for laboratory personnel
Goal	To improve the necessary work processes in the laboratory so that errors do not occur when producing the service or test result	To identify weaknesses or errors in the laboratory processes at the practice level that could cause poor patient service or test result
Objective	Aims to prevent errors by being proactive	Aims to identify and correct errors by being reactive
Action	Establishes a QA plan and accompanying generic processes using available QA tools, such as, Lean or Six Sigma	Finds and eliminates sources of errors in specific activities or practices so that the patient's requirements are continually met
Who is Responsible?	Everyone on the clinical laboratory team	The phlebotomist or laboratory person performing the activity
When implemented?	Quality assurance activities are determined by the team before work begins	Quality control is about adherence to requirements by the person performing the activity
Example of Activities	Development of standards and process checklists, project audits	Following the standards and using the checklists, monitoring performance, determining causes of errors

changes that prevent errors. Some strategies and tools for improving quality and patient safety—including failure modes and effects analysis (FMEA), Six Sigma, Lean, and root-cause analysis (RCA) are explained in Box 2-3.

> *Guidelines or directives are developed for all processes used and play a part in meeting TJC's commitment to continuously improve health care for the public.*

QUALITY INDICATORS

One of the most important aspects of setting up a QA ID and evaluation process is establishing indicators to monitor certain areas of patient care. **Quality indicators** must be measurable, well defined, objective, and specific. From available inpatient data, indicators can be selected that measure quality, adequacy, accuracy, timeliness, and effectiveness of patient care, along with

customer satisfaction. They are designed to look at areas of care that tend to cause problems. For example, an indicator on the Microbiology QA form shown in Figure 2-1 states: "Blood culture contamination rate will not exceed 3%." A contamination rate that increased beyond the pre-established threshold listed on the form would signify unacceptable performance, in which case action should be taken.

> **See the Microbiology Quality Assessment Form: Labeling Exercise 2-1, in the WORKBOOK to better understand quality indicators.**

THRESHOLDS AND DATA

Threshold values must be established for all quality indicators. A threshold value is a level of acceptable practice beyond which quality patient care cannot be assured. Exceeding this level may trigger intensive evaluation to see if there is a problem that needs to be

Box 2-3

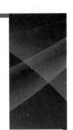

Quality/Process Improvement Tools

Failure Modes and Effects Analysis (FMEA)	• Systematic process to reduce the risk of harm to patients and employees by preventing failures rather than treating bad outcomes.
	• Asks the questions:
	• What could go wrong?
	• Why did it go wrong?
	• What would be the outcome if it did?
Six Sigma	• Structured and rigorous process use to evaluate preanalytic and postanalytic processes.
	• Monitors a process to minimize or eliminate waste.
	• Measures improvement by comparing the process effectiveness before improvement with the process capability after trying various solutions.
Lean Methodology	• Aims to improve patient safety and the quality of health care by eliminating waste in the form of unnecessary processes and redirecting efforts to the customer needs.
	• Strives to make every employee a problem solver so they can develop action plans that improved, simplified, and redesigned work processes.
	• Steps in this method depend on root-cause analysis to investigate errors and then improve quality and prevent similar errors.
Root-Cause Analysis (RCA)	• Formalized investigation and problem-solving approach used after an event or problem has occurred.
	• Focuses on identifying trends and understanding the underlying or root causes of an event.
	• Required by The Joint Commission
	• to be performed in response to all SEs and expects the organization to produce and implement an action plan that is designed to reduce future risk of events.
	• to monitor the effectiveness of those improvements.

corrected. During the evaluation process, data are collected and organized. Data sources include such information as patient records, laboratory results, incident reports, patient satisfaction reports, and direct patient observation. A corrective action plan is established if the data identify a problem or opportunity for improvement. An action plan defines what will change and when that change is expected. Even when the problem appears to be corrected, monitoring and evaluation continue to ensure that care is consistent and that quality continually improves.

PROCESS AND OUTCOMES

QA has traditionally looked at outcomes. Outcomes are in numbers only. For example, a phlebotomy outcome measurement may give the number of times that patient specimens were redrawn because the improper tube was used for collection. It is important to know how often this occurs, but it does not explain why it happened.

To improve an outcome, the process must be reviewed. This entails following the process from start to finish. As TJC suggests, it means standardizing the way performance is measured and activities are evaluated. In the previous example, it would mean looking at what the requester did at the time he or she decided the test was needed, how it was ordered, and how the laboratory processed the request until the time the results were on the patient's chart and in the hands of the person who ordered them. To ensure that the same process is always followed, there must be checks and controls on quality along the way. The use of checks and controls is called **quality control (QC)**.

QC DEFINED

QC is a component of a QA program and a form of procedural control. Phlebotomy QC involves using all available QC checks on every operational procedure or process to make certain it is performed correctly. In

HOSPITAL & HEALTH CENTER
QUALITY ASSESSMENT AND IMPROVEMENT TRACKING
CONFIDENTIAL A.R.S. 36-445 et. seq.

STANDARD OF CARE/SERVICE:

IMPORTANT ASPECT OF CARE/SERVICE:
LABORATORY SERVICES
COLLECTION/TRANSPORT

SIGNATURES:

_____
DIRECTOR

_____
MEDICAL DIRECTOR

_____
VICE PRESIDENT/ADMINISTRATOR

DEPARTMENTS:
DATA SOURCE(S):
METHODOLOGY: [X] RETROSPECTIVE   [   ] CONCURRENT
TYPE: [   ] STRUCTURE   [   ] PROCESS   [X] OUTCOME
PERSON RESPONSIBLE FOR:
• DATA COLLECTION: J. HERRIG
• DATA ORGANIZATION: J. HERRIG
• ACTION PLAN: J. HERRIG
• FOLLOW-UP: J. HERRIG
DATE MONITORING BEGAN: 1990
TIME PERIOD THIS MONITOR: 2ND QUARTER 2009
MONITOR DISCONTINUED BECAUSE:
FOLLOW-UP:

INDICATORS	THLD	ACT	PREV	CRITICAL ANALYSIS/EVALUATION	ACTION PLAN
Blood Culture contamination rate will not exceed 3%				**Population: All patients** All monthly indicators were under threshold, 3%	Share results and analysis with Lab staff and ER staff.
APR - # of Draws: 713 　　　# Contaminated: 13	3.00%	1.8%	1.2%	% Contamination from draws other than Line draws, by unit:	
MAY - # of Draws: 710 　　　# Contaminated: 23	3.00%	2.8%	2.3%	APR: ER = 4.7%　　Lab = 0.7% MAY: ER = 11.5%　　Lab = 1.0% JUN: ER = 8.6%　　Lab = 1.1%	
JUN - # of Draws: 702 　　　# Contaminated: 17	3.00%	2.4%	1.9%	ER was over threshold for each month of quarter.	
Total for 1st Quarter - 　　# of Draws: 2125 　　# Contaminated: 50	3.00%	2.4%	1.9%		

Figure 2-1 A microbiology quality assessment form.

phlebotomy, it is the responsibility of the person who supervises the phlebotomist to oversee QA and ensure that checks are being done and standards are being met. It is the responsibility of the phlebotomist to meet those standards at all times. Consistently following national standards for phlebotomy procedures is a means of controlling the quality of the results.

Areas of Phlebotomy Subject to Quality Assessment

PATIENT PREPARATION PROCEDURES

Quality assessment in laboratory testing actually starts before the specimen is collected in the preanalytical stage. To obtain a quality specimen, the patient must be prepared properly. Instructions on how to prepare a patient for testing can be found by checking the laboratory's Test Menu or Catalog which, in most cases, is electronically available on the web.

Check out Skills Drill 2-4 in the WORKBOOK. This exercise takes you to Quest Diagnostics web site so you can see their test menu online.

SPECIMEN COLLECTION PROCEDURES

Identification

Patient ID (as described in Chapter 8) is the most important aspect of specimen collection. Methods are being continually improved to ensure that all ID is done correctly. An example is the use of barcodes for patient information on ID bands, requisitions, and specimen labels. Barcode readers that are used to scan this information (Fig. 2-2) prior to collecting specimens substantially reduces human error.

TJC moved toward stricter patient ID requirements by their revision of NPSGs in 2009. It clearly states that patient ID using only the inpatient's arm bracelet does

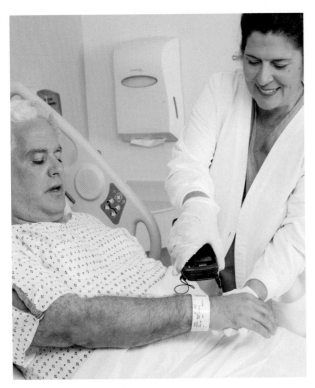

Figure 2-2 A nurse scans the patient ID band. (Courtesy of Siemens Medical Solutions, Malvern, PA.)

not meet the standard. Phlebotomist must "actively involve" patients in their ID process prior to any specimen collection.

Key Point A person doing phlebotomy must use at least two identifiers for patient identification. The patient's room number or physical location cannot be used as an identifier. For outpatients without ID bands, the agency requirements are met when the patient's spoken name is compared with the name on the requisition and the patient provides a second verbal identifier such as birth date or phone number.

According to JCAHO, acceptable "person-specific" identifiers include:
- The individual's name
- An assigned ID number
- Telephone number
- Date of birth
- Social security number
- Address
- Photograph

Electronic ID, such as barcode readers, meet the standard as long as the technology includes two or more identifiers since a barcoded wristband could be on the wrong patient.

Patient identifiers in the emergency department, if the patient is unresponsive, can be a temporary "name" and a medical record number or the assigned ED number until the formal ID is confirmed.

Equipment

Puncture Devices

Ensuring the quality and sterility of every needle and lancet is essential for patient safety. All puncture devices come in sealed, sterile containers and should be used only once. If the seal has been broken, the device should be put in a sharps container and a new one obtained. Manufacturing defects in needles, such as barbs and blunt tips, can be avoided before use by quickly inspecting the needle after unsheathing.

Evacuated Tubes

CLSI has established standards for evacuated tubes to help ensure specimen integrity. Manufacturers print expiration dates on each tube for QA (see Fig 7-22) and the lot numbers of the tubes are recorded when received in the laboratory. It is common practice to keep only a limited supply on hand to avoid tossing out tubes that were not used by the expiration date. Outdated tubes should never be used because they may not fill completely, causing dilution of the sample, distortion of the cell components, and erroneous results. In addition, anticoagulants in expired tubes may not work effectively, instead allowing small clots to form and thereby invalidating hematology and immunohematology test results. As part of QC, evacuated tubes should be checked occasionally for adequate vacuum and additive. Results of these and other QC checks should be documented.

Labeling

Labeling must be exact. Labeling requirements as outlined in Chapter 8 should be strictly followed. Inaccuracies, such as transposed letters or missing information, will result in the specimen being discarded. Computer labels (Fig. 2-3) normally contain correctly printed patient information. However, the correct label must be placed on the correct patient's specimen and the date, time of draw, and ID of the person collecting the sample must be noted. All blood containers and other types of specimens must be labeled in the patient's presence as stated in TJC NPSG Goal 01.

Key Point There have been cases where patient information on computer labels was incorrect because incorrect information had been entered into the computer upon patient admission. Proper patient ID procedures can catch such errors.

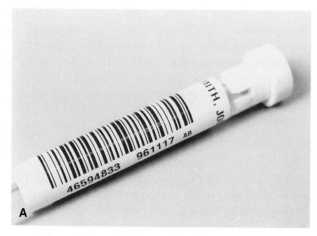

A

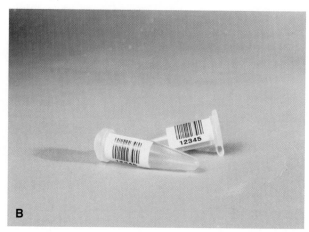

B

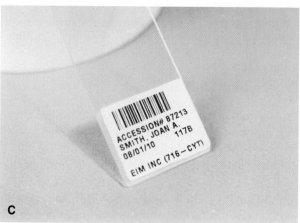

C

Figure 2-3 A: Specimen tube with bar code label. **B:** Micro-collection container with bar code label. **C:** Slide with bar code label. (Courtesy of Electronic Imaging Materials, Inc., Keene, NH.)

Technique

Proper phlebotomy technique must be carefully taught by a professional who understands the importance of following national standards and the reasons for using certain equipment or techniques. When a phlebotomist understands the rationale for maintaining the standards, high-quality specimens are ensured.

> 🔑 **Key Point** No matter how experienced phlebotomists may be, a periodic review of their techniques is necessary for quality assurance and performance improvement.

Collection Priorities

Specimen collection priorities must be stressed. The importance of knowing how to recognize which specimen request is the most critical or when a specimen involves special collection criteria (e.g., renins or therapeutic drug monitoring [TDM]) can save the patient unnecessary medication or additional testing. It may even shorten the patient's stay in the hospital because, in many instances, therapy is based on test values from specimens assumed to have been collected at the right time and in the proper manner.

Delta Checks

Delta checks help ensure quality in testing. A **delta check** compares current results of a laboratory test with previous results for the same test on the same patient. Although some variation is to be expected, a major difference in results would be flagged and could indicate an error that requires investigation.

Documentation

Documentation is critical in all areas of health care. Medical errors due to wrong information are prevalent and sometimes deadly.

> ⓘ In November 2010, the New England Journal of Medicine stated that 25% of patients admitted to a healthcare facility were actually harmed by the care they received. According to the Huffington Post, 2012, a new initiative by the Department of Health and Human Services called "Partnership for Patients: Better Care, Lower Costs," intends to reduce preventable injuries in US hospitals by 40%, saving 60,000 lives, by 2014.

Using the right PI tools and developing the correct documentation are essential for patient safety. Since there is no universal documentation template, forms used for CQI vary by institution. Today's technology allows electronically provided QC forms to be current and available for all personnel when needed.

Documentation can be used for legal purposes as long as it is legible and includes only standard abbreviations. All records kept in the process of providing health care are subject to review by TJC or other such agencies for the purpose of accreditation. Easily the most important of these is the patient's record.

THE PATIENT'S RECORD

The patient's record is a chronologic documentation of the medical care given. The law requires that medical records be kept on hospital patients, but it does not require physicians in private practice to keep such records, although most do so in the form of a clinical record. Every notation in the patient's medical or clinical record should be legible, factual, and an objective account of the patient, past and present. The basic reasons for maintaining accurate, up-to-date medical records are as follows:

- To provide an aid to the practice of medicine by documenting treatment and a plan for continued care.
- To provide an aid to communications between the physician and others involved with present and future care for the patient.
- To serve as a legal document that may be used in a court of law.
- To serve as a very valuable tool for helping the hospital evaluate performance outcomes. The patient's records include such information as a history of examinations, medical testing, laboratory reports, prescriptions written, and supplies used; these are all very informative for utilization review, a monitoring process for appropriate and cost-effective care.

> ⚠️ **CAUTION** For confidentiality reasons, access to a patient's medical record is restricted to those who have a verifiable need to review the information.

In 2009, the Health Information Technology for Economic and Clinical Health Act was passed. Two of the key provisions of the bill were the financial incentives to promote electronic record keeping and penalties for those who don't comply. Insurance companies, large medical facilities, and federal and state governments began encouraging the use of electronic medical records (EMRs) or electronic health records (EHRs).

In today's healthcare environment, EMR software and wireless tablets are a necessity for more efficient, cost-effective, quality care. More and more physicians, nurses, and other healthcare providers are using computer data entry for all patient interactions. With the recent health reforms, ACOs have found EMRs absolutely necessary to standardize and make accessible shared records. Studies have shown that EMRs improve the quality of care by reducing waste, liability, medication errors, adverse SEs, and duplication of information from general practice to the hospital.

TEST CATALOGS AND REFERENCE MANUALS

> 📖 **See Labeling Exercise 2-2 in the WORKBOOK for practice in reading a reference manual.**

Searchable online menus or catalogs are examples of QA documents made available to customers and blood collectors at all specimen collection sites. In an outpatient setting, like a clinic or physician's office, there is the option to receive the instruction in the form of a printed Reference Manual (Fig. 2-4). All of these documents detail how to prepare the patient and any additional information needed to collect a high-quality sample. They typically list: the test CPT code type of specimen and amount needed, special handling requirements, transport temperature and container type, and causes for specimen rejection.

THE PROCEDURE MANUAL

The **Procedure Manual** (Fig. 2-5) states the policies and procedures that apply to each test or practice performed in the laboratory. The Procedure Manual, another QA document, must be made available to all employees of the laboratory for standardization purposes. Accrediting agencies such as CAP and TJC demand that this manual be updated annually at a minimum. Box 2-4 lists typical information found in a procedure manual.

THE SAFETY MANUAL

The **Safety Manual** contains policies and procedures related to chemical, electrical, fire, and radiation safety; exposure control; and disaster plans as well as complete details on how to handle hazardous materials. OSHA regulations require every business to have a workplace safety manual. Organizations can receive hefty fines for not having such a manual available for employee use.

THE INFECTION PREVENTION AND CONTROL MANUAL

In today's healthcare environment emerging infectious diseases and drug-resistant organisms make managing

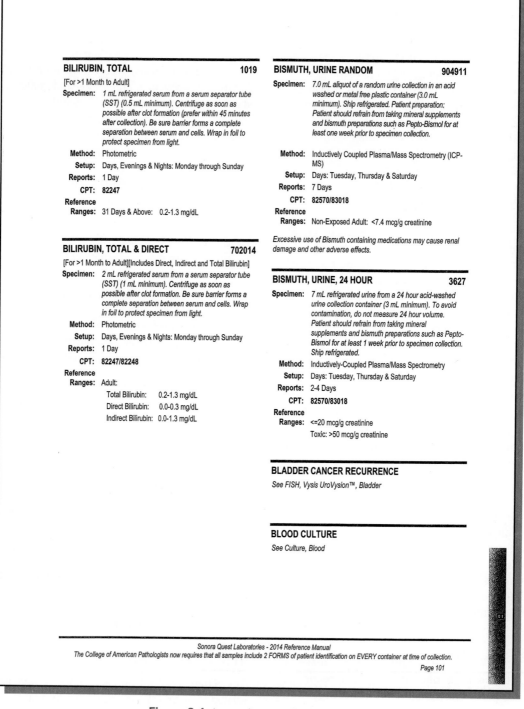

BILIRUBIN, TOTAL 1019

[For >1 Month to Adult]

Specimen: *1 mL refrigerated serum from a serum separator tube (SST) (0.5 mL minimum). Centrifuge as soon as possible after clot formation (prefer within 45 minutes after collection). Be sure barrier forms a complete separation between serum and cells. Wrap in foil to protect specimen from light.*

Method: Photometric

Setup: Days, Evenings & Nights: Monday through Sunday

Reports: 1 Day

CPT: **82247**

Reference Ranges: 31 Days & Above: 0.2-1.3 mg/dL

BILIRUBIN, TOTAL & DIRECT 702014

[For >1 Month to Adult][Includes Direct, Indirect and Total Bilirubin]

Specimen: *2 mL refrigerated serum from a serum separator tube (SST) (1 mL minimum). Centrifuge as soon as possible after clot formation. Be sure barrier forms a complete separation between serum and cells. Wrap in foil to protect specimen from light.*

Method: Photometric

Setup: Days, Evenings & Nights: Monday through Sunday

Reports: 1 Day

CPT: **82247/82248**

Reference Ranges: Adult:

Total Bilirubin:	0.2-1.3 mg/dL
Direct Bilirubin:	0.0-0.3 mg/dL
Indirect Bilirubin:	0.0-1.3 mg/dL

BISMUTH, URINE RANDOM 904911

Specimen: *7.0 mL aliquot of a random urine collection in an acid washed or metal free plastic container (3.0 mL minimum). Ship refrigerated. Patient preparation: Patient should refrain from taking mineral supplements and bismuth preparations such as Pepto-Bismol for at least one week prior to specimen collection.*

Method: Inductively Coupled Plasma/Mass Spectrometry (ICP-MS)

Setup: Days: Tuesday, Thursday & Saturday

Reports: 7 Days

CPT: **82570/83018**

Reference Ranges: Non-Exposed Adult: <7.4 mcg/g creatinine

Excessive use of Bismuth containing medications may cause renal damage and other adverse effects.

BISMUTH, URINE, 24 HOUR 3627

Specimen: *7 mL refrigerated urine from a 24 hour acid-washed urine collection container (3 mL minimum). To avoid contamination, do not measure 24 hour volume. Patient should refrain from taking mineral supplements and bismuth preparations such as Pepto-Bismol for at least 1 week prior to specimen collection. Ship refrigerated.*

Method: Inductively-Coupled Plasma/Mass Spectrometry

Setup: Days: Tuesday, Thursday & Saturday

Reports: 2-4 Days

CPT: **82570/83018**

Reference Ranges: <=20 mcg/g creatinine

Toxic: >50 mcg/g creatinine

BLADDER CANCER RECURRENCE

See FISH, Vysis UroVysion™, Bladder

BLOOD CULTURE

See Culture, Blood

Sonora Quest Laboratories - 2014 Reference Manual
The College of American Pathologists now requires that all samples include 2 FORMS of patient identification on EVERY container at time of collection.
Page 101

Figure 2-4 A page from a reference manual.

all aspects of infection control more critical then ever. The **Infection Prevention and Control Manual** outlines policies and procedures for all employees in all areas of the HCO and must be in compliance with federal regulations and accreditation requirements. The manual addresses such items as hand hygiene, precautions to take when dealing with patients or handling specimens, and how to handle accidental contamination, including procedures to be implemented following exposure incidents.

QUALITY ASSURANCE FORMS

Accreditation standards for agencies such as TJC require the laboratory to have available all documentation on QC checks. In the phlebotomy areas, these may include temperature

Patient Identification

Content Applies To:
The Best Clinic: Support Services, Division of Laboratory Medicine
Scope
This procedure applies to all Support Services areas involved with patient identification.
Purpose
Patient Identification is paramount in the laboratory setting. Not properly identifying a
patient seriously compromises patient safety. The purpose of this procedure is to provide
instructions on how to properly identify patients prior to specimen collection to ensure an
accurate match will be made to the laboratory order received.
Revision date: 1/22/2015
Synopsis of Change: Revised to include latest patient ID policies.

Procedure

Step	Action		Detail

01	Ask patient to state his/her first and last name and date of birth.		Identification of patient is required by using two patient identifiers before specimens are collected. Preferred patient identifiers are:
			o Full name (first, last and middle initial as needed)
			o Date of birth
			o MRN
			o Other acceptable identifiers:
			   o Address
			   o Legal photo ID
			   o Verification by a family member or caregiver

02	Compare and confirm information provided by the patient match the patient order received: o Inpatient – patient's armband and the LIS Soft PC/PDA o Outpatient – Cerner notification sheet and LIS Soft PC/PDA		
03	If no discrepancies found	Proceed with patient sample draw	Inpatient Venipuncture Collection Procedure **Or** Outpatient Venipuncture Collection Procedure
	If patient information requires correction	**Inpatient:** go to nurse to have information corrected **Outpatient:** Use *Correction of Patient Demographics Procedure*	

Figure 2-5 A page from a procedure manual.

logs for refrigerators and freezers used for specimen storage, centrifuge maintenance records, heat block temperature logs, event report forms, and incident reports.

Equipment Check Forms

In hospitals and clinics, the facilities department
uses a computerized system to monitor freezers and
refrigerators. Control checks on the centrifuge require

documentation of the maintenance periodically. Just
as for freezers and refrigerators, it is the responsibility
of the facilities or biomedical services department to
monitor centrifuges. In a smaller outpatient setting,
often called **Patient Service Center (PSC)**, the temperature logs and centrifuge information are kept on
paper log sheets and recorded daily by the phlebotomy
supervisor.

Box 2-4

Typical Information Found in a Procedure Manual

- Purpose of the procedure
- Policy
- Specimen type and collection method
- Equipment and supplies required
- Detailed step-by-step procedure
- Limitations and variables of the method

- Corrective actions
- Method validation
- Normal values and references
- Review and revision dates
- Approval signatures and dates

Internal Reports

Confidential incident and occurrence reports must be filled out when a problem occurs. These forms identify the problem, state the consequence, and describe the corrective action. An **Incident Report** is to be completed when an occupational injury or exposure, such as an accidental needle stick, has occurred, or a delayed medical condition has developed, no matter how minor. The report like the one in Figure 2-6 should be completed and submitted to the appropriate person even if medical treatment was not required.

An occurrence form is filled out for any errors made in the patient ID, specimen collection, handling or reporting of the results. This **Near Miss/Occurrence Report Form** (Fig. 2-7) would be used, for example, if a CBC result was reported out and then platelet clumps were found on the slide, causing the result to be inaccurate, or when an RN calls to say she incorrectly labeled the tube sent to the laboratory for chemistry tests. Basically this form is an audit trail. When the occurrence is completely documented, it is then reviewed by a supervisor to decide whether counseling is required, if the process is flawed, or other action is necessary.

These reports should state facts and not feelings. The function of such a report is not to place blame but to discover problems with the process and state the corrective action taken so that such an event does not happen again.

The QC document called the **Performance Improvement Plan** (Fig. 2-8) is used when counseling or suspension of an individual is necessary. The document states the deficiency, describes a specific action plan for improvement, and the next step if necessary.

Risk Management

Risk, defined as "the chance of loss or injury," is inherent in the healthcare environment. **Risk management** is an internal process focused on identifying and minimizing situations that pose risk to patients and employees. Risk can be managed in two ways: controlling risk to avoid incidents and paying for occurrences after they have happened. Generic steps in risk management involve ID of the risk, treatment of the risk using policies and procedures already in place, education of employees and patients, and evaluation of what should be done in the future.

From the beginning, laboratories have used some sort of QC system to manage certain risks and avoid unnecessary problems. When the final CLIA regulations were put into place in 2003, they set basic requirements for a QC program without taking into consideration that each clinical laboratory uses different instruments, different procedures, and their own staff in different ways. Soon it became evident that the national standards did not address all risks.

In 2011, CLSI published a new guideline, **Laboratory Quality Control Based on Risk Management (EP-23)**. This standard recognized the diversity in laboratories and the need for customization of QC plans. CLSI designed EP-23 as a guide for ensuring quality in each individual laboratory while keeping up with continuous changes in technology.

In 2014, CMS, the government division that oversees and administers laboratory regulations, incorporated key concepts from EP-23 into CLIA policies. This new addition to the existing CLIA quality system is called the **Individualized Quality Control Plan (IQCP)**. Up until this time, PI tools like Six Sigma, Lean, and RCA as described in Box 2-3 were plentiful, but there had been no comprehensive approach to QC until IQCP. Accrediting agencies, such as CAP and TJC immediately began incorporating IQCP into their survey process since QC issues were ranked as one of their most prominent deficiencies. CMS acknowledged that each IQCP would be unique since it is designed to fit the needs of only that particular laboratory. This individualized approach allows laboratories to use whatever PI tools deemed necessary to manage risk.

Risk factors in phlebotomy can be identified by looking at trends in reporting tools such as incident or occurrence reports as described previously. Proper investigation is initiated if a situation is identified that deviates from the normal. When new procedures that reduce risk are instituted, employees are informed immediately and instructed on what to do. Evaluation of occurrences, trends, and outcomes is essential throughout the process, so that errors can be identified and the appropriate changes made. Risk management procedures and other QA measures demonstrate the intent of a healthcare facility to adhere to national standards of good practice. The result is a noticeable reduction of legal issues involving

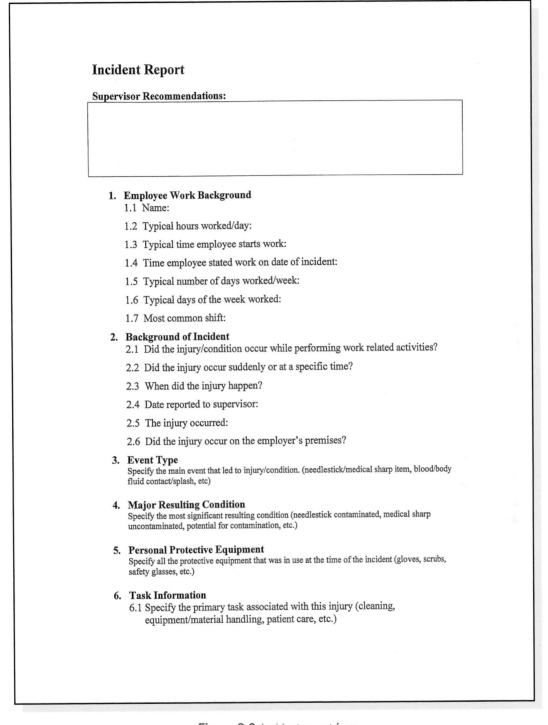

Figure 2-6 Incident report form.

the healthcare consumers as well as the facility's employees, even in such issues as sexual harassment and hostile work environment.

Sexual Harassment

Sexual harassment is a form of sex discrimination and therefore, violations fall under Title VII of the Civil Rights Act of 1964. Title VII is a federal law that makes it illegal to discriminate in employment on the basis of sex, race, color, national origin, and religion. Retaliation against someone who complains of sexual harassment or helps to investigate a claim is also prohibited under the Title VII. This law applies to any employer with 15 or more employees.

Sexual harassment is defined as persistent or offensive conduct related to a person's sex that negatively

---

Clinical Laboratory
Near Miss/Occurrence Report Form

Patient Name: _____   Patient Location: _____
Medical Rec. #: _____   Occurrence Date: _____ Occurrence Time: _____
Accession #: _____
Test (s): _____
Type of Spec.: _____
Problem Description: _____
_____
_____

Initial steps performed. Mark all that apply:

SPECIMEN INTEGRITY	RESULT (Process/Equipment/Environment)
____ Hemolysis ____ Clotted ____ QNS ____ Incorrect container ____ Leaking/contaminated ____ Transport time exceeded ____ Collected above IV ____ Fluid contaminated from line draw ____ Lipemia ____ Other	____ Repeat – same specimen, new specimen, previous specimen ____ Check patient history ____ Verify QC/instrument ____ Dilution error ____ Wrong cup/specimen/accession ____ Check ABO Acc# _____ ABO/RH_____ Acc# _____ ABO/RH_____ ____ Other:

SPECIMEN IDENTIFICATION	DISPOSITION
____ Unlabeled ____ Mislabeled (wrong) ____ Improperly labeled (alignment) ____ Transposed letters/numbers ____ Incomplete label ____ Incorrect collection time ____ Other:	____ Incorrect result ____ Procedure cancelled ____ Erroneous results corrected ____ Procedure credited ____ Notification to _____ date/time_____ _____ date/time_____ ____ Specimen recollected ____ Unlabeled/leaking specimen discarded ____ Mislabeled specimen in ERROR rack

PATIENT ORDER/INFORMATION	LABORATORY USE ONLY
____ Ordered on wrong patient ____ Wrong procedure ordered ____ Wrong encounter ____ Wrong date/time ____ Missing or incorrect requisition ____ Wrong therapy Other Departments affected by Near Miss Occurrence: ☐ No ☐ Yes	Date: _____ Employee Name: _____ Counseled By: _____ Repeat Error: Yes No Other Corrective Action Needed: Yes No ____ Written PIP ____ Final Written

	OFFICE USE ONLY
Occurrence by (username): _____ Report completed by: _____ Date: _____ Report Reviewed by: _____ Date: _____	Midas NMOR: _____ Date: _____ Midas Follow up: _____ Date: _____ Spec Mislabel: _____ Date: _____ FDA Report: _____ Date: _____

Figure 2-7 Near miss/occurrence report form.

---

affects a reasonable person's job. It is a regrettable fact that this type of harassment is a common problem in the workplace today.

🔑 **Key Point** It is important to note that sexual harassment should not be confused with another form of workplace harassment called hostile work environment. This hostile form of harassment involves some type of behavior or action that discriminates against a protected classification, such as age, religion, disability, or race. To be classified as a hostile work environment, the communication or behavior must be pervasive and seriously disrupt the employee's work or career progress.

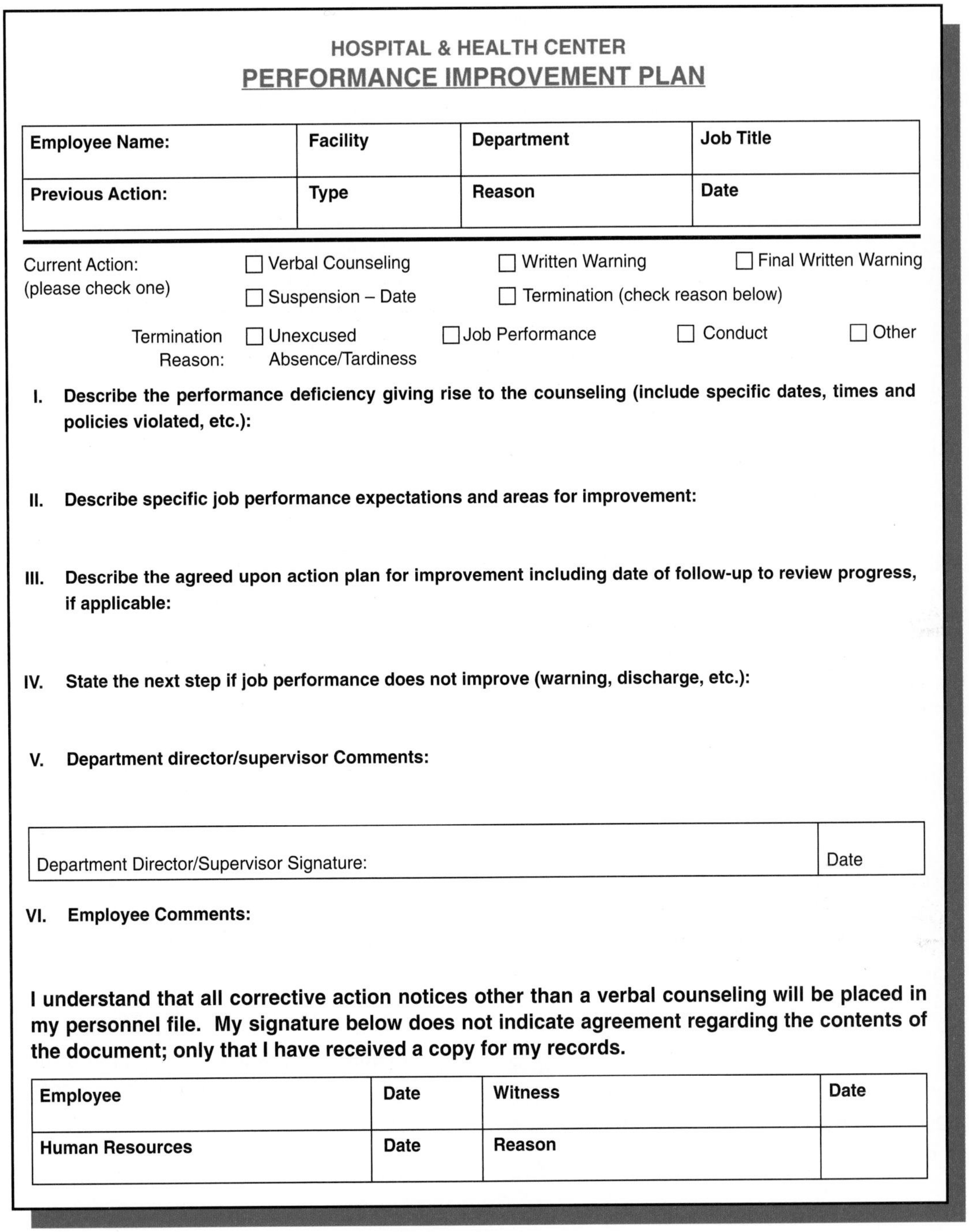

HOSPITAL & HEALTH CENTER
PERFORMANCE IMPROVEMENT PLAN

Employee Name:	Facility	Department	Job Title
Previous Action:	Type	Reason	Date

Current Action: (please check one)
☐ Verbal Counseling ☐ Written Warning ☐ Final Written Warning
☐ Suspension – Date ☐ Termination (check reason below)

Termination Reason:
☐ Unexcused Absence/Tardiness ☐ Job Performance ☐ Conduct ☐ Other

I. Describe the performance deficiency giving rise to the counseling (include specific dates, times and policies violated, etc.):

II. Describe specific job performance expectations and areas for improvement:

III. Describe the agreed upon action plan for improvement including date of follow-up to review progress, if applicable:

IV. State the next step if job performance does not improve (warning, discharge, etc.):

V. Department director/supervisor Comments:

Department Director/Supervisor Signature:	Date

VI. **Employee Comments:**

I understand that all corrective action notices other than a verbal counseling will be placed in my personnel file. My signature below does not indicate agreement regarding the contents of the document; only that I have received a copy for my records.

Employee	Date	Witness	Date
Human Resources	Date	Reason	

Figure 2-8 Performance improvement form.

Sexual harassment can occur in many different ways, but essentially, it happens when there is "unwelcome" conduct of a sexual nature that is cruel or invasive and undermines morale, affects productivity, and can create a hostile work environment.

Sexual harassment is not limited by gender and does not have to involve the opposite sex. The harasser is not always the victim's supervisor or superior. The person could be a co-worker or even someone not employed in the workplace. In the healthcare field, that person could even be a patient.

CAUTION Healthcare workers should be aware at all times of how they interact with patients to avoid being accused of any type of unwelcome conduct interpreted as sexual in nature.

When an employee experiences or witnesses harassment, he or she is responsible for reporting the occurrence to the appropriate person. Direct attempt at resolution, verbally or in writing, is encouraged. It must be made clear by the recipient to the other person involved that their action was unwelcome. Documentation of the interaction or copies of the correspondence should be kept. If the actions persist, a detailed log should be kept. Next, a meeting with the supervisor to file a complaint should be scheduled. If it is uncomfortable to report to a supervisor, then the Human Resources department that is usually responsible for handling such claims should be contacted.

Legal Issues

Technology, such as the Internet, has led to increased awareness and concern by the healthcare consumer. Today, litigation is common in the healthcare industry, where physicians and other healthcare providers were once considered above reproach. As healthcare providers go about their daily work, there are many activities that, if performed without reasonable care and skill, could result in a lawsuit. It has been proven in past lawsuits that persons performing phlebotomy can and will be held legally accountable for their actions. Although most legal actions against healthcare workers are **civil actions** in which the alleged injured party sues for monetary damages, willful actions by healthcare workers with the intent to produce harm or death can result in criminal charges. See Table 2-1 for a description of criminal and civil actions.

> (i) The same act may lead to both criminal and civil actions. For example, in assault and battery cases, a guilty defendant can face imprisonment by the state and also civil action in which the injured party tries to collect monetary damages.

> See Knowledge Drill 2-5 in the WORKBOOK to better understand the difference between criminal and civil actions.

Tort

The most common civil actions in health care are based on **tort law**. A tort is a wrongful act other than breach of contract committed against someone's person, property, reputation, or other legally protected right, for which the individual is entitled to damages awarded by the court. It is an act that is committed without a just cause and may be intentional (willful) or unintentional (accidental). The following list includes definitions of tort actions and related legal terminology.

- **Assault:** An act or threat causing another to be in fear of immediate battery (harmful touching). Battery does not necessarily have to follow an assault; however, the victim must believe the ability to carry out the threat is there.

- **Battery:** An intentional harmful or offensive touching of, or use of force on, another person without consent or legal justification. Legal justification would be, for example, when a mother gives permission to have blood drawn from her child. Intentional harm may range from permanent disfigurement to merely grabbing something out of another person's hand without permission. Battery is usually both a tort and a criminal offense.

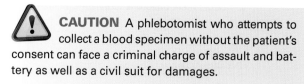 **CAUTION** A phlebotomist who attempts to collect a blood specimen without the patient's consent can face a criminal charge of assault and battery as well as a civil suit for damages.

- **Fraud:** A deceitful practice or false portrayal of facts either by words or by conduct, often done to obtain money or property. An example includes billing for services that have not been provided.

- **Invasion of privacy:** The violation of one's right to be left alone. It can involve a physical intrusion or the unauthorized publishing or release of private information, which can also be considered a breach of confidentiality.

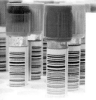

Table 2-1: Criminal and Civil Actions

Action	Definition	Punishment
Criminal	Concerned with laws designed to protect all members of society from unlawful acts by others; i.e., felonies and misdemeanors.	• A felony is a crime (i.e., murder, assault, and rape) punishable by death or imprisonment. • Misdemeanors are considered lesser offenses and usually carry a penalty of a fine or less than 1 year in jail.
Civil	Concerned with actions between two private parties, such as individuals or organizations; constitute the bulk of the legal actions dealt within the medical.	• Damages may be awarded in a court of law and result in monetary penalties, office, or other healthcare facilities.

Key Point Invasion of privacy by physical intrusion may be no more than opening the door and walking into a patient's room without asking permission to enter.

- **Breach of confidentiality:** The failure to keep privileged medical information private. An example is the unauthorized release of patient information such as laboratory results. This could lead to a lawsuit for medical malpractice if it caused harm to the patient, such as the loss of his or her job. Patient confidentiality is protected under state law.

- **Malpractice:** A type of negligence (described below) committed by a professional. The training and experience of the accused individual is taken into consideration when deciding whether an act resulting in injury should be labeled negligence or malpractice. A claim of malpractice implies that a greater standard of care was owed to the injured person than the "reasonable person" standard associated with negligence.

- **Negligence:** The failure to exercise **due care**, the level of care that a person of ordinary intelligence and good sense would exercise under the given circumstances. In other words, negligence is doing something that a *reasonable* person would *not* do, or *not* doing something that a *reasonable* person *would* do. If a medical procedure results in injury and there is no intent to injure, it is called negligence, and the injured person has the right to sue for damages. To claim negligence, the following must be present:
  1. A legal duty or obligation owed by one person to another
  2. A breaking or breach of that duty or obligation
  3. Harm done as a direct result of the action

- *Res ipsa loquitur:* A Latin phrase meaning "the thing speaks for itself," which applies to the rule of evidence in a case of negligence. When a breach of duty is so obvious that it does not need further explanation, it is said that the situation speaks for itself. For example, a homebound patient sitting on a kitchen barstool faints while having blood drawn and falls, hitting his head. A head injury develops that was obviously due to the fall. If a lawsuit results, the burden of proof is shifted to the phlebotomist, who must prove that he or she was not negligent.

- *Respondeat superior:* A Latin phrase that means "let the master respond." An employer is liable (legally responsible) for the actions of an employee, even though the employee is the one at fault. Thus, a tort action may be filed if a neglectful or intentional act of an employee results in some type of physical injury to a client. The key points in a claim of *respondeat*

superior are that the employee is working within the scope of employment and has had the proper training to perform the required duties.

Key Point If a neglectful act occurs while an employee is doing something that is not within his or her duties or training, the employee may be held solely responsible for that act.

- **Standard of care:** The normal level of skill and care that a healthcare practitioner would be expected to adhere to in order to provide due care for patients. This duty is established by standards of the profession and the expectations of society. It is the standard of care expected of everyone at all times; a failure to exercise due care is negligence. Employers are responsible for providing employees who possess the qualifications and training necessary to meet the standard of care and are ultimately liable if they do not.

- **Statute of limitations:** A law setting the length of time after an alleged injury in which the injured person is permitted to file a lawsuit. The time limit is specified in each state's medical malpractice law. The question for all parties involved is when does the clock start? The statute of limitations period typically begins when one of the following circumstances occurs:
  1. The day the alleged negligent act was committed
  2. When the injury resulting from the alleged negligence was actually discovered or should have been discovered by a reasonably alert patient
  3. The day the physician–patient relationship ended or the day of the last medical treatment in a series
  4. In the case of minors, often not until the minor reaches the age of majority

- **Vicarious liability:** Liability imposed by law on one person for acts committed by another. One example is employer liability under *respondeat superior,* explained above. Another example is employer liability for negligence by an independent contractor or consultant who was hired. This is based on the principle that the contractor or consultant is acting on behalf of the employer by virtue of the contract between them.

Key Point A hospital, as an employer, cannot escape liability for a patient's injury simply by subcontracting out various services to other persons and claiming it is not responsible because the party that caused the injury is not on its payroll.

Malpractice Insurance

Malpractice insurance compensates the insured in the event of malpractice liability. Individual workers are not typically targets of lawsuits because of *respondeat superior* or vicarious liability, both of which involve the "deep pockets" theory (let the one with the most money pay). They can, however, be named as codefendants, in which case the employer's malpractice insurance may not cover them. It is important for healthcare personnel to examine the possibility of a civil suit being brought against them and to consider carrying malpractice insurance. The decision to purchase this insurance should be based on financial considerations as well as legal ones. From the legal point of view, it may be desirable to be covered by a separate professional liability policy because the employer may give his or her insurer the right to recover damages from an employee who is found to be negligent. Healthcare personnel may be able to purchase malpractice insurance from their professional organizations.

Avoiding Lawsuits

The best insurance against lawsuits is to take steps to avoid them. A good way to avoid lawsuits is to consistently follow the guidelines listed in Box 2-5. Above all, always remember to respect the rights of patients. This gives them control over the situation and makes them less likely to feel that they have been treated poorly.

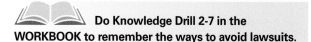 **Do Knowledge Drill 2-7 in the WORKBOOK to remember the ways to avoid lawsuits.**

Patient Consent

Obtaining the patient's consent before initiating a procedure is critical. There are a number of different types of patient consent including **informed consent, expressed consent, implied consent, HIV consent,** and **consent for minors**. It is important to be familiar with them all and **refusal of consent** as well.

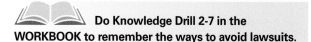 **When you have finished reading this section, do Matching 2-2 in the WORKBOOK to reinforce your understanding of the different types of consent.**

INFORMED CONSENT

- Implies voluntary and competent permission for a medical procedure, test, or medication.
- Requires that a patient be given adequate information regarding the method, risks, and consequences of a procedure before consenting to it.

Box 2-5

Guidelines to Avoid Lawsuits

- Acquire informed consent before collecting specimens.
  - Be meticulous when identifying patients and patient specimens.
  - Carefully monitor the patient before, during, and after venipuncture.
- Respect a patient's right to confidentiality.
- Strictly adhere to CLSI standards and other accepted procedures and practices.
- Use proper safety containers and devices.
- Listen and respond appropriately to the patient's requests.
- Accurately and legibly record all information concerning patients.
- Document incidents or occurrences.
- Participate in continuing education to maintain proficiency.
- Perform at the prevailing standard of care.
- Never perform procedures that you are not trained to do.

- Information must be given to the patient in nontechnical terms and in his or her own language, if possible, meaning an interpreter may be necessary.
- The patient's permission or consent must be obtained before initiating any medical procedure.
- Minors require consent of their parents or legal guardians.

EXPRESSED CONSENT

- Required for treatment that involves surgery, experimental drugs, or high-risk procedures.
- May be given verbally or in writing.
- Written consent gives the best possible protection for both the treatment provider and the patient, must be signed by both, and must be witnessed by a third party.
- Verbal consent for treatment should be followed by an entry in the patient's chart covering what was discussed with the patient.
- Consent should cover what procedures are going to be performed and should not be in a general form that allows the physician full authority to do whatever he or she wants to do.

When a general consent issue goes to court, the court typically takes the word of the patient as to what he or she understood was to take place.

IMPLIED CONSENT

- The patient's actions imply consent without a verbal or written expression of consent.
- Implied consent may be necessary in emergency procedures, such as CPR to save a person's life.
- Laws involving implied consent are enacted at the state level and may differ greatly from state to state.

Key Point If a phlebotomist tells a patient that he or she is going to collect a blood specimen and the patient holds out an arm, it is considered implied consent.

HIV CONSENT

- Legislation governing informed consent for HIV tests has been enacted in most states.
- Laws specify exactly what type of information must be given to inform the client properly.
- Generally speaking, the client must be advised on (a) the test and its purpose, (b) how the test might be used, and (c) the meaning of the test and its limitations.

CONSENT FOR MINORS

- As a general rule, a minor cannot give consent for the administration of medical treatment.
- Parental or guardian consent is required.
- Healthcare personnel who violate this rule are liable for assault and battery.

A minor is anyone who has not reached the age of majority as determined by state law.

REFUSAL OF CONSENT

- An individual has a constitutional right to refuse a medical procedure such as venipuncture.
- The refusal may be based on religious or personal beliefs and preferences.
- A patient who refuses medical treatment is normally required to verify the refusal in writing on a special form.

 Test yourself on the litigation process with the WORKBOOK exercise Knowledge Drill 2-6.

The Litigation Process

Litigation is the process used to settle legal disputes. Approximately 10% of malpractice lawsuits actually go to court. The rest are settled out of court, which can happen at any time prior to the final court decision. Malpractice litigation involves the following four phases:

- **Phase one** begins when an alleged patient incident occurs or the patient becomes aware of a prior possible injury.
- **Phase two** begins when the injured party or a family member consults an attorney. The attorney requests, obtains, and reviews copies of the medical records involved and decides whether to take the case. If the attorney thinks that malpractice has occurred and takes the case, an attempt to negotiate a settlement is made. If the case is not resolved by negotiation, a complaint is filed by the patient's attorney. Once a complaint is filed, the injured party becomes the **plaintiff** and the person or persons against whom the complaint is filed becomes the **defendant**. Both sides now conduct formal **discovery**, which involves taking depositions and interrogating parties involved. Giving a **deposition** is a process in which one party questions another under oath while a court reporter records every word. The plaintiff, the defendant, and expert witnesses for both sides may give depositions. Expert witnesses are persons who are asked to review medical records and give their opinion of whether or not the standard of care was met. A person who lies under oath while giving a deposition can be charged with perjury.
- **Phase three** is the trial phase, the process designed to settle a dispute before a jury. Both sides present their versions of the facts and the jury determines which version appears to be correct. If the jury decides in the plaintiff's favor, damages may be awarded. At this point, the lawsuit may proceed to phase four.
- **Phase four** begins with an appeal of the jury's decision. Although either side has the right to an appeal, the losing party is usually the one to choose this option.
- Phlebotomists concerned with CQI and safe practice reduce their exposure to malpractice litigation. With the rapid evolution of medicine and, more specifically, laboratory testing, safe practice includes the phlebotomist's responsibility to stay abreast of all changes to ensure the safe collection of quality specimens. This, in turn, directly affects the quality of clinical laboratory services.

Legal Cases Involving Phlebotomy Procedures

The following are examples of actual legal cases involving phlebotomy procedures. They serve as a reminder that phlebotomy is not an innocuous procedure and that failure to exercise due care can result in injury to the patient and legal consequences.

CASE 1: A NEGLIGENCE CASE SETTLED THROUGH BINDING ARBITRATION

A patient had a blood specimen collected at a physician's office. Blood had been collected from him at the same office on several prior occasions with no problem. The phlebotomist, who was new to the patient and seemed to be in a hurry, inserted the needle deeper into the arm and at a much steeper angle than the patient was used to. She redirected the needle several times before hitting the vein. A hematoma began to form. Meanwhile, the patient told the phlebotomist that he felt great pain, but the phlebotomist told him it would be over soon and continued the draw. The pain continued after the draw and the patient's arm later became bruised and swollen. The patient suffered permanent injury to a nerve from compression by the hematoma. The patient sued and was awarded unknown damages.

CASE 2: A NEGLIGENCE CASE SETTLED THROUGH BINDING ARBITRATION

A phlebotomist was sent to a woman's home to draw blood for insurance purposes. After missing twice, she made a third attempt, which was also unsuccessful. The phlebotomist commented that she thought "she hit a muscle." The client complained of pain and suffered immediate swelling and bruising in the form of a hematoma. For up to a year after the failed venipuncture attempts, the client had restricted use of her right arm and hand because of tingling and shocking sensations. It was determined that the client had suffered permanent damage to her arm because the phlebotomist was not sufficiently trained and failed to adhere to the standard of care. The client sued and was awarded $1 million in damages.

CASE 3: A NEGLIGENCE CASE SETTLED THROUGH BINDING ARBITRATION

A college student who had been studying for final examinations and had not eaten or slept well for 2 days went to an outpatient laboratory to have blood drawn. The phlebotomist failed to observe the student's anxiety and pallor or to listen to the student's concerns. Following the blood collection, the phlebotomist did not ask the patient how she was feeling or if she would like to lie down. As the student walked alone from the blood collection area, she fainted and fell against a stone threshold at the building's exit. She suffered multiple facial fractures as well as permanent scarring to her face; she also lost three front teeth. She was hospitalized for 2 weeks and missed her college examinations. The outpatient laboratory had not provided a bed for patients to use when feeling faint, nor had it set aside a separate room for emergency situations. The supervisor was not available on site at the time of the accident. The first aid administered to the student before the ambulance arrived was incorrect and resulted in additional harm. At arbitration, the student was awarded $1.5 million in damages.

CASE 4: CONGLETON VERSUS BATON ROUGE GENERAL HOSPITAL

The plaintiff went to donate blood at a hospital. She complained of pain during the procedure and the technician repositioned the needle twice. The technician offered to remove the needle but the plaintiff chose to complete the procedure. After completing the donation, she complained of numbness in her arm. Later evaluation by a neurologist indicated injury to the antebrachial cutaneous nerve. The plaintiff sued and was awarded unknown damages.

CASE 5: JURY VERDICT AFFIRMED ON APPEAL BY KENTUCKY SUPREME COURT

The plaintiff went to the hospital to have her blood drawn. The phlebotomist placed a tourniquet on the plaintiff's arm and then left the room to answer a phone call. When she returned approximately 10 minutes later, the plaintiff's arm was swollen and had changed color. The plaintiff experienced medical complications and sought treatment. After medical consultation, three physicians concluded that the plaintiff was experiencing nerve problems with her right arm that were related to the tourniquet incident. The plaintiff sued and was awarded $100,000 in damages.

Study and Review Questions

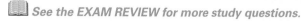 *See the EXAM REVIEW for more study questions.*

1. **Which of the following is the oldest and largest healthcare standards–setting body in the nation?**
   a. American Medical Association
   b. Center for Medicare and Medicaid
   c. College of American Pathologists
   d. The Joint Commission

2. **The CLIA federal regulations are administered by**
   a. CAP.
   b. CLSI.
   c. CMS.
   d. CoW.

3. **Which of the following are set up to monitor all areas of care that tend to cause problems?**
   a. Internal Report Forms
   b. Quality indicators
   c. Sentinel events
   d. Threshold values

4. **Proper patient identification means**
   a. actively involving patients in their own identification.
   b. asking a second person to verify your ID procedure.
   c. checking the requisition against the patient's room number.
   d. scanning patient ID bands with barcode readers only.

5. **What manual describes the necessary steps to follow in patient preparation for laboratory tests?**
   a. The Patient Record
   b. The Procedure Manual
   c. The Safety Manual
   d. The Test Catalog

6. **Which of the following can identify trends for risk management?**
   a. Delta checks
   b. Incident reports
   c. Safety data sheets
   d. Test menus

7. **Informed consent means that a**
   a. nurse has the right to perform a procedure on a patient even if the patient refuses.
   b. patient agrees to a procedure after being told of the consequences associated with it.
   c. patient has the right to look at all his or her medical records and test results.
   d. phlebotomist tells the patient why the test is ordered and the meaning of the results.

8. **A national organization that develops guidelines and sets standards for laboratory procedures is the**
   a. CAP.
   b. CLIAC.
   c. CLSI.
   d. NAACLS.

9. **A physician is sued for negligence due to the actions of an inexperienced, contracted phlebotomist hired to cover summer vacations. This is an example of**
   a. assault and battery.
   b. *res ipsa loquitur.*
   c. the statute of limitations.
   d. vicarious liability.

10. **A young adult comes to an outpatient lab to have his blood drawn. The phlebotomist refuses to draw this patient's blood because the patient**
    a. does not have insurance, but offers to pay cash.
    b. has never had his blood drawn before this time.
    c. has not reached the age of majority in the state.
    d. has not eaten breakfast and feels light-headed.

11. **The NPSGs are**
    a. CLSI's voluntary standards and guidelines.
    b. NAACLS national educational guidelines.
    c. Safety rules set down by CDC and OSHA.
    d. TJC's annual safety requirement goals.

12. **A delta check refers to**
    a. checking the wristband with the requisition.
    b. comparing current test results with previous one.
    c. documenting all of the results of the QC checks.
    d. reporting new infection control precautions.

13. **Blood culture contamination is a quality indicator for the**
    a. Environmental Services area.
    b. Infection Control Department.
    c. Microbiology Department.
    d. Specimen Processing area.

14. **Failure to exercise "due care" is**
    a. assault and battery.
    b. invasion of privacy.
    c. negligence.
    d. *res ipsa loquitur.*

15. **The statute of limitations timing can begin**
    a. on the day the negligent act took place.
    b. the first day in a series of medical treatments.
    c. the first day of consulting with a lawyer.
    d. a month after the injury was discovered.

Case Studies

 See the WORKBOOK for more case studies.

Case Study 2-1: Scope of Duty

A newly trained phlebotomist is sent to collect a blood specimen from a patient. The phlebotomist is an employee of a laboratory that contracts with the hospital to perform laboratory services, including specimen collection. The phlebotomist collects the specimen with no problems. Before the phlebotomist has a chance to leave the room, the patient asks for help to walk to the bathroom. The patient is a very large woman, but the phlebotomist lends an arm to help her. On the way to the bathroom, the patient slips on some liquid on the floor. The phlebotomist tries but is unable to prevent her from falling. The patient fractures her arm in the fall.

QUESTIONS

1. Was it wrong of the phlebotomist to try to help the patient? Explain why or why not.

2. Is the hospital liable for the patient's injury? Explain why or why not.

3. Can the phlebotomist be held liable for the patient's injuries? Explain why or why not.

Case Study 2-2: Quality Assurance in the ER

The phlebotomist arrives in ER to collect a specimen from a patient headed to surgery as quickly as possible to remove a spike from his head. The atmosphere is hectic because of the serious condition of the patient, but he is awake and able to talk. Sensing that time is of the essence, the phlebotomist only checks the wristband; verifies the patient's ID using the electronic barcode system, and proceeds to draw the blood. When the nurse arrives at the blood bank window to pick up the unit of blood for this patient, she notices that the information does not match with what is on her requisition.

QUESTIONS

1. What mistake did the phlebotomist make?

2. What does the NPSGs say about patient identification?

3. Why could this incident cause the hospital to be issued a Preliminary Denial of Accreditation?

Bibliography and Suggested Readings

American Hospital Association (AHA). http://www.aha.org

Clinical Laboratory Improvement Amendments (CLIA). http://www.cms.hhs.gov/clia/

Fremgen BF. *Medical Law and Ethics.* Upper Saddle River, NJ: Prentice Hall; 2011.

Kentucky Supreme Court, case #2003-SC-471-DG. *Baptist Healthcare Systems, Inc. D/B/A Central Baptist Hospital v Golda H. Miller et al.,* opinion rendered August 25, 2005.

Hughes RG, ed. *Patient Safety and Quality: An Evidence-Based Handbook for Nurses.* Rockville, MD; Agency for Healthcare Research and Quality (US); 2008.

Phillips LD. *Manual of I.V. Therapeutics,* 4th ed. Philadelphia, PA: FA Davis; 2005.

Sayles N. *Health Information Management Technology: An Applied Approach.* Chicago, IL: AHiMA; 2013.

The Joint Commission. http://www.jointcommission.org

Williams SJ. *Essentials of Health Services.* 3rd ed. New York, NY: Delmar Publishers; 2013.

Chapter 3

Infection Control, Safety, First Aid, and Personal Wellness

NAACLS Entry Level Competencies

2.00 Demonstrate knowledge of infection control and safety.

2.1 Identify policies and procedures for maintaining laboratory safety.

2.2 Demonstrate accepted practices for infection control, isolation techniques, aseptic techniques, and methods for disease prevention.

2.3 Comply with federal, state, and locally mandated regulations regarding safety practices.

9.9 List the causes of stress in the work environment and discuss the coping skills used to deal with stress in the work environment.

Key Terms

Do Matching Exercise 3-1 in the WORKBOOK to gain familiarity with these terms.

asepsis
BBP
Biohazard
CDC
chain of infection
engineering
  controls
EPA
fire tetrahedron
fomites
HAI
HBV
HCS

HCV
HICPAC
HIV
immune
infectious/
  causative
  agent
isolation
  procedures
microbe
neutropenic
NHSN
NIOSH

nosocomial
  infection
OSHA
parenteral
pathogenic
pathogens
percutaneous
permucosal
pictogram
PPE
reservoir
reverse
  isolation

SDS
standard
  precautions
susceptible host
transmission-
  based
  precautions
vector
  transmission
vehicle
  transmission
work practice
  controls

Objectives

Upon successful completion of this chapter, the reader should be able to:

1 Demonstrate knowledge of terminology and practices related to Infection Control and identify agencies associated with infection control precautions, procedures, and programs.

2 Identify key elements of the Blood-Borne Pathogen Standard and the Needlestick Safety and Prevention Act, and identify associated organizations.

3 Identify hazards, warning symbols, and safety rules related to the laboratory, patient areas, and biological, electrical, fire, radiation, and chemical safety, and discuss actions to take if incidents occur.

4 Recognize symptoms needing first aid and list the main points of the American Heart Association CPR and ECC guidelines.

5 Describe the role of personal wellness as it relates to nutrition, rest, exercise, stress management, and back protection.

Overview

This chapter covers infection control, safety, first aid, and personal wellness. A thorough knowledge in these areas is necessary for phlebotomists to protect themselves, patients, coworkers, and others from infection or injury, react quickly and skillfully in emergency situations, and stay healthy both physically and emotionally, all without compromising the quality of patient care. This chapter explains the process of infection, identifies the components of the chain of infection, lists required safety equipment, and describes infection control procedures. Also covered are biological, electrical, fire, radiation, and chemical hazards and the safety precautions, rules, and procedures necessary to eliminate or minimize them. First aid issues covered include control of external hemorrhage and how to recognize and treat shock victims. Wellness issues addressed include the prevention of back injury, benefits of exercise, and dealing with stress.

Infection Control

Although important advances have been made in understanding and treating infection, the threat of infection looms as large as ever. New enemies in the battle against infection emerge, and enemies that had once been conquered may become resistant to treatment, as in the case of *Mycobacterium tuberculosis* and methicillin-resistant *Staphylococcus aureus*. Blood collection personnel typically encounter numerous patients every day, many of whom may be harboring infectious microorganisms. Measures to prevent the spread of infection must be taken in the course of all patient encounters. This portion of the chapter explains the infection process and describes infection control measures needed to protect blood collection personnel, patients, staff, visitors, and those doing business within healthcare facilities. Infection control involves implementing procedures and policies that prevent infection; it starts with an understanding of the process of infection.

Infection

Infection is a condition that results when a microorganism (**microbe** for short) is able to invade the body, multiply, and cause injury or disease. Microbes include bacteria, fungi, protozoa, and viruses. Most microbes are nonpathogenic, meaning that they do not cause disease under normal conditions. Microbes that are **pathogenic** (causing or productive of disease) are called **pathogens**. We normally have many nonpathogenic microbes on our skin and in other areas such as the gastrointestinal (GI) tract. These microbes can become pathogens if they enter and multiply in areas of the body where they do not exist normally. Some microbes are pathogenic regardless of where they are found. Infections caused by pathogens can be local (restricted to a small area of the body) or systemic (sis-tem'ik), in which case the entire body is affected.

COMMUNICABLE INFECTIONS

Some pathogenic microbes cause infections that are **communicable** (able to spread from person to person); the diseases that result are called communicable diseases. An agency of the U.S. Department of Health and Human Services called the **Centers for Disease Control and Prevention (CDC)** is charged with the investigation and control of various diseases, especially those that are communicable and have epidemic potential. The CDC also develops guidelines and recommends safety precautions to protect healthcare workers and others from infection.

 Key Point The **National Institute for Occupational Safety and Health (NIOSH)**, which is part of the CDC, is responsible for conducting research and making recommendations for the prevention of work-related illness and injury.

NOSOCOMIAL AND HEALTHCARE-ASSOCIATED INFECTIONS

The term **nosocomial infection** is applied to patient infections acquired in hospitals. **Healthcare-associated infection (HAI)** is a newer term that applies to infections acquired during healthcare delivery in all healthcare settings, including home care. HAIs can result from contact with various sources, including infected personnel, other patients, visitors, and contaminated food, drugs, or equipment. An HAI prevalence survey of U.S. acute care hospitals conducted by the CDC in 2011, found that on any given day, about 1 in 25 patients has at least one HAI, and up to 1 in 9 end up dying from it. According to the Institute of Medicine 5% to 15% of patients in all types of U.S. healthcare facilities are exposed to and

Box 3-1

CDC List of Diseases and Organisms Found in Healthcare Settings

- *Acinetobacter*
- *Burkholderia cepacia*
- *Clostridium difficile*
- *Clostridium sordellii*
- Enterobacteriaceae (carbapenem-resistance)
- Gram-negative bacteria
- Hepatitis
- Human Immunodeficiency Virus (HIV/AIDS)
- Influenza
- Klebsiella
- Methicillin-resistant *Staphylococcus aureus* (MRSA)
- *Mycobacterium abscessus*
- Norovirus
- *Pseudomonas aeruginosa*
- *Staphylococcus aureus*
- Tuberculosis (TB)
- Vancomycin-intermediate *Staphylococcus aureus* (VISA)
- Vancomycin-resistant *Staphylococcus aureus* (VRSA)
- Vancomycin-resistant enterococci (VRE)

Reprinted from U.S. Department of Health and Human Services, Centers for Disease Control and Prevention. National Center for Emerging and Zoonotic Infectious Diseases (NCEZID), Division of Healthcare Quality Promotion (DHQP). *Diseases and Organisms in Healthcare Settings.* Accessed April 9, 2014, from http://www.cdc.gov/hai/organisms/organisms.html

contract an infection after admission. This results in an estimated 2 million infections and 90,000 associated deaths each year. (See Box 3-1 for a CDC list of diseases and organisms found in healthcare settings).

 Key Point According to the HAI prevalence survey, for the first time, the most common healthcare-associated pathogen was *Clostridium difficile* (*C. difficile* or *C. diff*), just barely surpassing *Staphylococcus aureus,* which had previously held the top spot.

The most widely used HAI tracking system is provided by the CDC **National Healthcare Safety Network (NHSN)**. Data provided by NHSN helps U.S. healthcare facilities eliminate HAIs by identifying problem areas and measuring progress of prevention efforts. HAI prevention efforts are also aided by the **Healthcare Infection Control Practices Advisory Committee (HICPAC)**, which provides the CDC with advice and guidance regarding the practice of infection control and prevention in healthcare settings, the updating of CDC guidelines, and the development of new CDC infection control guidelines.

Key Point The most common type of HAI reported to NHSN is urinary tract infection (UTI), accounting for over 30% of all HAIs.

ANTIBIOTIC-RESISTANT INFECTIONS

A core activity of the CDC is monitoring the magnitude, extent, and trends of antibiotic resistance, which is the ability of microbes to develop resistance to specific antibiotics, and a growing problem that is of great concern to public health. Antibiotic resistance leads to much suffering and increases a patient's risk of dying from once easily treatable infections.

Well-Established Antibiotic-Resistant Bacteria

Well-known enemies in the antibiotic resistance fight include the three of the most common HAI pathogens, *C. difficile* (*C. diff*), methicillin-resistant *Staphylococcus* (staph) *aureas* (MRSA), and *Enterococcus*. Some progress has been made in reducing infections caused by these bacteria, but they still pose a major threat and continue to be responsible for many HAIs.

C. diff, a type of intestinal bacteria that multiplies when patients are treated with antibiotics, is responsible for mild to very severe GI infections, and is the most commonly identified cause of diarrhea in healthcare settings. MRSA is responsible for many types of HAIs from skin, wound, and surgical site infections, to pneumonia and bloodstream infections that can be fatal.

i MRSA has also become a growing community concern in the United States, and according to the CDC, the most commonly identified antibiotic-resistant pathogen in many other areas of the world too.

Enterococcus bacteria are normally present in the digestive tract and female genital tract where they do not pose a threat to healthy individuals. They do however pose a serious threat to those more susceptible to infection such as the elderly, intensive care unit (ICU) patients, and those with chronic diseases such as diabetes or kidney failure. *Enterococcus* infections include bloodstream infections, wound and surgical site infections, and UTIs. About 30% of *Enterococcus* HAIs are vancomycin resistant enterococcus (VRE).

Multidrug-Resistant Gram-Negative Bacteria

The newest challenge in antibiotic resistance in the healthcare setting comes from multidrug-resistant gram-negative bacteria. Some of these bacteria are resistant to almost all available treatments. Of primary concern are bacteria that are resistant to a class of drugs called Carbapenems that have traditionally been considered the "last resort" for treating bacterial infections such as *Escherichia coli (E. coli),* which causes the majority of urinary tract infections, and *Klebsiella pneumonia,* which causes many types of HAIs. Other examples of drug-resistant gram-negative bacteria are *Acinetobacter baumannii,* responsible for many wound infections, and *Pseudomonas aeruginosa,* often the cause of bloodstream infections and pneumonia.

The Chain of Infection

Infection transmission requires the presence of a number of components, which make up what is referred to as the **chain of infection** (Fig. 3-1). The chain must be complete for an infection to occur. If the process of infection is stopped at any component or link in the chain, an infection is prevented. However, when a pathogen successfully enters a susceptible host, the chain is completed, the host becomes a new source of infectious microorganisms, and the process of infection continues.

Key Point A phlebotomist, whose duties involve contact with many patients, must be fully aware of the infection process and take precautions to prevent the spread of infection.

CHAIN OF INFECTION COMPONENTS

There are six key components or "links" in the chain of infection that must be present for an infection to occur. They are an **infectious agent, a reservoir, an exit pathway, a means of transmission, an entry pathway,** and **a susceptible host**.

Infectious Agent

The infectious agent, also called the **causative agent**, is the pathogenic microbe responsible for causing an infection.

Reservoir

The source of an infectious agent is called a reservoir. It is a place where the microbe can survive, grow, or

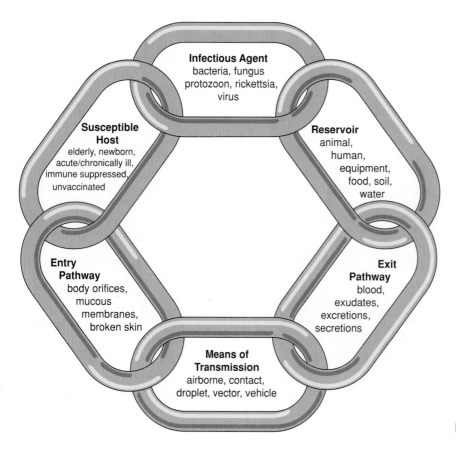

Figure 3-1 The chain of infection.

multiply. Reservoirs include humans, animals, food, water, soil, and contaminated articles and equipment. An individual or animal infected with a pathogenic microbe is called a reservoir host. Human reservoir hosts can be patients, personnel, or visitors and include those with an active disease, those incubating a disease, and chronic carriers of a disease. Another reservoir for potentially infectious microbes is a person's own normal flora (microorganisms that normally live on the skin and other areas of the human body).

Contaminated articles and equipment can be a major source of infectious agents. The ability of these inanimate objects to transmit infectious agents depends upon the amount of contamination, the **viability** or ability of the microbe to survive on the object, the **virulence** or degree to which the microbe is capable of causing disease, and the amount of time that has passed since the item was contaminated. For example, **hepatitis B virus (HBV)**, the virus that causes hepatitis B, is much more virulent than **human immunodeficiency virus (HIV)**, the virus that causes AIDS, because a smaller amount of HBV infective material is capable of causing disease. HBV is also more viable because it is capable of surviving longer on surfaces than HIV. However, if enough time elapses from the time of contamination until contact by a susceptible host, it is no longer alive and therefore unable to transmit disease.

Exit Pathway

An exit pathway is a way an infectious agent is able to leave a reservoir host. Infectious agents can exit a reservoir host in secretions from the eyes, nose, or mouth; exudates from wounds; tissue specimens; blood from venipuncture and skin puncture sites; and excretions of feces and urine.

Means of Transmission

The means of transmission is the method an infectious agent uses to travel from a reservoir to a susceptible individual. Means of infection transmission include **airborne, contact, droplet, vector,** and **vehicle.** The same microbe can be transmitted by more than one route.

Airborne Transmission

Airborne transmission involves dispersal of infectious agents that can remain infective for long periods of time in particles that are typically less than 5 μm in diameter and can be inhaled, such as droplet nuclei (residue of evaporated droplets). The particles, generated by sneezing, coughing, talking, and activities that produce aerosols, can remain suspended in the air or in dust particles and become widely dispersed and eventually inhaled by susceptible individuals who have not been anywhere near the infectious individual. Consequently, any patient with an airborne infection requires an **airborne infection isolation room (AIIR)**

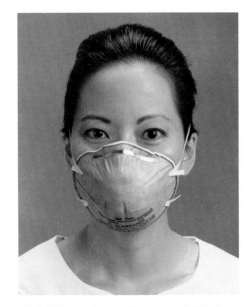

Figure 3-2 N95 respirator. (Courtesy of 3M Occupational Health and Environmental Safety Division. St. Paul, MN.)

that has special air handling and ventilation. Anyone who enters an AIIR should wear a NIOSH certified N95 (N category, 95% efficiency) or higher-level respirator (Fig. 3-2).

Key Point *Mycobacterium tuberculosis,* rubeola virus, and varicella virus are examples of infectious agents spread by airborne transmission.

Test your knowledge of Key Points with WORKBOOK Knowledge Drill 3-1.

Contact Transmission

Contact transmission is the most common means of transmitting infection. There are two types of contact transmission: direct and indirect. **Direct contact transmission** is the physical transfer of an infectious agent to a susceptible host through close or intimate contact such as touching or kissing. **Indirect contact transmission** can occur when a susceptible host touches contaminated objects such as patient bed linens, clothing, dressings, and eating utensils. It includes contact with phlebotomy equipment such as gloves, needles, specimen tubes, testing equipment, and trays. It also includes less obvious contaminated objects such as countertops, computer keyboards, phones, pens, pencils, doorknobs, and faucet handles. The transfer of infectious agents from contaminated hands to a susceptible host is also considered indirect contact transmission.

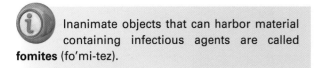 Inanimate objects that can harbor material containing infectious agents are called **fomites** (fo'mi-tez).

Droplet Transmission

Droplet transmission is the transfer of an infectious agent to the mucous membranes of the mouth, nose, or conjunctiva of the eyes of a susceptible individual via infectious droplets (particles 5 µm in diameter or larger) generated by coughing, sneezing, or talking or through procedures such as suctioning or throat swab collection.

Key Point Droplet transmission differs from airborne transmission in that droplets normally travel less than 10 feet and do not remain suspended in the air.

Vector Transmission

Vector transmission is the transfer of an infectious agent carried by an insect, arthropod, or animal. Examples of vector transmission include the transmission of West Nile virus by mosquitoes and bubonic plague (*Yersinia pestis*) by rodent fleas.

Vehicle Transmission

Vehicle transmission is the transmission of an infectious agent through contaminated food, water, or drugs. Examples of vehicle transmission are *Salmonella* infection from handling contaminated chicken and *Shigella* infection from drinking contaminated water.

Key Point The transmission of hepatitis viruses and HIV through blood transfusion is also considered vehicle transmission.

Entry Pathway

The entry pathway is the way an infectious agent is able to enter a susceptible host. Entry pathways include body orifices (openings); mucous membranes of the eyes, nose, or mouth; and breaks in the skin. Patients' entry pathways can be exposed during invasive procedures such as catheterization, venipuncture, fingersticks, and heel puncture. Entry pathways of healthcare personnel can be exposed during spills and splashes of infectious specimens or created by needlesticks and injuries from other sharp objects.

Susceptible Host

A **susceptible host** is someone with a decreased ability to resist infection. Factors that affect susceptibility include age, health, and immune status. For example, newborns are more susceptible to infection because their immune systems are still forming, and the elderly are more susceptible because their immune systems weaken with age. Disease, antibiotic treatment, immunosuppressive drugs, and procedures such as surgery, anesthesia, and insertion of catheters can all leave a patient more susceptible to infection. A healthy person who has received a vaccination against an infection with a particular virus or recovered from one has developed antibodies against that virus and is considered to be **immune**, or unlikely to develop the disease.

Key Point Individuals who are exposed to the hepatitis B virus (HBV) are less likely to contract the disease if they have previously completed an HBV vaccination series.

A microorganism that primarily infects individuals with weakened immune systems is called an opportunist. One classic opportunist that is becoming more and more of a threat is a type of bacterium called *Acinetobacter baumannii*. It is found most commonly in hospitals, infecting the chronically ill, the elderly, patients with HIV, and transplant patients.

BREAKING THE CHAIN OF INFECTION

Breaking the chain of infection involves stopping infections at the source, preventing contact with substances from exit pathways, eliminating means of transmission, blocking exposure to entry pathways, and reducing or eliminating the susceptibility of potential hosts. Examples of ways to break the chain and prevent infections are shown in Box 3-2.

Infection Control Programs

The Joint Commission requires every healthcare institution to have an infection control program responsible for protecting patients, employees, visitors, and anyone doing business within healthcare institutions from infection. A typical infection control program implements procedures aimed at breaking the chain of infection, monitors and collects data on all infections occurring within the institution, and institutes special precautions in the event of outbreaks of specific infections.

EMPLOYEE SCREENING AND IMMUNIZATION

An important way in which infection control programs prevent infection is through employee screening and

Box 3-2

Examples of Ways to Break the Chain of Infection

Ways Healthcare Workers Break the Chain

- Effective hand hygiene procedures
- Good nutrition, adequate rest, and reduction of stress
- Immunization against common pathogens
- Proper decontamination of surfaces and instruments
- Proper disposal of sharps and infectious waste
- Use of gloves and other personal protective equipment (PPE) when indicated
- Use of needle safety devices during blood collection

Ways Healthcare Institutions Break the Chain

- Infection control programs
- Insect and rodent control
- Isolation procedures

immunization programs. Screening for infectious diseases typically takes place prior to or upon employment and on a regular basis throughout employment. Employee screening tests typically include a tuberculosis (TB) test; employees with positive TB test results receive chest x-ray evaluations to determine their status. Screening tests may also include tests for diarrheal and skin diseases. Employees with certain conditions or infections may be subject to work restrictions. (Conditions requiring work restrictions are listed in Appendix D.)

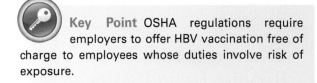 **Key Point** Tests for TB include the tuberculin skin test (TST), also called a PPD test after the purified protein derivative used, and a relatively new TB test called the QuantiFERON®-TB Gold (QFT-G) test that requires collection of a blood sample.

Immunizations typically required include current HBV; measles, mumps, rubella (MMR); diphtheria; and tetanus vaccinations or proof of immunity. Most employers provide vaccinations free of charge.

Key Point OSHA regulations require employers to offer HBV vaccination free of charge to employees whose duties involve risk of exposure.

EVALUATION AND TREATMENT

An infection control program also provides for the evaluation and treatment of employees who are exposed to infections on the job. This includes Occupational Safety and Health Administration (OSHA)-mandated confidential medical evaluation, treatment, counseling, and follow-up as a result of exposure to blood-borne pathogens.

SURVEILLANCE

Another major function of an infection control program is surveillance or monitoring. This involves closely watching patients and employees at risk of acquiring infections as well as collecting, evaluating, and distributing data on infections contracted by patients and employees. Infection control measures are updated and new policies instituted based on this information.

The CDC developed **The National Surveillance System For Healthcare Workers (NaSH)** to collaborate with healthcare facilities in the collection of information important in preventing occupational exposure and infection among healthcare workers.

Infection Control Practices

Since infectious microbes are invisible to the naked eye it is easy to forget that the healthcare environment can be teeming with them. Studies have shown that patient items and anything in the surrounding area such as chairs, privacy curtains, floors, night stands, and tray tables can be contaminated with potential pathogens. Many of the contaminating organisms can stay viable for weeks; some even for months. Consequently all healthcare workers (HCWs) must be mindful of contamination sources and take measures to prevent the spread of infection.

Key Point Good infection control practices prevent the spread of infection in the healthcare setting and to the community as well.

Box 3-3

Situations That Require Hand Hygiene Procedures

- Before and after each patient contact
- Between unrelated procedures on a patient such as wound care and drawing blood
- Before putting on gloves and after taking them off
- Before leaving the laboratory
- Before going to lunch or on break
- Before and after going to the restroom
- Whenever hands become visibly or knowingly contaminated

HAND HYGIENE

Hand hygiene is one of the most important means of preventing the spread of infection provided that it is achieved properly and when required. Hand hygiene measures include the frequent use of alcohol-based antiseptic hand cleaners or hand washing, depending upon the degree of contamination. It is important that all healthcare personnel learn proper hand hygiene procedures and recognize situations when they should be performed. Box 3-3 lists situations that require hand hygiene procedures.

Hand hygiene effectiveness can be reduced by the type and length of fingernails. Studies have shown that artificial nails harbor more pathogenic microbes than natural nails. Consequently many healthcare facilities ban the wearing of artificial nails for all who provide patient care.

Key Point The World Health Organization (WHO) consensus recommendations in the 2009 Guidelines on Hand Hygiene in Health Care are that HCWs do not wear artificial fingernails or extenders when having direct contact with patients and natural nails should be kept short (0.5 cm long or approximately 1/4 inch long).

Use of Alcohol-Based Antiseptic Hand Cleaners

CDC/HICPAC guidelines recommend the use of alcohol-based antiseptic hand cleaners (gels, foams, and rinses) in place of hand washing as long as the hands are not visibly soiled. These products have been shown to have superior **microbicidal** (destructive to microbes) activity. Sufficient cleaner must be used to cover all surfaces of the hands, including between the fingers, and the alcohol must be allowed to evaporate to achieve proper antisepsis. Studies have shown that alcohol-based cleaners can be used multiple times in a row, however, if hands become visibly soiled or feel as if something is on them they should be washed with soap and water. In addition, if hands are heavily contaminated with organic material and hand washing facilities are not available, it is recommended that hands be cleaned with detergent containing wipes, followed by the use of an alcohol-based antiseptic hand cleaner.

CAUTION The spores of some microbes such as *C. Diff* (*Clostridium difficile*) are not killed by alcohol-based hand cleaners. Patients known to be infected with such microbes will normally be in contact isolation with a sign posted to remind those who enter the room that washing hands with soap and water is required before leaving the room. See Figure 3-3.

Test your knowledge of proper hand washing procedure with WORKBOOK Skills Drill 3-3.

Hand Washing

There are different methods of hand washing, depending on the degree of contamination and the level of

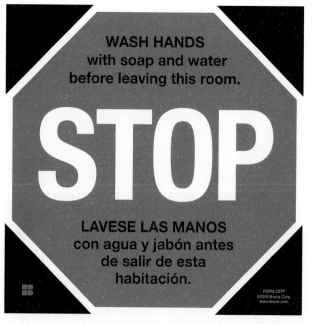

Figure 3-3 Stop sign reminder to wash hands with soap and water.

antimicrobial activity required. A routine hand washing procedure uses plain soap and water to mechanically remove soil and transient bacteria. According to the CDC, hand antisepsis requires the use of an antimicrobial soap to remove, kill, or inhibit transient microorganisms. A 2-minute surgical hand scrub uses an antimicrobial soap or equivalent to remove or destroy transient microorganisms and reduce levels of normal flora prior to surgical procedures. Proper routine hand washing procedure is described in Procedure 3-1.

thePoint. *View the Hand Washing/Hand Antisepsis video at http://thepoint.lww.com/McCall6e.*

USE OF PERSONAL PROTECTIVE EQUIPMENT

Protective clothing and other items worn by an individual to protect mucous membranes, airways, skin, and clothing from contact with infectious substances is called **personal protective equipment (PPE)**. PPE provides a barrier against infection. Used properly, it protects those wearing it. Disposed of properly, it prevents spread of infection to others. The type of PPE required depends upon the type of precautions required. (See Isolation Precautions) PPE includes the following.

thePoint. *View the Donning and Removal of Protective Equipment video at http://thepoint.lww.com/McCall6e.*

Procedure 3-1: Hand Washing Technique

PURPOSE: Decontaminate hands to prevent the spread of infection

EQUIPMENT: Liquid soap, disposable towels, trash can

Step	Explanation/Rationale
1. Stand back so that you do not touch the sink.	The sink may be contaminated.
2. Turn on the faucet and wet hands under warm running water.	Water should not be too hot or too cold and hands should be wet before applying soap to minimize drying, chapping, or cracking of hands from frequent hand washing.

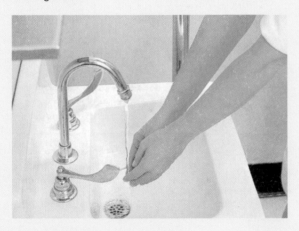

3. Apply soap and work up a lather.	A good lather is needed to reach all surfaces.
4. Scrub all surfaces, including between the fingers and around the knuckles.	Scrubbing is necessary to dislodge microorganisms from surfaces, especially between fingers and around knuckles.

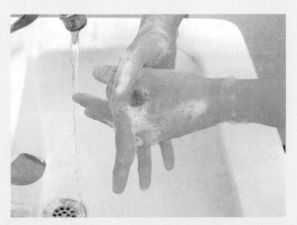

Procedure 3-1: Hand Washing Technique (Continued)

Step	Explanation/Rationale
5. Rub your hands together vigorously.	Friction helps loosen dead skin, dirt, debris, and microorganisms. (Steps 4 and 5 should take at least 20 seconds, about the time it takes to sing the ABCs or the happy birthday song two times from beginning to end).
6. Rinse your hands in a downward motion from wrists to fingertips. 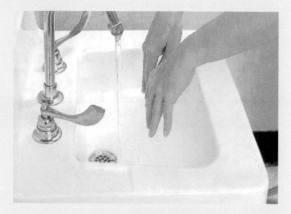	Rinsing with the hands downward allows contaminants to be flushed from the hands and fingers into the sink rather than flowing back up the arm or wrist.
7. Dry hands with a clean paper towel. 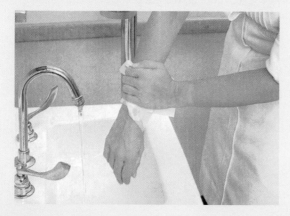	Hands must be dried thoroughly and gently to prevent chapping or cracking. Reusable towels can be a source of contamination.
8. Use a clean paper towel to turn off the faucet unless it is foot or motion activated.	Clean hands should not touch contaminated faucet handles.

Images from Kronenberger J, Woodson, D. *Lippincott Williams & Wilkins Clinical Medical Assisting.* 4th ed. Baltimore, MD: Lippincott Williams & Wilkins; 2012.

Gloves

Clean, nonsterile gloves are worn when collecting or handling blood and other body fluids, handling contaminated items, and touching nonintact skin or mucous membranes. Gloves should be pulled over the cuffs of gowns or lab coats to provide adequate protection. Three main reasons for wearing gloves are as follows:

- To prevent contamination of the hands when handling blood or body fluids or when touching mucous membranes or nonintact skin

- To reduce the chance of transmitting organisms on the hands of personnel to patients during invasive or other procedures that involve touching a patient's skin or mucous membranes

- To minimize the possibility of transmitting infectious microorganisms from one patient to another

Key Point Wearing gloves during phlebotomy procedures is mandated by the OSHA blood-borne pathogens standard.

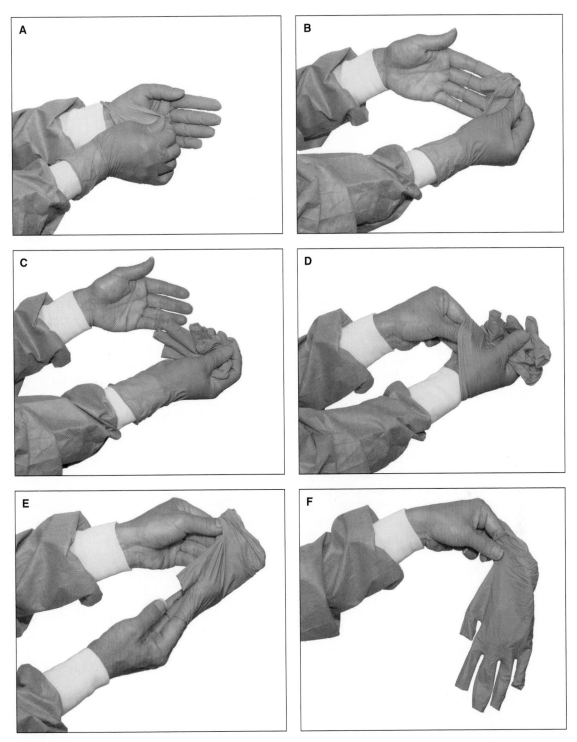

Figure 3-4 Glove removal. **A:** The outside of one glove is grasped below the wrist with the opposite gloved hand. **B:** The glove is pulled inside out, over the hand. **C:** The glove is pulled off the hand and held in the gloved hand. **D:** The fingers of the nongloved hand are slipped under the wrist of the remaining glove without touching the exterior surfaces. **E:** The glove is then pulled inside out over the hand so that the first glove ends up inside the second glove, with no exterior glove surfaces exposed. **F:** Contaminated gloves ready to be dropped into the proper waste receptacle.

Proper Glove Removal

After use, gloves must be removed in a manner that does not contaminate the hands, and then promptly discarded. To remove gloves properly (Fig. 3-4), grasp the outside of one glove below the wrist and pull it inside out and off the hand, ending up with it in the palm of the still-gloved hand. Slip fingers of the ungloved hand under the second glove at the wrist and pull it off the hand, ending with one glove inside the other with the contaminated surfaces inside.

> **Key Point** Glove use does not replace the need for hand hygiene. Hands should be sanitized immediately after glove removal and before going to another patient, back to the laboratory, or performing other duties.

Gowns

Clean, nonsterile, fluid-resistant gowns are worn by healthcare personnel to protect the skin and prevent contamination of clothing during patient-care activities in which splashes or sprays of blood or body fluids are possible or when entering isolation rooms (see Isolation Procedures). Sterile gowns are worn to protect certain patients (such as newborns and patients with compromised immune systems) from contaminants on the healthcare worker's clothing. Most gowns are made of disposable cloth or paper, are generous in size to adequately cover clothing, have long sleeves with knit cuffs, and fasten in the back.

Putting On and Removing Gowns

When putting on a gown, only inside surfaces of the gown should be touched. A properly worn gown has the sleeves pulled all the way to the wrist, and the gown overlapped and wrapped around the back, completely closed, and securely fastened at the neck and waist. To remove a gown, unfasten the ties, pull the gown away from the neck and shoulders by touching the inside only, and slide the arms out of the sleeves, turning the gown inside out. Hold the gown away from the body, fold or roll it into a bundle, and discard in a waste container.

Lab Coats and Scrubs

Lab coats, like gowns, are worn to protect skin and prevent soiling of healthcare workers' clothing during patient-care activities in which splashes or sprays of blood or body fluids are possible. They are required attire for most phlebotomy situations. Lab coats used for specimen collection and handling are generally made of fluid-resistant cotton or synthetic material, have long sleeves with knit cuffs, and come in both reusable and disposable styles.

> **Key Point** Lab coats worn as PPE must not be worn on break, in the cafeteria or other nonpatient areas, or outside the hospital.

Scrubs are considered street clothes and not PPE unless they are put on at work and removed before leaving work. Scrubs worn home can carry microbes with them, including *C. difficile* spores, which can survive for months on surfaces.

> **Key Point** Scrubs or other pants that touch the floor can easily pick up infectious material. According to CLSI laboratory safety guidelines, pants worn by laboratory personnel should be 1 to 1½ inches off of the floor to prevent contamination.

Masks, Face Shields, and Goggles

A mask is worn to protect against droplets generated by coughing or sneezing. To put on a mask, place it over your nose and mouth. Adjust the metal band (if applicable) to fit snugly over your nose. For masks with ties, fasten the top ties around the upper portion of your head; then tie the lower ones at the back of your neck. If the mask has elastic fasteners, slip them around your ears. A face shield or a mask and goggles are worn to protect the eyes, nose, and mouth from splashes or sprays of body fluids. If an activity requires goggles, it also requires a mask. Some masks have plastic eye shields attached.

> **CAUTION** Masks should be for one use only. If hung around the neck for reuse they can become reservoirs for bacteria and viruses.

Respirators

NIOSH-approved N95 respirators (Fig. 3-2) are required when entering rooms of patients with pulmonary TB and other diseases with airborne transmission. Respirators must fit snugly with no air leaks.

thePoint: *See the Donning and Removal of Protective Equipment video at http://thepoint.lww.com/McCall6e.*

SEQUENCE FOR DONNING AND REMOVING PPE

When donning (putting on) a complete set of PPE such as gown, mask, and gloves, the gown is put on first (Fig. 3-5A). The mask or respirator, if indicated, is put on next, making certain it covers the nose and mouth (Fig. 3-5B). If goggles or face shield are required, they are put on after the mask or respirator. Gloves are put on last and pulled over the cuffs of the gown (Fig. 3-5C).

Except for a respirator, protective clothing worn in isolation rooms is removed at the door before leaving the patient room or anteroom. Protective items must be removed in an aseptic (sterile or pathogen free) manner to prevent contamination of the wearer, and promptly

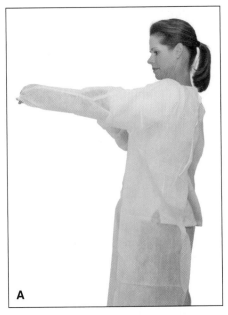
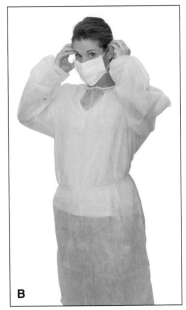
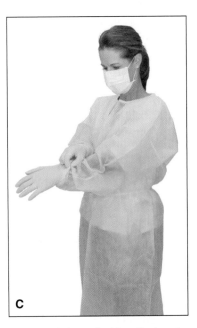

Figure 3-5 Protective clothing. **A:** Phlebotomist slips arms into a protective gown. **B:** A mask is applied by slipping the elastic band over the ears. **C:** Gloves are put on last and pulled over the gown cuffs.

discarded. Gloves are removed first, being careful not to touch contaminated surfaces with ungloved hands. Goggles or face shields can be removed next, touching only the headband or ear pieces. The gown is then removed by pulling it from the shoulders toward the hands so that it turns inside out. It must be held away from the body and rolled into a bundle before discarding. The mask is removed last touching only the strings. A respirator is removed touching only the elastic band, and only after leaving the patient's room and closing the door. Hands must then be immediately decontaminated.

At one time protective clothing worn in isolation required double bagging after removal. With the advent of standard precautions (See Guideline for Isolation Precautions later in this chapter) double bagging is no longer recommended unless a bag containing contaminated items is visibly contaminated on the outside or contamination has soaked through the bag.

ASEPSIS AND ASEPTIC TECHNIQUE

Asepsis is a condition of being free of contamination or germs (microbes) that could cause disease. Something that is free of disease causing microbes (i.e., pathogens) is said to be aseptic. **Aseptic technique** is a healthcare practice used to reduce the chance of microbial contamination with the goal of protecting patients from infection and preventing the spread of infection.

Key Point Any patient is potentially susceptible to infection, although those with certain conditions such as severe burns or immune system disorders are more vulnerable.

Aseptic techniques important to blood collection personnel include:
- following proper hand hygiene procedures
- keeping supplies within easy reach to prevent dropping them
- opening equipment packages in a way that avoids contamination
- prompt and safe disposal of contaminated equipment
- prompt cleanup up of infectious material
- wearing gloves and other PPE when indicated

NURSERY AND NEONATAL ICU INFECTION CONTROL TECHNIQUE

Newborns are more susceptible to infections than healthy older children and adults because their immune systems are not yet fully developed. Consequently, anyone who enters the nursery or other neonatal unit should use special infection control techniques. No one is allowed to enter if they have symptoms of illness such as cough, chills, or fever. Typical nursery and neonatal ICU infection control technique includes the following:
- Wash hands thoroughly and put on clean gloves.
- Gather only those items necessary to perform the specimen collection.

- Leave the blood collection tray or cart outside the nursery.
- Remove gloves, decontaminate hands, and put on new gloves between patients.

Isolation Procedures

One way in which an infection control program minimizes the spread of infection is through the establishment of **isolation procedures**. Isolation procedures separate patients with certain transmissible infections from contact with other patients and limit their contact with hospital personnel and visitors. Isolating a patient requires a doctor's order and is implemented either to prevent the spread of infection from a patient who has or is suspected of having a contagious disease or to protect a patient whose immune system is compromised. Patients are most commonly isolated in a private room. A card or sign indicating the type of isolation along with a description of required precautions is typically posted on the patient's door. A cart containing supplies needed to enter the room or care for the patient is typically placed in the hall outside the door.

> ⚠️ **CAUTION** Different types of isolation require the use of different types of PPE. Follow the directions on the precaution sign on the patient's door or check with the patient's nurse if instructed to do so, before entering an isolation room.

PROTECTIVE/REVERSE ISOLATION

Protective or **reverse isolation** is used for patients who are highly susceptible to infections. In this type of isolation, protective measures are taken to keep healthcare workers and others from transmitting infection to the patient rather than vice versa. Patients who may require protective isolation include those with suppressed or compromised immune function, such as burn patients, organ transplant patients, AIDS patients, and **neutropenic** (having a low neutrophil count) chemotherapy patients.

 A neutrophil is a type of white blood cell.

UNIVERSAL PRECAUTIONS

At one time isolation systems required a diagnosis or the suspicion of a transmissible disease to be instituted. Precautions were based on either the type of disease or its mode of transmission and often resulted in over isolation and increased costs. This changed when the CDC instituted an infection control strategy called **Universal Precautions (UP)** after reports of healthcare

workers being infected with HIV through needlesticks and other exposures to HIV-contaminated blood. Under UP, the blood and certain body fluids of *all* individuals were considered potentially infectious. This changed the focus of infection control from prevention of patient-to-patient infection transmission, to prevention of patient-to-personnel transmission, and was a required part of an overall infection control plan.

BODY SUBSTANCE ISOLATION

Shortly after the introduction of UP, another system called **Body Substance Isolation (BSI)** gained acceptance. The intent of BSI was to isolate workers from pathogens. BSI was also followed for *every* patient, but went beyond UP by requiring that gloves be worn when in contact with *any* moist body substance.

GUIDELINE FOR ISOLATION PRECAUTIONS

Widespread variation in the use of UP or BSI, confusion over which body fluids required precautions, lack of agreement on the importance of hand washing after glove use, and the need for additional precautions to prevent transmission of infectious agents in addition to blood-borne pathogens led to the Guideline for Isolation Precautions in Hospitals, developed and issued jointly by the CDC and HICPAC.

This guideline, which has been updated and expanded to include precautions for preventing transmission of infectious agents in all healthcare settings, contains two tiers of precautions. The first tier, **standard precautions**, specifies precautions to use in caring for all patients regardless of diagnosis or presumed infection status. The second tier, **transmission-based precautions**, specifies precautions to use for patients either suspected or known to be infected with certain pathogens transmitted by airborne, droplet, or contact routes. The guideline also lists specific clinical conditions that are highly suspicious for infection and specifies appropriate transmission-based precautions to use for each, in addition to standard precautions, until a diagnosis can be made.

Standard Precautions

Standard precautions (Fig. 3-6) are to be used in the care of all patients and constitute the number one strategy for prevention of HAIs. This blanket approach is necessary because a large percentage of individuals with infectious diseases do not have symptoms, and may not even know they have a disease. Standard precautions combine the major features of UP and BSI to minimize the risk of infection transmission from both recognized and unrecognized sources. Standard precautions apply to blood, *all* body fluids (including all secretions and excretions

STANDARD PRECAUTIONS

FOR INFECTION CONTROL

Assume that every person is potentially infected or colonized with an organism that could be transmitted in the healthcare setting.

Hand Hygiene

Avoid unnecessary touching of surfaces in close proximity to the patient.

When hands are visibly dirty, contaminated with proteinaceous material, or visibly soiled with blood or body fluids, wash hands with soap and water.

If hands are not visibly soiled, or after removing visible material with soap and water, decontaminate hands with an alcohol-based hand rub. Alternatively, hands may be washed with an antimicrobial soap and water.

Perform hand hygiene:

Before having direct contact with patients.
After contact with blood, body fluids or excretions, mucous membranes, nonintact skin, or wound dressings.
After contact with a patient's intact skin (e.g., when taking a pulse or blood pressure or lifting a patient).
If hands will be moving from a contaminated body site to a clean body site during patient care.
After contact with inanimate objects (including medical equipment) in the immediate vicinity of the patient.
After removing gloves.

Personal protective equipment (PPE)

Wear PPE when the nature of the anticipated patient interaction indicates that contact with blood or body fluids may occur.

Before leaving the patient's room or cubicle, remove and discard PPE.

Gloves

Wear gloves when contact with blood or other potentially infectious materials, mucous membranes, nonintact skin, or potentially contaminated intact skin (e.g., of a patient incontinent of stool or urine) could occur.

Remove gloves after contact with a patient and/or the surrounding environment using proper technique to prevent hand contamination. Do not wear the same pair of gloves for the care of more than one patient.

Change gloves during patient care if the hands will move from a contaminated body site (e.g., perineal area) to a clean body site (e.g., face).

Gowns

Wear a gown to protect skin and prevent soiling or contamination of clothing during procedures and patient-care activities when contact with blood, body fluids, secretions, or excretions is anticipated.

Wear a gown for direct patient contact if the patient has uncontained secretions or excretions.

Remove gown and perform hand hygiene before leaving patient's environment.

Mouth, nose, eye protection

Use PPE to protect the mucous membranes of the eyes, nose and mouth during procedures and patient-care activities that are likely to generate splashes or sprays of blood, body fluids, secretions and excretions.

During aerosol-generating procedures wear one of the following: a face shield that fully covers the front and sides of the face, a mask with attached shield, or a mask and goggles.

Respiratory Hygiene/Cough Etiquette

Educate healthcare personnel to contain respiratory secretions to prevent droplet and fomite transmission of respiratory pathogens, especially during seasonal outbreaks of viral respiratory tract infections.

Offer masks to coughing patients and other symptomatic persons (e.g., persons who accompany ill patients) upon entry into the facility.

Patient-Care equipment and instruments/devices

Wear PPE (e.g., gloves, gown), according to the level of anticipated contamination, when handling patient-care equipment and instruments/devices that are visibly soiled or may have been in contact with blood or body fluids.

Care of the environment

Include multi-use electronic equipment in policies and procedures for preventing contamination and for cleaning and disinfection, especially those items that are used by patients, those used during delivery of patient care, and mobile devices that are moved in and out of patient rooms frequently (e.g., daily).

Textiles and laundry

Handle used textiles and fabrics with minimum agitation to avoid contamination of air, surfaces and persons.

Figure 3-6 Standard precautions signs. (Courtesy Brevis Corp., Salt Lake City, UT.)

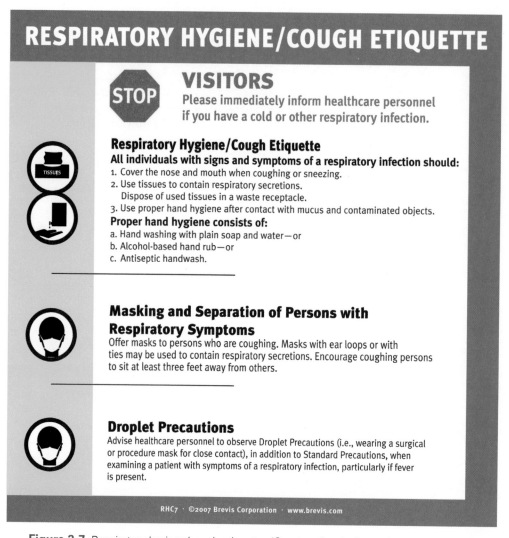

Figure 3-7 Respiratory hygiene/cough etiquette. (Courtesy Brevis Corp., Salt Lake City, UT.)

except sweat, whether or not they contain visible blood), nonintact skin, and mucous membranes. Standard precautions include hand hygiene procedures and depending on the type of exposure to body fluids anticipated, the use of PPE such as gloves, gowns, and masks.

Key Point An update to the isolation precautions guideline added respiratory hygiene/cough etiquette as a standard precaution. (See Fig. 3-7) This precaution applies to all who enter a healthcare setting and includes covering the mouth and nose with tissue when coughing, prompt disposal of used tissues, hand hygiene after contact with respiratory secretions, and 3 feet of separation from persons with respiratory infections.

Transmission-Based Precautions

Transmission-based precautions are to be used for patients known or suspected to be infected or colonized with highly transmissible or epidemiologically (related to the study of epidemics) significant pathogens that require special precautions in addition to standard precautions. Table 3-1 lists clinical conditions that warrant transmission-based precautions pending diagnosis. Common diseases and conditions that require transmission-based precautions are listed in Table 3-2. Precautions may be combined for diseases that have more than one means of transmission. There are three types of transmission-based precautions:

- **Airborne precautions** (Fig. 3-8) or the equivalent, which must be used in addition to standard precautions for patients known or suspected to be infected with microorganisms transmitted by airborne droplet nuclei (particles smaller than 5 µm)
- **Droplet precautions** (Fig. 3-9) or the equivalent, which must be used in addition to standard precautions for patients known or suspected to be infected with microorganisms transmitted by droplets (particles larger than 5 µm), generated when a patient

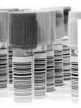

Table 3-1: Clinical Conditions Warranting Transmission-Based Precautions Pending Confirmation of Diagnosis

Condition	Potential Pathogen	Precaution
Diarrhea		
Acute diarrhea with a likely infectious cause in an incontinent or diapered patient	Enteric pathogen	Contact
Diarrhea in an adult with a history of broad-spectrum or long-term antibiotics	*Clostridium Difficile*	Contact
Meningitis	*Neisseria meningitidis*	Droplet
Rash for Inflamed Skin Eruptions		
Petechial/ecchymotic with fever	*Neisseria meningitidis*	Droplet
Vesicular	Varicella	Airborne and contact
Maculopapular	Rubeola (measles)	Airborne
Respiratory Infections		
Cough/fever/upper lobe pulmonary infiltrate in an HIV-negative patient and a patient at low risk for HIV infection	*Mycobacterium tuberculosis*	Airborne
Cough/fever/pulmonary infiltrate in any lung location in an HIV-infected patient and at high risk for HIV infection	*M. tuberculosis*	Airborne
Paroxysmal or severe persistent cough during periods of pertussis activity	*Bordetella pertussis*	Droplet
Respiratory infections, particularly bronchiolitis and croup, in infants and young children	Respiratory syncytial virus or parainfluenza virus	Contact
Risk of Multidrug-Resistant Microorganisms		
History of infection or colonization with multidrug-resistant organisms	Resistant bacteria	Contact
Skin, wound, or urinary tract infection in a patient with a recent hospital or nursing home stay in a facility where multidrug-resistant organisms are prevalent	Resistant bacteria	Contact
Skin or Wound Infection		
Abscess or draining wound that cannot be covered	*Staphylococcus aureus* Group A streptococcus	Contact

talks, coughs, or sneezes and during certain procedures such as suctioning

- **Contact precautions** (Fig. 3-10) or the equivalent, which must be used in addition to standard precautions when a patient is known or suspected to be infected or colonized with epidemiologically important microorganisms that can be transmitted by direct contact with the patient or indirect contact with surfaces or patient-care items

conditions must be ensured by employers as mandated by the Occupational Safety and Health Act and enforced by the **OSHA**. Even so, biological, electrical, radiation, and chemical hazards are encountered in a healthcare setting, often on a daily basis. It is important for the phlebotomist to be aware of the existence of hazards and know the safety precautions and rules necessary to eliminate or minimize them. General lab safety rules are listed in Box 3-4. Safety rules to follow when in patient rooms and other patient areas are listed in Box 3-5.

Safety

Providing quality care in an environment that is safe for employees as well as patients is a concern that is foremost in the minds of healthcare providers. Safe working

Biosafety

Biosafety is a term used to describe the safe handling of biological substances that pose a risk to health.

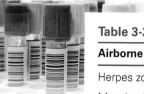

Table 3-2: Transmission-Based Precautions for Common Diseases and Conditions

Airborne Precautions	Droplet Precautions	Contact Precautions
Herpes zoster (shingles)[a]	Adenovirus infection[b]	Adenovirus infection[b]
Measles (rubeola)	Diphtheria (pharyngeal)	Cellulitis (uncontrolled drainage)
Pulmonary tuberculosis	*Haemophilus influenzae meningitis*	*Clostridium difficile*
Varicella (chickenpox)	Influenza	Conjunctivitis (acute viral)
	Meningococcal pneumonia	Decubitus ulcer (infected, major)
	Meningococcal sepsis	Diphtheria (cutaneous)
	Mumps (infectious parotitis)	Enteroviral infections[a]
	Mycoplasma pneumoniae	Herpes zoster (shingles)[a]
	Neisseria meningitidis	Impetigo
	Parvovirus B19	Parainfluenza virus
	Pertussis (whooping cough)	Pediculosis (lice)
	Pneumonic plague	Respiratory syncytial virus
	Rubella (German measles)	Rubella (congenital)
	Scarlet fever[b]	Scabies
		Varicella (chickenpox)

[a]Widely disseminated or in immunocompromised patients.
[b]Infants and children only.

Box 3-4

General Laboratory Safety Rules

- *Never* eat, drink, smoke, or chew gum in the laboratory. *Never* put pencils or pens in the mouth.
- *Never* place food or beverages in a refrigerator used for storing reagents or specimens.
- *Never* apply cosmetics, handle contact lenses, or rub eyes in the laboratory.
- *Never* wear long chains, large or dangling earrings, or loose bracelets.
- *Always* wear a fully buttoned lab coat when engaged in lab activities. *Never* wear a lab coat to lunch, on break, or when leaving the lab to go home. *Never* wear personal protective equipment outside the designated area for its use.
- *Always* tie back hair that is longer than shoulder length.
- *Always* keep finger nails short and well manicured. *Do not* wear nail polish or artificial nails. *Never* bite nails or cuticles.
- *Always* wear a face shield when performing specimen processing or any activity that might generate a splash or aerosol of bodily fluids.

Biological hazards can be encountered in a healthcare setting on a daily basis. Healthcare personnel must be able to recognize them in order to take the precautions necessary to eliminate or minimize exposure to them.

 Have some fun finding biohazard exposure route terms in the WORKBOOK Knowledge Drill 3-2.

BIOHAZARD

Anything harmful or potentially harmful to health is called a **biohazard** (short for biological hazard) and should be identified by a **biohazard symbol** (Fig. 3-11). Because most laboratory specimens have the potential to contain infectious agents, they are considered biohazards.

BIOHAZARD EXPOSURE ROUTES

There are many routes by which healthcare workers can be exposed to biohazards. Ingestion is probably the most easily recognized, but routes other than the digestive tract, referred to as **parenteral** (par-en'ter-al) routes, can also result in biohazard exposure. The most common biohazard exposure routes are as follows.

Airborne

Biohazards can become airborne and inhaled when splashes, aerosols, or fumes are generated. Aerosols

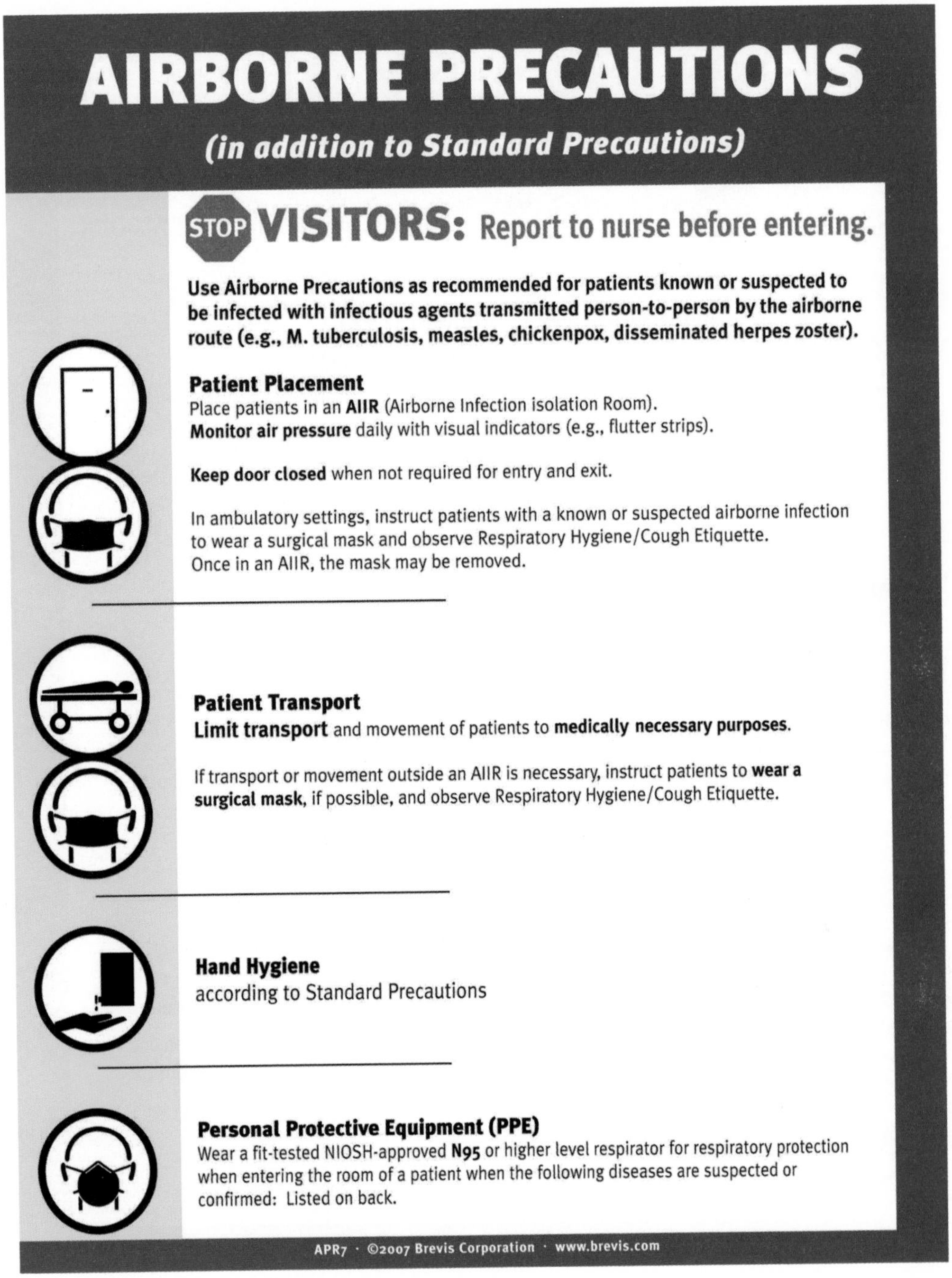

AIRBORNE PRECAUTIONS
(in addition to Standard Precautions)

STOP **VISITORS:** Report to nurse before entering.

Use Airborne Precautions as recommended for patients known or suspected to be infected with infectious agents transmitted person-to-person by the airborne route (e.g., M. tuberculosis, measles, chickenpox, disseminated herpes zoster).

Patient Placement
Place patients in an **AIIR** (Airborne Infection isolation Room).
Monitor air pressure daily with visual indicators (e.g., flutter strips).

Keep door closed when not required for entry and exit.

In ambulatory settings, instruct patients with a known or suspected airborne infection to wear a surgical mask and observe Respiratory Hygiene/Cough Etiquette.
Once in an AIIR, the mask may be removed.

Patient Transport
Limit transport and movement of patients to **medically necessary purposes**.

If transport or movement outside an AIIR is necessary, instruct patients to **wear a surgical mask**, if possible, and observe Respiratory Hygiene/Cough Etiquette.

Hand Hygiene
according to Standard Precautions

Personal Protective Equipment (PPE)
Wear a fit-tested NIOSH-approved **N95** or higher level respirator for respiratory protection when entering the room of a patient when the following diseases are suspected or confirmed: Listed on back.

APR7 · ©2007 Brevis Corporation · www.brevis.com

Figure 3-8 Airborne precautions signs. (Courtesy Brevis Corp., Salt Lake City, UT.)

and splashes can be created when specimens are centrifuged, when tube stoppers are removed, and when specimen aliquots are being prepared. Dangerous fumes can be created if chemicals are improperly stored, mixed, or handled. Patients with airborne diseases can transmit infection to workers unless N95 respirators are worn when caring for them. Protection against airborne biohazard exposure includes following safe handling practices, wearing appropriate PPE, and working behind safety shields or splash guards.

Ingestion

Biohazards can be ingested if healthcare workers neglect to sanitize hands before handling food, gum, candy, cigarettes, or drinks. Other activities that can lead to ingestion of biohazards include covering the mouth with hands instead of tissue when coughing or sneezing, biting nails, chewing on pens or pencils, and licking fingers when turning pages in books. Frequent hand sanitization, avoiding hand-to-mouth activities, and refraining from holding items in the mouth or chewing on them

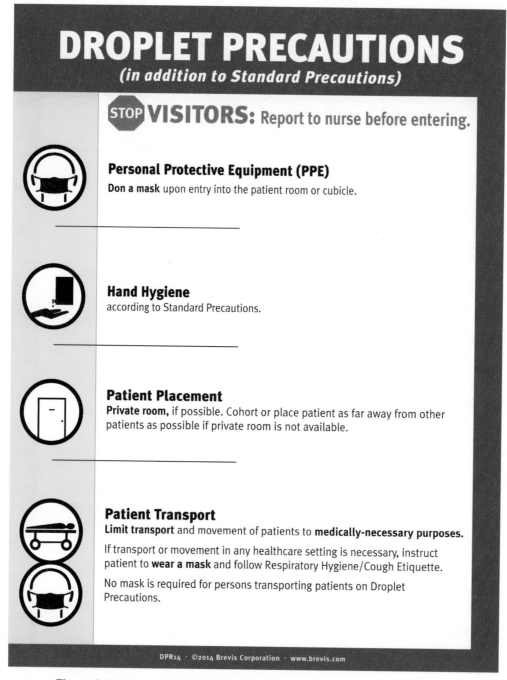

Figure 3-9 Droplet precautions signs. (Courtesy Brevis Corp., Salt Lake City, UT.)

provides the best defense against accidental ingestion of biohazardous substances.

Nonintact Skin

Biohazards can enter the body through visible and invisible pre-existing breaks in the skin such as abrasions, burns, cuts, scratches, sores, dermatitis, and chapped skin. Defects in the skin should be covered with waterproof (nonpermeable) bandages to prevent contamination, even when gloves are worn.

Percutaneous

Percutaneous (through the skin) exposure to biohazardous microorganisms in blood or body fluid occurs through intact (unbroken) skin as a result of accidental needlesticks and injuries from other sharps including broken glass and specimen tubes. Ways to reduce the chance of percutaneous exposure include using needle safety devices properly, wearing heavy-duty utility gloves when cleaning up broken glass, and never handling broken glass with the hands.

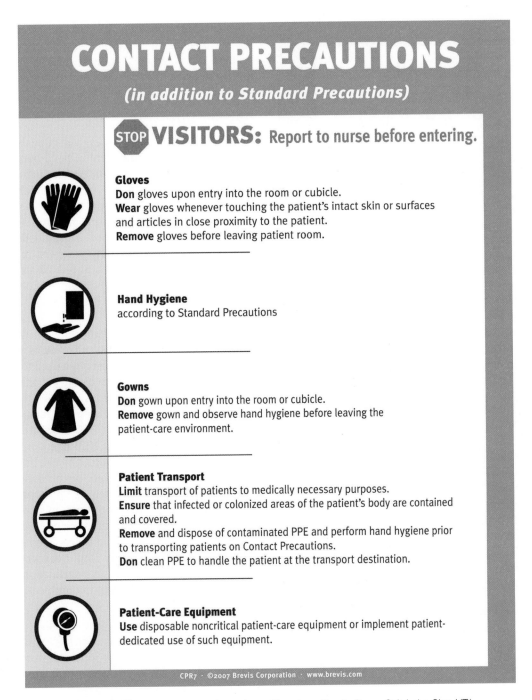

CONTACT PRECAUTIONS
(in addition to Standard Precautions)

STOP VISITORS: Report to nurse before entering.

Gloves
Don gloves upon entry into the room or cubicle.
Wear gloves whenever touching the patient's intact skin or surfaces and articles in close proximity to the patient.
Remove gloves before leaving patient room.

Hand Hygiene
according to Standard Precautions

Gowns
Don gown upon entry into the room or cubicle.
Remove gown and observe hand hygiene before leaving the patient-care environment.

Patient Transport
Limit transport of patients to medically necessary purposes.
Ensure that infected or colonized areas of the patient's body are contained and covered.
Remove and dispose of contaminated PPE and perform hand hygiene prior to transporting patients on Contact Precautions.
Don clean PPE to handle the patient at the transport destination.

Patient-Care Equipment
Use disposable noncritical patient-care equipment or implement patient-dedicated use of such equipment.

CPR7 · ©2007 Brevis Corporation · www.brevis.com

Figure 3-10 Contact precautions signs. (Courtesy Brevis Corp., Salt Lake City, UT.)

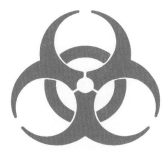

Figure 3-11 The biohazard symbol.

See how well you know your airborne and blood-borne pathogens with WORKBOOK Knowledge Drill 3-6.

Permucosal

Permucosal (through mucous membranes) exposure occurs when infectious microorganisms and other biohazards enter the body through the mucous membranes

Box 3-5

Safety Rules When in Patient Rooms and Other Patient Areas

- Avoid running. It is alarming to patients and visitors and may cause an accident.
- Be careful entering and exiting patient rooms; housekeeping equipment, dietary carts, x-ray machines, and other types of equipment may be just inside the door or outside in the hall.
- Do not touch electrical equipment in patient rooms while drawing blood. Electrical shock can pass through a phlebotomist and the needle and shock the patient.
- Follow standard precautions when handling specimens.
- Properly dispose of used and contaminated specimen collection supplies and return all other equipment to the collection tray before leaving the patient's room.
- Replace bedrails that were let down during patient procedures.
- Report infiltrated IVs or other IV problems to nursing personnel.
- Report unresponsive patients to nursing personnel.
- Report unusual odors to nursing personnel.
- Watch out for and report food, liquid, and other items spilled on the floor to appropriate personnel.

of the mouth and nose and the conjunctiva of the eyes in droplets generated by sneezing or coughing, splashes, and aerosols and by rubbing or touching the eyes, nose, or mouth with contaminated hands. The chance of permucosal exposure can be reduced by following procedures to prevent exposure to splashes and aerosols and avoiding rubbing or touching the eyes, nose, or mouth.

BLOOD-BORNE PATHOGENS

The term **blood-borne pathogen (BBP)** is applied to any infectious microorganism present in blood and other body fluids and tissues. Such pathogens, which can be present in a patient's body fluids even if there are no symptoms of disease, are among the most significant biohazards faced by healthcare workers. Although HBV, **hepatitis C virus (HCV)**, and HIV tend to receive the most attention,

BBPs include other hepatitis viruses; cytomegalovirus (CMV); *Treponema pallidum*, the microbe that causes syphilis, the microbes that cause malaria and relapsing fever; the agent that causes Creutzfeldt–Jakob disease; and more recently, West Nile virus.

HBV and HDV

Hepatitis B (once called serum hepatitis) is caused by HBV, a potentially life-threatening blood-borne pathogen that targets the liver. (*Hepatitis* means "inflammation of the liver.") It has been the most frequently occurring laboratory-associated infection and the major occupational hazard in the healthcare industry, although the rate of infection has dropped substantially since the advent of HBV immunization programs in the 1980s. Anyone infected with HBV is at risk of also acquiring hepatitis D (delta) virus (HDV), which is able to multiply only in the presence of HBV.

HBV Vaccination

The best defense against HBV infection is vaccination. The vaccination schedule most often used for adults is a series of three equal intramuscular injections of vaccine: an initial dose, a second dose 1 month after the first, and a third dose 6 months following the initial dose. The vaccine also protects against HDV since it can only be contracted concurrently with HBV infection. Success of immunization and proof of immunity can be determined 1 to 2 months after the last vaccination dose by a blood test that detects the presence of the hepatitis B surface antibody (anti-HBs) in the person's serum. OSHA requires employers to offer the vaccine free to employees within 10 working days of being assigned to duties with potential BBP exposure. Employees who refuse the vaccination must sign and date a declination (statement of refusal) form, which is kept in their personnel file.

> (i) The most commonly used hepatitis B vaccine does not contain live virus and poses no risk of transmitting HBV, which was a problem of earlier vaccines.

HBV Exposure Hazards

HBV can be present in blood and other body fluids such as urine, semen, cerebrospinal fluid (CSF), and saliva. It can survive up to a week in dried blood on work surfaces, equipment, telephones, and other objects. In a healthcare setting, it is primarily transmitted through needlesticks (a single needlestick can transmit HBV) and other sharps injuries and contact with contaminated equipment, objects, surfaces, aerosols, spills, and splashes. In nonmedical settings, it is transmitted primarily through sexual contact and sharing of dirty needles.

Symptoms of HBV Infection

HBV symptoms resemble flu symptoms but generally last longer. They include fatigue; loss of appetite; mild fever; muscle, joint, and abdominal pain; nausea; and vomiting. Jaundice appears in about 25% of cases. About 50% of those infected show no symptoms. Some individuals become carriers who can pass the disease on to others. Carriers have an increased risk of developing cirrhosis of the liver and liver cancer. Active HBV infection is confirmed by detection of hepatitis B surface antigen (HBsAg) in an individual's serum.

Hepatitis C Virus

Hepatitis C, caused by infection with HCV, has become the most widespread chronic blood-borne illness in the United States. The virus, discovered in 1988 by molecular cloning, was found to be the primary cause of non-A, non-B hepatitis. No vaccine is currently available, although research and development of a vaccine is underway.

HCV Exposure Hazards

HCV is found primarily in blood and serum, less frequently in saliva, and seldom in urine and semen. It can enter the body in the same manner as HBV. However, infection primarily occurs after large or multiple exposures. As in the case of HBV, sexual contact and needle sharing are the primary means of transmission in non-medical settings.

Symptoms of HCV Infection

HCV symptoms are similar to those of HBV infection, although only 25% to 30% of infections even cause symptoms. As with HBV, chronic and carrier states exist that can lead to cirrhosis of the liver and liver cancer. In fact, HCV infection is a leading indication for liver transplantation. HCV antibodies usually appear in a patient's serum from 4 to 10 weeks after infection occurs.

Human Immunodeficiency Virus

HIV attacks the body's immune system, causing acquired immunodeficiency syndrome (AIDS) by leaving the body susceptible to opportunistic infections. Opportunistic infections are caused by organisms that would not ordinarily be pathogens to a normal healthy individual. HIV infection has a poor prognosis and is of great concern to healthcare workers.

HIV Exposure Hazards

HIV has been isolated from blood, semen, saliva, tears, urine, CSF, amniotic fluid, breast milk, cervical secretions, and tissue of infected persons. The risk to healthcare workers, however, is primarily through exposure to blood. HIV can enter the body through all the same routes as the hepatitis viruses.

Symptoms of HIV Infection

The incubation phase of HIV infection is thought to range from a few weeks up to a year or more. Initial symptoms are mild to severe flu-like symptoms. During this phase, the virus enters the T lymphocytes (T lymphs or helper T cells), triggering them to produce multiple copies of the virus. The virus then enters a seemingly inactive incubation phase while hiding in the T lymphs. Certain conditions reactivate the virus, which slowly destroys the T lymphs. Once the T lymph count is reduced to 200 or fewer per milliliter of blood, the patient is officially diagnosed as having AIDS, the third and final phase of infection. In this phase, the immune system deteriorates significantly and opportunistic infections take hold. Two symptoms of AIDS are hairy leukoplakia, a white lesion on the tongue, and Kaposi sarcoma, a cancer of the capillaries that produces bluish-red nodules on the skin. End stages of AIDS are characterized by deterioration of the nervous system leading to neurological symptoms and dementia.

OSHA BLOOD-BORNE PATHOGENS STANDARD

The OSHA **Blood-Borne Pathogens (BBP) Standard** was promulgated (put into force) when it was concluded that healthcare employees face a serious health risk from occupational exposure to blood and other body fluids and tissues. Enforcement of the standard, which is mandated by federal law, and for which OSHA is also responsible, is intended to reduce the chance of occupational exposure to BBPs. The standard requires implementation of **engineering controls** and **work practice controls** to prevent exposure incidents, availability and use of PPE, special training, medical surveillance, and the availability of vaccination against HBV for all at-risk employees. Although exposure to BBPs is still a serious issue, the incidence of occupationally acquired Hepatitis B infection has declined since the BBP Standard was put in to force.

Key Point Although the incidence of work-related HIV infection is relatively low, CDC studies have shown that phlebotomy procedures were involved in approximately 50% of the HIV exposures that have occurred so far in healthcare settings.

Key Point Engineering controls are devices that isolate or remove a BBP hazard. Work practice controls are practices that change the way tasks are performed to reduce the likelihood of BBP exposure.

NEEDLESTICK SAFETY AND PREVENTION ACT

The **Needlestick Safety and Prevention Act** imposed additional requirements on healthcare employers concerning sharps procedures in order to further reduce healthcare worker exposure to blood-borne pathogens. The act directed OSHA to revise the BBP standard in the following four key areas:

- Revision and updating of the exposure control plan
- Solicitation of employee input in selecting engineering and work practice controls
- Modification of definitions relating to engineering controls
- New record-keeping requirements, including the requirement to keep a sharps injury log.

> (i) According to safeneedle.org there are 384,000 needlestick injuries to U.S. hospital healthcare professionals every year.

EXPOSURE CONTROL PLAN

To comply with the OSHA standard, employers must have a written exposure control plan. The plan must be reviewed and updated at least annually to document the evaluation and implementation of safer medical devices. Nonmanagerial employees with risk of exposure must be involved in the identification, review, and selection of engineering and work practice controls and their participation must be documented. Key elements of an exposure control plan are shown in Box 3-6.

BBP EXPOSURE ROUTES

Occupational exposure to blood-borne pathogens can occur if any of the following happens while a healthcare worker is performing his or her duties.

- The skin is pierced by a contaminated needle or sharp object.
- Blood or other body fluid splashes into the eyes, nose, or mouth.
- Blood or other body fluid comes in contact with a cut, scratch, or abrasion.
- A human bite breaks the skin.

EXPOSURE INCIDENT PROCEDURE

An exposure incident requires immediate attention for the most promising outcome in the event that the exposure involves a BBP. The immediate response by the employee in the event of an exposure incident includes the following:

- Needlestick or other sharps injury: Carefully remove shards of glass or other objects that may be embedded in the wound and wash the site with soap and water for a minimum of 30 seconds.

> 🔑 **Key Point** There is currently no scientific evidence that squeezing the wound or cleaning with an antiseptic reduces the transmission of BBPs. Cleaning with bleach or other caustic agents is not recommended.

- Mucous membrane exposure: Flush the site (i.e., eyes, nose, or mouth) with water or sterile saline for a minimum of 10 minutes. Use an eyewash station (Fig. 3-12) if available to adequately flush a splash to the eyes. Remove contact lenses as soon as possible and disinfect them before reuse or discard.
- Report the incident to the immediate supervisor.
- Report directly to a licensed healthcare provider for a medical evaluation, treatment if required, and counseling (see Box 3-7 for key elements of a postexposure medical evaluation).

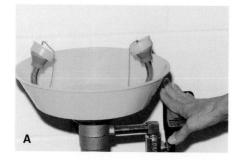 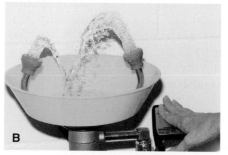

Figure 3-12 Eyewash basin. **A:** Press the lever at the right side of the basin. **B:** The stream of water forces the caps from the nozzles. Lower your face and eyes into the stream and continue to wash the area until the eyes are clear. (Reprinted with permission from Kronenberger J. *Lippincott Williams and Wilkins' Comprehensive Medical Assisting*. 4th ed. Baltimore, MD: Lippincott Williams & Wilkins; 2012.)

Box 3-6

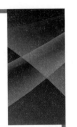

Key Elements of an Exposure Control Plan

1. An exposure determination: A list of all job categories and tasks with potential BBP exposure
2. Methods of implementation and compliance including:
   - A *universal precautions statement* requiring all employees to observe UP or the equivalent.
   - *Engineering controls,* such as sharps disposal containers, self-sheathing needles, sharps with engineered sharps injury protections, and needleless systems that isolate or remove the BBP hazard.
   - *Work practice controls* that reduce likelihood of exposure by altering the way tasks are performed. Examples include policies that require hand washing after glove removal and prohibit eating, drinking, smoking, or applying cosmetics in laboratory work areas.
   - *PPE or barrier protection devices* such as gloves, gowns, lab coats, aprons, face shields, masks, and resuscitation mouthpieces that minimize the risk of BBP infection. Disposable PPE and laundry service for reusable PPE must be provided to the employee at no cost.
   - *Housekeeping schedule and methods* that require decontamination of work surfaces at least once a day and after any contact with blood or other potentially infectious material with 1:10 bleach solution or other EPA-approved disinfectant.
3. Hepatitis B vaccine and postexposure follow-up procedures.
4. Communication of hazards to employees in the form of:
   - *Warning labels and signs* attached to containers of potentially infectious material, including refrigerators and freezers where infectious material may be stored. Labels must be predominantly fluorescent orange or orange-red, containing a biohazard symbol and the word "biohazard." Red bags or containers may be substituted for labels.
   - *BBP training and information* provided to employees at no cost and during working hours when first assigned to tasks with risk of exposure. A copy of the BBP standard and an explanation of its contents readily available to employees. Provision for annual training within 1 year of initial training.
5. Record-keeping requirements include:
   - *Medical records:* A requirement for the employer to maintain confidential medical records on each employee with occupational exposure. Records must include the employee's name, social security number, and HBV vaccination status.
   - *Training records:* A requirement for the employer to maintain records of training sessions that include the content, the qualifications of persons conducting them, and the names and titles of persons attending.
   - *Sharps injury log:* A requirement for the employer to keep a log of injuries from contaminated sharps. The log entry should include where and how the incident occurred, and the type and brand of device involved. Information recorded must protect employee confidentiality.

Box 3-7

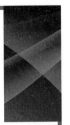

Key Elements of a Postexposure Medical Evaluation

The employee's blood is tested for HIV in an accredited laboratory.
- The source patient's blood is tested for HIV and HBV, with the patient's permission.
- If the source patient refuses testing, is HBV-positive, or is in a high-risk category, the employee may be given immune globulin or an HBV vaccination.
- If the source patient is HIV-positive, the employee is counseled and tested for HIV infection immediately and at periodic intervals, normally 6 weeks, 12 weeks, 6 months, and 1 year after exposure.

The employee may be given azidothymidine (AZT) or other HIV therapy.
- The exposed employee is counseled to be alert for acute retroviral syndrome (acute viral symptoms) within 12 weeks of exposure.

Procedure 3-2: Cleanup Procedures for Blood and Other Body Fluid Spills

Type of Spill	Cleanup Procedure
Small spill (a few drops)	Carefully absorb spill with a paper towel or similar material Discard material in biohazard waste container Clean area with appropriate disinfectant
Large spill	Use a special clay or chlorine-based powder to absorb or gel (thicken) the liquid Scoop or sweep up absorbed or thickened material Discard material in a biohazard waste container Wipe spill area with appropriate disinfectant
Dried spills	Moisten spill with disinfectant (avoid scraping, which could disperse infectious organisms into the air) Absorb spill with paper towels or similar material Discard material in biohazard waste container Clean area with appropriate disinfectant
Spills involving broken glass	Wear heavy-duty utility gloves (Never handle broken glass with your hands) Scoop or sweep up material Discard in biohazard sharps container Clean area with appropriate disinfectant

Key Point Free confidential medical evaluation following an exposure incident is required by OSHA regulations. If postexposure treatment is recommended, it should be started as soon as possible.

SURFACE DECONTAMINATION

OSHA requires surfaces in specimen collection and processing areas to be decontaminated by cleaning them with a 1:10 bleach solution or other disinfectant approved by the **Environmental Protection Agency (EPA)**, a government agency whose mission is to protect health and the environment by implementing and enforcing environmental laws. Bleach solutions should be prepared daily. Cleaning must take place at the end of each shift or whenever a surface is visibly contaminated. Gloves should be worn when cleaning.

CLEANUP OF BODY FLUID SPILLS

Special EPA-approved chemical solutions and kits are available for cleanup of blood and other body fluid spills and for disinfecting surfaces. Gloves must be worn during the cleaning process. Cleanup procedures, which vary slightly depending upon the type and size of spill (see Procedure 3-2), should concentrate on absorbing the material without spreading it over a wider area than the original spill. Disposable cleanup materials must be discarded in a biohazard waste container. Reusable cleanup materials should be properly disinfected after use.

BIOHAZARD WASTE DISPOSAL

Nonreusable items contaminated with blood or body fluids are biohazardous waste and must be disposed of in special containers or bags marked with a biohazard symbol. Filled biohazard waste containers require special handling prior to decontamination and disposal. OSHA, EPA, and state and local agencies regulate biohazard waste disposal.

Electrical Safety

Fire and electrical shock are potential hazards associated with the use of electrical equipment. Knowledge of the proper use, maintenance, and servicing of electrical equipment such as centrifuges can minimize hazards associated with their use. Box 3-8 contains guidelines for electrical safety.

Box 3-8

Electrical Safety

- *Avoid* the use of extension cords.
- *Do not* attempt to make repairs to equipment if you are not trained to do so.
- *Do not* handle electrical equipment with wet hands or when standing on a wet floor.
- *Do not* overload electrical circuits.
- *Do not* touch electrical equipment in patient rooms, especially when in the process of drawing blood. An electrical shock could pass through the phlebotomist and the needle and shock the patient.
- *Inspect* cords and plugs for breaks and fraying. Make certain all electrical cords have three-prong plugs and that the third prong (grounding prong) is functional.
- *Know* the location of the circuit breaker box.
- *Unplug* and do not use equipment that is malfunctioning.
- *Unplug* equipment that has had liquid spilled in it. Do not plug in again until the spill has been cleaned up and you are certain the wiring is dry.
- *Unplug* equipment when you are servicing it, including when you are replacing a light bulb.

Actions to Take If Electrical Shock Occurs

- Shut off the source of electricity.
- If the source of electricity cannot be shut off, use non-conducting material (e.g., hand inside a glass beaker) to remove the source of electricity from the victim.
- Call for medical assistance.
- Start cardiopulmonary resuscitation if indicated.
- Keep the victim warm.

Fire Safety

All employees of any institution should be aware of procedures to follow in case of fire. They should know where fire extinguishers are located and how to use them. They should know where the fire blankets (Fig. 3-13) are kept and how to use them or heavy toweling to smother clothing fires. They should know the location of emergency exits and be familiar with evacuation routes. Fire spreads rapidly and it is important for

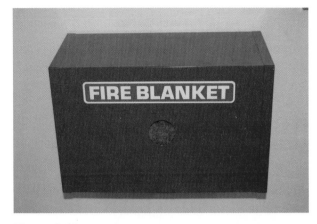

Figure 3-13 Fire blanket storage box.

employees to know the basics of what to do and also what not to do if a fire occurs so they can react quickly and appropriately. Box 3-9 lists dos and don'ts to follow if a fire occurs.

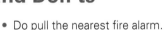 **Test your classes of fire knowledge and express your creativity with color. Do WORKBOOK Matching Exercise 3-3.**

FIRE COMPONENTS

Four components, present at the same time, are necessary for fire to occur. Three of the components, *fuel* (combustible material), *heat* to raise the temperature of the material until it ignites or catches fire, and *oxygen* to

Box 3-9

Fire Safety Dos and Don'ts

- Do pull the nearest fire alarm.
- Do call the fire department.
- Do attempt to extinguish a small fire.
- Do close all doors and windows if leaving the area.
- Do smother a clothing fire with a fire blanket or have the person roll on the floor in an attempt to smother the fire.
- Do crawl to the nearest exit if there is heavy smoke present.
- Don't panic.
- Don't run.
- Don't use elevators.

Fire Tetrahedron

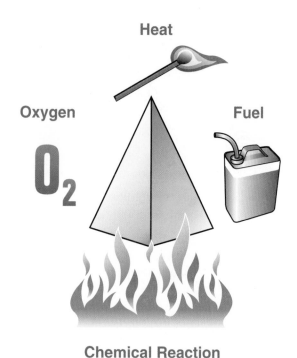

Figure 3-14 Fire tetrahedron.

maintain combustion or burning have traditionally been referred to as the fire triangle. The fourth component, the chemical reaction that produces fire, actually creates a **fire tetrahedron** (Fig. 3-14). Basic fire safety involves keeping the components apart to prevent fire or removing one or more of the components to extinguish (i.e., put out) a fire. Fire extinguishers work by removing one or more fire components. There are different types of fire extinguishers, depending on the class of fire involved.

CLASSES OF FIRE

Five classes of fire are now recognized by the **National Fire Protection Association (NFPA)**. Classification is based on the fuel source of the fire. The five classes are as follows:

- *Class A* fires occur with ordinary combustible materials, such as wood, papers, or clothing, and require water or water-based solutions to cool or quench the fire to extinguish it.
- *Class B* fires occur with flammable liquids and vapors, such as paint, oil, grease, or gasoline, and require blocking the source of oxygen or smothering the fuel to extinguish.
- *Class C* fires occur with electrical equipment and require nonconducting agents to extinguish.
- *Class D* fires occur with combustible or reactive metals, such as sodium, potassium, magnesium, and

lithium, and require dry powder agents or sand to extinguish (they are the most difficult fires to control and frequently lead to explosions).
- *Class K* fires occur with high-temperature cooking oils, grease, or fats and require agents that prevent splashing and cool the fire as well as smother it.

Memory Jogger The following are ways to remember each fire classification.
- Class A fires occur with ordinary combustible materials; emphasize the "a" when saying the word "ordinary."
- Class B fires occur with flammable liquids; emphasize the "b" when saying the word "flammable."
- Class C fires are electrical fires; emphasize the "c" when saying the word "electrical."
- Class D fires occur with combustible or reactive metals; keep in mind that when you say the word "metal" quickly, it sounds like "medal," which has a "d" in it, and medals are commonly made of metal.
- Class K fires occur with cooking oils or fats in kitchens, which begins with a "k."

FIRE EXTINGUISHERS

There is a fire extinguisher class (Fig. 3-15) that corresponds to each class of fire except class D. Class D fires present unique problems and are best left to firefighting personnel to extinguish. Using the wrong type of fire extinguisher on a fire can be dangerous. Consequently, some fire extinguishers are multipurpose to eliminate the confusion of having several different types of extinguishers. Multipurpose extinguishers are the type most frequently used in healthcare institutions. Common fire extinguisher classes and how they typically work are as follows:

- *Class A extinguishers* use soda and acid or water to cool the fire.
- *Class B extinguishers* use foam, dry chemical, or carbon dioxide to smother the fire.
- *Class C extinguishers* use dry chemical, carbon dioxide, halon, or other nonconducting agents to smother the fire.
- *Class ABC (multipurpose) extinguishers* use dry chemical reagents to smother the fire. They can be used on class A, B, and C fires.
- *Class K extinguishers* use a potassium-based alkaline liquid specifically formulated to fight high-temperature grease, oil, or fat fires by cooling and smothering them without splashing. Some class K extinguishers can also be used on class A, B, and C fires.

CLASS & SYMBOL	INTENDED USE	ICON	TYPE OF EXTINGUISHER	OPERATION
A Ordinary Combustibles	Fires involving ordinary combustible materials such as cloth, wood, rubber, paper, and many plastics.	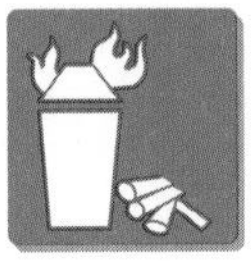	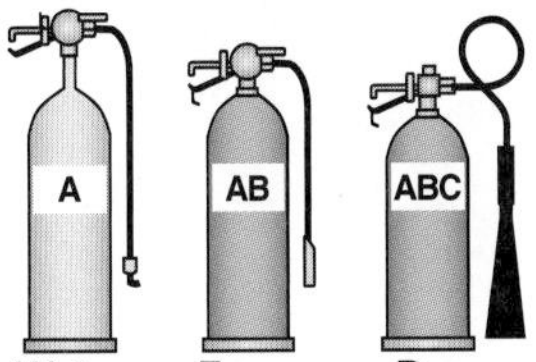 Water Foam Dry chemical	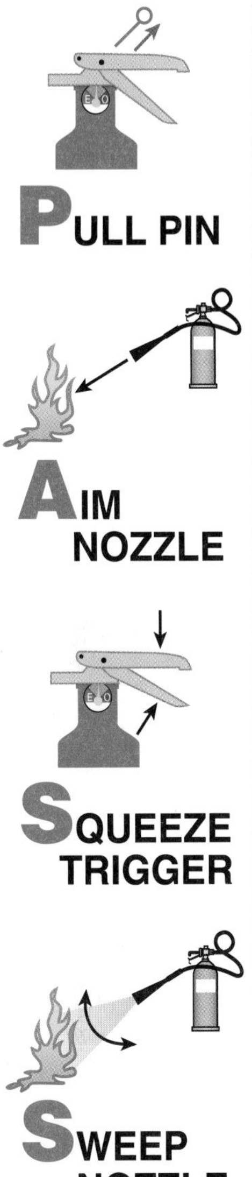 **P**ULL PIN
B Flammable Liquids	Fires involving flammable liquids and vapors, such as grease, gasoline, oil, and oil-based paints.	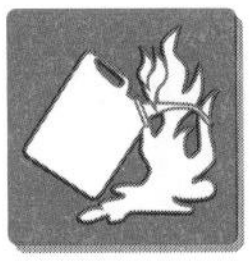	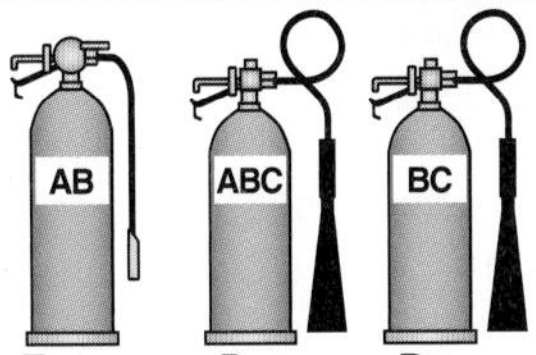 Foam Dry chemical Dry chemical	**A**IM NOZZLE
C Electrical Equipment	Fires involving electrical equipment such as appliances, tools, or other equipment that is plugged into an electricity source.	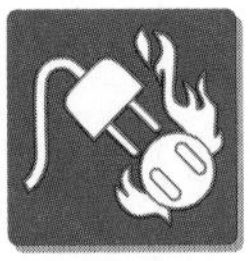	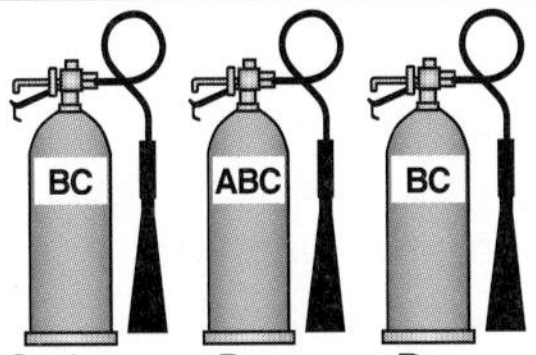 Carbon dioxide Dry chemical Dry chemical	**S**QUEEZE TRIGGER
D Combustible Metals	Fires involving combustible, reactive, or flammable metals.	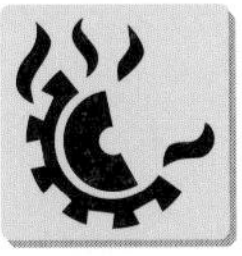	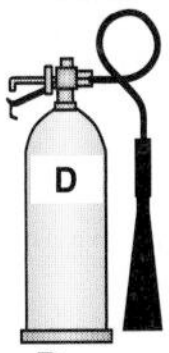 Dry powder	
K Cooking Oils	Fires involving high temperature cooking oils, grease or fat such as vegetable oils, animal oils, or fats typically found in commercial kitchens.	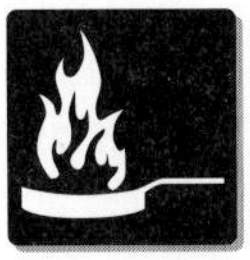	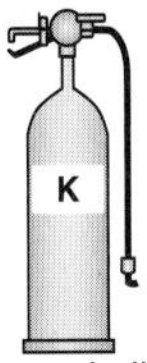 Potassium-based alkaline liquid	**S**WEEP NOZZLE

Figure 3-15 Classes of fire extinguishers. (Symbols reprinted with permission from NFPA 10, Portable Fire Extinguishers, Copyright © 2007, National Fire Protection Association. This reprinted material is not the complete and official position of the NFPA on the referenced subject, which is represented only by the standard in its entirety.)

Memory Jogger The NFPA code word for the order of action in the event of fire is RACE, where the letters stand for the following:

R = *Rescue* individuals in danger.

A = *Alarm:* activate the fire alarm.

C = *Confine* the fire by closing all doors and windows.

E = *Extinguish* the fire with the nearest suitable fire extinguisher.

Radiation Safety

The principles involved in radiation exposure are *distance, shielding,* and *time.* This means that the amount of radiation you are exposed to depends upon how far you are from the source of radioactivity, what protection you have from it, and how long you are exposed to it. Exposure time is important because radiation effects are cumulative.

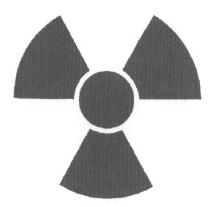

Figure 3-16 The radiation hazard symbol.

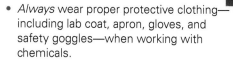

Box 3-10

General Rules for Chemical Safety

- *Always* wear proper protective clothing—including lab coat, apron, gloves, and safety goggles—when working with chemicals.
- *Always* use proper chemical cleanup materials when cleaning up chemical spills.
- *Never* store chemicals above eye level.
- *Never* add water to acid.
- *Never* indiscriminately mix chemicals together.
- *Never* store chemicals in unlabeled containers.
- *Never* pour chemicals into dirty containers, especially containers previously used to store other chemicals.
- *Never* use chemicals in ways other than their intended use.

Key Point Those working in areas where there may be high levels of radioactivity are required to wear a dosimeter badge, which records accumulated radiation exposure. Badge readings must be checked by the appropriate authority at regular intervals.

A clearly posted **radiation hazard symbol** (Fig. 3-16) is required in areas where radioactive materials are used and on cabinet or refrigerator doors where radioactive materials are stored. In addition, radioactive reagents and specimens must be labeled with a radiation hazard symbol. A radiation hazard symbol on a patient's door signifies that a patient has been treated with radioactive isotopes.

A phlebotomist may encounter radiation hazards when collecting specimens from patients who have been injected with radioactive dyes, when collecting specimens from patients in the radiology or nuclear medicine departments, and when delivering specimens to radioimmunoassay sections of the laboratory. The phlebotomist should be aware of institutional radiation safety procedures, recognize the radiation hazard symbol, and be cautious when entering areas where the symbol is displayed.

CAUTION Because radiation is particularly hazardous to a fetus, pregnant employees should avoid areas displaying the radiation symbol, patients who have recently been injected with radioactive dyes, and specimens collected from patients while radioactive dye is still in their systems.

Chemical Safety

A phlebotomist may come in contact with hazardous chemicals when using cleaning reagents, adding preservatives to 24-hour urine containers, or delivering specimens

to the laboratory. Inappropriate use of chemicals can have dangerous consequences. For example, mixing bleach with other cleaning compounds can release dangerous gases. In addition, many chemicals are potent acids, such as the hydrochloric acid (HCl) used as a urine preservative, or alkalis, both of which can cause severe burns. Container labels provide important information regarding the contents and should always be read carefully before use. See Box 3-10 for general chemical safety rules.

CAUTION An important chemical safety rule to remember when dealing with acids and other liquids is *never* add water or other liquids to an acid, as it can cause an explosive type reaction. If a mixture containing both is to be made, always add the acid to the other liquid.

Memory Jogger Think of the letters "AAA" to remember the safety rule "always add acid."

OSHA HAZARD COMMUNICATION STANDARD

OSHA developed the **Hazard Communication (HazCom) Standard (HCS)** to protect employees who may be exposed to hazardous chemicals. According to

Box 3-11

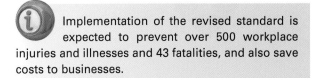

GHS Elements Incorporated into the Hazcom Standard Update

1. Harmonized signal word: one of two new signal words to specify the severity of the hazard; "Danger" if the hazard is severe, or "Warning" if the hazard is less severe.

2. GHS pictogram: a symbol with other graphic elements (e.g., a border, background pattern, or color) meant to communicate specific information about the hazard. An individual pictogram is a symbol on a white background within a red diamond-shaped frame

3. Hazard statement: a statement for each class and category that describes the nature of the hazard, and the hazard degree, if applicable.

4. Precautionary statement: a statement describing measures to take to minimize or prevent adverse effects of exposure or improper handling or storage.

5. Supplier identification: name, address, and phone number of manufacturer or supplier

the law, all chemicals must be evaluated for health hazards, and all chemicals found to be hazardous must be labeled as such and the information communicated to employees. The HCS was recently revised to align it with the Globally Harmonized System of Classification and Labeling of Chemicals (GHS) that is being promoted for use worldwide. The intent of the revised HCS standard is to increase employee safety by providing consistent, easily understandable information concerning the safe handling and use of hazardous chemicals. Important GHS elements that will have been incorporated into the Hazcom Standard label requirements by June 1, 2016 are shown in Box 3-11.

Key Point The HCS is known as "the right to know" law because the labeling requirement gives employees the right to know about chemical hazards they encounter in the workplace. The GHS changes to the HCS now give employees the ability to better understand the chemical hazards they may face.

Major HCS changes include the following:

- Specific criteria for classification of health and physical hazards.
- New labeling requirements
- New **safety data sheet (SDS)** requirements
- Required employee training in the new label elements and SDS format

Implementation of the revised standard is expected to prevent over 500 workplace injuries and illnesses and 43 fatalities, and also save costs to businesses.

HazCom Labeling Requirements

All chemical manufacturers must comply with GHS labeling requirements. In addition to the identity of a chemical, the label of a hazardous chemical must include a precautionary statement and a GHS hazard statement, signal word, and **pictogram** for each hazard class and category. A signal word specifies the severity of the hazard faced. There are two GHS signal words: "Danger" if the hazard is severe, or "Warning" if the hazard is less severe. A pictogram is an easily recognized and universally accepted symbol that alerts users to the type of chemical hazard they may face. The pictograms are diamond-shaped, framed with a red border, and have a white background on which the symbol is displayed. The revised HCS designates eight specific GHS hazard category pictograms for use on labels (Fig. 3-17).

There is a ninth pictogram for environmental hazards. It is not required by OSHA because environmental hazards are not within OSHA's jurisdiction.

Safety Data Sheets

In addition to the labeling requirement, the revised HCS requires chemical manufacturers, distributors, or importers to supply customers with a GHS standardized 16 section **safety data sheet (SDS)** (formerly called an MSDS or material safety data sheet) for every hazardous chemical. Like the MSDS the new SDS communicates general and precautionary information about the hazard to users. However, the information will now be consistent for every chemical manufacturer or distributor in that the headings of information sections and the order the sections are presented will always be the same. The required SDS sections are shown in Box 3-12.

HCS Pictograms and Hazards

Health Hazard

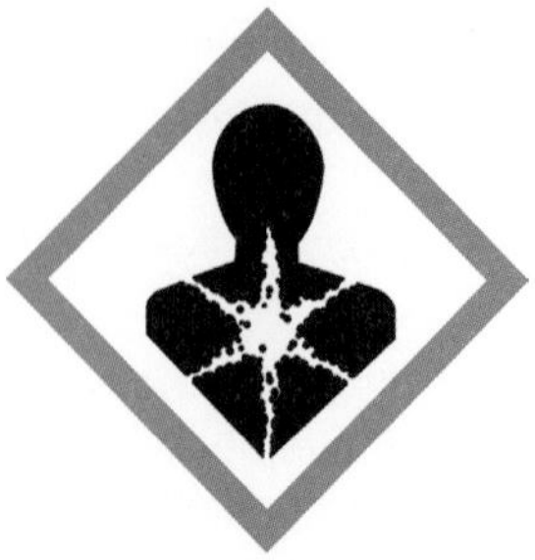

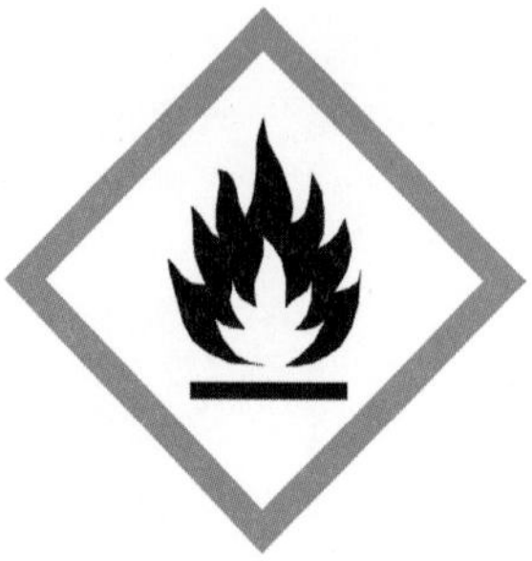

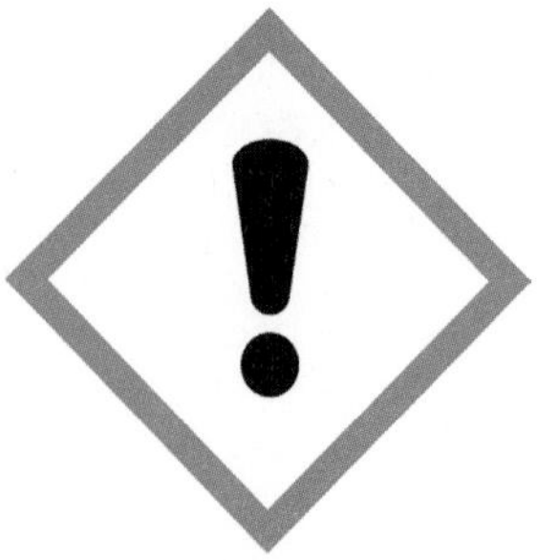

- Carcinogen
- Mutagenicity
- Reproductive Toxicity
- Respiratory Sensitizer
- Target Organ Toxicity
- Aspiration Toxicity

Flame

- Flammables
- Pyrophorics
- Self-Heating
- Emits Flammable Gas
- Self-Reactives
- Organic Peroxides

Exclamation Mark

- Irritant (skin and eye)
- Skin Sensitizer
- Acute Toxicity
- Narcotic Effects
- Respiratory Tract Irritant
- Hazardous to Ozone Layer (Nonmandatory)

Gas Cylinder

- Gases Under Pressure

Corrosion

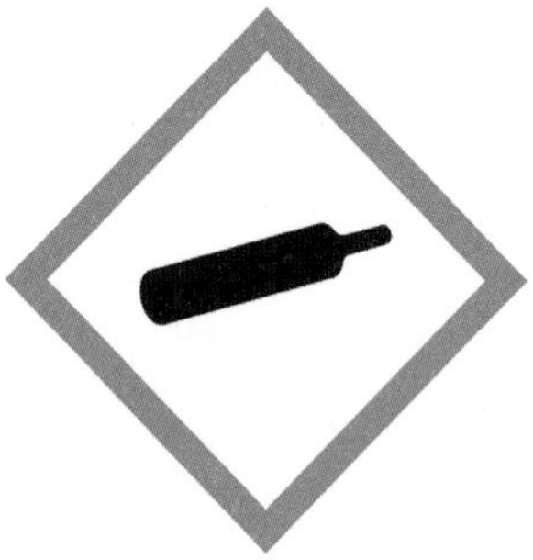

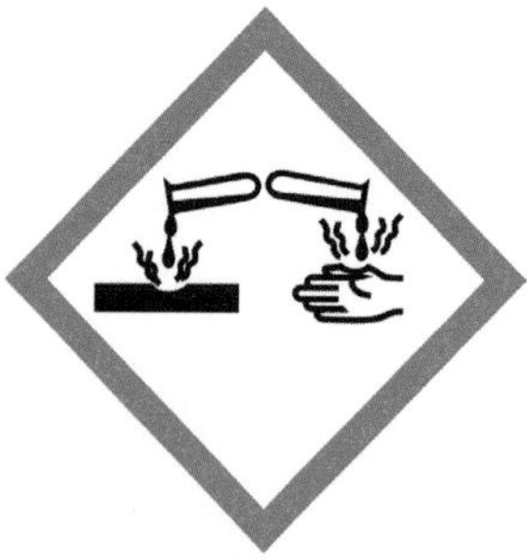

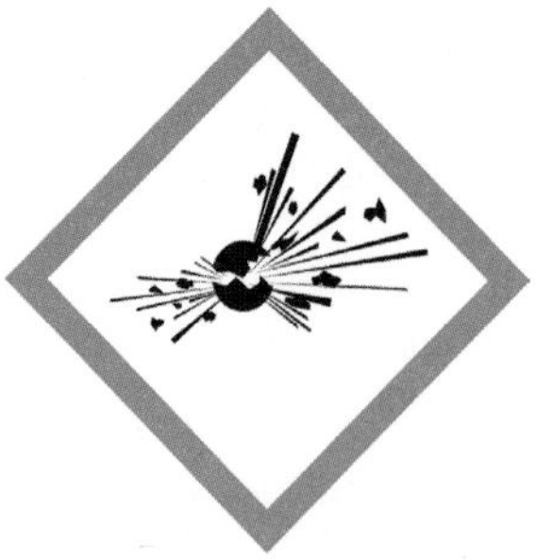

- Skin Corrosion/Burns
- Eye Damage
- Corrosive to Metals

Exploding Bomb

- Explosives
- Self-Reactives
- Organic Peroxides

Flame Over Circle

- Oxidizers

Environment
(Nonmandatory)

- Aquatic Toxicity

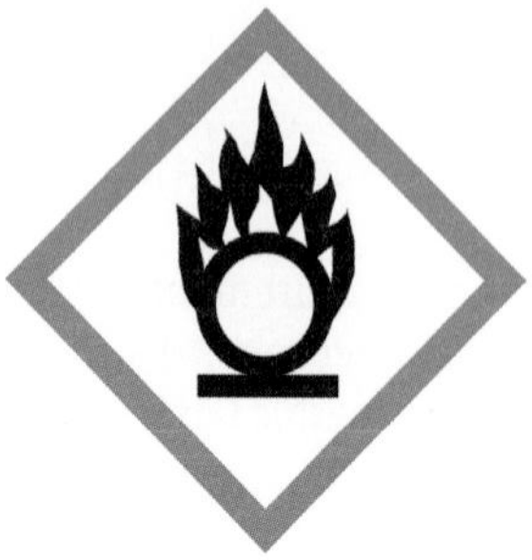

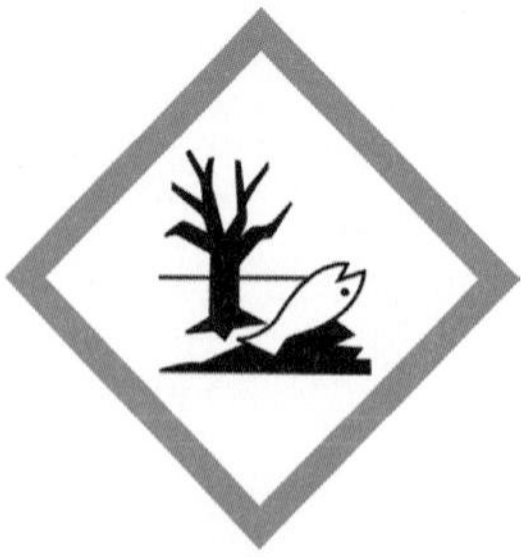

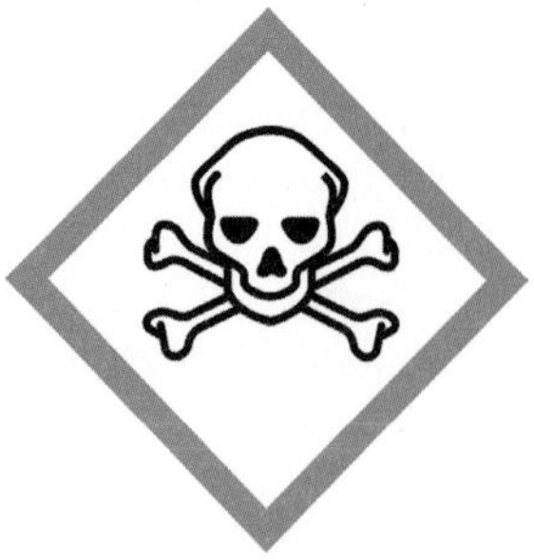

Skull and Crossbones

- Acute Toxicity (fatal or toxic)

Figure 3-17 HCS hazard category pictograms.

Box 3-12

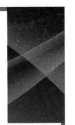

SDS Sections

Sections required by OSHA:

- *Section 1. Identification*—will include the product identifier, how the chemical is to be used and any restrictions, the supplier's contact information plus an emergency phone number.

- *Section 2. Hazard Identification*—will include the GHS classification of the substance and the pictogram or the name of the symbol.

- *Section 3. Composition and Information on Ingredients*—will include the chemical identity, its common name and synonyms, and the chemical abstract service (CAS) number.

- *Section 4. First Aid Measures*—will describe routes of exposure such as inhalation, skin and eye contact, and ingestion. It also will indicate any immediate medical attention and special treatment that is needed.

- *Section 5. Fire-fighting Measures*—will include extinguishing media and special protective equipment and precautions for fire fighters.

- *Section 6. Accidental Release Measures*—will include emergency procedures and any environmental precautions, including methods and materials for containment and cleaning up.

- *Section 7. Handling and Storage*—will include the safe handling and storage of the chemical including any incompatibilities.

- *Section 8. Exposure Controls/Personal Protection*—will include occupational or biological exposure limit values, engineering controls, and personal protective equipment.

- *Section 9. Physical and Chemical Properties*—will include the chemical appearance, melting or freezing point, boiling range, flash point, evaporation rate, flammability, vapor pressure and density, solubility, and autoignition and decomposition temperatures.

- *Section 10. Stability and Reactivity*—will describe the chemical's stability. It will also indicate conditions to avoid such as static discharge, shock or vibration, incompatible materials, and hazardous decomposition products.

- *Section 11. Toxicological Information*—will include a description of the toxicological effects of the chemical including routes of exposure, symptoms related to the physical, chemical, and toxicological characteristics, as well as effects from short- and long-term exposure.

Sections that may be included, but are not required by OSHA:

- *Section 12. Ecological Information*—will include ecotoxicity, persistence, and degradability, bioaccumulative potential, mobility in soil, and any other adverse effects.

- *Section 13. Disposal Considerations*—will include a description of the waste residues, their safety handling, and the disposal of any contaminated packaging.

- *Section 14. Transport Information*—will include the United Nations (UN) number, the United States proper shipping name, hazard classes, packing group, if applicable, if it is a marine pollutant and any special precautions for transport or conveyance either within or outside the facility's premises.

- *Section 15. Regulatory Information*—will include safety, health, and environmental regulations for the chemical.

- *Section 16. Other Information*—may include any relevant information that is not covered by the other 15 sections and may include the date of preparation or last revision of the SDS.

Key Point Employers are required to obtain the SDS of every hazardous chemical present in the workplace and to make all SDSs readily accessible to employees either by electronic means or hard copy.

DEPARTMENT OF TRANSPORTATION LABELING SYSTEM

Hazardous materials may have additional labels of precaution, including a Department of Transportation (DOT) symbol incorporating a United Nations hazard classification number and symbol (Table 3-3). The DOT labeling

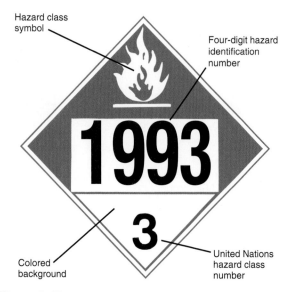

Figure 3-18 Example of a DOT hazardous material label.

system uses a diamond-shaped warning sign (Fig. 3-18) containing the United Nations hazard class number, the hazard class designation or four-digit identification number, and a symbol representing the hazard.

NATIONAL FIRE PROTECTION ASSOCIATION LABELING SYSTEM

Another hazardous material rating system (Fig. 3-19) was developed by the NFPA to label areas where hazardous chemicals and other materials are stored, thus alerting firefighters in the event of a fire. This system uses a diamond-shaped symbol divided into four quadrants. Health hazards are indicated in a blue diamond on the left, the level of fire hazard is indicated in the upper quadrant in a red diamond, stability or reactivity hazards are indicated in a yellow diamond on the right, and other specific hazards are indicated in a white quadrant on the bottom.

SAFETY SHOWERS AND EYEWASH STATIONS

The phlebotomist should know the location of and be instructed in the use of safety showers and eyewash stations (Fig. 3-20) in the event of a chemical spill or splash to the eyes or other body parts. The affected parts should be flushed with water for a minimum of 15 minutes, followed by a visit to the emergency room for evaluation.

CHEMICAL SPILL PROCEDURES

Chemical spills require cleanup using special kits (Fig. 3-21) containing absorbent and neutralizer materials. The type of materials used depends upon the type of chemical spilled. An indicator in the cleanup materials detects when the materials have been neutralized and are safe for disposal. The EPA regulates chemical disposal.

First Aid

The ability to recognize and react quickly and skillfully to emergency situations may mean the difference between life and death for a victim. First aid is something that can usually be carried out by a bystander with minimal or even no supplies or medical equipment.

> **Do you know the meaning of the elements that make up the word hemorrhage? Test yourself with WORKBOOK Skills Drill 3-2.**

External Hemorrhage

According to current American Red Cross guidelines, hemorrhage (abnormal or profuse bleeding) from an obvious wound can be effectively controlled by firmly applying direct pressure to the wound until bleeding stops or EMS rescuers arrive. Pressure should be applied using cloth or gauze, with additional material added if bleeding continues. It is acceptable to use an elastic bandage to hold the compress in place as long as pressure is applied to the bandage. Standard precautions should be followed.

> **⚠ CAUTION** The original compress should not be removed when adding additional ones because removal can disrupt the clotting process.

Previous guidelines added elevating the affected part above the level of the heart and, if efforts to control bleeding were ineffective, use of arterial pressure points. The effects of elevation have not been studied and pressure points have been found to have little effect. Consequently these procedures are no longer recommended. Using a tourniquet to control bleeding can be harmful and is also not recommended. A tourniquet should be used only as a last resort to save a life after all other means to control bleeding are unsuccessful, as may occur with an **avulsion** (a tearing away or amputation of a body part) or a severely mangled or crushed body part.

Shock

A state of shock results when there is insufficient return of blood flow to the heart, resulting in an inadequate supply of oxygen to all organs and tissues of the body. Numerous conditions including hemorrhage, heart attack, trauma, and drug reactions can lead to some degree of shock. Because shock can be a life-threatening situation, symptoms must be recognized and dealt with immediately.

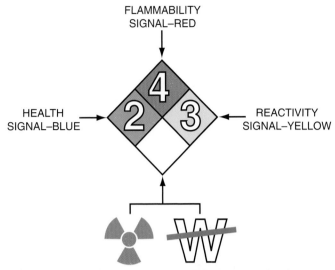

Identification of Health Hazard Color Code: **BLUE**		Identification of Flammability Color Code: **RED**		Identification of Reactivity (Stability) Color Code: **YELLOW**	
	Type of possible injury		Susceptibility of materials to burning		Susceptibility to release of energy
SIGNAL		SIGNAL		SIGNAL	
4	Materials that on very short exposure could cause death or major residual injury even though prompt medical treatment was given.	4	Materials that will rapidly or completely vaporize at atmospheric pressure and normal ambient temperature, or that are readily dispersed in air and that will burn readily.	4	Materials that in themselves are readily capable of detonation or of explosive decomposition or reaction at normal temperatures and pressures.
3	Materials that on short exposure could cause serious temporary or residual injury even though prompt medical treatment was given.	3	Liquids and solids that can be ignited under almost all ambient temperature conditions.	3	Materials that in themselves are capable of detonation or explosive reaction but require a strong initiating source or that must be heated under confinement before initiation or that react explosively with water.
2	Materials that on intense or continued exposure could cause temporary incapacitation or possible residual injury unless prompt medical treatment is given.	2	Materials that must be moderately heated or exposed to relatively high ambient temperatures before ignition can occur.	2	Materials that in themselves are normally unstable and readily undergo violent chemical change but do not detonate. Also, materials that may react violently with water or that may form potentially explosive mixtures with water.
1	Materials that on exposure would cause irritation but only minor residual injury even if no treatment is given.	1	Materials that must be preheated before ignition can occur.	1	Materials that in themselves are normally stable, but that can become unstable at elevated temperatures and pressures or that may react with water with some release of energy, but not violently.
0	Materials that on exposure under fire conditions would offer no hazard beyond that of ordinary combustible material.	0	Materials that will not burn.	0	Materials that in themselves are normally stable, even under fire exposure conditions, and that are not reactive with water.

Figure 3-19 National Fire Protection Association 704 marking system example and explanation.

COMMON SYMPTOMS OF SHOCK

It is important to be able to recognize the symptoms of shock in order to respond quickly and appropriately. Common symptoms of shock include:

- Pale, cold, clammy skin
- Rapid, weak pulse
- Increased, shallow breathing rate
- Expressionless face and staring eyes

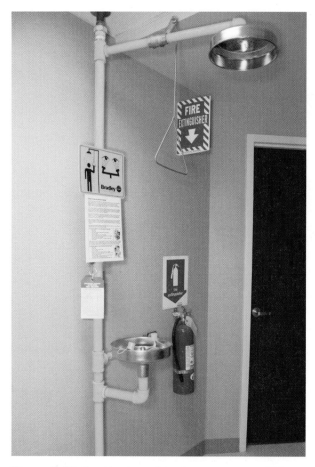

Figure 3-20 Combination safety shower and eyewash.

FIRST AID FOR SHOCK

When providing first aid to a victim of shock, be sure to do the following:

1. Maintain an open airway for the victim.
2. Call for assistance.
3. Keep the victim lying down with the head lower than the rest of the body.

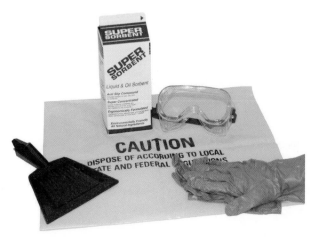

Figure 3-21 Spill cleanup kit.

4. Attempt to control bleeding or other cause of shock if known.
5. Keep the victim warm until help arrives.

> ⚠️ **CAUTION** *Never* give fluids if the patient is unconscious or semiconscious or has injuries likely to require surgery and anesthesia.

Cardiopulmonary Resuscitation and Emergency Cardiovascular Care

Most healthcare institutions require their personnel to be certified in cardiopulmonary resuscitation (CPR). Consequently, most phlebotomy programs require it as a prerequisite or corequisite or include it as part of the course. The American Heart Association (AHA) recommends the 6- to 8-hour Basic Life Support (BLS) Healthcare Provider Course for those in healthcare professions. The course includes instruction in how to perform CPR on victims of all ages, use of an automated external defibrillator (AED), and how to remove a foreign body airway obstruction. Certification is good for 2 years.

AMERICAN HEART ASSOCIATION CPR AND ECC GUIDELINES

The current AHA guidelines for CPR and Emergency Cardiovascular Care (ECC) aim to simplify lay rescuer training, and stress the need for early chest compressions for victims of sudden cardiac arrest. Untrained bystanders are now encouraged to provide Hands-Only™ (compressions only) CPR. Trained lay rescuers, if able, still provide compressions and ventilations; however, the latest guidelines call for them to start chest compressions before opening the airway or initiating rescue breathing. Consequently, the previous ABCs (airway, breathing, compressions) of CPR taught in BLS courses have been replaced with CAB (compressions, airway, breathing), except for CPR on newborns. The guidelines also place increased emphasis on high-quality CPR that includes:

A compression rate of at least 100 per minute (formerly it was *approximately* 100 per minute)

An adult compression depth of at least 5 cm (2 inches)

An infant and child compression depth is one-third of the anterior–posterior diameter of the chest; approximately 4 cm (1.5 inches) for infants and 5 cm (2 inches) for children

Allowing complete chest recoil between compressions

Minimizing interruptions in chest compressions (trying to limit them to less than 10 seconds)

Avoiding excessive ventilation (BLS single rescuer compression-to-ventilation ratio stays at 30:2)

AHA ECC ADULT CHAIN OF SURVIVAL

The AHA ECC adult chain of survival is a five-step course of action used to aid victims of sudden cardiac arrest that can optimize their chance of survival and recovery. The links in the chain are:

1. Immediate **recognition** of cardiac arrest and activation of the emergency response system
2. Early **CPR** with an emphasis on chest compressions
3. Rapid **defibrillation**
4. Effective **advanced life support**
5. Integrated **postcardiac arrest care**

Personal Wellness

"The doctor of the future will give no medicine but will interest his patients in the care of the human frame, in diet, and in the cause and prevention of disease."
—Thomas Edison

Today, personal wellness is more popular than ever. It seems as if wellness businesses are popping up on every street corner, and small to large companies are seeing the value in implementing wellness programs. Personal wellness is not just about what you eat, it requires a holistic approach, one that meets the physical, emotional, social, spiritual, and economic needs. Integrative Nutrition, the world's largest nutrition school, offers a Food Pyramid that incorporates this holistic approach to wellness (Fig. 3-22).

 Holistic comes from the Greek word *Holos,* which means *to heal.*

Our most serious health threats today are chronic illnesses such as heart disease or cancer—diseases that we have the power to prevent. The good news is that prevention has become a greater focus now than ever before. Insurance plans must now provide free preventive services to all members as part of Health Care Reform. By taking aim at prevention and creating a well balanced life through knowledge, self-awareness and self-care, personal wellness is something most everyone can achieve.

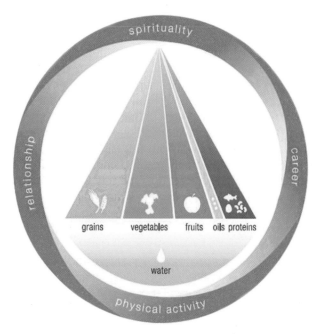

Figure 3-22 Holistic food pyramid. © 2007–2012 Integrative Nutrition, Inc. Reprinted with permission. No further copying and/or republication is permitted.

Proper Nutrition

"Let thy food be thy medicine, and thy medicine be thy food."
—Hippocrates, the father of medicine, 500 B.C.

Nutrition has been defined as the "act or process of nourishing." In other words, a food is nutritious if it supplies the nutrients the body needs "to promote growth and repair and maintain vital processes." The basic purpose of nutrition is to keep us alive, but more importantly, good nutrition provides what the body needs for energy and day-to-day functioning.

Physical health requires eating well. In this fast-paced world, few of us receive the nutrition we need. Much of the food found on the shelves of a typical American grocery store is so highly processed and chemically altered that it has very little nutritional value and does not promote healthy bodies. The American Institute for Cancer Research (AICR) has published a recommended diet to reduce the risk of cancer. They suggest that a person choose a predominantly plant-based diet rich in a variety of vegetables, fruits, legumes, and minimally processed starchy staple foods. A healthy diet contains the widest possible variety of natural foods. It provides a good balance of carbohydrates, fat, protein, vitamins, minerals, and fiber.

Key Point In general, it is best to eat whole foods in their natural state. Avoid processed foods with chemical additives or sweeteners as much as possible.

Rest and Exercise

Personal wellness requires a nutritious diet, exercise, and getting the right amount of rest. Healthcare workers often complain of fatigue (physical or mental exhaustion). Fatigue brought on by physical causes is typically relieved by sleep. Lack of rest and sleep can lead to medical problems. The typical frantic pace in healthcare facilities today makes it especially important to get the required hours of sleep and to take breaks during the day to rest, refresh, and stay fit. With smart phones occupying free moments and allowing us to take our work everywhere, there seem to be very few moments of peace, quiet, and relaxation even when not at work.

Studies show that being physically fit increases the chance of staying healthy and living longer. The most accurate measurements of fitness consist of evaluating three components—strength (the ability to carry, lift, push, or pull a heavy load), flexibility (the ability to bend, stretch, and twist), and endurance (the ability to maintain effort for an extended period of time). Some activities, such as the increasingly popular sport of cycling (Fig. 3-23), incorporate all of those components and is a great way to pedal away workplace stress. No single measurement of performance classifies a person as fit or unfit. If a person becomes breathless after climbing a flight of stairs or hurrying to catch a bus but is otherwise healthy, clearly he or she could benefit from some form of conditioning or exercise.

Exercise contributes to improved quality of life on a day-to-day basis. It strengthens the immune system, increases energy, and reduces stress by releasing substances called endorphins, which create a peaceful state. People who exercise tend to relax more completely, even when under stress. Regular physical activity also appears to reduce symptoms of depression and anxiety and to increase the ability to perform daily tasks. Walking requires no special equipment and is a form of exercise that can easily be incorporated into almost anyone's life.

> 🔑 **Key Point** According to the American Heart Association if activity during work is low to moderate, a 30-minute brisk walk or similar exercise daily can improve blood pressure, and reduce the risk of heart disease and type 2 diabetes.

Weight training is suggested as an excellent strength exercise. Studies have shown that using weights can build bone mass, even in the very elderly. Using your own body as a weight by doing push ups, pull ups, or wall sits is an easy way to weight train without equipment. For flexibility, yoga and Pilates are two forms of exercise that emphasize bending, stretching, and twisting. In choosing an exercise activity, it is most important is to pick one that is enjoyable so that you will be more apt to do it routinely.

Personal Hygiene

Personal wellness includes good personal hygiene. Personal hygiene communicates a strong impression about an individual. It is important to shower or bathe and use deodorant on a regular basis. Teeth should be brushed and mouthwash used more than once a day if possible. Hair should be clean and neatly combed. Fingernails should be clean, short, and neatly trimmed. A fresh, clean appearance without heavily scented lotions or colognes portrays health and instills confidence in employees and their patients and employers as well.

> 🔑 **Key Point** Phlebotomists should pay special attention to personal hygiene not only for optimal health, but also because their job involves close patient contact.

thePoint *View the Poor and Good Workplace Ergonomics for Phlebotomy and Proper Lifting Technique videos at http://thepoint.lww.com/McCall6e.*

Back Protection

To lead an active and healthy life, you need a healthy back. The spine is designed to withstand everyday movement, including the demands of exercise. Improper lifting and poor posture habits, however, can cause weaknesses. It is estimated that back injuries account for approximately 20% of all workplace injuries and

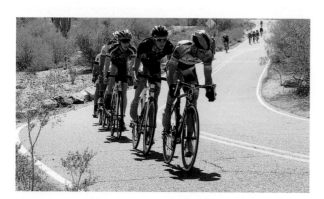

Figure 3-23 Cyclists compete in road race.

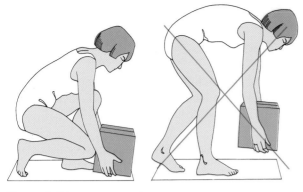

Figure 3-24 Lifting techniques.

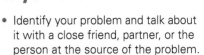

> ## Ways to Control Stress
>
> - Identify your problem and talk about it with a close friend, partner, or the person at the source of the problem.
> - Learn to relax throughout the day—close your eyes, relax your body, and clear your mind.
> - Exercise regularly—develop a consistent exercise routine that you can enjoy.
> - Avoid making too many changes at once—plan for the future to avoid simultaneous major changes.
> - Spend at least 15 minutes a day thoroughly planning the time you have.
> - Set realistic goals—be practical about what you can accomplish.
> - Avoid procrastination by tackling the most difficult job first.

illnesses. Lower back pain is a costly health problem that affects both industry and society in general. Strategies to prevent back injuries include instruction concerning back mechanics and lifting techniques (Fig. 3-24), lumbar support, and exercise. Exercise promotes strong backs; it improves back support and directly benefits the disks in the spinal column. Stress can make a person vulnerable to back problems because of muscle spasms. Keeping back muscles flexible with exercise can alleviate this stress reaction.

Key Point Healthcare workers are at risk for back injury because of activities they are required to do (e.g., lift and move patients) and because of the stressful environment often associated with healthcare today.

Stress Management

Stress is a condition or state that results when physical, chemical, or emotional factors cause mental or bodily tension. It challenges our ability to cope or adapt. Stress is sometimes useful, keeping us alert and increasing our energy when we need it. Persistent or excessive stress, on the other hand, can be harmful.

Evidence suggests that "negative stress" (such as an emergency or an argument) has a damaging effect on personal wellness. Stressful situations are more likely to be damaging if they cannot be predicted or controlled. This fact is particularly apparent where job stress is concerned. Highly demanding jobs are much more stressful

if an individual has no control over the workload, as is often the case in healthcare. Stress is more likely to have adverse effects on an individual if social support is lacking or there are personal or financial concerns. Although the signs of stress may not be immediately apparent, different organs and systems throughout the body are being affected. The immune system may be weakened, and other symptoms such as hypertension, ulcers, migraines, and nervous breakdowns may eventually result.

In today's hectic lifestyle and especially in healthcare environment, it is necessary to manage stress to maintain personal wellness. Box 3-13 lists ways to deal with stress.

Key Point The easiest way to reduce stress in the moment is to pause wherever you are and take three deep and mindful breaths. Deep breathing has a positive effect on the nervous system and relaxes the body.

Study and Review Questions

📖 *See the EXAM REVIEW for more study questions.*

1. **Which of the following situations involves an HAI?**
   a. A man has a bladder infection upon hospital admission.
   b. An employee contracts hepatitis B from a needlestick.
   c. A patient in ICU has an incision that becomes infected.
   d. A baby in the nursery has a congenital herpes infection.

2. **Reverse isolation may be used for**
   a. a patient with the measles.
   b. an adult patient with the flu.
   c. a patient with tuberculosis.
   d. a patient with severe burns.

3. **The single most important means of preventing the spread of infection is**
   a. proper hand antisepsis.
   b. keeping clothes clean.
   c. wearing a mask.
   d. wearing gloves.

4. **The most frequently occurring lab-acquired infection is**
   a. hepatitis B.
   b. HIV infection.
   c. syphilis.
   d. tuberculosis.

5. **To destroy transient microorganisms when washing hands, use**
   a. antiseptic soap.
   b. bleach solution.
   c. plain soap.
   d. all of the above.

6. **In the event of a body fluid splash to the eyes, the victim should immediately**
   a. call 911 so the paramedics will come.
   b. flush eyes with water for 10 minutes.
   c. go to the emergency room.
   d. wipe the eyes with a tissue.

7. **Which of the following items is PPE?**
   a. Biohazard bag
   b. Countertop shield
   c. Nonlatex gloves
   d. Sharps container

8. **Which of the following examples of potential exposure to blood-borne pathogens involves a parenteral route of transmission?**
   a. Chewing gum while collecting blood specimens
   b. Eating a snack while accessing specimens
   c. Licking fingers while turning lab manual pages
   d. Rubbing the eyes while processing specimens

9. **Surfaces in the specimen collection and processing area should be cleaned with**
   a. 70% isopropyl alcohol.
   b. 1:10 bleach solution.
   c. soap and water.
   d. any of the above.

10. **Which of the following is a proper way to clean up a small blood spill that has dried on a countertop?**
    a. Moisten it with a disinfectant and carefully absorb it with a paper towel.
    b. Rub it with an alcohol pad, then wipe the area with a clean alcohol pad.
    c. Scrape it into a biohazard bag and wash the surface with soap and water.
    d. Use a disinfectant wipe and scrub it in ever-increasing concentric circles.

11. **Distance, time, and shielding are principles of**
    a. BBP safety.
    b. electrical safety.
    c. fire safety.
    d. radiation safety.

12. **Safe working conditions are mandated by**
    a. CDC.
    b. HazCom.
    c. HICPAC.
    d. OSHA.

13. **A globally harmonized signal word signifies the**
    a. identity of the chemical.
    b. reactivity of the chemical.
    c. severity of a hazard faced.
    d. type of hazard involved.

14. According to the HAI prevalence survey the most common HAI pathogen is
   a. *Acinetobacter baumannii.*
   b. *Clostridium difficile.*
   c. *Mycobacterium tuberculosis.*
   d. *Staphylococcus aureus.*

15. When exiting an isolation room, this item of PPE must be removed outside the room.
   a. Gloves
   b. Gown
   c. Mask
   d. Respirator

Case Studies

 See the WORKBOOK for more case studies.

Case Study 3-1: An Accident Waiting to Happen

A female blood drawer works alone in a clinic. It is almost time to close for lunch when a patient arrives for a blood test. The blood drawer is flustered because she has a special date for lunch. She is dressed up for the occasion, wearing a nice dress and high heels. She looks nice except for a large scratch on her left wrist, which she got while playing with her cat that morning. She quickly draws the patient's blood. As she turns to put the specimen in a rack, she slips and falls, and one of the tubes breaks. She does not get cut, but blood splashes everywhere, including on her left wrist.

QUESTIONS

1. What is the first thing the phlebotomist should do?

2. How did the phlebotomist's actions contribute to this accident?

3. What should she have done that might have prevented the exposure, despite the tube breaking?

4. What type of exposure did she receive?

Case Study 3-2: Hitch-Hiking Microbes

You are one of only two phlebotomists working this holiday. You are very busy and hardly have time to sanitize your hands, much less remember to put your lab coat back on over your scrubs for every draw. Besides, you are too warm with it on. Everyone you have drawn in the ER today seems to have the flu or some sort of diarrhea or stomach issue. As soon as your shift is over, you head straight home. No time to change clothes before you have to fix dinner for the family, but you do take a few minutes to throw your feet up in the recliner and relax. Your 18-month old, Daren, crawls onto your lap to snuggle. Four days later Daren ends up at Urgent Care because diarrhea and vomiting have made him very dehydrated.

QUESTIONS

1. Daren's illness is similar to those of the ER patients. Why might this be?

2. If the contamination came from an ER patient, identify three ways his illness could have been avoided.

3. Would this be considered an HAI?

 Time to try your luck at the crossword in the WORKBOOK.

Bibliography and Suggested Readings

Carrico R, Costello P. Clean Spaces, Healthy Patients, Association for Professionals in Infection Control and Epidemiology (AIPC), March 26, 2012.

CDC. Rutala W, Weber D, HICPAC. Guideline for Disinfection and Sterilization in Healthcare Facilities. Department of Health and Human Services, Centers for Disease Control and Prevention. 2008.

CDC. Guidelines for Hand Hygiene in Health Care Settings, Vol. 51/ No. RR-16. MMWR. October 25, 2002; reviewed 2011.

CDC. Guidelines for Preventing Transmission of Mycobacterium tuberculosis in Health-Care Facilities. Department of Health and Human Services, Centers for Disease Control and Prevention. MMWR. December 30, 2005.

Clinical and Laboratory Standards Institute, M29-A3. *Protection of Laboratory Workers from Occupationally Acquired Infections; Approved Guideline.* 3rd ed. Wayne, PA: CLSI/NCCLS; 2005.

Clinical and Laboratory Standards Institute, GP17-A3. *Clinical Laboratory Safety; Approved Guideline.* 3rd ed. Wayne, PA: CLSI; 2012.

Healthcare Infection Control Practices Advisory Committee (HICPAC) and CDC. 2007 Guideline for Isolation Precautions in Hospitals. Centers for Disease Control and Prevention; 2007.

Jabbar U, Leischner J, Kasper D, Gerber R, Sambol SP, Parada JP, Johnson S, Gerding DN. Effectiveness of alcohol-based hand rubs for removal of Clostridium difficile spores from hands. *Infect Control Hosp Epidemiol.* 2010;31(6):565–570.

MRSA Contaminates Hospital Privacy Curtains, Physician's Weekly, September 23, 2011.

National fire protection association (NFPA). National Fire Codes. www.nfpa.org. Accessed April 10, 2014.

Occupational Safety and Health Administration (OSHA) Brief: Hazard Communication Standard Safety Data Sheets. 29 CFR 1910.1200(g), 2012.

Occupational Safety and Health Administration. Hazard Communication Standard: Occupational. 29CFR Part 1910.1200. Washington, DC: OSHA; 1986. Revised 2012.

Occupational Safety and Health Administration. Occupational exposure to bloodborne pathogens: final rule. 29CFR Part 1910.1030. Washington, DC: OSHA; 1991.

Occupational Safety and Health Administration. Occupational Exposure to Bloodborne Pathogens: Needlestick and Other Sharps Injuries: Final Rule. 29 CFR Part 1910, Docket No. H370 A, RIN 1218-AB85. Washington, DC: OSHA; 2001.

Siegel JD, Rhinehart E, Jackson M, Chiarello L, The Healthcare Infection Control Practices Advisory Committee (HICPAC). *Guideline for Isolation Precautions: Preventing Transmission of Infectious Agents in Healthcare Settings. Department of Health and Human Services, Centers for Disease Control and Prevention;* 2007.

United Nations Globally Harmonized System of Classification and Labeling of Chemicals (GHS), 5th revised edition, United Nations, New York and Geneva, 2013.

World Health Organization, WHO. Guidelines on Hand Hygiene in Health Care, 2009.

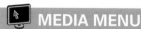

MEDIA MENU

Online Ancillaries (at http://thepoint.lww.com/McCall6e)

- Videos:
  - Donning and Removal of Protective Equipment
  - Hand Washing/Hand Antisepsis
  - Poor and Good Workplace Erognomics for Phlebotomy
  - Proper Lifting Technique
- Interactive exercises and games, including Look and Label, Word Building, Body Building, Roboterms, Crossword Puzzles, Quiz Show, and Concentration
- Audio flash cards and flashcard generator
- Audio glossary

Internet Resources

- College of American Pathologists: http://www.cap.org
- National Fire Protection Association: http://www.nfpa.org
- OSHA's Hazard Communication website: http://www.osha.gov/dsg/hazcom/index.html
- Occupational Safety and Health Administration: http://www.osha.gov/dcsp/osp/statestandards.html
- Occupational Safety and Health Administration: http://www.osha.gov/hospitals
- http://www.osha.gov/dcsp/osp/statestandards.html.
- U.S. Department of Health and Human Services, Centers for Disease Control and Prevention: http://www.cdc.gov
- U.S. Department of Health and Human Services, Centers for Disease Control and Prevention, 2007 Guideline for Isolation Precautions: Preventing Transmission of Infectious Agents in Healthcare Settings: http://www.cdc.gov/ncidod/dhqp/pdf/guidelines/Isolation2007.pdf

Other Resources

- McCall R, Tankersley C. *Student Workbook for Phlebotomy Essentials, 6th ed.* (Available for separate purchase).
- McCall R, Tankersley C. *Phlebotomy Exam Review, 6th ed.* (Available for separate purchase).

Unit II

Overview of the Human Body

Chapter 4

Medical Terminology

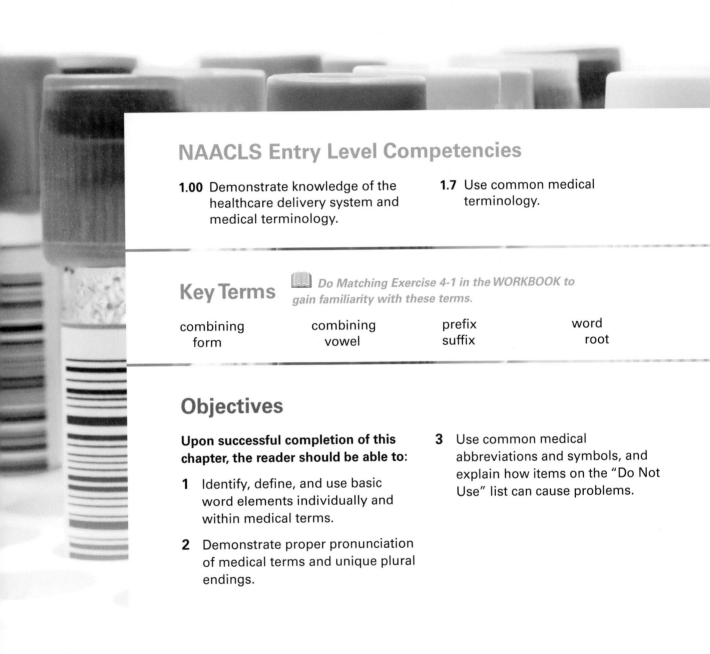

NAACLS Entry Level Competencies

1.00 Demonstrate knowledge of the healthcare delivery system and medical terminology.

1.7 Use common medical terminology.

Key Terms

📖 *Do Matching Exercise 4-1 in the WORKBOOK to gain familiarity with these terms.*

combining form

combining vowel

prefix
suffix

word root

Objectives

Upon successful completion of this chapter, the reader should be able to:

1 Identify, define, and use basic word elements individually and within medical terms.

2 Demonstrate proper pronunciation of medical terms and unique plural endings.

3 Use common medical abbreviations and symbols, and explain how items on the "Do Not Use" list can cause problems.

Overview

Medical terminology is a special vocabulary of scientific and technical terms used in the healthcare professions to speak and write effectively and precisely. It is based on an understanding of three basic word elements (word roots, prefixes, and suffixes) that are often derived from Greek and Latin words. Most medical terms are formed from two or more of these elements. If the meanings of the word elements are known, the general meaning of most medical terms can be established (although the actual definition may differ slightly). This chapter covers the three basic word elements, related elements called combining vowels and combining forms, unique plural endings, and pronunciation guidelines for medical terms. Common abbreviations and symbols used in health care, including those found on the Joint Commission's "Do Not Use" lists, are also covered.

Key Point To determine the meaning of a medical term, it is generally best to start with the suffix, then go to the prefix, and identify the meaning of the word root or roots last.

Modern medicine was founded by the Greeks and influenced by Latin, the universal language at the time. Consequently, many medical terms are derived from Greek or Latin words. For example, many surgical or diagnosis terms are derived from Greek words, and many anatomical terms have a Latin origin. New terms are often of English origin because English is now considered the universal language.

Word Roots

A **word root** (sometimes called a word stem) is the subject of a medical term and the foundation upon which the term is built. The meaning of a medical term is established by analyzing the other word elements, such as prefixes and suffixes attached to the word root.

Key Point A word root typically indicates a tissue, organ, body system, color, condition, substance, or structure. For example, the word root *phleb* means "vein," a body structure.

Some medical terms have more than one word root. The term *thrombophlebitis* is made up of the word root *phleb* and the word root *thromb* meaning "clot." In a few instances, a root will have several very different meanings. For example, the root *ped* appears in words derived from both Greek and Latin words for "foot" and the Greek word for "child." In addition, some words containing *ped* are derived from the Latin term *pediculus*, meaning "louse." To establish the meaning of the root in these cases consider the context in which the word is used. Table 4-1 lists common medical word roots.

Key Point Occasionally there will be both a Greek and Latin word root with the same meaning. For example, the Greek root *nephr* and the Latin root *ren* both mean "kidney."

Prefixes

A **prefix** is a word element that comes before a word root. A prefix modifies the meaning of the word root by adding information such as presence, absence, location, number, or size.

Example: A/   NUCLEAR
              prefix   root
              (without)   (nucleus)

The prefix *a-* means "without." The word root *nuclear* means nucleus. The word *anuclear* means "without a nucleus." Table 4-2 lists common medical prefixes.

Suffixes

A **suffix** is a word ending. It follows a word root and either changes or adds to the meaning of the word root. The best way to determine the meaning of a medical term is to first identify the meaning of the suffix.

Example: GASTR/   IC
              root   suffix
              (stomach)   (pertaining to)

The word root *gastr* means "stomach." The suffix *-ic* means "pertaining to." The word *gastric* means "pertaining to the stomach." Table 4-3 lists common medical suffixes.

Key Point When a suffix begins with "rh," the "r" is doubled, as in *hemorrhage.* When a suffix is added to a word ending in "x," the "x" is changed to a "g" or "c," as in *pharynx* becoming *pharyngeal* and *thorax* becoming *thoracic.* When a suffix begins with a vowel and the word root ends in the same vowel, one is dropped as in *carditis.*

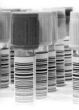

Table 4-1: Common Medical Word Roots

Root	Meaning	Example	Root	Meaning	Example
adip	fat	adipose	hepat	liver	hepatitis
aer	air	aerobic	hist	tissue	histology
angi	vessel	angiogram	kerat	hard, cornea	keratinized
arteri	artery	arteriosclerosis	leuk	white	leukocyte
arthr	joint	arthritis	lip	fat	lipemia
bar	weight	bariatric	melan	black	melanoma
bili	bile	bilirubin	morph	form	morphology
bronch	bronchus	bronchitis	my	muscle	myalgia
bucc	cheek	buccal	myel	bone marrow, or spinal cord	osteomyelitis
carcin	cancer	carcinogenic			
cardi	heart	electrocardiogram	nat	birth	natal
cephal	head	cephalic	necr	death	necrosis
chondr	cartilage	osteochondritis	nephr	kidney	nephritis
coron	crown, circle	coronary	neur	nerve	neurology
crin	to secrete	endocrine	onc	tumor	oncologist
cry	cold	cryoglobulin	oste	bone	osteoporosis
cubit	elbow	antecubital	path	disease	pathogen
cutane	skin	percutaneous	ped	child	pediatric
cyan	blue	cyanotic	phag	eat, swallow	phagocytic
cyst	bladder	cystitis	phleb	vein	phlebotomy
cyt	cell	cytology	pneumon	air, lung	pneumonia
cyte	cell	erythrocyte	prandi	meal	postprandial
derm	skin	dermis	pub	pubic	suprapubic
dermat	skin	dermatitis	pulmon	lung	pulmonary
encephal	brain	encephalitis	ren	kidney	renal
enter	intestines	enteritis	scler	hard	sclerotic
erythr	red	erythema	sphygm	pulse	sphygmomanometer
esophag	esophagus	esophagitis	squam	flat, scale	squamous
estr	female	estrogen	thorac	chest	thoracic
fibrin	fiber	fibrinolysis	thromb	clot	thrombosis
gastr	stomach	gastrointestinal	tox	poison	toxicology
gluc	sugar, glucose	glucose	ur, urin	urine	urinalysis
glyc	sugar, glucose	glycolysis	vas	vessel	vascular
hem	blood	hemolysis	ven	vein	venipuncture
hemat	blood	hematology	viscer	organ	visceral

Table 4-2: Common Medical Prefixes

Prefix	Meaning	Example	Prefix	Meaning	Example
a-, an-, ar-	without	arrhythmia	hypo-	low, under	hypoglycemia
ab-	away from	abduct	intra-	within	intramuscular
ana-	again, upward, back	anabolism	inter-	between	intercellular
aniso-	unequal	anisocytosis	iso-	equal, same	isothermal
ante	before, in front of	antecubital	later-	side	lateral
anti-	against	antiseptic	macro-	large, long	macrocyte
auto-	self	autologous	mal-	poor	malnutrition
bi-	two	bicuspid	medi-	middle	medial
bio-	life	biology	micro-	small	microcyte
brady-	slow	bradycardia	mid-	middle	midline
cata-	down	catabolism	mono-	one	mononuclear
cyan-	blue	cyanotic	neo-	new	neonatal
dia-	across, through	diapedesis	per-	through	percutaneous
dorso-	back	dorsal	peri-	around	pericardium
dys-	difficult	dyspnea	poly-	many, much	polyuria
endo-	in, within	endothelium	post-	after	postprandial
epi-	on, over, upon	epidermis	pre-	before	prenatal
erythr-	red	erythrocyte	semi-	half	semilunar
exo-	outside	exocrine	sub-	below, under	subcutaneous
extra-	outside	extravascular	supra-	above	suprapubic
hetero-	different	heterosexual	tachy-	rapid, fast	tachycardia
homo-	same	homogeneous	tri-	three	tricuspid
homeo-	same	homeostasis			
hyper	too much, high	hypertension			

Combining Vowels/Forms

A **combining vowel** is a vowel ("o" is the most common, followed by "i") that is added between two word roots or a word root and a suffix to make pronunciation easier. A word root combined with a vowel is called a **combining form**.

Key Point A combining vowel is not normally used when a suffix starts with a vowel. However, a combining vowel is kept between two word roots, even if the second word root begins with a vowel.

Example 1:

GASTR /O/	ENTER /O/	LOGY
word root	word root	suffix
combining	combining	
vowel	vowel	
(combining form)	(combining form)	
(stomach)	(intestines)	(study of)

The two word roots are combined by the vowel "o" to ease pronunciation, even though the second root *enter* begins with a vowel. The vowel "o" is also used between the word root *enter* and the suffix *-logy*. The term gastroenterology means "study of the stomach and intestines." The combining forms created are *gastro* and *entero*.

Example 2:

PHLEB/	ITIS
root	suffix
(vein)	(inflammation)

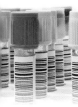

Table 4-3: Common Medical Suffixes

Suffix	Meaning	Example	Suffix	Meaning	Example
-ac, -al	pertaining to	cardiac, neural	-meter	instrument that measures or counts	thermometer
-algia	pain	neuralgia	-ole	small	arteriole
-ar, -ary	pertaining to	muscular, urinary	-oma	tumor	hepatoma
-ase	enzyme	lipase	-ose	pertaining to	adipose
-centesis	surgical puncture to remove a fluid	thoracentesis	-osis	abnormal condition	necrosis
-cyte	cell	erythrocyte	-ous	pertaining to	cutaneous
-ectomy	excision, removal	appendectomy	-oxia	oxygen level	hypoxia
-emia	blood condition	anemia	-pathy	disease	cardiomyopathy
-gram	recording, writing	electrocardiogram	-penia	deficiency	leukopenia
-ia	state or condition	hemophilia	-pnea	breathing	dyspnea
-iatr	treatment	pediatric	-poiesis	formation	hemopoiesis
-ic, -tic	pertaining to	thoracic	-rrhage	burst forth/excessive flow	hemorrhage
-ism	condition or state of	hypothyroidism	-spasm	twitch, involuntary muscle movement	arteriospasm
-ist	one who specializes in	pharmacist	-stasis	stopping, controlling, standing	hemostasis
-itis	inflammation	tonsillitis	-tomy	cutting, incision	phlebotomy
-ium	structure, tissue	pericardium	-ule	small	venule
-logist	specialist in the study of	cardiologist			
-logy	study of	histology			
-lysis	breakdown, destruction	hemolysis			

Check your knowledge of the word elements by doing Labeling Exercise 4-1, Knowledge Drill 4-2 (Scrambled Words), and Skills Drill 4-2 (Word Building) activities in the WORKBOOK.

Because the suffix *-itis* begins with a vowel, a combining vowel is not used after the word root *phleb*. Phlebitis means "inflammation of a vein."

Discrepancies in the Classification of Word Elements

Medical terminology texts sometimes vary in the way they classify the word elements of medical terms. Also, some word elements may be classified one way in one term and a different way in another. For example, the word element *erythr*, which means "red," is classified as a word root in the term *erythema*. It functions as a prefix, however, in the word *erythrocyte*, which means "red

blood cell." Either way, the meaning of the word part is basically the same.

Key Point It is more important to be able to identify the meaning of a word element than to identify its classification.

Unique Plural Endings

Identify the singular or plural forms of words listed in Labeling Exercise 4-2 in the WORKBOOK.

The plural forms of some medical terms follow English rules. Others have **unique plural endings** that follow the rules of the Greek or Latin from which they originated. It is important to evaluate medical terms individually to determine the correct plural form. Table 4-4 lists the unique plural forms of typical singular medical term endings.

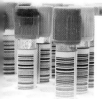

Table 4-4: Unique Plural Endings

Word Ending	Plural Ending	Singular Example	Plural Example
-a	-ae	vena cava	vena cavae (ka've)
-en	-ina	lumen	lumina (lu'min-a)
-ex, -ix	-ices	appendix	appendices (a-pen'di-sez)
-is	-es	crisis	crises (kri'sez)
-nx	-nges	phalanx	phalanges (fa-lan'-jez)
-on	-a	protozoon	protozoa (pro"to-zo'a)
-um	-a	ovum	ova (o'va)
-us	-i	nucleus	nuclei (nu'kle-i)

Pronunciation

Medical terms must be pronounced properly to convey the correct meaning, which can be changed by even one mispronounced syllable. Basic English pronunciation rules apply to most medical terms, and some may have more than one acceptable pronunciation. For example, hemophilia can be pronounced "he mo filé e a" or "hem o filé e a." In addition, some terms that are spelled differently are pronounced the same. For example, *ilium,* which means "hipbone," is pronounced the same as *ileum,* which means "small intestine." These terms can be confused when spoken rather than written. Verifying spelling eliminates confusion. General pronunciation guidelines are found in Table 4-5.

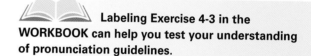

Labeling Exercise 4-3 in the WORKBOOK can help you test your understanding of pronunciation guidelines.

Abbreviations and Symbols

To save time, space, and paperwork, it is common practice in the healthcare professions to use abbreviations and symbols (such as objects and signs) to shorten words and phrases. Some of the most common abbreviations related to healthcare and healthcare acts, agencies, and organizations, are listed in Tables 4-6 and 4-7 respectively. Healthcare-related symbols are listed in Table 4-8.

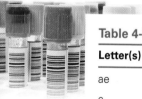

Table 4-5: General Pronunciation Guidelines

Letter(s)	Pronunciation Guideline	Example(s)
ae	Pronounce the second vowel only	chordae
c	Sounds like "s" when it precedes "e," "i," or "y" (in terms of Greek or Latin origin)	cell, circulation, cytology
	Has a hard sound when it precedes other vowels	capillary, colitis, culture
g	Sounds like "j" when it precedes "e," "i," or "y" (in terms of Greek or Latin origin)	genetic, *Giardia*, gyrate
	Has a hard sound when it precedes other vowels	gallbladder, gonad, gut
ch	Often pronounced like a "k"	chloride, cholesterol
e	May be pronounced separately when at the end of a term	syncope, diastole
es	May be pronounced as a separate syllable when at the end of a term	nares
i	Pronounce like "eye" when at the end of a plural term	fungi, nuclei
ph	Pronounce with an "f" sound	pharmacy
pn	Pronounce the "n" sound only when at the start of a term	pneumonia
	Pronounce both letters separately when in the middle of a term	dyspnea, apnea
ps	pronounce like "s"	pseudopod, psychology

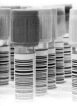

Table 4-6: Common Healthcare-Related Abbreviations

Abbreviation	Meaning	Abbreviation	Meaning
ABGs	arterial blood gases	CML	chronic myelogenous leukemia
ABO	blood group system	CNS	central nervous system
a.c.	before meals	c/o	complains of
ACTH	adrenocorticotropic hormone	CO_2	carbon dioxide
ADH	antidiuretic hormone	COPD	chronic obstructive pulmonary disease
ad lib	as desired	CPR	cardiopulmonary resuscitation
AIDS	acquired immunodeficiency syndrome	Crit	hematocrit (see HCT)
alb	albumin	C-section	cesarean section
ALL	acute lymphocytic leukemia	CSF	cerebrospinal fluid
ALT	alanine transaminase (see SGPT)	CT scan	computed tomography scan
AML	acute myelocytic leukemia	CVA	cerebrovascular accident (stroke)
Aq	water (aqua)	CXR	chest x-ray
AST	aspartate aminotransferase (see SGOT)	D	day
ASO	antistreptolysin O	DIC	disseminated intravascular coagulation
AV	atrioventricular	Diff	differential count of white blood cells
b.i.d.	twice a day (*bis in die*)	Dil	dilute
bili	bilirubin	DKA	diabetic acidosis (ketoacidosis)
BMP	basic metabolic profile	DNA	deoxyribonucleic acid
BP	blood pressure	DOB	date of birth
BS	blood sugar	DVT	deep venous thrombosis
BUN	blood urea nitrogen	Dx	diagnosis
Bx	biopsy	ECG	electrocardiogram
$\bar{c}$	with (*cum*)	ECHO	echocardiogram
C	celsius; centigrade	ECU	emergency care unit
C & S	culture & sensitivity	ED	emergency department
Ca	calcium	EEG	electroencephalogram
CABG	coronary artery bypass graft	EKG	electrocardiogram
CAD	coronary artery disease	EMG	electromyogram
CAT	computed axial tomography	ENT	ear, nose, and throat
CBC	complete blood count	Eos	eosinophils
cc	cubic centimeter	ER	emergency room
CCU	coronary (cardiac) care unit	ESR/sed rate	erythrocyte sedimentation rate
Chem	chemistry	ETOH	ethyl alcohol
Chemo	chemotherapy	exc	excision
CHF	congestive heart failure	F	Fahrenheit
Chol	cholesterol	FBS	fasting blood sugar
CK	creatine kinase	Fe	iron
cm	centimeter	FH	family history

(*continued*)

Table 4-6: Common Healthcare-Related Abbreviations (Continued)

Abbreviation	Meaning	Abbreviation	Meaning
FS	frozen section	LDL	low-density lipoprotein
FSH	follicle-stimulating hormone	LE	lupus erythematosus (lupus)
FUO	fever of unknown origin	LH	luteinizing hormone
Fx	fracture	LP	lumbar puncture
GH	growth hormone	lymphs	lymphocytes
GI	gastrointestinal	lytes	electrolytes
gluc	glucose	M	meter
Gm, gm, g	gram	Mcg	microgram
GTT	glucose tolerance test	MCH	mean corpuscular hemoglobin
GYN	gynecology	MCHC	mean corpuscular hemoglobin concentration
h	hour	MCV	mean corpuscular volume
HAV	hepatitis A virus	Mets	metastases
Hb, Hgb	hemoglobin	Mg	milligram
HBsAg	hepatitis B surface antigen	Mg^{++}	magnesium
HBV	hepatitis B virus	MI	myocardial infarction
HCG	human chorionic gonadotropin	ML	milliliter
HCL	hydrochloric acid	Mm	millimeter
HCT/Hct	hematocrit (see crit)	Mono	monocyte
HCV	hepatitis C virus	MRI	magnetic resonance imaging
HDL	high-density lipoprotein	MS	multiple sclerosis
Hg	mercury	Na^+	sodium
HGB/hgb	hemoglobin	Neg	negative
HH (H & H)	hemoglobin and hematocrit	NG	nasogastric
HIV	human immunodeficiency virus	NKA	no known allergy
h/o	history of	noc	night
H_2O	water	NPO	nothing by mouth (*nil per os*)
h.s.	at bedtime (*hora somni*)	NSAID	nonsteroidal anti-inflammatory drug
hx	history	O_2	oxygen
ICU	intensive care unit	OB	obstetrics
ID	identification, intradermal	O&P	ova and parasite
IM	intramuscular	OP	outpatient
IP	inpatient	OR	operating room
IV	intravenous	Oz	ounce
IVP	intravenous pyelogram	$\bar{p}$	after
K^+	potassium	P	pulse; phosphorus
Kg	kilogram	PaO_2	partial pressure of oxygen
L	left, liter	PAP	papanicolaou test (smear)
Lat	lateral	Path	pathology
lb	pound	p.c.	after meals
LD/LDH	lactic dehydrogenase		

Table 4-6: Common Healthcare-Related Abbreviations (Continued)

Abbreviation	Meaning	Abbreviation	Meaning
PCO_2	partial pressure of carbon dioxide	SC, SQ	subcutaneous
Peds	pediatrics	sed rate	erythrocyte sedimentation rate (ESR)
PET	positron emission tomography	segs	segmented white blood cells
pH	hydrogen ion concentration (measure of acidity or alkalinity)	SGOT	serum glutamic–oxaloacetic transaminase (see AST)
PKU	phenylketonuria	SGPT	serum glutamic–pyruvic transaminase (see ALT)
PLT	platelet	SLE	systemic lupus erythematosus
PMNs	polymorphonuclear leukocytes	sol	solution
PNS	peripheral nervous system	SpGr	specific gravity
p/o	postoperative	Staph	staphylococcus
p.o.	orally (per os)	STAT, stat	immediately (*statum*)
polys	polymorphonuclear leukocytes	STD	sexually transmitted disease
pos	positive	Strep	streptococcus
post-op	after operation	Sx	symptoms
PP	postprandial (after a meal)	T	temperature
PPBS	postprandial blood sugar	T_3	triiodothyronine (a thyroid hormone)
PPD	purified protein derivative (TB test)	T_4	thyroxine (a thyroid hormone)
pre-op	before operation	TB	tuberculosis
prep	prepare for	T cells	lymphocytes from the thymus
PRN, prn	as necessary (*pro re nata*)	T&C	type and crossmatch (type & x)
protime	Prothrombin time	TIA	transient ischemic attack
PSA	Prostate-specific antigen	TIBC	total iron binding capacity
pt	patient	TPN	total parenteral nutrition (intravenous feeding)
PT	prothrombin time/physical therapy	TPR	temperature, pulse, and respiration
PTT	partial thromboplastin time	Trig	triglycerides
PVC	premature ventricular contraction	TSH	thyroid-stimulating hormone
QNS, q.n.s.	quantity not sufficient	Tx	treatment
R	right	UA, ua	urinalysis
RA	rheumatoid arthritis	URI	upper respiratory infection
RBC	red blood cell or red blood count (also rbc)	UTI	urinary tract infection
req	requisition	UV	ultraviolet
RIA	radioimmunoassay	VCU	voiding cystourethrogram
R/O	rule out	VD	venereal disease
RPR	rapid plasma reagin	W̶	water reactive
RT	respiratory therapy	WBC, wbc	white blood cell
RR	recovery room	wd	wound
Rx	treatment	WT, wt	weight
s̄	without	y/o	years old
SA	sinoatrial		
SAD	seasonal affective disorder		

Table 4-7: Abbreviations for Healthcare-Related Acts, Agencies, and Organizations

Abbreviation	Meaning	Abbreviation	Meaning
AABB	American Association of Blood Banks	DOT	Department of Transportation
ACA	Affordable Care Act	EPA	Environmental Protection Agency
ACO	Accountable Care Organizations	FDA	Food and Drug Administration
AHA	American Hospital Association	FFA	Federal Aviation Administration
AHCCCS	Arizona Health Care Cost Containment System	HCFA	Health Care Financing Administration
AICR	American Institute for Cancer Research	HICPAC	Heatlhcare Infection Control Practices Advisory Committee
ASCLS	American Society for Clinical Laboratory Sciences	HIPAA	Health Insurance Portability and Accountability Act
ASM	American Society for Microbiology	HMO	Health Maintenance Organization
ASTM	American Society for Testing and Materials, International	HHS	Health and Human Services
CAP	College of American Pathologists	MCO	Managed Care Organization
CDC	Centers for Disease Control and Prevention	NAACLS	National Accrediting Agency for Clinical Laboratory Sciences
CIC	Connectivity Industry Consortium	NFPA	National Fire Protection Association
CLIA	Clinical Laboratory Improvement Act (1967)	NIA	National Institute on Aging
		NIDA	National Institute on Drug Abuse
CLIAC	Clinical Laboratory Improvement Act Committee	NIH	National Institute for Health
CLSI	Clinical Laboratory Standards Institute	NIOSH	National Institute for Occupational Safety and Health
CMS	Centers for Medicare and Medicaid Services	PHS	Public Health Services
		PPACA	Patient Protection and Affordable Care Act
DHHS	Department of Health & Human Services	PPO	Preferred Provider Organization

Table 4-8: Common Healthcare-Related Symbols

Symbol	Meaning	Symbol	Meaning
α	alpha	>	greater than
β	beta	≥	equal to or greater than
δ	delta	±	plus or minus, positive or negative
γ	gamma	®	registered trademark
λ	lambda	™	trademark
∞	infinity	#	number, pound
μ	micron	%	percent
μg	microgram (mcg)	Δ	heat
+	plus, positive	♀	female
−	minus, negative	♂	male
=	equals	↑	increase
<	less than	↓	decrease
≤	equal to or less than		

Official "Do Not Use" List[1]

Do Not Use	*Potential Problem*	**Use Instead**
U, u (unit)	Mistaken for "0" (zero), the number "4" (four) or "cc"	Write "unit"
IU (International Unit)	Mistaken for IV (intravenous) or the number 10 (ten)	Write "International Unit"
Q.D., QD, q.d., qd (daily)	Mistaken for each other	Write "daily"
Q.O.D., QOD, q.o.d, qod (every other day)	Period after the Q mistaken for "I" and the "O" mistaken for "I	Write "every other day"
Trailing zero (X.0 mg)*	Decimal point is missed	Write X mg
Lack of leading zero (.X mg)		Write 0.X mg
MS	Can mean morphine sulfate or magnesium sulfate	Write "morphine sulfate"
MSO_4 and $MgSO_4$	Confused for one another	Write "magnesium sulfate"

[1] Applies to all orders and all medication-related documentation that is handwritten (including free-text computer entry) or on pre-printed forms.

***Exception:** A "trailing zero" may be used only where required to demonstrate the level of precision of the value being reported, such as for laboratory results, imaging studies that report size of lesions, or catheter/tube sizes. It may not be used in medication orders or other medication-related documentation.

Figure 4-1 Official "Do Not Use" List, © The Joint Commission, 2013. Reprinted with permission.

The Joint Commission's "Do Not Use" List

To help reduce the number of medical errors related to incorrect interpretation of terminology, the Joint Commission created a list of dangerous abbreviations, symbols, and acronyms that must be included on a **"Do Not Use" list** (Fig. 4-1) by every organization it accredits.

According to a September 2013 article in the *Journal of Patient Safety*, it is estimated that between 210,000 and 400,000 deaths in the United States each year are caused by preventable medical errors.

The list applies to all orders and all medication-related documentation that is handwritten, entered on computer, or written on preprinted forms. The list applies to handwritten laboratory reports but printed and electronic laboratory reports are exempted. Laboratories are also exempted from the ban on the use of a trailing zero (a zero to the right of a decimal point) because in reporting laboratory test results the precision of a numeric value is often indicated by the digits after the decimal point, even if the trailing digit is a zero. For example, it would be acceptable to report a serum potassium level as 4.0 mEq/L, rather than 4 mEq/L.

The True/False activity in Knowledge Drill 4-3 in the WORKBOOK will help you test your overall knowledge of this chapter.

Study and Review Questions

 See the EXAM REVIEW for more study questions.

1. **A prefix**
   a. comes before a word root and modifies its meaning.
   b. establishes the basic meaning of a medical term.
   c. follows a word root and adds to or changes its meaning.
   d. makes pronunciation of the term easier.

2. **Which part of gastr/o/enter/o/logy is the suffix?**
   a. enter
   b. gastr
   c. logy
   d. o

3. **Which one of the following organizations writes guidelines for laboratory practices?**
   a. ACA
   b. CLSI
   c. HCFA
   d. PHS

4. **What does the suffix -algia mean?**
   a. between
   b. condition
   c. disease
   d. pain

5. **The plural form of atrium is**
   a. atri.
   b. atria.
   c. atrial.
   d. atrices.

6. **The medical term for red blood cell is**
   a. erythrocyte.
   b. hepatocyte.
   c. leukocyte.
   d. thrombocyte.

7. **Cystitis means**
   a. blueness of the skin.
   b. cellular infection.
   c. inflammation of the bladder.
   d. pertaining to a cell.

8. **The "e" is pronounced separately in**
   a. diastole.
   b. syncope.
   c. systole.
   d. all of the above.

9. **The abbreviation NPO means**
   a. negative patient outcome.
   b. new patients only.
   c. no parenteral output.
   d. nothing by mouth.

10. **Which of the following abbreviations is on the Joint Commission "Do Not Use" list?**
    a. cc
    b. IU
    c. mL
    d. UTI

Case Studies

See the WORKBOOK for more case studies.

Case Study 4-1: Lab Orders

A physician orders ASAP blood cultures on an ER patient with a diagnosis of FUO.

QUESTIONS

1. When should the blood cultures be collected?
2. Where is the patient located?
3. What does the diagnosis abbreviation FUO mean?

Case Study 4-2: Misinterpreted Instructions

A phlebotomy student is doing a clinical rotation with a laboratory in a medical clinic. A patient comes in for a TB test. The phlebotomist in charge thinks that it would be a good learning experience for the student to administer the test. The student is a little reluctant. The phlebotomist tells her not to worry, writes out the instructions shown below, and goes about processing specimens that are ready to be centrifuged. Phlebotomist's instructions:

Choose a clean site on the inside of the arm below the elbow.

Draw .1 mL TB antigen into a tuberculin syringe.

Insert the needle just under the skin, and pull back the plunger slightly.

If you don't see blood slowly inject the antigen under the skin, remove the needle, but do not hold pressure or bandage the site.

The student filled the syringe with antigen. As she was injecting it into the patient, a large wheal started to form. She got scared and called the phlebotomist, who noticed that half the 1-mL syringe contained antigen. She instructed the student to pull the needle out immediately, telling her that she had used too much antigen.

QUESTIONS

1. Why would the student have used too much antigen?
2. How could the mistake have been prevented?
3. What else could have prevented the error?
4. What effect might the error have on the patient?

Bibliography and Suggested Readings

James JT. A new evidence-based estimate of patient harms associated with hospital care. *J Patient Saf.* 2013;9(3):122–128.

Mosby's Dictionary of Medicine, Nursing & Health Professions. 9th ed. St. Louis, MO: Mosby/Elsevier; 2012.

Stedman's Medical Dictionary for the Health Professions and Nursing. 7th ed. Philadelphia, PA: Lippincott Williams & Wilkins; 2011.

*Stedman's Medical Abbreviations, Acronyms * Symbols.* 5th ed. Philadelphia, PA: Lippincott Williams & Wilkins; 2012.

Venes D. *Taber's Cyclopedic Medical Dictionary.* 22nd ed. Philadelphia, PA: FA Davis; 2013.

Willis M. *Medical Terminology, Quick and Concise.* Philadelphia, PA: Lippincott Williams & Wilkins; 2009.

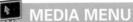

MEDIA MENU

Online Ancillaries (at http://thepoint.lww.com/McCall6e)
- Interactive exercises and games, including Look and Label, Word Building, Body Building, Roboterms, Crossword Puzzles, Quiz Show, and Concentration
- Audio flash cards and flashcard generator
- Audio glossary

Internet Resources
- American Association of Medical Assistants, CMA (AAMA) Practice Exam: Medical Terminology: http://www.aama-ntl.org/becomeCMA/practice_term.aspx
- Des Moines University, Medical Terminology Course: http://www.dmu.edu/medterms/
- The Joint Commission's Do Not Use List: http://www.jointcommission.org/about_us/patient_safety_fact_sheet.aspx
- Sheppard Software, Vocabulary Games: http://www.sheppardsoftware.com/web_games_vocab_med.htm

Other Resources
- McCall R, Tankersley C. *Student Workbook for Phlebotomy Essentials.* 6th ed. (Available for separate purchase).
- McCall R, Tankersley C. *Phlebotomy Exam Review.* 6th ed. (Available for separate purchase).

Chapter 5

Human Anatomy and Physiology Review

NAACLS Entry Level Competencies

3.0 Demonstrate basic understanding of the anatomy of the main body systems and anatomic terminology in order to relate major areas of the clinical laboratory to general pathologic conditions associated with the body systems.

3.1 Describe the basic functions of each of the main body systems, and demonstrate basic knowledge of the circulatory (see Chapter 6), urinary, and other body systems necessary to perform assigned specimen collection.

Key Terms

Do Matching Exercise 5-1 in the WORKBOOK to gain familiarity with these terms.

acidosis	body plane	gametes	pituitary gland
alkalosis	bursae	hemopoiesis	prone/pronation
alveoli	cartilage	homeostasis	proximal
anabolism	catabolism	hormones	sagittal plane
anatomic	diaphragm	meninges	supine/
position	distal	metabolism	supination
anatomy	dorsal	mitosis	surfactant
anterior	endocrine	nephron	synovial fluid
avascular	glands	neuron	transverse
axons	exocrine glands	phalanges	plane
body cavities	frontal plane	physiology	ventral

Objectives

Upon successful completion of this chapter, the reader should be able to:

1 Demonstrate basic knowledge of the terminology, functions, and organization of the body.

2 Describe functions, identify components or major structures, and correctly use terminology associated with each body system.

3 List disorders and diagnostic tests commonly associated with each body system.

Overview

The human body consists of over 30 trillion cells, 206 bones, 700 muscles, approximately 5 L of blood, and about 25 miles of blood vessels. To fully appreciate the workings of this wonder, it is necessary to have a basic understanding of human **anatomy** (structural composition) and **physiology** (function). A fundamental knowledge of human anatomy and physiology (A&P) is an asset to anyone working in a healthcare setting and especially helps the phlebotomist understand the nature of the various disorders of the body, the rationale for the laboratory tests associated with them, and the importance of the role that laboratory tests play in monitoring body system functions and diagnosing disorders. This chapter covers general body organization and function, anatomical terminology, and the functions, structures, disorders, and diagnostic tests associated with nine body systems. Because of its special importance to phlebotomy, a 10th system (circulatory) is covered separately in Chapter 6.

Key Point The medical science and specialty practice concerned with all aspects of disease—including the characteristics, causes, and effects of disease on the structure and function of the body—is called pathology, and the medical professional trained in this area is called a pathologist.

Body Positions

ANATOMIC POSITION

The human body can be described in a number of different ways. For consistency in describing the direction or the location of a given point of the body, medical personnel normally refer to the body as if the patient was in the **anatomic position**, regardless of actual body position. A person in the **anatomic position** is standing erect, with feet parallel, arms at the sides, and eyes and palms facing forward.

OTHER POSITIONS

Two other body positions of particular importance to a blood drawer are **supine**, in which the patient is lying horizontal on the back with the face up, and **prone**, the opposite of supine, in which the patient is lying face down. The term *prone* also describes the hand with the palm facing down, a position sometimes used during blood collection.

The act of turning the hand so that the palm faces down is called **pronation**. The act of turning the palm to face upward is called **supination**.

Memory Jogger A way to equate supine with lying down is to think of the *ine* as in *recline*. To remember that a person who is supine is *face up,* look for the word *up* in supine.

Body Planes

A **body plane** (Fig. 5-1) is a flat surface resulting from a real or imaginary cut through a body in the normal anatomical position. Areas of the body are often referred to according to their location with respect to one of the following body planes:

- **Frontal (coronal) plane:** divides the body vertically into front and back portions.
- **Midsagittal (medial) plane:** divides the body vertically into equal right and left portions.
- **Sagittal plane:** divides the body vertically into right and left portions.
- **Transverse plane:** divides the body horizontally into upper and lower portions.

A procedure called computed tomography (CT) produces x-rays in a transverse plane of the body. Magnetic resonance imaging (MRI) can produce images of the body in all three planes using electromagnetic waves instead of x-rays.

Body Directional Terms

Areas of the body are also identified using **directional terms** (Fig. 5-2). Directional terms describe the relationship of an area or part of the body with respect to the rest of the body or body parts. Directional terms are often paired with a term that means the opposite. Table 5-1 lists common paired directional terms.

Can you find this and other key points in Knowledge Drill 5-1 in the WORKBOOK?

Key Point Directional terms are relative positions in respect to other parts of the body. For example, the ankle can be described as **distal** to the leg and **proximal** to the foot.

Body Cavities

Various organs of the body are housed in large, hollow spaces called **body cavities** (Fig. 5-3). Body cavities are

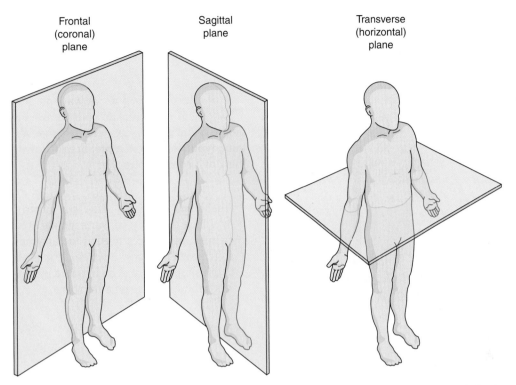

Figure 5-1 Body planes of division. (Reprinted with permission from Cohen BJ. *Memmler's the Human Body in Health and Disease*. 12th ed. Philadelphia, PA: Lippincott Williams & Wilkins; 2013:9.)

divided into two groups, dorsal and ventral, according to their location within the body.

- **Dorsal (posterior) cavities** are located in the back of the body and include the **cranial cavity**, which houses the brain, and the **spinal cavity**, which encases the spinal cord.

- **Ventral (anterior) cavities** are located in the front of the body and include the **thoracic cavity**, which houses primarily the heart and lungs; the **abdominal cavity**, which houses numerous organs including the stomach, liver, pancreas, gallbladder, spleen, and kidneys; and the **pelvic cavity**, which houses primarily the urinary bladder and reproductive organs.

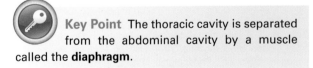 **See how well you can identify body planes, directional terms, and cavities in Labeling Exercises 5-1, 5-2, and 5-3 in the WORKBOOK.**

Key Point The thoracic cavity is separated from the abdominal cavity by a muscle called the **diaphragm**.

Body Functions
HOMEOSTASIS

The human body constantly strives to maintain its internal environment in a state of equilibrium or balance. This balanced or "steady state" condition is called **homeostasis** (ho'me-o-sta'sis), which literally translated means "standing the same." The body maintains homeostasis by compensating for changes in a process that involves feedback and regulation in response to internal and external changes.

Table 5-1: Common Paired Directional Terms

Directional Term and Meaning	Paired or Related Term and Meaning
Anterior (ventral): to the front of the body	Posterior (dorsal): to the back of the body
External (superficial): on or near the surface of the body	Internal (deep): within or near the center of the body
Medial: toward the midline or middle of the body	Lateral: toward the side of the body
Palmar: concerning the palm of the hand (opposite term is dorsal)	Plantar: concerning the sole of the foot (opposite term is dorsal)
Proximal: nearest to the center of the body, origin, or point of attachment	Distal: farthest from the center of the body, origin, or point of attachment
Superior (cranial): higher, or above or toward the head	Inferior (caudal): beneath, or lower or away from the head

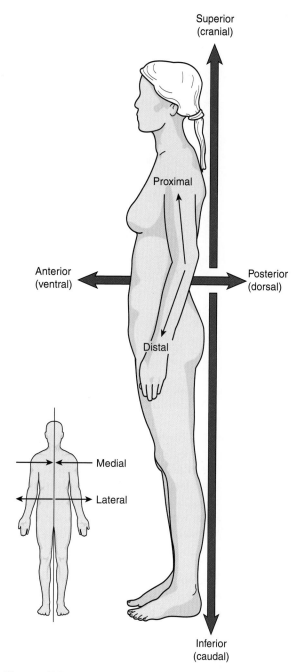

Figure 5-2 Directional terms. (Adapted with permission from Cohen BJ. *Memmler's the Human Body in Health and Disease.* 12th ed. Philadelphia, PA: Lippincott Williams & Wilkins; 2013:8.)

METABOLISM

Metabolism (me-tab'o-lizm) is the sum of all the physical and chemical reactions necessary to sustain life. There are two primary processes of metabolism: catabolism and anabolism.

- **Catabolism** (kah-tab'o-lizm) is a destructive process by which complex substances are broken down into simple substances, usually with the release of energy. An example is the conversion of carbohydrates in

food into the glucose needed by the cells and the subsequent glycolysis or breakdown of glucose by the cells to produce energy.

Memory Jogger A way to equate catabolism with breakdown is to remember that it begins with *cat* just like *catastrophe*. When something (your car, for example) breaks down, you often think of it as a catastrophe.

- **Anabolism** (ah-nab'o-lizm) is a constructive process by which the body converts simple compounds into complex substances needed to carry out the cellular activities of the body. An example is the body's ability to use simple substances provided by the bloodstream to synthesize or create a hormone.

Body Organization

CELLS

The cell (Fig. 5-4) is the basic structural unit of all life. The human body consists of trillions of cells, responsible for all the activities of the body. There are many categories of cells, and each category is specialized to perform a unique function. No matter what their function, however, all cells have the same basic structural components (Table 5-2).

Complete Labeling Exercise 5-4 in the WORKBOOK to enhance your ability to identify cellular structures.

Key Point Most cells are able to duplicate themselves, which allows the body to grow, repair, and reproduce itself. When a typical cell duplicates itself, the DNA doubles and the cell divides by a process called **mitosis** (mi-to'sis).

TISSUES

Tissues are groups of similar cells that work together to perform a special function. There are four basic types of normal tissue: connective, **epithelial**, muscle, and nerve.

- Connective tissue supports and connects all parts of the body and includes **adipose** (fat) tissue, **cartilage**, bone, and blood.
- Epithelial (ep-i-the'le-al) tissue covers and protects the body and lines organs, vessels, and cavities.
- Muscle tissue contracts to produce movement.
- Nerve tissue has the ability to transmit electrical impulses.

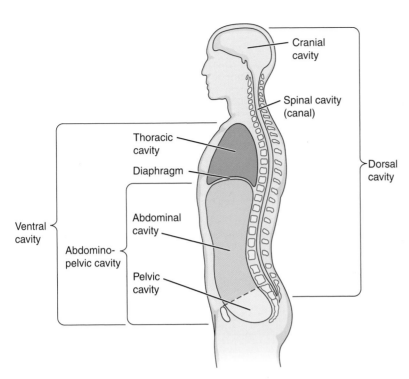

Figure 5-3 Lateral view of body cavities. (Reprinted with permission from Cohen BJ. *Memmler's the Human Body in Health and Disease*. 12th ed. Philadelphia, PA: Lippincott Williams & Wilkins; 2013:11.)

(i) A scar is made up of fibrous tissue that has replaced normal tissue destroyed by disease or injury.

ORGANS

Organs are structures composed of tissues that function together for a common purpose.

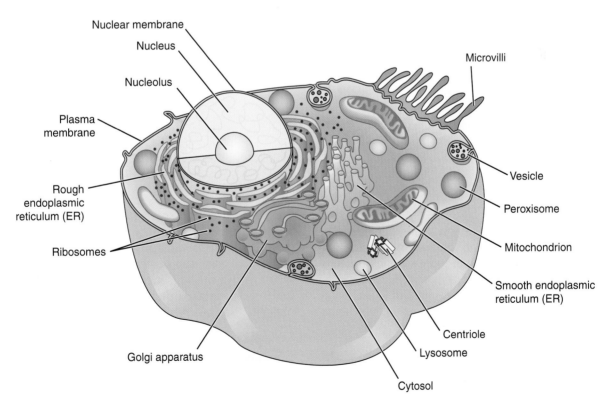

Figure 5-4 Cell diagram. (Reprinted with permission from Cohen BJ. *Memmler's the Human Body in Health and Disease*. 12th ed. Philadelphia, PA: Lippincott Williams & Wilkins; 2013:39.)

Table 5-2: Basic Structural Components of Cells

Component	Description	Function
Plasma membrane	Outer layer of a cell	Encloses the cell and regulates what moves in and out of it
Microvilli	Small projections on the cell membrane of certain cells	Increase surface area for absorption
Nucleus	Large, dark-staining organelle near the center of the cell and composed of DNA and protein	The command center of the cell that contains the chromosomes or genetic material
Nucleolus	Small body in the nucleus that is primarily RNA, DNA, and protein	Makes ribosomes
Chromosomes	Long strands of DNA organized into units called genes, occurring in humans in 23 identical pairs (46 individual)	Govern all cell activities, including reproduction
Cytoplasm	Substance within a cell composed of fluid (cytosol) and various organelles and inclusions	Site of numerous cellular activities
Organelles	Specialized structures within the cytoplasm	Varied, distinct functions depending on the type
Centrioles	Rod-shaped bodies close to the nucleus	Assist chromosome separation during cell division
Endoplasmic reticulum (ER)	Network of either smooth or rough tubular membranes. Rough ER has ribosomes attached.	Smooth ER plays a role in lipid synthesis. Rough ER sorts proteins and creates complex compounds from them.
Golgi apparatus	Layers of membranes	Makes, sorts, and prepares protein compounds for transport
Lysosomes	Small sacs of digestive enzymes	Digest substances within the cell
Peroxisomes	Enzyme-containing organelles	Destroy harmful substances
Mitochondria	Oval- or rod-shaped organelles	Play a role in energy production
Ribosomes	Tiny bodies that exist singly, in clusters, or attached to ER	Play a role in assembling proteins from amino acids
Vesicles	Small pouches in the plasma membrane	Store substances and move them in or out of the cell
Surface organelles	Structures that project from certain cells	Move the cell or move fluids around the cell
Cilia	Small hair-like projections	Waving motion moves fluids around the cell
Flagellum	Whip-like extension found on sperm	Propels the sperm toward an egg

Body Systems

Body systems are structures and organs that are related to one another and function together. There are a number of different ways to group organs and structures together, and the number of body systems may vary in different textbooks. The following are 9 of 10 commonly recognized body systems. The 10th system, the circulatory system, is discussed in greater detail in Chapter 6.

INTEGUMENTARY SYSTEM

Functions

The skin and accessory structures within it form the integumentary system. **Integument** (in-teg'u-ment) means "covering" or "skin." The skin (Fig. 5-5), the largest organ of the body, is the cover that protects the body from bacterial invasion, dehydration, and the harmful rays of the sun. Structures within the skin help regulate body temperature, eliminate small amounts of waste through sweat, receive environmental stimuli (sensation of heat, cold, touch, and pain), and manufacture vitamin D from sunlight.

Structures

The integumentary system consists of the skin and associated structures referred to as appendages (Table 5-3), which include **exocrine glands** (oil and sweat glands), hair, and nails. It also includes blood vessels, nerves, and sensory organs within the skin.

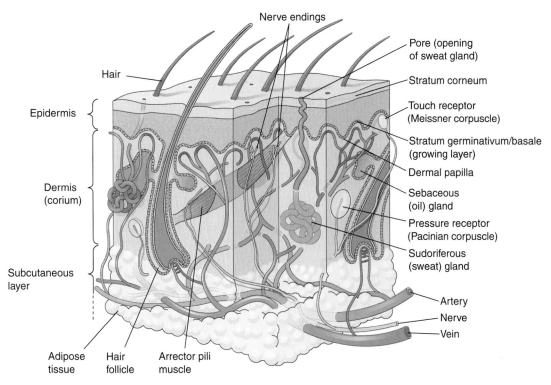

Figure 5-5 Cross section of the skin. (Adapted with permission from Cohen BJ. *Memmler's the Human Body in Health and Disease.* 12th ed. Philadelphia, PA: Lippincott Williams & Wilkins; 2013:112.)

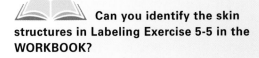 **Can you identify the skin structures in Labeling Exercise 5-5 in the WORKBOOK?**

Skin Layers

There are two main layers of the skin, the **epidermis** (ep'i-der'mis) and the **dermis**. The dermis lies on top of a layer of **subcutaneous** tissue.

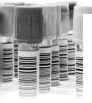

Table 5-3: Skin Appendages

Appendage	Description	Function
Hair	Nonliving material primarily composed of keratin (ker'a-tin), a tough protein	Protection
Hair follicles	Sheaths that enclose hair and contain a bulb of cells at the base from which hair develops	Produce hair
Arrector pili	Tiny, smooth muscles attached to hair follicles	Responsible for the formation of "goose bumps" as they react to pull the hair upstraight when a person is cold or frightened When the muscle contracts, it presses on the nearby sebaceous gland, causing it to release sebum to help lubricate the hair and skin
Nails	Nonliving keratin material that grows continuously as new cells form from the nail root	Protect the fingers and toes and help grasp objects
Sebaceous (oil) glands	Glands connected to hair follicles; called oil glands because they secrete an oily substance called sebum (se'bum)	Sebum helps lubricate the skin and hair to keep it from drying out
Sudoriferous (sweat) glands	Coiled dermal structures with ducts that extend through the epidermis and end in a pore on the skin surface	Produce perspiration, a mixture of water, salts, and waste

Epidermis

The epidermis is the outermost and thinnest layer of the skin. It is primarily made up of **stratified** (layered), **squamous** (flat, scale-like) epithelial cells. The epidermis is **avascular**, meaning it contains no blood or lymph vessels. The only living cells of the epidermis are in its deepest layer, the **stratum germinativum** (ger-mi-na-ti'vum), also called stratum **basale** (ba'sal'e), which is the only layer where mitosis (cell division) occurs. It is also where the skin pigment **melanin** is produced. Cells in the stratum germinativum are nourished by diffusion of nutrients from the dermis. As the cells divide, they are pushed toward the surface, where they gradually die from lack of nourishment and become **keratinized** (hardened), which helps thicken and protect the skin.

Dermis

The dermis, also called corium or true skin, is the inner layer of the skin. It is much thicker than the epidermis and is composed of elastic and fibrous connective tissue. Elevations called **papillae** (pa-pil'e) and resulting depressions in the dermis where it joins the epidermis give rise to the ridges and grooves that form fingerprints. This area is often referred to as the **papillary dermis**. The dermis contains blood and lymph vessels, nerves, **sebaceous** (se-ba'shus) and **sudoriferous** (su-dor-if'er-us) **glands**, and **hair follicles**. These structures can also extend into the subcutaneous layer.

Subcutaneous

The **subcutaneous** (beneath the skin) **layer** is composed of connective and adipose (fat) tissue that connects the skin to the surface muscles.

> (i) Aging causes thinning of the epidermis, dermis, and subcutaneous layer. This makes the skin more translucent and fragile and leaves the blood vessels less well protected. As a result the elderly bruise more easily.

Disorders and Diagnostic Tests

Examples of disorders and diagnostic tests associated with the integumentary system are listed in Box 5-1.

MUSCULAR SYSTEM

Functions

The muscular system gives the body the ability to move, maintain posture, and produce heat. It also plays a role in organ function and blood circulation. Muscle cells have the ability to contract, which produces muscle movement. Muscle tone, a steady partial contraction of muscles, helps the body maintain posture. Muscle cell metabolism produces heat as a by-product.

Box 5-1

Examples of Integumentary System Disorders and Diagnostic Tests

Integumentary System Disorders

Acne (ak'ne): inflammatory disease of sebaceous glands and hair follicles

Dermatitis (der"ma-ti'tis): skin inflammation

Decubitus ulcers (bed sores): Necrosis of the skin and underlying tissue due to constant pressure or friction at the site

Fungal infections: invasion of the skin, hair, or nails by fungi such as tinea (e.g., ringworm)

Herpes (her'pez): eruption of blisters (e.g., fever blisters or cold sores) usually caused by a virus

Impetigo (im-pe-ti'go): contagious skin infection caused by *Staphylococcus aureus* or group A streptococci

Keloid (ke'loyd): elevated overgrowth of scar tissue at a wound or incision site

Pediculosis (pe-dik"u-lo'sis): lice infestation

Pruritus (proo-ri'tus): itching

Psoriasis (so-ri'a-sis): chronic skin condition of unknown origin characterized by clearly defined red patches of scaly skin

Skin cancer (kan'ser): (e.g., basal cell, squamous, and melanoma); uncontrolled growth of malignant cells

Tests for Integumentary System Disorders

- Biopsy
- Microbiology cultures
- Skin scrapings for fungal culture
- Skin scrapings for KOH (potassium hydroxide) preparation
- Tissue cultures

> 🔑 **Key Point** Skeletal muscle movement helps keep blood moving through your veins. For example, moving your arms helps move blood from your fingertips back to your heart.

Structures

The muscular system includes all the muscles of the body, of which there are three types: cardiac, skeletal, (Fig. 5-6) and smooth (visceral). Muscle type (Fig. 5-7) is determined by location, **histological** (microscopic) cellular characteristics, and how muscle action is controlled (Table 5-4).

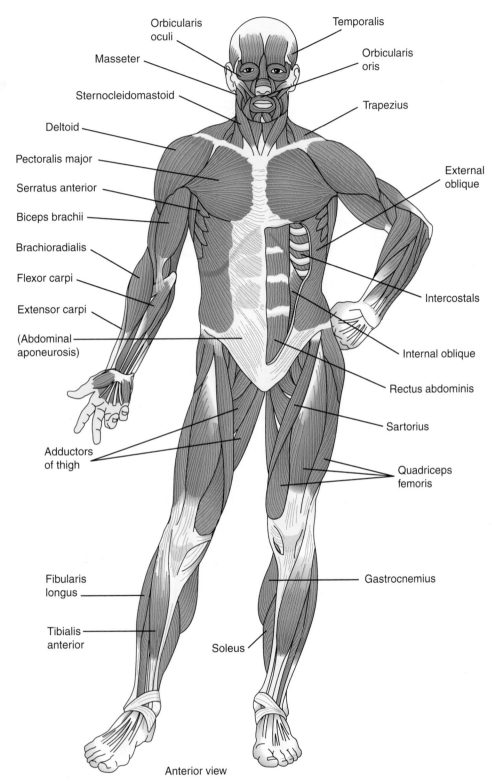

Orbicularis oculi

Temporalis

Masseter

Orbicularis oris

Sternocleidomastoid

Trapezius

Deltoid

Pectoralis major

External oblique

Serratus anterior

Biceps brachii

Brachioradialis

Flexor carpi

Extensor carpi

Intercostals

(Abdominal aponeurosis)

Internal oblique

Rectus abdominis

Sartorius

Adductors of thigh

Quadriceps femoris

Fibularis longus

Gastrocnemius

Tibialis anterior

Soleus

Anterior view

Figure 5-6 Muscular system: superficial skeletal muscles, anterior view. Associated structures are labeled in parentheses. (Reprinted with permission from Cohen BJ. *Memmler's the Human Body in Health and Disease.* 12th ed. Philadelphia, PA: Lippincott Williams & Wilkins; 2013:173.)

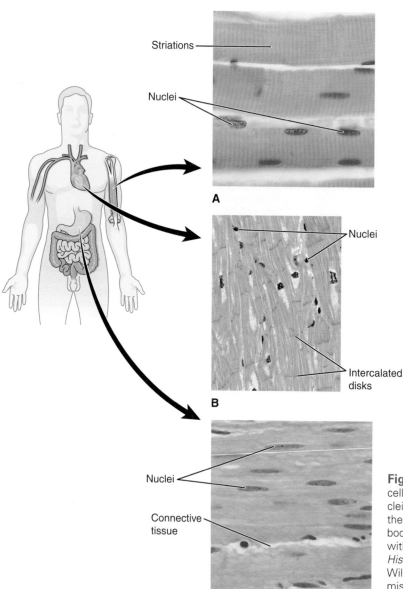

Striations

Nuclei

A

Nuclei

Intercalated disks

B

Nuclei

Connective tissue

C

Figure 5-7 Muscle tissue. **A:** Skeletal muscle cells have bands (striations) and multiple nuclei. **B:** Cardiac muscle makes up the wall of the heart. **C:** Smooth muscle is found in soft body organs and in vessels. (**A** and **C** reprinted with permission from Cormack DH. *Essential Histology.* 2nd ed. Philadelphia, PA: Lippincott Williams & Wilkins; 2001; **B** reprinted with permission from Gartner LP, Hiatt JL. *Color Atlas of Histology.* 4th ed. Baltimore, MD: Lippincott Williams & Wilkins; 2005.)

Table 5-4: Comparison of the Different Types of Muscle

	Smooth	Cardiac	Skeletal
Location	Walls of hollow organs, vessels, respiratory passageways	Walls of the heart	Attached to bones
Cell characteristics	Tapered at each end, branching networks, nonstriated	Branching networks; special membranes (intercalated disks) between cells; single nucleus; lightly striated	Long and cylindrical; multinucleated; heavily striated
Control	Involuntary	Involuntary	Voluntary
Action	Produces peristalsis; contracts and relaxes slowly; may sustain contraction	Pumps blood out of heart; self-excitatory but influenced by nervous system and hormones	Produces movement at joints; stimulated by nervous system; contracts and relaxes rapidly

Check out Labeling Exercise 5-6 in the WORKBOOK to help strengthen your muscular system knowledge.

Find the name of a muscle type in the WORKBOOK scrambled words drill (Knowledge Drill 5-2).

Disorders and Diagnostic Tests

Examples of disorders and diagnostic tests associated with the muscular system are listed in Box 5-2.

SKELETAL SYSTEM

Functions

The skeletal system is the framework that gives the body shape and support, protects internal organs, and along with the muscular system provides movement

Box 5-2

Examples of Muscular System Disorders and Diagnostic Tests

Muscular System Disorders

Atrophy (at'ro'fe): a decrease in size (wasting) of a muscle usually due to inactivity
Muscular dystrophy (dis'tro'fe) (MD): genetic disease in which muscles waste away or atrophy
Myalgia (mi'al'je'ah): painful muscle
Tendonitis (ten'dun i'tis): inflammation of muscle tendons, usually due to overexertion

Tests for Muscular System Disorders

- Antinuclear antibody (ANA)
- Autoimmune profile
- Cold agglutinin titer, quantitative
- Creatine
- Creatine kinase (CK), total plus isoenzymes
- Electromyography
- Lactic acid
- Lactate dehydrogenase (LD/LDH)
- Myoglobin
- Tissue biopsy or culture

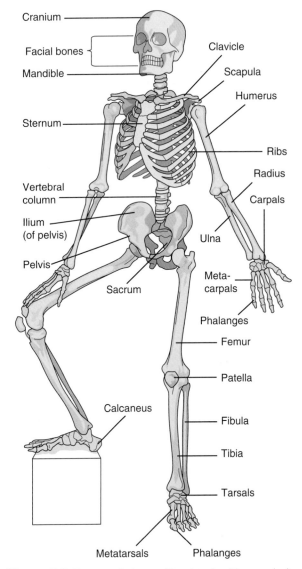

Figure 5-8 Human skeleton. (Reprinted with permission from Cohen BJ. *Memmler's the Human Body in Health and Disease.* 12th ed. Philadelphia, PA: Lippincott Williams & Wilkins; 2013:132.)

and leverage. It is also responsible for calcium storage and **hemopoiesis** (he'mopoy-e'sis) or **hematopoiesis** (hem'a-to-poy-e'sis), the production of blood cells, which normally occurs in the bone marrow.

Structures

Structures of the skeletal system include all the bones (206), joints, and supporting connective tissue that form the skeleton (Fig. 5-8).

Test your bone identification skills with Labeling Exercise 5-7 in the WORKBOOK.

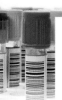

Table 5-5: Classification of Bones by Shape

Bone Shape	Examples
Flat	Rib bones and most skull (cranial) bones
Irregular	Back bones (vertebrae) and some facial bones
Long	Leg (femur, tibia, fibula), arm (humerus, radius, ulna), and hand bones (metacarpals, phalanges)
Short	Wrist (carpals) and ankle bones (tarsals)

Bones

Bones are a special type of dense connective tissue consisting of bone cells (mature bone cells are called osteocytes) surrounded by hard deposits of calcium salts. They are living tissue with their own network of blood vessels, lymph vessels, and nerves. Bones can be classified by shape into four groups, as shown in Table 5-5.

> **Key Point** Bones of particular importance in capillary blood collection are the distal **phalanx** of the finger and the **calcaneus** or heel bone of the foot.

Joints

A joint is the junction or union between two or more bones. Freely movable joints have a cavity that contains a viscid (sticky), colorless liquid called **synovial fluid**. Some joints have a small sac nearby called a **bursa** (bur'sa) (pl. bursae) (bur'se) that is filled with synovial fluid. Bursae help ease movement over and around areas subject to friction, such as prominent joint parts or where tendons pass over bone.

Disorders and Diagnostic Tests

Examples of disorders and diagnostic tests associated with the skeletal system are listed in Box 5-3.

NERVOUS SYSTEM

Functions

The nervous system (Fig. 5-9) controls and coordinates activities of the various body systems by means of electrical impulses and chemical substances sent to and received from all parts of the body. The nervous system has two functional divisions, the somatic nervous system and the autonomic nervous system, identified by the type of control (voluntary or involuntary), and according to the type of tissue stimulated (Table 5-6).

Box 5-3

Examples of Skeletal System Disorders and Diagnostic Tests

Skeletal System Disorders

Arthritis (ar-thri"tis): joint disorder characterized by joint inflammation, pain, and swelling

Bone tumor: abnormal growth of bone tissue

Bursitis (bur-si"tis): inflammation of a bursa (fluid-filled sac near a joint)

Gout (gowt): a painful form of arthritis precipitated by deposits of needle-like uric acid crystals in the joints and surrounding tissues as a result of faulty uric acid metabolism

Osteomyelitis (os'te-o-mi'el-i'tis): inflammation of the bone (especially the marrow), caused by bacterial infection

Osteochondritis (os'te-o-kon-dri'tis): inflammation of the bone and cartilage

Osteoporosis (os'te-por-o'sis): disorder involving loss of bone density

Rickets (rik'ets): abnormal bone formation indirectly resulting from lack of vitamin D needed for calcium absorption

Tests for Skeletal System Disorders

- Alkaline phosphatase (ALP) (bone-specific)
- Calcium (ionized)
- C-telopeptide
- Erythrocyte sedimentation rate (ESR)
- Osteocalcin
- Phosphorus
- Rheumatoid arthritis test (RA latex)
- Synovial fluid analysis
- Uric acid, serum, and 24-hour urine
- Vitamin D

Structures

The fundamental unit of the nervous system is the **neuron** (Fig. 5-10). The two main structural divisions of the nervous system are the **central nervous system (CNS)** and the **peripheral nervous system (PNS)**.

 Exercise your brain by doing Labeling Exercise 5-9 in the WORKBOOK.

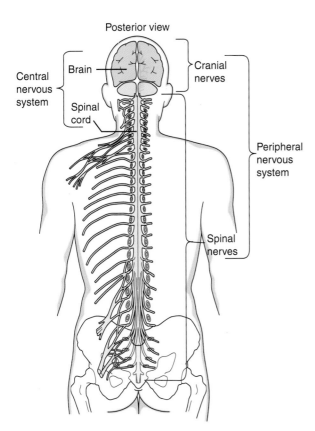

Figure 5-9 Structural divisions of the nervous system. (Reprinted with permission from Cohen BJ. *Memmler's the Human Body in Health and Disease.* 12th ed. Philadelphia, PA: Lippincott Williams & Wilkins; 2013:192.)

Neurons

Neurons are highly complex cells capable of conducting messages in the form of impulses that enable the body to interact with its internal and external environment. Neurons have a cell body containing a nucleus and organelles typical of other cells, but are distinguished by unique thread-like fibers called **dendrites** (from Gr. *dendra* meaning "tree") and **axons** that extend out from the cell body. Dendrites carry messages to the nerve cell body, while axons carry messages away from it.

Central Nervous System

The CNS consists of the brain, the nervous system command center that interprets information and dictates responses, and the spinal cord. Every part of the body

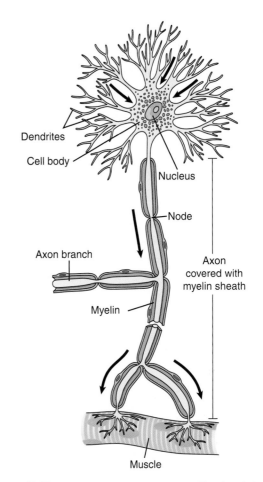

Figure 5-10 Diagram of a motor neuron. The break in the axon denotes length; the *arrows* show the direction of the nerve impulse. (Reprinted with permission from Cohen BJ. *Memmler's the Human Body in Health and Disease.* 12th ed. Philadelphia, PA: Lippincott Williams & Wilkins; 2013:193.)

is in direct communication with the CNS by means of its own set of nerves, which come together in one large trunk that forms the spinal cord.

The brain and spinal cord are surrounded and cushioned by a cavity filled with a clear, plasma-like fluid called **cerebrospinal** (ser'e-bro-spi'nal) **fluid** (CSF). The cavity is completely enclosed and protected by three layers of connective tissue called the **meninges** (me-nin'jez). When CSF is needed for testing, a physician performs a **lumbar puncture** (spinal tap) to enter the cavity and obtain a CSF sample.

Table 5-6: Functional Nervous System Divisions

Division	Function	Type of Control	Tissue Stimulated
Autonomic	Conducts impulses that affect activities of the organs, vessels, and glands	Involuntary	Cardiac muscle, smooth muscle, and glands
Somatic	Conducts impulses that allow an individual to consciously control skeletal muscles	Voluntary	Skeletal muscle

Lumbar puncture involves inserting a hollow needle into the space between the third and fourth lumbar vertebrae. There is no danger of injuring the spinal cord with the needle in this area because the spinal cord ends at the first lumbar vertebra.

Peripheral Nervous System

The PNS consists of all the nerves that connect the CNS to every part of the body. Two main types of nerves are **motor** or **efferent** (ef′fer-ent) **nerves** and **sensory** or **afferent** (a′fer-ent) **nerves.**

- Motor nerves carry impulses from the CNS to organs, glands, and muscles.
- Sensory nerves carry impulses to the CNS from sensory receptors in various parts of the body.

Disorders and Diagnostic Tests

Examples of nervous system disorders and diagnostic tests are listed in Box 5-4.

ENDOCRINE SYSTEM

Functions

The word **endocrine** comes from the Greek words *endon,* meaning "within" and *krinein,* meaning "to secrete." The endocrine system (Fig. 5-11) consists of a group of ductless glands called **endocrine glands** that secrete substances called **hormones** directly into the bloodstream. Hormones are powerful chemical substances that have a profound effect on many body processes such as metabolism, growth and development, reproduction, personality, and the ability of the body to react to stress and resist disease.

Structures

Endocrine system structures include various hormone-secreting glands and other organs and structures that have endocrine function. The **pituitary (pi-tu′i-tar-ee) gland** is often called the master gland of this system because it secretes hormones that stimulate the other glands. However, release of hormones by the pituitary is actually controlled by chemicals called releasing hormones sent from the hypothalamus of the brain. Table 5-7 lists the various hormone-secreting glands and organs, their location in the body, the major hormones they secrete, and the principal function of each hormone.

 Identify the endocrine glands and have fun too with Labeling Exercise 5-10 in the WORKBOOK.

Box 5-4

Examples of Nervous System Disorders and Diagnostic Tests

Nervous System Disorders

Amyotrophic (a-mi″-o-tro′fik) lateral sclerosis (skle-ro′sis) (ALS): a disease involving muscle weakness and atrophy due to degeneration of portions of the brain and spinal cord

Encephalitis (en-sef-a-li′tis): inflammation of the brain

Epilepsy (ep′l-lep′se): recurrent pattern of seizures

Hydrocephalus (hi′dro-sef″a-lus): accumulation of cerebrospinal fluid in the brain

Meningitis (men-in-ji′tis): inflammation of the membranes of the spinal cord or brain

Multiple sclerosis (MS): disease involving destruction of the myelin sheath of CNS nerves

Neuralgia (nu′ral′je′a): severe pain along a nerve

Parkinson disease: chronic nervous disease characterized by fine muscle tremors and muscle weakness

Shingles (shing′gelz): acute eruption of herpes blisters along the course of a peripheral nerve

Tests for Nervous System Disorders

- Acetylcholine receptor antibody
- Cerebrospinal fluid (CSF) analysis
- Cell count
- Glucose
- Protein
- Culture
- Cholinesterase
- Dilantin (phenytoin)
- Electroencephalogram (EEG)
- Serotonin

Interesting facts about hormones:

- Adrenal hormones adrenaline and noradrenaline are known as the "fight-or-flight" hormones because of their effects when the body is under stress. They act by increasing blood pressure, heart activity, metabolism, and glucose release, permitting the body to do an extraordinary amount of work.

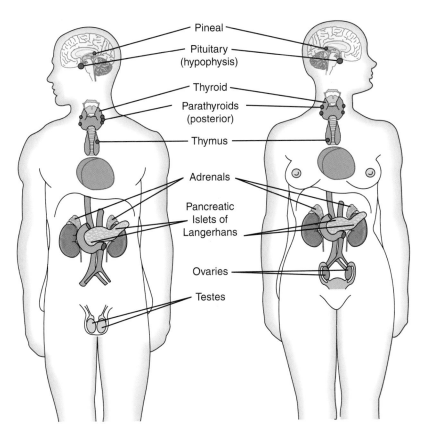

Figure 5-11 Endocrine system. (Adapted with permission from Cohen BJ. *Memmler's the Human Body in Health and Disease.* 12th ed. Philadelphia, PA: Lippincott Williams & Wilkins; 2013:267.)

- Because the pineal hormone melatonin plays a role in promoting sleep, travelers sometimes take melatonin pills to help overcome the effects of jet lag brought on by crossing different time zones.
- Production of thyroid hormones requires the presence of adequate amounts of iodine in the blood. Iodine was first added to salt to prevent goiter, an enlargement of the thyroid gland sometimes caused by the lack of iodine in the diet.

Other Structures with Endocrine Function

There are a number of other body structures with endocrine function. For example,

- the heart ventricles secrete a hormone called B-type natriuretic peptide (BNP) in response to volume expansion and pressure overload.
- the kidneys secrete erythropoietin (e-rith'ro-poy'e-tin) (EPO), which stimulates red blood cell production when oxygen levels are low.
- the lining of the stomach secretes a hormone that stimulates digestion.
- the placenta secretes several hormones that function during pregnancy.

Key Point Pregnancy tests are based on a reaction with a hormone called **human chorionic** (ko-re-on'ik) **gonadotropin** (gon-ah-do-tro'pin) (hCG) secreted by embryonic cells that eventually give rise to the placenta.

Disorders and Diagnostic Tests

Endocrine disorders are most commonly caused by tumors, which can cause either **hypersecretion** (secreting too much) or **hyposecretion** (secreting too little) by the gland. Diagnostic tests typically involve measuring hormone levels specific to the gland known or thought to be affected. Examples of diagnostic tests associated with the endocrine system are listed in Box 5-5.

DIGESTIVE SYSTEM

Functions

The digestive system (Fig. 5-12) provides the means by which the body takes in food, breaks it down into usable components for absorption, and eliminates waste products from this process.

Structures

The digestive system components form a continuous passageway called the digestive or **gastrointestinal (GI)**

Table 5-7: Endocrine Glands

Gland	Location	Hormone	Principal Function
Pituitary (pi-tu'i-tar-ee)	In the brain	Adrenocorticotropic (ad-re'no-kor'ti-ko-trop'ik) hormone (ACTH)	Stimulates the adrenal glands
		Antidiuretic (an'ti-di-u-ret'ik) hormone (ADH)	Decreases urine production
		Follicle-stimulating hormone (FSH)	Stimulates development of ova and sperm and the secretion of reproductive hormones
		Growth hormone (GH)	Regulates growth
		Thyroid-stimulating hormone (TSH)	Controls thyroid activity
Pineal (pin'eal)	In the brain, posterior to the pituitary	Melatonin	Helps set diurnal (daily) rhythm with levels lowest around noon and peaking at night; thought to play a role in seasonal affective disorder (SAD)
Thyroid (thi'royd)	In the throat near the larynx	Calcitonin (kal'si-to'nin)	Lowers blood calcium levels
		Triiodothyronine (tri-i-o-do-thi'ro-nin) or T_3	Increases metabolic rate
		Thyroxine (thi-roks'in) or T_4	Increases metabolic rate
Parathyroids (par-a-thi'royds)	In the throat behind the thyroid gland, two on each side	Parathyroid hormone (PTH)	Regulates calcium exchange between blood and bones; increases blood calcium levels
Thymus (thi'mus)	In the chest behind the sternum (breastbone)	Thymosin (thi'mo-sin)	Promotes maturation of specialized WBCs called T lymphocytes (T cells) and the development of immunity
Adrenals	One on top of each kidney	Epinephrine (ep-I-nef'rin), also called adrenalin (a-dren'a-lin)	Increases blood pressure, heart rate, metabolism, and release of glucose
		Norepinephrine, also called noradrenaline	Increases blood pressure, heart rate, metabolism, and release of glucose
		Cortisol (kor'ti-sol)	Active during stress, aids carbohydrate, protein, and fat metabolism
		Aldosterone (al-dos'ter-on)	Helps the kidneys regulate sodium and potassium in the bloodstream
Islets (i'lets) of Langerhans (lahng'er-hanz)	Pancreas	Insulin	Needed for movement of glucose into the cells and decreases blood glucose levels
		Glucagon (gloo'ka-gon)	Increases blood glucose levels by stimulating the liver to release glucose (stored as glycogen) into the bloodstream
Testes	Scrotum	Testosterone (tes-tos'ter-on)	Stimulates growth and functioning of the male reproductive system and development of male sexual characteristics
Ovaries	Pelvic cavity	Estrogens (es'tro-jens)	Stimulate growth and functioning of the female reproductive system and development of female sexual characteristics
		Progesterone (pro'jes-ter-on)	Prepares the body for pregnancy

Box 5-5

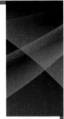

Examples of Endocrine System Disorders and Diagnostic Tests

Endocrine System Disorders

Pituitary Disorders

Acromegaly (ak'ro'meg'a'le): overgrowth of the bones in the hands, feet, and face caused by excessive GH in adulthood.

Diabetes insipidus (di'a'be'tez in'sip'id'us): condition characterized by increased thirst and urine production caused by inadequate secretion of ADH, also called vasopressin (vas'o'pres'in).

Dwarfism: condition of being abnormally small, one cause of which is growth hormone (GH) deficiency in infancy.

Gigantism: excessive development of the body or of a body part due to excessive GH.

Thyroid Disorders

Congenital hypothyroidism: insufficient thyroid activity in a newborn, either from a genetic deficiency or maternal factors such as lack of dietary iron during pregnancy.

Cretinism (kre'tin-izm): severe untreated congenital hypothyroidism in which the development of the child is impaired, resulting in a short, disproportionate body, thick tongue and neck, and mental handicap.

Goiter (goy'ter): enlargement of the thyroid gland.

Hyperthyroidism (Graves disease): condition characterized by weight loss, nervousness, and protruding eyeballs, due to an increased metabolic rate caused by excessive secretion of the thyroid gland.

Hypothyroidism: condition characterized by weight gain and lethargy due to a decreased metabolic rate caused by decreased thyroid secretion.

Myxedema (hypothyroid syndrome): condition characterized by anemia, slow speech, mental apathy, drowsiness, and sensitivity to cold resulting from decreased thyroid function.

Parathyroid Disorders

Kidney stones and bone destruction caused by hypersecretion of the parathyroids.

Muscle spasms and convulsions caused by hyposecretion of the parathyroids.

Adrenal Disorders

Addison disease: condition characterized by weight loss, dehydration, and hypotension (abnormally low blood pressure) caused by decreased glucose and sodium levels due to hyposecretion of the adrenal glands.

Aldosteronism: condition characterized by hypertension (high blood pressure) and edema caused by excessive sodium and water retention due to hypersecretion of aldosterone.

Cushing syndrome: condition characterized by a swollen, "moon-shaped" face and redistribution of fat to the abdomen and back of the neck caused by the excess of cortisone.

Pancreatic Disorders

Diabetes mellitus (di'a'be'tez mel-i-tus): a condition in which there is impaired carbohydrate, fat, and protein metabolism due to the deficiency of insulin.

Diabetes mellitus type I or insulin-dependent diabetes mellitus (IDDM): type of diabetes in which the body is unable to produce insulin. It is often called juvenile-onset diabetes because it usually appears before 25 years of age.

Diabetes mellitus type II or non–insulin-dependent diabetes mellitus (NIDDM): type of diabetes in which the body is able to produce insulin, but either the amount produced is insufficient or there is impaired use of the insulin produced. This type occurs predominantly in adults.

Hyperglycemia (hi"per-gli-se'me-a): increased blood sugar that often precedes diabetic coma if not treated.

Hyperinsulinism: too much insulin in the blood due to excessive secretion of insulin or an overdose of insulin (insulin shock).

Hypoglycemia (hi"po'gli'se'me'a): abnormally low glucose (blood sugar) often due to hyperinsulinism.

Tests for Endocrine System Disorders

- Adrenocorticotropic hormone (ACTH)
- Aldosterone
- Antidiuretic hormone (ADH)
- Cortisol
- Erythropoietin

- Glucagon
- Glucose tolerance test (GTT)
- Glycosylated hemoglobin
- Growth hormone (GH)
- Insulin level

- Thyroid function studies:
  - T_3 (Triiodothyronine)
  - T_4 (Thyroxine)
  - TSH (Thyroid-stimulating hormone)

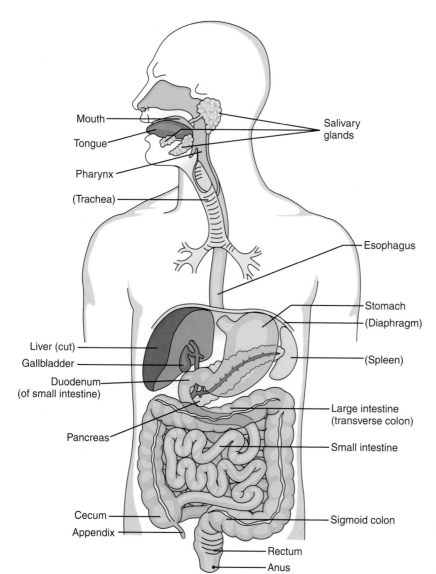

Mouth

Tongue

Pharynx

(Trachea)

Salivary glands

Esophagus

Stomach

(Diaphragm)

Liver (cut)

Gallbladder

Duodenum
(of small intestine)

(Spleen)

Pancreas

Large intestine
(transverse colon)

Small intestine

Cecum

Appendix

Sigmoid colon

Rectum

Anus

Figure 5-12 Digestive system. (Reprinted with permission from Cohen BJ. *Memmler's the Human Body in Health and Disease.* 12th ed. Philadelphia, PA: Lippincott Williams & Wilkins; 2013:413.)

tract, which extends from the mouth to the anus through the **pharynx, esophagus**, stomach, and small and large intestines.

> Grab your colored markers and do **Labeling Exercise 5-11 in the WORKBOOK to help you learn digestive system structures.**

Accessory Organs and Structures

The digestive system also includes and is assisted by a number of accessory organs and structures: lips, teeth, tongue, **salivary glands, liver, pancreas,** and **gallbladder**.

Accessory Organ Functions

The lips, teeth, and tongue help chew and swallow food. Salivary glands secrete saliva, which moistens food and

begins the process of starch digestion. Digestive functions of the liver include glycogen storage, protein catabolism, detoxifying harmful substances, and secreting bile needed for fat digestion. Bile is concentrated and stored in the gallbladder. The pancreas secretes insulin and glucagon and produces digestive enzymes, including **amylase, lipase,** and **trypsin**.

Disorders and Diagnostic Tests

Examples of disorders and diagnostic tests associated with the GI tract and accessory organs of the digestive system are listed in Box 5-6.

> Stomach ulcers, a common digestive system disorder, are sometimes caused by the *Helicobacter pylori* (*H. pylori*) microorganism and are treated with antibiotics in addition to antacids.

Box 5-6

Examples of Digestive System Disorders and Diagnostic Tests

Digestive System Disorders

Appendicitis (a'pen'di'si'tis): inflammation of the appendix

Cholecystitis (ko'le'sis'ti'tis): inflammation of the gallbladder

Colitis (ko'li'tis): inflammation of the colon

Diverticulosis (di'ver'tik'u'lo'sis): pouches in the walls of the colon

Gastritis (gas'tri'tis): inflammation of the stomach lining

Gastroenteritis (gas'tro'en'ter'i'tis): inflammation of the stomach and intestinal tract

Hepatitis (hep'a'ti'tis): inflammation of the liver

Pancreatitis (pan'kre'a'ti'tis): inflammation of the pancreas

Peritonitis (per'i'to'ni'tis): inflammation of the abdominal cavity lining

Ulcer: open sore or lesion

Tests for Digestive System Disorders

Tests for Gastrointestinal Tract Disorders

- C-urea breath test
- Fecal fat
- Gastric analysis
- Occult blood
- Ova and parasites (O&P)
- Serum gastrin analysis
- Stool analysis

Tests for Accessory Organ Disorders

- Ammonia
- Amylase
- Bilirubin (bili)
- Carcinoembryonic antigen (CEA)
- Carotene
- Cholesterol
- Complete blood count (CBC)
- Glucose
- Glucose tolerance test (GTT)
- Lipase
- Triglycerides

REPRODUCTIVE SYSTEM

Functions

The reproductive system (Fig. 5-13) produces the **gametes** (gam'eets), **sex** or **germ cells,** that are needed to form a new human being. In males, the gametes are called **spermatozoa** (sper'mat-o-zo'a), or sperm. In females, the gametes are called **ova** (o'va), or eggs. Reproduction occurs when an **ovum** (singular of ova) is fertilized by a sperm.

Key Point Two chromosomes (called X and Y) determine gender. Every egg contains an X chromosome only. Every sperm contains either an X or a Y chromosome. If an egg is fertilized by a sperm containing an X chromosome, the XX chromosome combination will result in a female fetus. If an egg is fertilized by a sperm containing a Y chromosome, the XY chromosome combination will result in a male fetus.

Structures

The reproductive system consists of glands called **gonads** (go'nads) and their associated structures and ducts. The gonads manufacture and store the gametes and produce hormones that regulate the reproductive process.

Structures of the female reproductive system include the ovaries (female gonads), fallopian (fa-lo'pe-an) tubes, uterus, cervix, vagina, and vulva.

Boost your ability to identify reproductive system structures by doing Labeling Exercise 5-12 in the WORKBOOK.

The PAP smear, a procedure used to diagnose cervical cancer, is named after George Papanicolaou, who developed the technique.

Structures of the male reproductive system include the testes (male gonads), seminal vesicles, prostate, epididymis (ep'i-did'i-mis), vas deferens (vas def'er-enz), seminal ducts, urethra, penis, spermatic cords, and scrotum.

Disorders and Diagnostic Tests

Examples of disorders and diagnostic tests associated with the reproductive system are listed in Box 5-7.

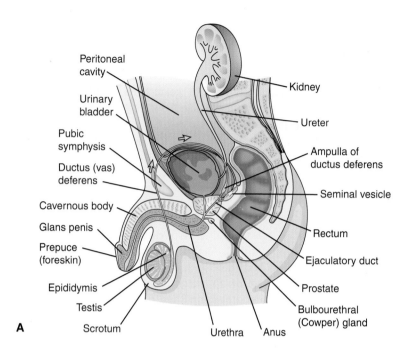

Peritoneal cavity

Urinary bladder

Pubic symphysis

Ductus (vas) deferens

Cavernous body

Glans penis

Prepuce (foreskin)

Epididymis

Testis

Scrotum

Urethra

Anus

Kidney

Ureter

Ampulla of ductus deferens

Seminal vesicle

Rectum

Ejaculatory duct

Prostate

Bulbourethral (Cowper) gland

A

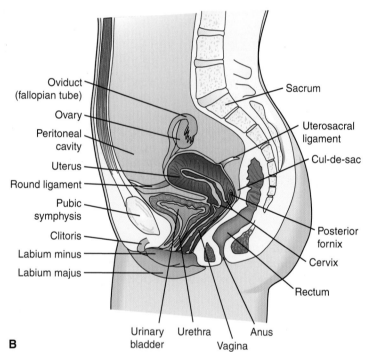

Oviduct (fallopian tube)

Ovary

Peritoneal cavity

Uterus

Round ligament

Pubic symphysis

Clitoris

Labium minus

Labium majus

Sacrum

Uterosacral ligament

Cul-de-sac

Posterior fornix

Cervix

Rectum

Urinary bladder

Urethra

Vagina

Anus

B

Figure 5-13 Reproductive system. **A:** Male. **B:** Female. (Reprinted with permission from Cohen BJ. *Memmler's the Human Body in Health and Disease.* 12th ed. Philadelphia, PA: Lippincott Williams & Wilkins; 2013:515, 523.)

URINARY SYSTEM

Functions

The urinary system (Fig. 5-14) filters waste products from the blood and eliminates them from the body. It also plays an important role in the regulation of body fluids. Activities of the urinary system result in the creation and elimination of urine.

Structures

The main structures of the urinary system are two **kidneys,** two **ureters,** a **urinary bladder,** and a **urethra.**

> **Labeling Exercise 5-14 in the WORKBOOK can help you learn the urinary system structures.**

The kidneys are bean-shaped organs located at the back of the abdominal cavity, just above the waistline, one on each side of the body. The kidneys help maintain water and electrolyte balance and eliminate urea (a waste product of protein metabolism). They also produce EPO, a hormone that stimulates red blood cell

Box 5-7

Examples of Reproductive System Disorders and Diagnostic Tests

Reproductive System Disorders

Cervical cancer: cancer of the cervix
Infertility: lower than normal ability to reproduce
Ovarian cancer: cancer of the ovaries
Ovarian cyst: a usually nonmalignant growth
in an ovary
Prostate cancer: cancer of the prostate gland
Sexually transmitted diseases (STDs):
diseases such as syphilis, gonorrhea, and
genital herpes, which are usually transmit-
ted by sexual contact
Uterine cancer: cancer of the uterus

Tests for Reproductive System Disorders

- Acid phosphatase
- Estrogen
- Follicle-stimulating hormone (FSH)
- Human chorionic gonadotropin (hCG)
- Luteinizing hormone (LH)
- Microbiological cultures
- PAP smear
- Prostate-specific antigen (PSA)
- Rapid plasmin reagin (RPR)
- Testosterone
- Viral tissue studies

production, and the enzyme renin, which plays a role in regulating blood pressure.

 Electrolytes include sodium, potassium, chloride, bicarbonate, and calcium ions; they are essential to normal nerve, muscle, and heart activities.

The basic working unit of the kidney is the **nephron**, of which each kidney contains nearly a million. As blood travels through a nephron, water and dissolved substances including wastes are filtered from it through a tuft of capillaries called the **glomerulus** (pl. glomeruli). The resulting glomerular filtrate travels through other structures within the nephron, where water and essential amounts of substances such as sodium, potassium, and calcium are reabsorbed into the bloodstream. The remaining filtrate is called urine.

Urine is transported from the kidney via a narrow tube called a ureter, and delivered to the urinary bladder, located in the anterior portion of the pelvic cavity. There it is stored until voided (emptied from the bladder to the outside of the body through a single tube called the urethra).

Key Point Blood creatinine is a measure of kidney function because creatinine is a waste product removed from the blood by the kidneys. If kidney function declines, creatinine accumulates in the blood.

Disorders and Diagnostic Tests

Examples of disorders and diagnostic tests associated with the urinary system are listed in Box 5-8.

Box 5-8

Urinary System Disorders and Diagnostic Tests

Urinary System Disorders

Cystitis (sis-ti'tis): bladder inflammation
Kidney stones: uric acid, calcium phosphate,
or oxalate stones in the kidneys, ureter, or
bladder
Nephritis (nef-ri'tis): inflammation of the kidneys
Renal (re'nal) failure: sudden and severe
impairment of renal function
Uremia (u-re'me-a): impaired kidney function
with a buildup of waste products in the blood
Urinary (u'ri-nar"e) tract infection (UTI): infection
involving urinary system organs or ducts

Tests for Urinary System Disorders

- Albumin
- Carnitine, total and free
- Creatinine clearance
- Creatinine, serum
- Creatinine, 24-hour urine
- Electrolytes
- Glomerular filtration rate, estimated (eGFR)
- Intravenous pyelography (IVP)
- Kidney function profile
- Osmolality, serum and urine
- Renal biopsy
- Renin activity
- Urea nitrogen, serum
- Urinalysis (UA), routine profile
- Urine culture, comprehensive
- Urine culture and sensitivity (C&S)

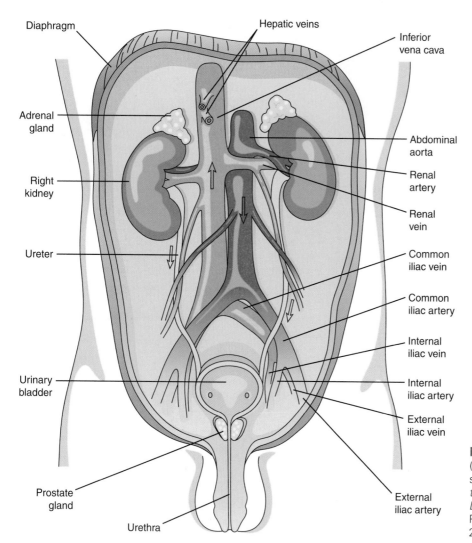

Diaphragm
Hepatic veins
Inferior vena cava
Adrenal gland
Abdominal aorta
Renal artery
Right kidney
Renal vein
Ureter
Common iliac vein
Common iliac artery
Internal iliac vein
Internal iliac artery
Urinary bladder
External iliac vein
Prostate gland
External iliac artery
Urethra

Figure 5-14 Urinary system (male). (Reprinted with permission from Cohen BJ. *Memmler's the Human Body in Health and Disease.* 12th ed. Philadelphia, PA: Lippincott Williams & Wilkins; 2013:490.)

Knowledge Drill 5-3 in the WORKBOOK will help you see how well you are grasping knowledge of the body systems.

RESPIRATORY SYSTEM

Functions

The respiratory system (Fig. 5-15A) delivers a constant supply of oxygen (O_2) to all the cells of the body and removes carbon dioxide (CO_2), a waste product of cell metabolism. This is accomplished with the help of the circulatory system through respiration.

Respiration

Respiration permits the exchange of the gases O_2 and CO_2 between the blood and the air and involves two processes, **external respiration** and **internal respiration**. External respiration occurs as a person breathes in and air travels to the lungs where O_2 from the air enters the bloodstream in the lungs. At the same time,

CO_2 leaves the bloodstream in the lungs and is breathed into the air as the person exhales. During internal respiration, O_2 leaves the bloodstream and enters the cells in the tissues, and CO_2 from the cells enters the bloodstream. The circulatory system is the means by which O_2 is transported from the lungs to the tissues and CO_2 is transported from the tissues to the lungs.

Although the nose is the main airway for external respiration, some air enters and leaves through the mouth.

Gas Exchange and Transport

During normal external respiration (Fig. 5-16), O_2 and CO_2 are able to diffuse (go from an area of higher concentration to an area of lower concentration) through the walls of the air sacs and the capillaries of the lungs. Blood in lung capillaries is low in O_2 and high in CO_2. Therefore, O_2 from the alveoli diffuses into the capillaries

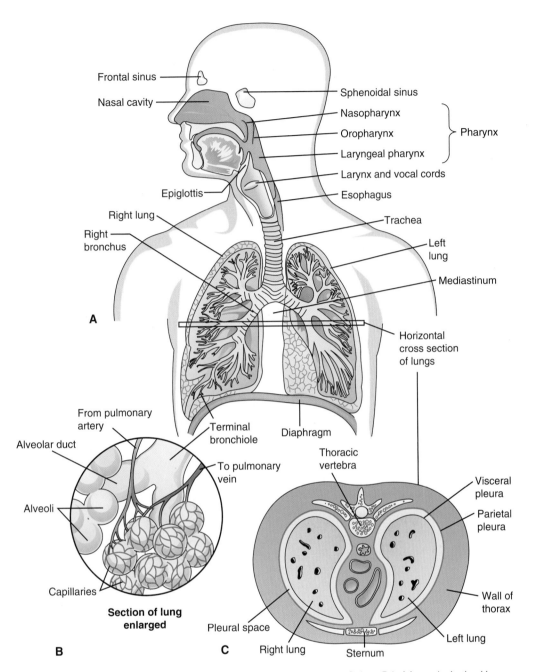

Figure 5-15 Respiratory system. (Adapted with permission from Cohen BJ. *Memmler's the Human Body in Health and Disease.* 12th ed. Philadelphia, PA: Lippincott Williams & Wilkins; 2013:403.)

while CO_2 diffuses from the capillaries (Figs. 5-15B and 5-16A) into the alveoli to be expired (breathed out).

thePoint. *View the Gas Exchange in Alveoli and Oxygen Transport animations at http://thepoint.lww. com/McCall6e.*

The amount of O_2 that can be dissolved in the blood plasma is not enough to meet the needs of the body. Fortunately, hemoglobin (a protein in red blood cells) is able to bind O_2, increasing the amount the blood can carry by more than 70%. Consequently, very little of the

O_2 that diffuses into the lung capillaries dissolves in the plasma, most of it binds to hemoglobin molecules. O_2 combined with hemoglobin is called **oxyhemoglobin**.

Hemoglobin can also bind with CO_2. When it does, it is called **carbaminohemoglobin**. About 20% of CO_2 from the tissues is carried to the lungs in this manner. Approximately 10% is carried as gas dissolved in the blood plasma. The remaining 70% is carried as **bicarbonate ion,** which is formed in the red blood cells and released into the blood plasma. In the lungs, the bicarbonate ion reenters the red blood cells and is

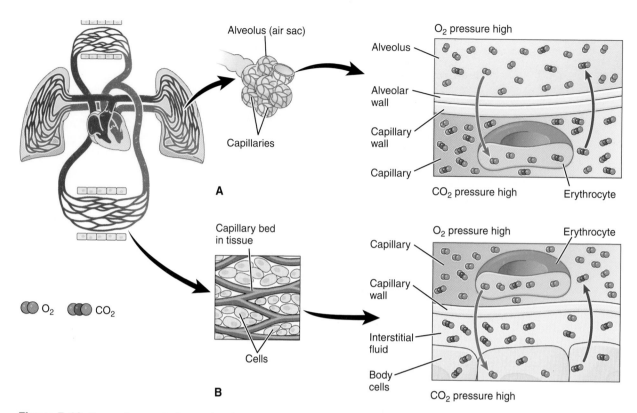

Figure 5-16 Gas exchange. **A:** External exchange between the alveoli and the blood. Oxygen diffuses into the blood and carbon dioxide diffuses out, based on concentration of the two gases in the alveoli and the blood. **B:** Internal exchange between the blood and the cells. Oxygen diffuses out of the blood and into the tissues, while carbon dioxide diffuses from the cells into the blood. (Reprinted with permission from Cohen BJ. *Memmler's the Human Body in Health and Disease*. 12th ed. Philadelphia, PA: Williams & Wilkins; 2013:410.)

released as CO_2 again, which diffuses into the alveoli and is exhaled by the body.

Whether oxygen associates (combines) with or disassociates (releases) from hemoglobin depends upon the partial pressure (P) of each gas. Partial pressure is the pressure exerted by one gas in a mixture of gases. Oxygen combines with hemoglobin in the lungs, where the **partial pressure of oxygen (Po_2)** is increased, and releases from hemoglobin in the tissues, where the Po_2 is decreased. Carbon dioxide combines with hemoglobin in the tissues, where the **partial pressure of carbon dioxide (Pco_2)** is increased, and releases from hemoglobin in the lungs, where the Pco_2 is decreased.

Acid–Base Balance

CO_2 levels play a major role in the acid–base (pH) balance of the blood. If CO_2 levels increase, blood pH decreases (i.e., becomes more acidic), which can lead to a dangerous condition called **acidosis**. The body responds by increasing the rate of respiration (hyperventilation) to increase O_2 levels. Prolonged hyperventilation causes a decrease in CO_2, resulting in an increase in pH (i.e., the blood is more alkaline) and a condition called **alkalosis**. During normal respiratory function, the bicarbonate ion acts as a buffer to keep the blood pH within a steady range from 7.35 to 7.45.

Structures

Respiratory Tract

The major structures of the respiratory system are the nose, **pharynx** (throat), **larynx** (voice box), **trachea** (windpipe), **bronchi**, and **lungs**. These structures form the respiratory tract, a continuous pathway for the flow of air to and from the air sacs in the lungs. Table 5-8 describes the major respiratory tract structures in the order of the flow of air to the lungs.

> **Test your ability to identify respiratory system structures with Labeling Exercise 5-15 in the WORKBOOK.**

Lungs

The human body has two lungs, a right with three lobes and a left with only two lobes, which leaves space for the heart. The lungs are encased in a thin double-layered membrane called the **pleura**. A tiny space between the layer that covers the lungs and the one that lines the inner thoracic cavity is called the **pleural space** or cavity (See Fig. 5-15C).

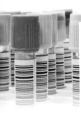

Table 5-8: Major Structures of Respiratory Tract

Structure	Description/Function	Flow of Air to the Lungs
Nose	Provides the main airway for respiration; warms, moistens, and filters air; provides a resonance chamber for the voice; and contains receptors for the sense of smell	Air enters the nose through the nares (nostrils) and passes through the nasal cavities into the pharynx
Pharynx	A funnel-shaped passageway that receives food from the mouth and delivers it to the esophagus and air from the nose and carries it into the larynx. (A thin, leaf-shaped structure called the epiglottis covers the entrance of the larynx during swallowing.)	Air enters the upper end of the pharynx, called the nasopharynx, and exits via the laryngeal pharynx that opens into the larynx
Larynx	The enlarged upper end of the trachea that houses the vocal cords, the ends of which mark the division between the upper and lower respiratory tracts	Air passes through the larynx into the lower trachea
Trachea	A tube that extends from the larynx into the upper part of the chest and carries air to the lungs	Air moves through the trachea into the bronchi in the lungs
Lungs	Organs that house the bronchial branches and the alveoli where gas exchange takes place	Air moves throughout the lungs within the bronchi
Bronchi (singular, bronchus)	Two airways that branch off the lower end of the trachea and lead into the lungs; one branch each into the left and right lungs, where they subdivide into secondary bronchi that divide into smaller and smaller branches	Air moves through the branches of the bronchi, referred to as the *bronchial tree,* until it reaches the terminal bronchioles
Terminal bronchioles	The smallest divisions of the bronchi, the ends of which contain the alveoli	Air flows out of the terminal bronchioles into the alveoli
Alveoli (singular, alveolus)	Tiny air sacs covered with blood capillaries where the exchange of gases in the lungs takes place	Oxygen leaves the alveoli and enters the capillaries. Carbon dioxide leaves the capillaries and enters the alveoli to be expired

Fluid within the pleural cavity (pleural fluid) helps keep the lungs expanded by reducing surface tension. It also helps prevent friction as the lungs expand and contract.

Alveoli

The **alveoli** (al-ve'o-li) (singular alveolus) are tiny air sacs in the lungs where the exchange of oxygen and carbon dioxide takes place. The walls of the alveoli are a single layer of squamous (flat) epithelial cells surrounded by a thin membrane. The thinness of the walls allows gases to easily pass between the alveoli and the blood in the tiny capillaries that cover them. Because the thin walls would ordinarily be prone to collapse,

they have a coating of fluid called **surfactant** that lowers the surface tension (or pull) on the walls and helps to stabilize them.

 Key Point A deficiency of surfactant in premature infants causes the alveoli to collapse, leading to a condition called **infant respiratory distress syndrome,** or IRDS. Premature infants can be given animal-derived or synthetic surfactant through inhalation in an effort to treat this life-threatening condition.

Disorders and Diagnostic Tests

Examples of disorders and diagnostic tests associated with the respiratory system are listed in Box 5-9.

Box 5-9

Examples of Respiratory System Disorders and Diagnostic Tests

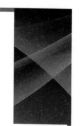

Respiratory System Disorders

Apnea (ap'ne'ah): a temporary cessation of breathing

Asthma (az'ma): difficulty in breathing accompanied by wheezing caused by spasm or swelling of the bronchial tubes

Bronchitis (brong-ki'tis): inflammation of the mucous membrane of the bronchial tubes

Cystic fibrosis (sis'tik fi-bro'sis): genetic endocrine disease causing an excess production of mucus

Dyspnea (disp'ne'ah): difficult or labored breathing

Emphysema (em'fi-se'ma): chronic obstructive pulmonary disease (COPD)

Hypoxia (hi'pok'se'ah): deficiency of oxygen

Infant respiratory distress syndrome (IRDS): severe impairment of respiratory function in the newborn due to a lack of surfactant in the baby's lungs

Pleurisy (ploo'ris-e): inflammation of the pleural membrane

Pneumonia (nu-mo'ne-a): inflammation of the lungs

Pulmonary edema (pul'mo-ne-re e-de'ma): accumulation of fluid in the lungs

Respiratory syncytial (sin'si'shal) virus: major cause of respiratory distress in infants and children

Rhinitis (ri-ni'tis): inflammation of the nasal mucous membranes

Tonsillitis (ton-sil-i'tis): infection of the tonsils

Tuberculosis (tu-ber"ku-lo'sis) (TB): infectious respiratory system disease caused by the bacteria *Mycobacterium tuberculosis*

Upper respiratory infection (URI): infection of the nose, throat, larynx, or upper trachea such as that caused by a cold virus

Tests for Respiratory System Disorders

- Acid fast bacillus (AFB) culture/smear
- Arterial blood gases (ABG)
- Capillary blood gases (CBG)
- Complete blood count (CBC)
- Cocci (IgG/IgM)
- Drug levels

- Electrolytes (lytes)
- Microbiology cultures
- Pleuracentesis
- Skin tests: PPD (tuberculin or TB test)
- Sputum culture
- Bronchial washings

Study and Review Questions

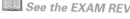 *See the EXAM REVIEW for more study questions.*

1. **The transverse plane divides the body**

   a. diagonally into upper and lower portions.

   b. horizontally into upper and lower portions.

   c. vertically into front and back portions.

   d. vertically into right and left portions.

2. **Proximal is defined as**

   a. away from the middle.

   b. closest to the middle.

   c. farthest from the center.

   d. nearest to the point of attachment.

3. **The process by which the body maintains a state of equilibrium is**

   a. anabolism.

   b. catabolism.

   c. homeostasis.

   d. venostasis.

4. **Which part of a cell contains the chromosomes or genetic material?**

   a. Cytoplasm

   b. Golgi apparatus

   c. Nucleus

   d. Organelles

5. **What type of muscle lines the walls of blood vessels?**
   a. Cardiac
   b. Skeletal
   c. Striated
   d. Visceral

6. **Which of the following is an accessory organ of the digestive system?**
   a. Heart
   b. Liver
   c. Lung
   d. Ovary

7. **Evaluation of the endocrine system involves**
   a. blood gas studies.
   b. drug monitoring.
   c. hormone determinations.
   d. spinal fluid analysis.

8. **The spinal cord and brain are covered by protective membranes called**
   a. meninges.
   b. neurons.
   c. papillae.
   d. viscera.

9. **Sudoriferous glands are**
   a. connected to hair follicles.
   b. endocrine system structures.
   c. referred to as sweat glands.
   d. responsible for goose bumps.

10. **Most gas exchange between blood and tissue takes place in the**
    a. arterioles.
    b. capillaries.
    c. pulmonary vein.
    d. venules.

Case Studies

 See the WORKBOOK for more case studies.

Case Study 5-1: Body System Structures and Disorders

A college student found that she was studying many hours a day after she arrived home and did most of it on the floor leaning on her elbows. She found no time to exercise except weekends, when she hit the pavement for 10 or more miles both days because she loved running and had been a marathon runner in the past. On Monday mornings, she would experience pain in her leg muscles and tendons. After a few months, she noticed a very large fluid-filled sac on her elbow.

QUESTIONS

1. What are the names of the conditions she is experiencing in her leg muscles and tendons?
2. What is that fluid-filled sac on her elbow called and why is it there?
3. What most likely caused her problems?

Case Study 5-2: Body Systems, Disorders, Diagnostic Tests, and Directional Terms

A phlebotomist responded to a call from the ER to collect stat glucose and insulin levels on a patient. The patient was unconscious, but the patient's husband granted permission for the blood draw. The patient had an IV in the left arm and a pulmonary function technician had just collected ABGs in the right wrist, so the phlebotomist elected to draw the sample distal to the IV.

QUESTIONS

1. What body systems of the patient are being evaluated?
2. What is most likely wrong with the patient?
3. Where did the phlebotomist collect the specimen?

Bibliography and Suggested Readings

Cohen BJ. *Memmler's the Human Body in Health and Disease.* 12th ed. Philadelphia, PA: Lippincott Williams & Wilkins; 2013.

Cohen BJ, Taylor JJ. *Memmler's Structure and Function of the Human Body.* 10th ed. Philadelphia, PA: Lippincott Williams & Wilkins; 2013.

Fischbach FT, Dunning MB. *Laboratory Diagnostic Tests.* 9th ed. Philadelphia, PA: Lippincott Williams & Wilkins; 2014.

Herlihy B. *The Human Body in Health and Illness.* 4th ed. Philadelphia, PA: Saunders; 2011.

Moore KL, Argur AM, Dalley AF. *Clinically Oriented Anatomy.* 7th ed. Philadelphia, PA: Wolters Kluwer/Lippincott Williams & Wilkins; 2014.

Stedman's Medical Dictionary for the Health Professions and Nursing. 7th ed. Philadelphia, PA: Lippincott Williams & Wilkins; 2011.

Turgeon ML. *Linne & Ringsrud's Clinical Laboratory Science: The Basics and Routine Techniques.* 6th ed. St. Louis, MO: Mosby/Elsevier; 2011.

Venes MD. *Taber's Cyclopedic Medical Dictionary.* 22nd ed. Philadelphia, PA: Davis; 2013.

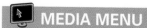

MEDIA MENU

Online Ancillaries (at http://thepoint.lww.com/McCall6e)
- Animations:
- Gas Exchange in Alveoli
- Oxygen Transport
- Interactive exercises and games, including Look and Label, Word Building, Body Building, Roboterms, Crossword Puzzles, Quiz Show, and Concentration
- Audio Flash Cards and Flashcard Generator
- Audio Glossary

Internet Resources
- Anatomy Arcade. http://www.anatomyarcade.com
- GetBodySmart.com. http://www.getbodysmart.com/ap/site/resourcelinks/links.html
- free-ed.net™, free education on the Internet. http://www.free-ed.net/free-ed/FreeEdmain01.asp
- Human Anatomy online. http://ect.downstate.edu/courseware/haonline/index.htm
- National Institute of Diabetes and Digestive and Kidney Diseases. http://www2.niddk.nih.gov/

Other Resources
- McCall R, Tankersley C. *Student Workbook for Phlebotomy Essentials.* 6th ed. (Available for separate purchase.)
- McCall R, Tankersley C. *Phlebotomy Exam Review.* 6th ed. (Available for separate purchase.)

Chapter 6

The Circulatory System

NAACLS Entry Level Competencies

3.00 Demonstrate basic understanding of the anatomy and physiology of body systems and anatomic terminology in order to relate major areas of the clinical laboratory to general pathologic conditions associated with the body systems.

3.1 Describe the basic functions of each of the main body systems, and demonstrate basic knowledge of the circulatory, urinary, and other body systems necessary to perform assigned specimen collection.

3.2 Identify the veins of the arms and hands on which phlebotomy is performed.

3.3 Explain the functions of the major constituents of blood, and differentiate between whole blood, serum, and plasma.

3.4 Define hemostasis.

3.5 Describe the stages of coagulation.

3.6 Discuss the properties of arterial blood, venous blood, and capillary blood.

Key Terms

Do Matching Exercise 6-1 in the WORKBOOK to gain familiarity with these terms.

antecubital
arrhythmia
atria
basilic vein
blood pressure
cardiac cycle
cephalic vein
coagulation
cross match

diastole
ECG/EKG
erythrocyte
extrinsic
fibrinolysis
hemostasis
intrinsic
leukocyte

median cubital
vein
plasma
pulmonary
circulation
serum
sphygmoma-
nometer

systemic
circulation
systole
thrombin
thrombocyte
vasoconstriction
ventricles

Objectives

Upon successful completion of this chapter, the reader should be able to:

1 Demonstrate basic knowledge of the terminology, structures, functions, organization, and processes of the circulatory system.

2 Discuss the cardiac cycle, how an ECG tracing relates to it, the origins of heart sounds and pulse rates, and how to take and interpret blood pressure readings.

3 Distinguish between the different types of blood vessels and blood components, and describe the structure and function of each, identify blood types and explain their importance, and trace the flow of blood throughout the circulatory system.

4 Name and locate major arm and leg veins and evaluate the suitability of each for venipuncture.

5 List the disorders and diagnostic tests of the circulatory system.

Overview

The **circulatory system** carries oxygen and food to the cells of the body and carries carbon dioxide and other wastes away from the cells to the excretory organs, kidneys, lungs, and skin. It also aids in the coagulation process, assists in defending the body against disease, and plays an important role in the regulation of body temperature. A thorough knowledge of this system is especially important to the phlebotomist, who must access it to collect blood specimens for analysis. It also helps the phlebotomist appreciate the importance of the many tests associated with it. This chapter covers the two main components of the circulatory system—the cardiovascular system (heart, blood vessels, and blood) and the lymphatic system (lymph vessels, lymph nodes, and lymph) and describes the structures, functions, disorders, and diagnostic tests associated with them, including the coagulation process, which helps protect the system from blood loss.

The Heart

The heart (Fig. 6-1) is the major structure of the circulatory system. It is the "pump" that circulates blood throughout the body. It is located in the center of the thoracic cavity between the lungs, with the apex (tip) pointing down and to the left of the body.

HEART STRUCTURE

The heart is a four-chambered, hollow, muscular organ that is slightly larger than a man's closed fist. It is surrounded by a thin fluid-filled sac called the **pericardium** (per'i-kar'de-um), and its walls have three distinct layers. The heart has two sides, a right and a left. Each side has two chambers, an upper and a lower. One-way valves between the chambers help prevent the backflow of blood and keep it moving through the heart in the right direction. The right and left chambers are separated from each other by partitions called **septa** (singular, **septum**).

> After you finish this section, grab some colored pencils and check out WORKBOOK Labeling Exercise 6-1.

Layers

The three layers of the heart (Table 6-1) are the **epicardium** (ep'-i-kar'de-um), the thin outer layer; the **myocardium** (mi-o-kar'de-um), the middle muscle layer; and **endocardium** (en'do-kar'de-um), the thin inner layer.

Chambers

The upper chambers on each side of the heart are called **atria** (a'tre-a), and the lower chambers are called **ventricles** (ven'trik-ls). The atria (singular, atrium) are receiving chambers, and the ventricles are pumping or delivering chambers. The location and function of the chambers of the heart are described in Table 6-2.

Valves

The valves at the entrance to the ventricles are called **atrioventricular** (a'tre-o-ven-trik'u-lar) **(AV) valves**.

> ⓘ The atrioventricular valves are attached to the walls of the ventricles by thin threads of tissue called **chordae** (kor'de) **tendineae** (ten-din'e-e), which keep the valves from flipping back into the atria.

The valves that exit the ventricles are called **semilunar** (sem'e-lu'nar) **valves** because they are crescent-shaped like a half moon (*semi* is Latin for *half; luna* is Latin for *moon*). See Table 6-3 to read more about the location, description, and function of the valves.

> ⓘ The term mitral valve comes from its resemblance to a miter, the pointed, two-sided hat worn by bishops.

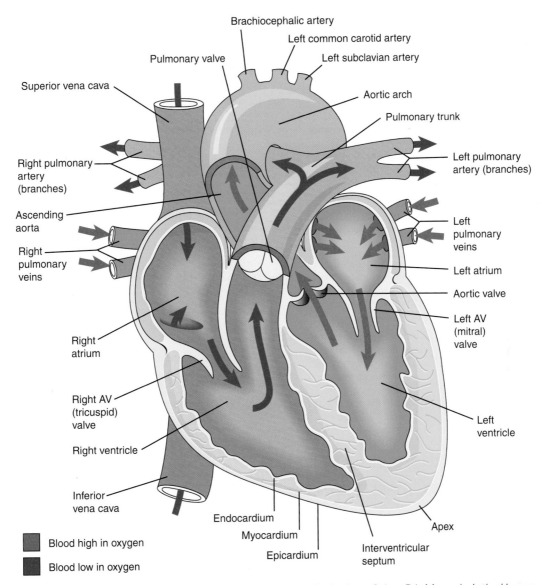

Figure 6-1 The heart and great vessels. (Adapted with permission from Cohen BJ. *Memmler's the Human Body in Health and Disease*. 12th ed. Philadelphia, PA: Lippincott Williams & Wilkins; 2013:314.)

Septa

There are two partitions separating the right and left sides of the heart. The partition that separates the right and left atria is called the **interatrial** (in-ter-a'tre-al) **septum**. The partition that separates the right and left ventricles is called the **interventricular** (in-ter-ven-trik'u-lar) **septum**. Each septum consists mostly of myocardium.

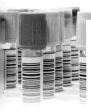

Table 6-1: Layers of the Heart

Layer	Location	Description	Function
Epicardium	Outer layer of the heart	Thin, serous (watery) membrane that is continuous with the lining of the pericardium	Covers the heart and attaches to the pericardium
Myocardium	Middle layer of the heart	Thick layer of cardiac muscle	Contracts to pump blood into the arteries
Endocardium	Inner layer of the heart	Thin layer of epithelial cells that is continuous with the lining of the blood vessels	Lines the interior chambers and valves

Table 6-2: Chambers of the Heart

Chamber	Location	Function
Right atrium	Upper right chamber	Receives deoxygenated blood from the body via both the superior (upper) vena cava (ve'na ka'va) and inferior (lower) vena cava (plural, venae cavae) and pumps it into the right ventricle.
Right ventricle	Lower right chamber	Receives blood from the right atrium and pumps it into the pulmonary artery, which carries it to the lungs to be oxygenated.
Left atrium	Upper left chamber	Receives oxygenated blood from the lungs via the pulmonary veins and pumps it into the left ventricle.
Left ventricle	Lower left chamber	Receives blood from the left atrium and pumps it into the aorta (a-or'ta). The walls of the left ventricle are nearly three times as thick as those of the right ventricle owing to the force required to pump the blood into the arterial system.

Coronary Circulation

The heart muscle does not receive nourishment or oxygen from blood passing through the heart. It receives its blood supply via the right and left **coronary (also called cardiac) arteries**, which branch off of the aorta, just beyond the aortic semilunar valve.

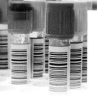 Corona means circle or crown. It is said that the coronary arteries are so named because they encircle the heart like a crown.

Any impairment of the coronary circulation is a dangerous situation. Partial obstruction of a coronary artery or one of its branches can reduce blood flow to a point where it is not adequate to meet the oxygen needs of the heart muscle, a condition called myocardial **ischemia** (is-kee'me-ah). Complete obstruction or prolonged ischemia leads to **myocardial** (mi'o-kar'de-al) **infarction** (MI) or "heart attack," because of necrosis (ne-kro'sis) or death of the surrounding tissue from lack of oxygen.

The buildup of fatty plaque from a condition called atherosclerosis can lead to severe narrowing of coronary arteries. This condition is sometimes treated by using a coronary bypass procedure. In this surgical procedure, a vein (commonly the saphenous vein from the leg) is grafted onto the artery to divert the blood around the affected area.

Coronary (cardiac) veins return oxygen-poor blood from the heart muscle back to the heart. Most coronary veins merge into a structure called the coronary sinus, which delivers the blood to the right atrium. Some coronary veins empty directly into one of the chambers of the heart.

HEART FUNCTION

Cardiac Cycle

thePoint **View the Cardiac Cycle animation at http://thepoint.lww.com/McCall6e.**

One complete contraction and subsequent relaxation of the heart lasts about 0.8 seconds and is called a **cardiac cycle**. The contracting phase of the cardiac cycle is called **systole** (sis'to-le), and the relaxing phase is called **diastole** (di-as'to-le).

Table 6-3: Heart Valves

Valve	Location	Description	Function
Right AV valve (also called the tricuspid [tri-kus'pid] valve)	Between the right atrium and right ventricle	Has three cusps (flaps), hence the name *tricuspid*	Closes when the right ventricle contracts and prevents blood from flowing back into the right atrium
Left AV valve (also called the bicuspid or mitral valve)	Between the left atrium and left ventricle	Has two cusps, hence the name *bicuspid*	Closes when the left ventricle contracts and prevents blood from flowing back into the left atrium
Right semilunar valve (also called pulmonary or pulmonic valve)	At the entrance to the pulmonary artery	Has three half-moon–shaped cusps	Closes when the right ventricle relaxes and prevents blood from flowing back into the right ventricle
Left semilunar valve (also called aortic valve)	At the entrance to the aorta	Has three half-moon–shaped cusps	Closes when the left ventricle relaxes and prevents blood from flowing back into the left ventricle

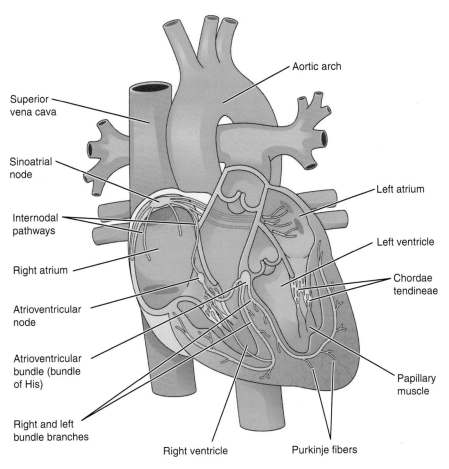

Aortic arch

Superior vena cava

Sinoatrial node

Internodal pathways

Right atrium

Atrioventricular node

Atrioventricular bundle (bundle of His)

Right and left bundle branches

Right ventricle

Left atrium

Left ventricle

Chordae tendineae

Papillary muscle

Purkinje fibers

Figure 6-2 The electrical conduction system of the heart. The sinoatrial (SA) node, the atrioventricular (AV) node, and specialized fibers conduct electrical energy that stimulates the heart muscle to contract. (Adapted with permission from Cohen BJ. *Memmler's the Human Body in Health and Disease.* 12th ed. Philadelphia, PA: Lippincott Williams & Wilkins; 2013:318.)

Electrical Conduction System

To be effective at pumping blood, the heart's contractions must be synchronized (coordinated) so that both atria contract simultaneously, followed by contraction of both ventricles. Synchronization is achieved by means of specialized muscle cells that form the electrical conduction system (Fig. 6-2). Instead of contracting, these cells act like nerve tissue in that they initiate and distribute electrical impulses throughout the myocardium to coordinate the cardiac cycle. These specialized tissues create an electrical conduction system pathway that includes two tissue masses called nodes and a network of specialized fibers that branch throughout the myocardium. Cardiac contraction is initiated by an electrical impulse generated from the **sinoatrial** (sin'o-a'tre-al) **node**, or SA node, also called the **pacemaker**, at the start of the pathway. The electrical conduction system pathway is described in Table 6-4.

Table 6-4: The Electrical Conduction System Pathway

Structure	Location	Function
Sinoatrial (SA) node	Upper wall of the right atrium	Begins the heartbeat by generating the electrical pulse that travels through the muscles of both atria, causing them to contract simultaneously and push blood through the atrioventricular (AV) valves into the ventricles
Internodal pathway fibers	Wall of the right atrium	Relay the impulse to the AV node
AV node	Bottom of the right atrium in the interatrial septum	Picks up the impulse, slows it down while the atria finish contracting, and then relays it through the AV bundle (bundle of His)
AV bundle (bundle of His)	Top of the interventricular septum	Relays impulse throughout the ventricular walls by means of bundle branches and Purkinje fibers. This causes the ventricles to contract, forcing blood through the semilunar valves. Both atria and ventricles relax briefly before the entire cycle starts again

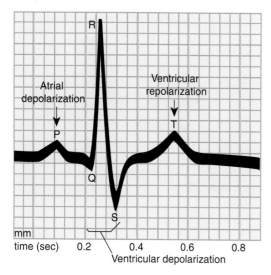

Figure 6-3 A normal ECG tracing showing one cardiac cycle. (Reprinted with permission from Cohen BJ. *Memmler's the Human Body in Health and Disease*. 12th ed. Philadelphia, PA: Lippincott Williams & Wilkins; 2013:325.)

The SA node is called the pacemaker because it sets the basic pace or rhythm of the heartbeat.

Electrocardiogram

An **electrocardiogram** (**ECG**, formerly also known as an **EKG**) is a graphic record of the heart's electrical activity during the cardiac cycle. An ECG is produced by a machine called an electrograph, which records the electrical currents corresponding to each event in heart muscle contraction. Electrical impulses are recorded as waves when electrodes (leads or wires) are placed on the skin at specific locations. The recording is called an ECG tracing (Fig. 6-3). The P wave of the tracing represents the activity of the atria and is usually the first wave seen. The QRS complex (a collection of three waves), along with the T wave, represents the activity of the ventricles. An ECG is useful in diagnosing damage to the heart muscle and abnormalities in the heart rate.

Origin of the Heart Sounds (Heartbeat)

As the ventricles contract (systole), the atrioventricular valves close, resulting in the first heart sound: a long, low-pitched sound commonly described as a "lubb." The second heart sound comes at the beginning of ventricular relaxation (diastole) and is due to the closing of the semilunar valves. It is shorter and sharper and described as a "dupp." Abnormal heart sounds are called **murmurs** and are often due to faulty valve action.

Heart Rate and Cardiac Output

The **heart rate** is the number of heartbeats per minute. The normal adult heart rate averages 72 beats per minute. The volume of blood pumped by the heart in 1 minute is called the **cardiac output** and averages 5 L per minute.

An irregularity in the heart's rate, rhythm, or beat is called an **arrhythmia** (ah-rith'me-ah). A slow rate, less than 60 beats per minute, is called **bradycardia** (brad'e-kar'de-ah). A fast rate, over 100 beats per minute, is called **tachycardia** (tak'e-kar'de-ah). Extra beats before the normal beat are called **extrasystoles**. Rapid, uncoordinated contractions are called **fibrillations** and can result in lack of pumping action.

Pulse

The **pulse** is the palpable rhythmic throbbing caused by the alternating expansion and contraction of an artery as a wave of blood passes through it. It is created as the ventricles contract and blood is forced out of the heart and through the arteries. In normal individuals, the pulse rate is the same as the heart rate. The pulse is most easily felt by compressing the radial artery on the thumb side of the wrist.

Blood Pressure

Blood pressure is the force (pressure) or tension exerted by the blood on the walls of blood vessels. It is commonly measured in a large artery (such as the brachial artery in the upper arm) using a **sphygmomanometer** (sfig'mo-mah-nom'e-ter), more commonly known as a blood pressure cuff. Blood pressure results are expressed in millimeters of mercury (mm Hg) and are read from a manometer that is either a gauge or a mercury column, depending upon the type of blood pressure cuff used. The two components of blood pressure measured are:

- **Systolic** (sis-tol'ik) **pressure:** the pressure in the arteries during contraction of the ventricles
- **Diastolic** (di-as-tol'ik) **pressure:** the arterial pressure during relaxation of the ventricles

A blood pressure reading is expressed as the systolic pressure over the diastolic pressure. The American Heart Association defines normal blood pressure as less than 120 over 80 mm Hg, which is written 120/80 mm Hg.

A brachial blood pressure reading is taken by placing a blood pressure cuff around the upper arm and a stethoscope over the brachial artery. The cuff is inflated until the brachial artery is compressed and the blood flow is cut off. Then the cuff is slowly deflated until the first heart sounds are heard with the stethoscope. The pressure reading at this time is the systolic pressure. The cuff is then slowly deflated until a muffled sound is heard. The pressure at this time is the diastolic pressure.

HEART DISORDERS AND DIAGNOSTIC TESTS

Examples of disorders and diagnostic tests associated with the heart are shown in Box 6-1.

Box 6-1

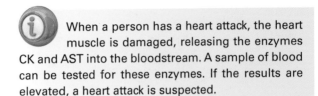

Heart Disorders and Diagnostic Tests

Examples of Heart Disorders

Angina pectoris (an'-ji'na pek'to-ris): also called ischemic heart disease (IHD); pain on exertion caused by inadequate blood flow to the myocardium from the coronary arteries

Aortic stenosis (a-or'tik ste-no'sis): narrowing of the aorta or its opening

Bacterial endocarditis (en'do-kar-di'tis): an infection of the lining of the heart, most commonly caused by streptococci

Congestive heart failure (CHF): impaired circulation due to inadequate pumping of a diseased heart, resulting in fluid buildup (edema) in the lungs or other tissues

Myocardial infarction (MI): heart attack or death of heart muscle due to obstruction (occlusion) of a coronary artery

Myocardial ischemia (is-kee'me-ah): insufficient blood flow to meet the needs of the heart muscle

Pericarditis (per-i-kar-di'tis): inflammation of the pericardium

Examples of Tests for Heart Disorders

- Arterial blood gases (ABGs)
- Aspartate aminotransferase (AST) or serum glutamic oxaloacetic transaminase (SGOT)
- Cholesterol
- Creatine kinase (CK)
- Creatine kinase (CK)-MB
- Digoxin
- Electrocardiogram (ECG or EKG)
- Lactate dehydrogenase (LD)
- Microbial cultures
- Myoglobin
- Potassium (K)
- Triglycerides
- Troponin T (TnT)

When a person has a heart attack, the heart muscle is damaged, releasing the enzymes CK and AST into the bloodstream. A sample of blood can be tested for these enzymes. If the results are elevated, a heart attack is suspected.

The Vascular System

FUNCTIONS

The vascular system is the system of blood vessels that, along with the heart, forms the closed loop through which blood is circulated to all parts of the body. There are two divisions to this system, the pulmonary circulation and the systemic circulation.

The Pulmonary Circulation

The **pulmonary circulation** carries blood from the right ventricle of the heart to the lungs to remove carbon dioxide and pick up oxygen; the oxygenated blood is then returned to the left atrium of the heart.

The Systemic Circulation

The **systemic circulation** serves the rest of the body, carrying oxygenated blood and nutrients from the left ventricle of the heart to the body cells and then returning to the right atrium of the heart with blood carrying carbon dioxide and other waste products of metabolism from the cells.

STRUCTURES

The structures of the vascular system are the various blood vessels that, along with the heart, form the closed system through which blood flows. Blood vessels are tube-like structures capable of expanding and contracting. According to information from the Arizona Science Center, the human vascular system has around 250,000 miles of blood vessels, 95% of which are capillaries, which make up what is called the capillary bed. The rest are arteries and veins.

Arteries

Arteries (Fig. 6-4) are blood vessels that carry blood away from the heart. They have thick walls because the blood that moves through them is under pressure from the contraction of the ventricles. This pressure creates a pulse that can be felt, distinguishing the arteries from the veins.

Key Point When arterial blood is collected by syringe, the pressure normally causes the blood to "pump" or pulse into the syringe under its own power.

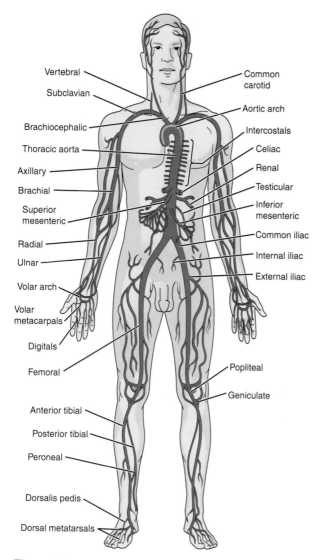

Figure 6-4 The principal arteries of the body. (Adapted with permission from Cohen BJ. *Memmler's the Human Body in Health and Disease*. 12th ed. Philadelphia, PA: Lippincott Williams & Wilkins; 2013:341.)

Systemic arteries carry oxygenated (oxygen-rich) blood away from the heart to the tissues. Because it is oxygen-rich, or full of oxygen, normal systemic arterial blood is bright red.

Key Point The pulmonary artery is the only artery that carries deoxygenated, or oxygen-poor, blood. It is part of the pulmonary circulation and carries deoxygenated blood from the heart to the lungs. It is classified as an artery because it carries blood away from the heart.

The smallest branches of arteries that join with the capillaries are called **arterioles** (ar-te're-olz). The largest artery in the body is the **aorta**. It is approximately 1 inch (2.5 cm) in diameter.

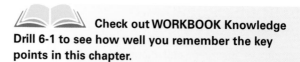 **Check out WORKBOOK Knowledge Drill 6-1 to see how well you remember the key points in this chapter.**

Veins

Veins (Fig. 6-5) are blood vessels that return blood to the heart. Veins carry blood that is low in oxygen (deoxygenated or oxygen-poor) except for the pulmonary vein, which carries oxygenated blood from the lungs back to the heart. Because systemic venous blood is oxygen-poor, it is much darker and more bluish-red than normal arterial blood.

The walls of veins are thinner than those of arteries because the blood is under less pressure than arterial blood. Since the walls are thinner, veins can collapse more easily than arteries. Blood is kept moving through

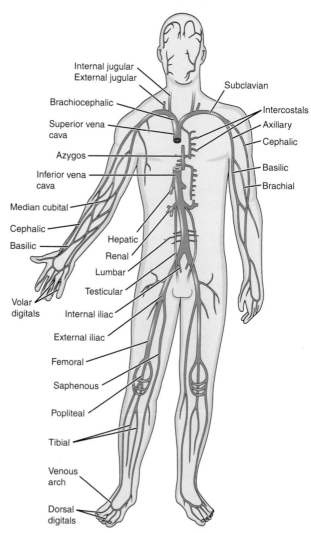

Figure 6-5 The principal veins of the body. (Adapted with permission from Cohen BJ. *Memmler's the Human Body in Health and Disease*. 12th ed. Philadelphia, PA: Lippincott Williams & Wilkins; 2013:343.)

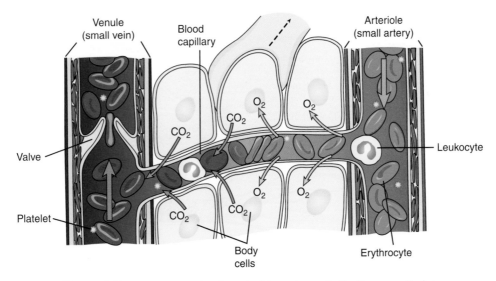

Venule (small vein)
Blood capillary
Arteriole (small artery)
Valve
O_2
CO_2
CO_2
O_2
Leukocyte
CO_2
O_2
O_2
Platelet
CO_2
CO_2
Erythrocyte
Body cells

Figure 6-6 The oxygen and carbon dioxide exchange in the tissue capillaries.

veins by skeletal muscle movement, valves that prevent the backflow of blood, and pressure changes in the abdominal and thoracic cavities during breathing.

The smallest veins at the junction of the capillaries are called **venules** (ven'ulz). The largest veins in the body are the **venae cavae** (singular, **vena cava**). The longest veins in the body are the **great saphenous** (sa-fe'nus) **veins** in the leg.

Capillaries

Capillaries are microscopic, one-cell–thick vessels that connect the arterioles and venules, forming a bridge between the arterial and venous circulation. Blood in the capillaries is a mixture of both venous and arterial blood. In the systemic circulation, arterial blood delivers oxygen and nutrients to the capillaries. The thin capillary walls allow the exchange of oxygen for carbon dioxide and nutrients for wastes between the cells and the blood (Fig. 6-6). Carbon dioxide and wastes are carried away in the venous blood. In the pulmonary circulation, carbon dioxide is delivered to the capillaries in the lungs and exchanged for oxygen.

the**Point**. *View the Gas Exchange in Alveoli and Oxygen Transport animations at http://thepoint.lww. com/McCall6e.*

BLOOD VESSEL STRUCTURE

Arteries and veins are composed of three main layers. The thickness of the layers varies with the size and type of blood vessel. Figure 6-7 shows a cross section of an artery and a vein as seen through a microscope. Capillaries are composed of a single layer of endothelial cells enclosed in a basement membrane. (See Fig. 6-8 for a comparison diagram of artery, vein, and capillary structure.)

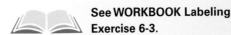

See **WORKBOOK** Labeling Exercise 6-3.

Layers

- **Tunica** (tu'ni-ka) **adventitia** (ad'ven-tish'e-a): the outer layer of a blood vessel, sometimes called the tunica externa. It is made up of connective tissue and is thicker in arteries than in veins.

- **Tunica media:** the middle layer of a blood vessel. It is made up of smooth muscle tissue and some elastic fibers. It is much thicker in arteries than in veins.

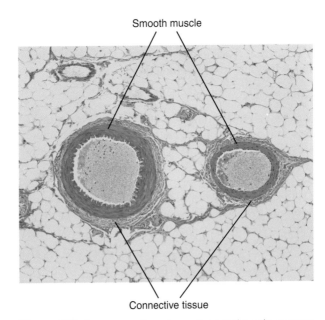

Smooth muscle

Connective tissue

Figure 6-7 A cross section of an artery and a vein as seen through a microscope. (Reprinted with permission from Cormack DH. *Essential Histology*. 2nd ed. Philadelphia, PA: Lippincott Williams & Wilkins; 2001.)

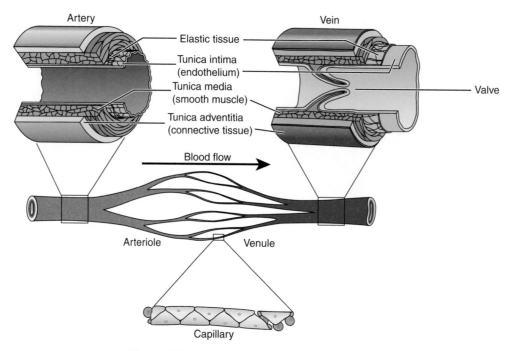

Figure 6-8 The artery, vein, and capillary structure.

- **Tunica intima** (in'ti-ma): the inner layer or lining of a blood vessel, sometimes called the tunica interna. It is made up of a single layer of endothelial cells with an underlying basement membrane, a connective tissue layer, and an elastic internal membrane.

 Tunica (Latin for "coat" or "sheath") means a coat or layer of tissue.

Lumen

The internal space of a blood vessel through which the blood flows is called the **lumen** (lu'men).

Valves

Venous valves are thin membranous leaflets composed primarily of epithelium similar to that of the semilunar valves of the heart. (A venous valve can be seen within the vein in Fig. 6-8.) Most of the venous system flows against the pull of gravity. As blood is moved forward by the movement of skeletal muscle, for example, the valves help keep it flowing toward the heart by allowing blood to flow in only one direction (see Fig. 6-9).

thePoint. *View the Venous Valve Action animation at http://thepoint.lww.com/McCall6e.*

🔑 **Key Point** The presence of valves within veins is a major structural difference between arteries and veins.

THE FLOW OF BLOOD

The network of arteries, veins, and capillaries forms the pathway for the flow of blood (Fig. 6-10) throughout the body; it allows for the delivery of oxygen and nutrients to the body cells and the removal of carbon dioxide and other waste products of metabolism. The order of vascular flow starting with the return of oxygen-poor blood to the heart is shown in Box 6-2.

PHLEBOTOMY-RELATED VASCULAR ANATOMY

Antecubital Fossa

Antecubital (an'te-ku'bi-tal) means "in front of the elbow." **Fossa** means a shallow depression. The **antecubital (AC) fossa** is the shallow depression in the arm that is anterior to (in front of) and below the bend of the elbow. It is the first-choice location for venipuncture because several major arm veins lie close to the surface in this area, making them relatively easy to locate and penetrate with a needle. These major superficial veins are referred to as **antecubital veins**. The anatomical arrangement of antecubital veins varies slightly from person to person; however, two basic vein distribution arrangements, referred to as the H- and M-shaped patterns are seen most often.

ⓘ The venous distribution patterns are so named because the major antecubital veins on the arm resemble the shape of either an "H" or an "M."

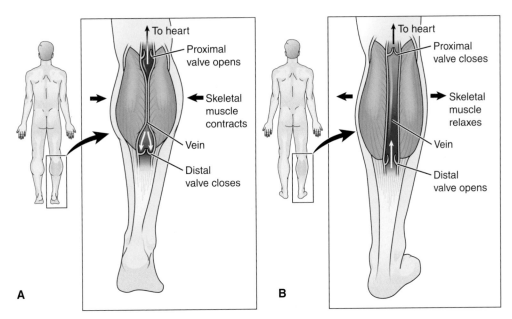

Figure 6-9 The role of skeletal muscles and valves in blood return. **A:** Contracting skeletal muscle compresses the vein and drives blood forward, opening the proximal valve, while the distal valve closes to prevent backflow of blood. **B:** When the muscle relaxes again, the distal valve opens and the proximal valve closes until blood moving in the vein forces it open again. (Reprinted with permission from Cohen BJ. *Memmler's the Human Body in Health and Disease*. 12th ed. Philadelphia, PA: Lippincott Williams & Wilkins; 2013:348.)

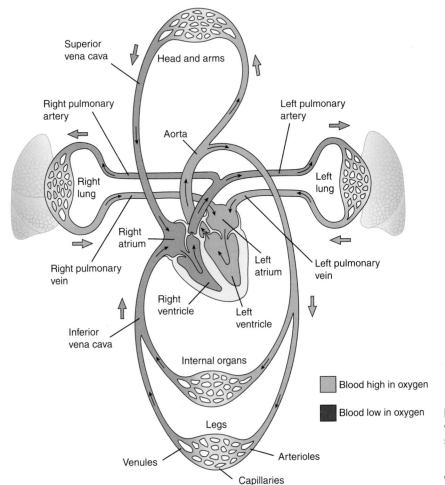

Figure 6-10 A representation of the vascular flow. (Reprinted with permission from Cohen BJ. *Memmler's the Human Body in Health and Disease*. 12th ed. Philadelphia, PA: Lippincott Williams & Wilkins; 2013:336.)

Box 6-2

The Flow of Blood

- Oxygen-poor blood is returned to the heart via the superior and inferior (upper and lower) venae cavae and enters the right atrium of the heart.
- Contraction of the right atrium forces the blood through the tricuspid valve into the right ventricle.
- Contraction of the right ventricle forces the blood through the pulmonary semilunar valve into the pulmonary artery.
- Blood flows through the pulmonary artery to the capillaries of the lungs, where carbon dioxide is released from the red blood cells and exchanged for oxygen through the walls of the alveoli.
- Oxygen-rich blood flows back to the heart via the pulmonary veins and enters the left atrium.
- Contraction of the left atrium forces the blood through the bicuspid valve into the left ventricle.
- Contraction of the left ventricle forces the blood through the aortic semilunar valve into the aorta.
- The blood travels throughout the body by way of the arteries, which branch into smaller and smaller arteries, the smallest of which are the arterioles.
- The arterioles connect with the capillaries, where oxygen, water, and nutrients from the blood diffuse through the capillary walls to the cells. At the same time, carbon dioxide and other end products of metabolism enter the bloodstream.
- The capillaries connect with the smallest branches of veins (venules).
- The venules merge into larger and larger veins until the blood returns to the heart by way of the superior or inferior vena cava, and the cycle starts again.

Key Point The brachial artery and several major arm nerves pass through the AC fossa so it is important to prioritize vein selection in either pattern to minimize risk of accidentally puncturing these structures if needle insertion is inaccurate.

WORKBOOK Labeling Exercises 6-5 and 6-6 will help you learn the names and locations of the AC veins.

H-Pattern Antecubital Veins

The H-shaped venous distribution pattern (Fig. 6-11) is displayed by approximately 70% of the population and includes the median cubital vein, cephalic vein, and basilic vein, described as follows:

- **Median cubital vein:** Located near the center of the antecubital area, it is the preferred, and thus first choice, vein for venipuncture in the H-shaped pattern. It is typically larger, closer to the surface, better anchored, and more stationary than the others, making it the easiest and least painful to puncture and the least likely to bruise. Performing venipuncture on this vein is least likely to injure nerves or the brachial artery. However, the most medial, or inner, aspect of this vein should be avoided as it overlies the brachial artery and several major nerves.

- **Cephalic vein:** Located in the lateral aspect of the antecubital area, it is the second-choice vein for venipuncture in the H-shaped pattern. It is often harder to palpate than the median cubital but is fairly well anchored and often the only vein that can be palpated (felt) in obese patients. The most lateral portions of the cephalic vein, however, should be avoided to prevent accidental injury to the **lateral cutaneous nerve**, sometimes called the lateral antebrachial cutaneous nerve.

- **Basilic vein:** A large vein located on the medial aspect (inner side) of the antecubital area, it is the last-choice vein for venipuncture in either venous distribution pattern. It is generally easy to palpate but is not as well anchored and rolls more easily, increasing the possibility of accidental puncture of the **median nerve** (a major arm nerve), the anterior or posterior branch of the **medial cutaneous nerve** (also called the medial antebrachial cutaneous nerve), or the brachial artery, all of which commonly underlie this area. Punctures in this area also tend to be more painful and to bruise more easily. This vein should not be chosen unless no other vein in either arm is suitable for venipuncture.

M-Pattern Antecubital Veins

The veins that form the M-shaped venous distribution pattern (Fig. 6-12) include the cephalic vein, median vein, median cephalic vein, median basilic vein, and basilic vein. The veins most commonly used for venipuncture in this distribution pattern are described as follows:

- **Median vein** (also called the **intermediate antebrachial vein**): Located near the center of the antecubital area, it is the first choice for venipuncture in the M-shaped pattern because it is well anchored, tends to be less painful to puncture, and is not as close to major nerves or arteries as the others, making it generally the safest one to use. The median vein and the lateral aspect of the median cubital vein overlie a fibrous membrane called the bicipital aponeurosis, which offers some protection to

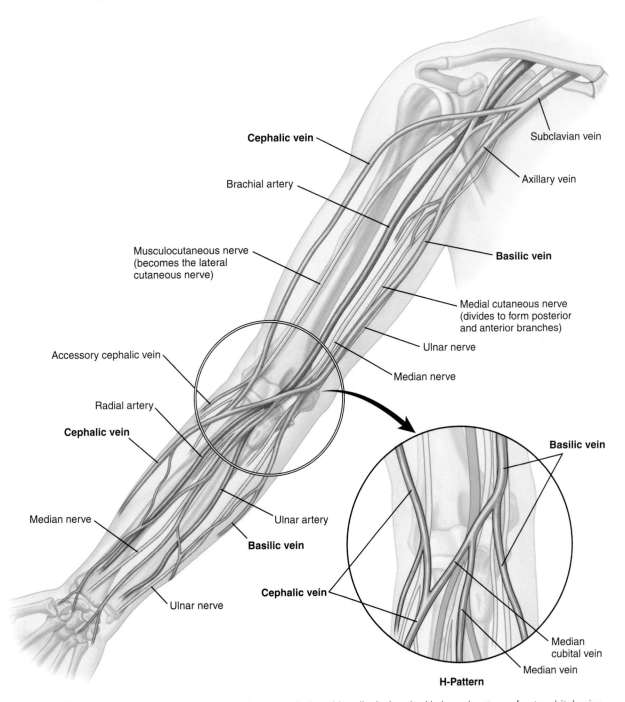

Figure 6-11 The principal veins of the right arm in anatomical position displaying the H-shaped pattern of antecubital veins.

underlying structures such as nerves and arteries. According to CLSI, an attempt should be made to locate one of these veins on either arm before an alternate AC vein is considered.

- **Median cephalic vein** (also called the **intermediate cephalic vein**): Located in the lateral aspect of the antecubital area, it is the second choice for venipuncture in the M-shaped pattern because it is accessible, and is for the most part located away from major nerves or arteries, making it generally safe to puncture. It is also less likely to roll and relatively less painful to puncture. As with the cephalic vein,

the most lateral portions of the median cephalic vein should be avoided to prevent accidental injury to the lateral cutaneous nerve. This vein should not be chosen unless the median or median cephalic veins of both arms have been ruled out.

- **Median basilic vein** (also called the **intermediate basilic vein**): Located in the medial aspect of the antecubital area, it is the last choice for venipuncture in the M-shaped pattern (even though it may appear more accessible) because it is more painful to puncture and, like the basilic vein, is located near the median nerve and the anterior and posterior branches

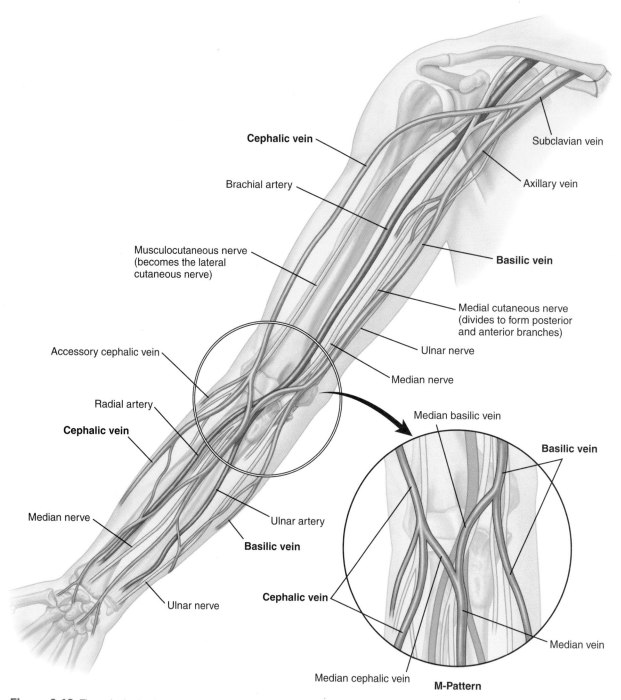

Figure 6-12 The principal veins of the right arm in anatomical position displaying the M-shaped pattern of antecubital veins.

of the medial cutaneous nerve and the brachial artery. As with the basilic vein, this vein should not be chosen unless no other vein in either arm is suitable for venipuncture.

⚠️ **CAUTION** The greatest chance of nerve injury is associated with venipuncture in the most medial and lateral portions of the antecubital fossa.

🔑 **Key Point** Vein location differs somewhat from person to person, and you may not see the exact textbook pattern. The important thing to remember is to choose a prominent vein that is well fixed and does not overlie a pulse, which indicates the presence of an artery and the potential presence of a major nerve.

Dorsal Forearm, Wrist, and Hand Veins

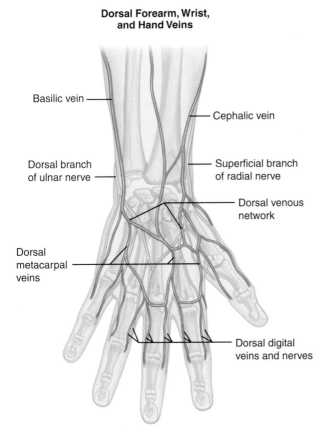

Figure 6-13 Right dorsal forearm, wrist, and hand veins.

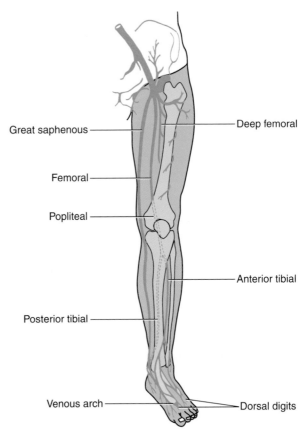

Figure 6-14 The major leg and foot veins.

Other Arm and Hand Veins

According to CLSI, although the larger and fuller median, median cubital, cephalic, and median cephalic veins are used most frequently, veins on the back of the hand and wrist are also acceptable for venipuncture (Fig. 6-13). Veins on the side of the wrist above the thumb must not be used as nerve injury could occur in this area.

 CAUTION Veins on the underside of the wrist are never acceptable for venipuncture.

Leg, Ankle, and Foot Veins

Because of the potential for significant medical complications such as phlebitis or thrombosis, veins of the leg, ankle, and foot (Fig. 6-14) must not be used for venipuncture without permission from the patient's physician. Puncture of the femoral vein is performed only by physicians or specially trained personnel.

Arteries

Arteries are not used for routine blood collection. Arterial puncture requires special training to perform, is more painful and hazardous to the patient, and is generally limited to the collection of arterial blood gas

(ABG) specimens for the evaluation of respiratory function. Arterial puncture for ABG collection is explained in Chapter 12.

VASCULAR SYSTEM DISORDERS AND DIAGNOSTIC TESTS

Examples of disorders and diagnostic tests associated with the vascular system are shown in Box 6-3.

The Blood

Blood has been referred to as "the river of life," as it flows throughout the circulatory system delivering nutrients, oxygen, and other substances to the cells and transporting waste products away from the cells for elimination.

BLOOD COMPOSITION

Blood is a mixture of fluid and cells; it is about five times thicker than water, salty to the taste, and slightly alkaline, with a pH of about 7.4 (pH is the degree of acidity or alkalinity on a scale of 1 to 14, with 7 being neutral). In vivo (in the living body), the fluid

Box 6-3

Examples of Vascular System Disorders and Diagnostic Tests

Vascular System Disorders

Aneurysm (an'u-rizm): a localized dilation or bulging in the wall of a blood vessel, usually an artery

Arteriosclerosis (ar-te're-o-skle-ro'sis): thickening, hardening, and loss of elasticity of artery walls

Atherosclerosis (ath'er-o'skle-ro'sis): a form of arteriosclerosis involving thickening of the intima of the artery due the buildup of plaque (lipid–calcium deposits)

Disseminated intravascular coagulation (DIC): pathological widespread clotting and fibrinolysis in which coagulation factors are consumed to such an extent that bleeding occurs

Embolism: obstruction of a blood vessel by an embolus

Embolus (em'bo-lus): a blood clot, part of a blood clot, or other mass of undissolved matter circulating in the bloodstream

Hemorrhoids: varicose veins in the rectal area

Phlebitis (fle-bi'tis): inflammation of a vein

Thrombophlebitis (throm'bo-fle-bi'tis): inflammation of a vein along with thrombus (blood clot) formation

Thrombus: a blood clot in a blood vessel or organ

Varicose veins (varices): swollen, knotted superficial veins

Tests for Vascular System Disorders

- D-dimer
- Fibrin degradation products (FDP)
- Lipoproteins
- Prothrombin time (PT)
- Partial thromboplastin time (PTT/APTT)
- Triglycerides

Key Point Testing personnel typically prefer specimens that contain roughly 2½ times the amount of sample required to perform the test; so the test can be repeated if needed, with some to spare. Consequently, a test that requires 1 mL of serum or plasma would require a 5-mL blood specimen because only half the specimen will be fluid, while a test that requires 1 mL of whole blood would require a 2½-mL specimen.

Plasma

Normal plasma is a clear, pale-yellow fluid that is approximately 91% water (H_2O) and 9% solutes, which are substances dissolved or suspended in the water. The composition of the solute portion includes the following:

- Gases, such as oxygen (O_2), carbon dioxide (CO_2), and nitrogen (N).
- Minerals such as sodium (Na), potassium (K), calcium (Ca), and magnesium (Mg). Sodium helps maintain fluid balance, pH, and calcium and potassium balance is necessary for normal heart action. Potassium is essential for normal muscle activity and the conduction of nerve impulses. Calcium is needed for proper bone and tooth formation, nerve conduction, and muscle contraction. In addition, calcium is essential to the clotting process.
- Nutrients to supply energy. Plasma nutrients include carbohydrates, such as glucose; and lipids (fats), such as triglycerides; and cholesterol.
- Proteins, such as albumin, which is manufactured by the liver and functions to help regulate osmotic pressure, or the tendency of blood to attract water; antibodies, which combat infection; and fibrinogen, which is also manufactured by the liver and functions in the clotting process.
- Waste products of metabolism such as blood urea nitrogen (BUN), creatinine, and uric acid.
- Other substances such as vitamins, hormones, and drugs.

Formed Elements

Erythrocytes

Erythrocytes (e-rith'ro-sites), or red blood cells (RBCs) (Fig. 6-15), are the most numerous cells in the blood, averaging 4.5 to 5 million per cubic millimeter of blood. Their main function is to carry oxygen from the lungs to the cells. They also carry carbon dioxide from the cells back to the lungs to be exhaled.

Key Point The main component of RBCs is **hemoglobin** (Hgb or Hb), an iron-containing pigment that enables them to transport oxygen and carbon dioxide and also gives them their red color.

portion of the blood is called **plasma**; the cellular portion is referred to as the **formed elements**. The average adult weighing 70 kg (approximately 154 pounds) has a blood volume of about 5 L (5.3 quarts), of which approximately 55% is plasma and 45% is formed elements. Accordingly, approximately one-half of a blood specimen will be serum or plasma and the other half will be blood cells.

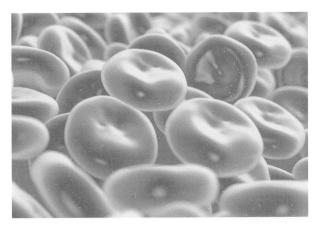

Figure 6-15 Red blood cells as seen under a scanning electron microscope. (Reprinted with permission from Cohen BJ. *Memmler's the Human Body in Health and Disease.* 12th ed. Philadelphia, PA: Lippincott Williams & Wilkins; 2013:290.)

RBCs are produced in the bone marrow. They are formed with a nucleus, which they lose as they mature and enter the bloodstream. Normally a few **reticulocytes** (re-tik'u-lo-sits), or **"retics"** (immature RBCs that still contain remnants of material from their nuclear stage), also enter the bloodstream. Mature RBCs have a lifespan of approximately 120 days, after which they begin to disintegrate and are removed from the bloodstream by the spleen and liver. They are described as anuclear (having no nuclei), biconcave (indented from both sides) disks approximately 7 to 8 µm in diameter. RBCs have **intravascular** (within blood vessels) function, which means that they do their job within the bloodstream.

Leukocytes

Leukocytes, or white blood cells (WBCs), contain nuclei. The average adult has from 5,000 to 10,000 WBCs per cubic millimeter of blood. WBCs are formed in the bone marrow and lymphatic tissue. They are said to have **extravascular** (outside the blood vessels) function because they are able to leave the bloodstream and do their job in the tissues. WBCs may appear in the bloodstream for only 6 to 8 hours but reside in the tissues for days, months, or even years. The lifespan of WBCs varies with the type.

ⓘ The process by which WBCs are able to slip through the walls of the capillaries to enter the tissues is called **diapedesis** (di'a-ped-e'sis). Dia (Greek for through), ped from "pedan" (leap), esis (condition or state).

The main function of WBCs is to neutralize or destroy pathogens. Some accomplish this by **phagocytosis** (fag'o-si-to'sis), a process in which a pathogen or foreign matter is surrounded, engulfed, and destroyed by the WBC. (WBCs also use phagocytosis to remove disintegrated tissue.) Some WBCs produce antibodies that destroy pathogens indirectly or release substances that attack foreign matter.

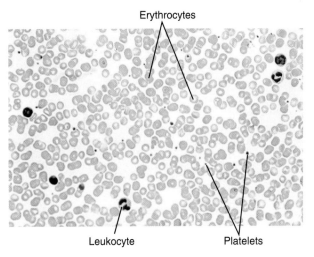

Figure 6-16 Blood cells in a stained blood smear as seen under a microscope. (Reprinted with permission from Eroschenko VP. *diFiore's Atlas of Histology.* Philadelphia, PA: Lippincott Williams & Wilkins; 2013:5.)

There are different types of WBCs, each identified by its size, the shape of the nucleus, and whether or not there are granules present in the cytoplasm when the cells in a blood smear are stained with a special blood stain called Wright stain (Fig. 6-16). WBCs containing easily visible granules are called **granulocytes** (gran'u-lo-sites'). WBCs that lack granules or have extremely fine granules that are not easily seen are called **agranulocytes**.

📖 **Unscramble the name for a type of WBC in WORKBOOK Knowledge Drill 6-2.**

Granulocytes

Granulocytes can be differentiated by the color of their granules when stained with Wright stain. There are three types of granulocytes: **neutrophils, eosinophils** ("eos"), and **basophils** ("basos"). Neutrophils are normally the most numerous type of WBC in adults. A typical neutrophil is **polymorphonuclear,** meaning its nucleus has several lobes or segments, and is also called a "poly," "PMN," or "seg" for short.

🔑 **Key Point** The presence of increased numbers of neutrophils is associated with bacterial infection.

Agranulocytes

There are two types of agranulocytes: **monocytes** ("monos") and **lymphocytes** ("lymphs"). Lymphocytes are normally the second most numerous type of WBC and the most numerous agranulocyte. Two main types of lymphocytes are **T lymphocytes** and **B lymphocytes.** Monocytes are the largest WBCs. (The various types of granulocytes and agranulocytes are shown and described in Table 6-5.)

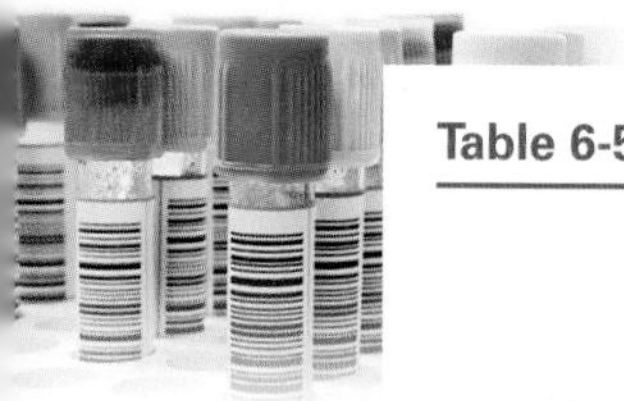

Table 6-5: Normal Leukocytes (White Blood Cells) (WBCs)

WBC Types	Relative Percentage of Total WBCs (Adult)	Description	Function	Lifespan
Granulocytes (nucleus is segmented)				
Neutrophils (nu'tro-fils) 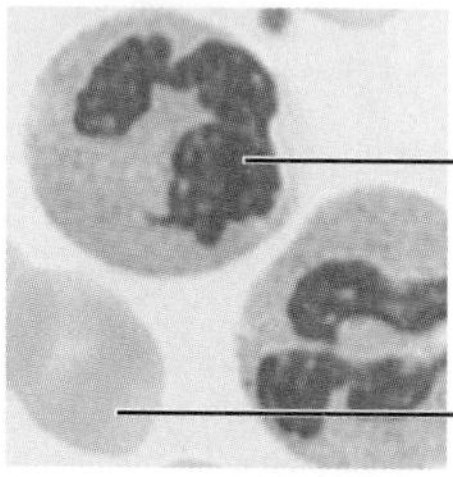	54–62%	Most numerous type of WBC. Segmented or multilobed nucleus. Fine-textured lavender-staining granules.	Destroy pathogens by phagocytosis.	6 hours to a few days
Eosinophils (e'o-sin'o-fils) 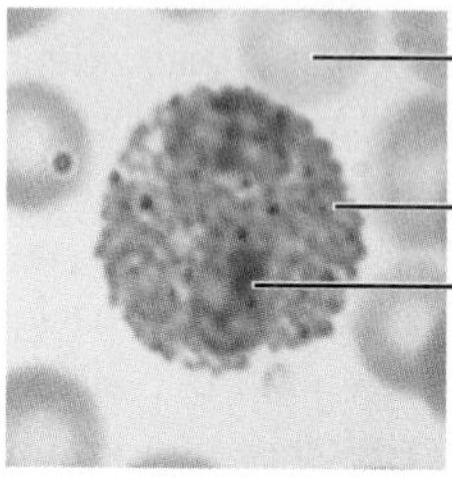	Up to 3%	Bead-like granules that stain bright orange-pink. Two-lobed nucleus.	Ingest and detoxify foreign protein; help turn off immune reactions; increase with allergies and parasite (e.g., pinworm) infestations.	8–12 days
Basophils (ba'so-fils) 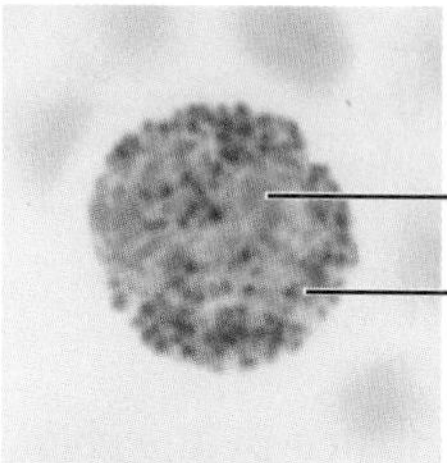	Less than 1%	Least numerous type of WBC: Large dark blue-black staining granules that often obscure a typically S-shaped nucleus.	Release histamine and heparin, which enhance the inflammatory response.	Thought to live several days
Agranulocytes (nucleus is unsegmented)				
Lymphocytes 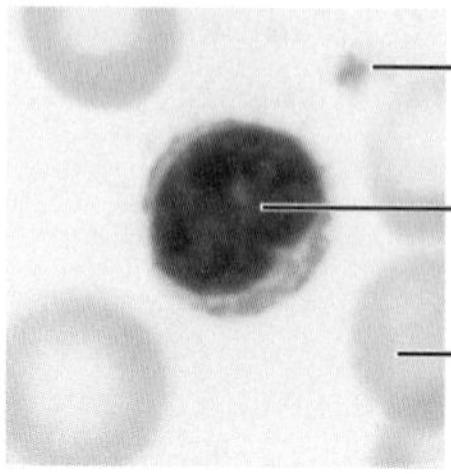	25–38%	Second most numerous type of WBC; typically has a large, round, dark-purple nucleus that occupies most of the cell and is surrounded by a thin rim of pale-blue cytoplasm.	T lymphocytes directly attack infected cells; B lymphocytes give rise to plasma cells that produce immunoglobulins (antibodies) that are released into the bloodstream to circulate and attack foreign cells.	Varies from a few hours to a number of years
Monocytes 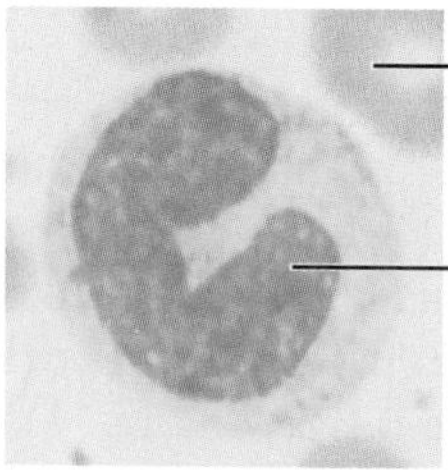	3–7%	Largest WBC; fine, gray-blue cytoplasm and a large, dark-staining nucleus.	Destroy pathogens by phagocytosis; first line of defense in the inflammatory process.	Several months

Neutrophils image labels: Nucleus, Erythrocyte

Eosinophils image labels: Erythrocyte, Granules, Nucleus

Basophils image labels: Nucleus, Granules

Lymphocytes image labels: Platelet, Nucleus, Erythrocyte

Monocytes image labels: Erythrocyte, Nucleus

Monocytes are sometimes called macrophages after they leave the bloodstream.

Thrombocytes

Thrombocytes (throm'bo-sits), better known as **platelets** (Fig. 6-17A), are the smallest of the formed elements. Platelets are actually parts of a large cell called a **megakaryocyte** (meg'a-kar'e-o-sit') (Fig. 6-17B), which is found in the bone marrow. The number of platelets in the blood (platelet count) of the average adult ranges from 150,000 to 400,000 per cubic millimeter. Platelets are essential to **coagulation** (the blood-clotting process) and are the first cell on the scene when an injury occurs (see "Hemostasis," below). The lifespan of a platelet is about 10 days.

BLOOD TYPE

An individual's blood type (also called blood group) is inherited and is determined by the presence or absence of certain proteins called antigens on the surface of the red blood cells. Some blood-type antigens cause formation of antibodies (also called agglutinins) to the opposite blood type. Some antibodies to blood-type antigens are preformed in the blood. (A person will not normally have or produce antibodies against his or her own RBC antigens.) If a person receives a blood transfusion of the wrong type, the antibodies may react with the donor RBCs and cause them to **agglutinate** (a-gloo'tin-ate), or clump together (Fig. 6-18), and **lyse** (līs)—that is,

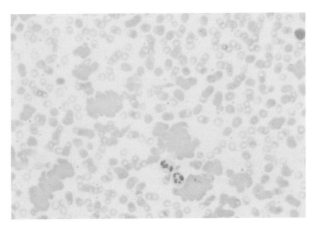

Figure 6-18 Stained blood smear with *a number of large clumps* of agglutinated red blood cells. (Reprinted with permission from Anderson S, Poulsen K. *Anderson's Atlas of Hematology.* 2nd ed. Philadelphia, PA: Lippincott Williams & Wilkins; 2013.)

to hemolize or disintegrate. Such an adverse reaction between donor cells and a recipient, which can be fatal, is called a **transfusion reaction.** The most commonly used method of blood typing recognizes two blood group systems: the ABO system and the Rh factor system.

ABO Blood Group System

The **ABO blood group system** recognizes four blood types, A, B, AB, and O, based on the presence or absence of two antigens identified as A and B. An individual who is type A has the A antigen, type B has the B antigen, type AB has both antigens, and type O has neither A nor B. Type O is the most common type, and type AB is the least common.

Unique to the ABO system are preformed antibodies in a person's blood that are directed against the opposite blood type. Type A blood has an antibody (agglutinin) directed against type B, called anti-B. A person with type B has anti-A, type O has both anti-A and anti-B, and type AB has neither. Table 6-6 shows the antigens and antibodies present in the four ABO blood types.

Individuals with type AB blood were once referred to as universal recipients because they have neither A nor B antibody to the RBC antigens and can theoretically receive any ABO type blood. Similarly, type O individuals were once called universal donors because they have

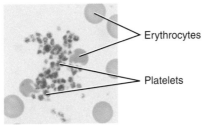

A Platelets

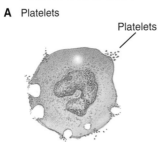

B Megakaryocyte

Figure 6-17 Platelets (thrombocytes) **A:** Platelets in a stained blood smear. **B:** A megakaryocyte releases platelets. (Reprinted with permission from Cohen BJ. *Memmler's the Human Body in Health and Disease.* 12th ed. Philadelphia, PA: Lippincott Williams & Wilkins; 2013:294.)

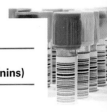

Table 6-6: ABO Blood Group System

Blood Type	RBC Antigen	Plasma Antibodies (Agglutinins)
A	A	Anti-B
B	B	Anti-A
AB	A and B	Neither anti-A nor anti-B
O	Neither	Anti-A and anti-B

neither A nor B antigen on their RBCs, and in an emergency, their blood can theoretically be given to anyone. However, type O blood does contain plasma antibodies to both A and B antigens, and when given to an A- or B-type recipient, it can cause a mild transfusion reaction. To avoid reactions, patients are usually given type-specific blood, even in emergencies.

Rh Blood Group System

The **Rh blood group system** is based upon the presence or absence of an RBC antigen called the D antigen, also known as **Rh factor.** An individual with the D antigen present on red blood cells is said to be positive for the Rh factor, or **Rh-positive** (Rh+). An individual whose RBCs lack the D antigen is said to be **Rh-negative** (Rh-). A patient must receive blood with the correct Rh type as well as the correct ABO type. Approximately 85% of the population is Rh+.

Unlike the ABO system, antibodies to the Rh factor (anti-Rh antibodies) are not preformed in the blood of Rh- individuals. However, an Rh- individual who receives Rh+ blood can become sensitized. This means that the individual may produce antibodies against the Rh factor. In addition, an Rh- woman who is carrying an Rh+ fetus may become sensitized by the RBCs of the fetus, most commonly by leakage of the fetal cells into the mother's circulation during childbirth. This may lead to the destruction of the RBCs of a subsequent Rh+ fetus, because Rh antibodies produced by the mother can cross the placenta into the fetal circulation. When this occurs, it is called **hemolytic disease of the newborn (HDN)**.

(i) An unsensitized Rh- woman can be given Rh immune globulin (RhIg), such as RhoGam, at certain times during her pregnancy and soon after an Rh+ baby's birth. RhIg will destroy Rh+ fetal cells that may have entered her bloodstream and thus prevent sensitization.

Compatibility Test/Cross Match

Other factors in an individual's blood can cause adverse reactions during a blood transfusion, even with the correct ABO- and Rh-type blood. Consequently, a test to determine if the donor unit of blood and the blood of the patient recipient are compatible (suitable to be mixed together) is performed using patient serum and cells as well as serum and cells from the donor unit. This test is called a **compatibility test** or **cross match**.

BLOOD SPECIMENS

Serum

Blood that has been removed from the body will coagulate or clot within 30 to 60 minutes. The clot consists of the blood cells enmeshed in a fibrin network (see "Hemostasis and Coagulation" later in this chapter). The remaining fluid portion is called **serum** and can be separated from the clot by centrifugation (spinning the clotted blood at very high speed in a machine called a centrifuge). See Figure 6-19B. Normal fasting serum is a clear, pale-yellow fluid. Serum has the same composition as plasma except that it does not contain fibrinogen,

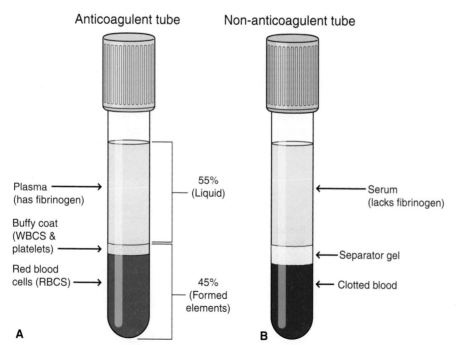

Anticoagulent tube   Non-anticoagulent tube

Plasma (has fibrinogen)

Buffy coat (WBCS & platelets)

Red blood cells (RBCS)

55% (Liquid)

45% (Formed elements)

Serum (lacks fibrinogen)

Separator gel

Clotted blood

A   B

Figure 6-19 Blood specimens. **A:** Separated whole-blood specimen. **B:** Centrifuged, clotted, serum specimen.

because the fibrinogen was used in the formation of the clot. Many laboratory tests are performed on serum, especially chemistry and immunology tests.

Plasma

Not all tests can be performed on serum. For example, most coagulation tests cannot be performed on serum because the coagulation factor fibrinogen and many of the other coagulation factors are used up in the process of clot formation. Some chemistry tests, such as ammonia and potassium, cannot be performed on serum because clotting releases these substances from the cells into the serum, which would lead to inaccurate test results. In addition, some chemistry test results are needed stat (immediately) in order to respond to emergency situations; having to wait 30 minutes or more for a specimen to clot before centrifuging it to get serum would be unacceptable. If clotting is prevented, however, coagulation factors and other substances affected by clotting are preserved, and the specimen can be centrifuged immediately.

Blood can be prevented from clotting by adding a substance called an anticoagulant (see "Anticoagulants," Chapter 7). Adding an anticoagulant initially creates a whole-blood specimen. When a whole-blood specimen is centrifuged (or allowed to stand for a prolonged period of time), it separates into three distinct layers (Fig. 6-19A): a bottom layer of red blood cells; a thin, fluffy-looking, whitish-colored middle layer of WBCs and platelets referred to as the **buffy coat**; and a top layer of liquid called plasma, which can be separated from the cells and used for testing. Normal fasting plasma is a clear to slightly hazy pale-yellow fluid visually indistinguishable from serum. Many laboratory tests can be performed on either serum or plasma.

Key Point The major difference between plasma and serum is that plasma contains fibrinogen, while serum does not.

Test your ability to identify layers of a separated whole-blood specimen with WORKBOOK Labeling Exercise 6-10.

Whole Blood

Some tests, including most hematology tests and some chemistry tests such as glycohemoglobin, cannot be performed on serum or plasma. These tests must be performed on **whole blood** (blood in the same form as it is in the bloodstream). This means that the blood specimen must not be allowed to clot or separate. To obtain a whole-blood specimen, it is necessary to add

an anticoagulant. In addition, because the components will separate if the specimen is allowed to stand undisturbed, the specimen must be mixed for a minimum of 2 minutes immediately prior to performing the test.

> (i) Some tests (e.g., glucose) can be performed on serum, plasma, or whole blood, depending upon the type of testing equipment used.

BLOOD DISORDERS AND DIAGNOSTIC TESTS

Examples of disorders and diagnostic tests associated with the blood are listed in Box 6-4.

Hemostasis and Coagulation

The ability of the body to stop the bleeding following a vascular injury is critical to maintaining life. **Hemostasis** (he'mo-sta'sis), which means the arrest or stoppage of bleeding (the opposite term is hemorrhage), is the body response that stops the loss of blood after an injury. It does this without affecting the flow of blood within the rest of the vascular system. The hemostatic process requires the coordinated interaction of endothelial cells that line the blood vessels, platelets, other blood cells, plasma proteins, calcium ions, and the coagulation (clotting) process.

> (i) Coagulation is the conversion of a liquid such as blood into a semisolid gel called a clot.

COAGULATION

Normal blood coagulation is a critical component of hemostasis that requires the activation of a series of proteins called **coagulation factors** (Table 6-7). These factors are designated by Roman numerals that were assigned in the order of discovery, not the order in which they become activated. (Activated factors have a lowercase "a" added to the Roman numeral). The coagulation factors can be divided into three categories: enzyme precursors, cofactors, and substrates. See Box 6-5.

> 🔑 **Key Point** Fibrinogen (factor I) is the main coagulation substrate. It is a precursor protein that is acted upon by the main coagulation enzyme, **thrombin** (factor IIa), to form fibrin, an elastic thread-like protein.

Box 6-4

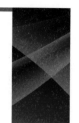

Examples of Blood Disorders and Diagnostic Tests

Blood Disorders

Anemia: an abnormal reduction in the number of RBCs in the circulating blood

Leukemia: disorder involving the multiplication of immature forms of WBCs in the blood

Leukocytosis: an abnormal increase in WBCs in the circulating blood

Leukopenia: an abnormal decrease in WBCs

Polycythemia: an abnormal increase in RBCs

Thrombocytosis: increased number of platelets

Thrombocytopenia: decreased number of platelets

Tests for Blood Disorders

- ABO and Rh type
- Bone marrow examination
- Complete blood count (CBC)
- Cross match
- Differential (diff)
- Eosinophil (Eos) count
- Erythrocyte sedimentation rate (ESR)
- Ferritin

- Hematocrit (Hct)
- Hemoglobin (Hb or Hgb)
- Hemogram
- Indices (MCH, MCV, MCHC)
- Iron (Fe)
- Reticulocyte (retic) count
- Total iron-binding capacity (TIBC)

Coagulation Pathways

Each activated factor activates another factor in what has been traditionally described as a cascade or water-fall involving two pathways:

- The **extrinsic**, or tissue factor (TF), pathway. *Extrinsic* means "originating outside." The extrinsic pathway is so named because it is initiated (started) by TF, which is normally outside the bloodstream or vascular system. (TF, also called thromboplastin and factor III, is present in the membranes of cells outside the vascular bed.)

- The **intrinsic**, or contact-activation, pathway. *Intrinsic* means "originating within." The intrinsic pathway is so named because it involves coagulation factors circulating within the bloodstream that are activated when they contact the surfaces of certain cells.

Key Point The prothrombin test (PT) is used to evaluate extrinsic pathway function and monitor coumarin therapy. The activated partial thromboplastin test (aPTT) is used to evaluate the intrinsic coagulation pathway and monitor heparin therapy.

Both pathways eventually join to form a common pathway that ends in the formation of a fibrin-reinforced blood clot. It was once thought that both pathways were separate, of equal importance, and activated independently both in a test tube (in vitro) and in the living body (in vivo). The separate pathway cascade model of coagulation does describe reactions that occur in a test tube and is important in the evaluation of coagulation through laboratory testing. The cascade model does not, however, adequately explain in vivo coagulation.

Blood collected in a tube that does not contain an anticoagulant clots because the intrinsic pathway is activated when the blood comes in contact with the tube or clot activator particles. In addition, the clotting process can be initiated by the extrinsic pathway before the blood enters the tube by tissue injury from the draw and thromboplastin (tissue factor) drawn into the needle.

Cell-Based In Vivo Coagulation

It is now known that the coagulation pathways have different jobs in the body during hemostasis. The extrinsic pathway is responsible for initiating the coagulation process.

The intrinsic pathway is responsible for producing large amounts of thrombin on the surface of activated platelets. (See Fig. 6-20 for a diagram of in vivo coagulation activation.) Because the majority of the process involves the formation of coagulation factor complexes (combinations) on cell surfaces it is called

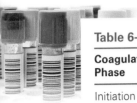

Table 6-7: Coagulation Phases, Factors, and Action Involved

Coagulation Phase	Factors Involved	Action Involved
Initiation	vWF TF II IIa VII VIIa X Xa IX IXa V Va	• Endothelial cell damage exposes collagen, von Willebrand factor (vWF), and tissue factor (TF) to circulating blood. • Platelets stick to vWF and collagen in a process called platelet adhesion, become partially activated, and undergo limited degranulation. This generates a small amount of thrombin (IIa) from prothrombin (II). • TF initiates the extrinsic coagulation pathway by activating factor VII and creating a TF/VIIa complex. • TF/VIIa complex activates small amounts of factor X to Xa and factor IX to IXa. • Factor Xa activates factor V and creates a Xa/Va complex on the surface of TF-bearing cells. This too results in the generation of a small amount of thrombin from prothrombin. • Thrombin binds to platelet surface receptors. • The platelets become fully activated, change shape, completely degranulate, and stick to one another in a process called platelet aggregation. • Some of the thrombin converts fibrinogen to soluble fibrin. • Platelet adhesion, aggregation, and fibrin generation result in formation of the primary platelet plug.
Amplification	V Va VIII VIIIa vWF XIa X Xa II IIa	• Cofactors V and VIII bound to platelets during platelet activation are activated by thrombin to factors Va and VIIIa. • Factor Va cleaves factor VIII from the VIII/vWF complex, allowing vWF to cause additional platelet adhesion and aggregation. • Factor XIa binds to factor VIIIa to form a complex that activates factor X on platelet surfaces. • Factor Xa and factor II bind to factor Va, forming a prothrombinase complex that starts mass conversion of prothrombin (II) to thrombin (IIa).
Propagation	IXa XIa Va XIII XIIIa	• Factor IXa activated during initiation binds to factor VIIIa on platelet surfaces creating a IXa/VIIIa complex. More factor IXa is supplied by factor XIa bound to platelet surfaces. • The factor IXa/VIIIa complex supplies factor Xa directly on the platelet surfaces. • Factor Xa quickly complexes with the factor Va bound to platelets during amplification. • The complex creates a prothrombin-converting capacity on the platelets, which creates the thrombin burst needed to trigger conversion of factor XIII to factor XIIIa. • Factor XIIIa cross links soluble fibrin into insoluble fibrin. • Insoluble fibrin reinforces and stabilizes the secondary hemostatic plug or blood clot.

Box 6-5

Three Categories of Coagulation Factors

Enzyme precursors: precursor proteins that become enzymes when activated. (Enzymes are active proteins that bring about chemical changes in other substances.)

Cofactors: proteins that accelerate enzymatic reactions in the coagulation process.

Substrates: substances that are acted upon and changed by enzymes.

a cell-based model of coagulation. Cell-based coagulation is described in terms of three overlapping phases: **initiation, amplification,** and **propagation,** all involving production of thrombin. (See Table 6-7.)

THE HEMOSTATIC PROCESS IN VIVO

Ongoing daily repair of vessels keeps the hemostatic process active at a low level all the time as cells die and are replaced. Therefore, when a blood vessel is injured, it can immediately begin to repair the damage. This involves four interrelated responses formerly referred to as stages. The responses are: (1) vasoconstriction; (2) formation of a primary **platelet plug** in the injured area; (3) progression, if needed, to a stable blood clot called the secondary

Coagulation Activation

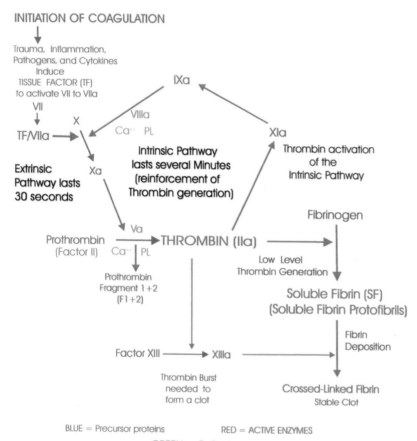

INITIATION OF COAGULATION

Trauma, Inflammation,
Pathogens, and Cytokines
Induce
TISSUE FACTOR (TF)
to activate VII to VIIa

VII

TF/VIIa ⟶

X

VIIIa
Ca⁺⁺ PL

IXa

XIa

Intrinsic Pathway
lasts several Minutes
(reinforcement of
Thrombin generation)

Thrombin activation
of the
Intrinsic Pathway

Extrinsic
Pathway lasts
30 seconds

Xa

Va

Prothrombin
(Factor II)

Ca⁺⁺ PL

THROMBIN (IIa)

Fibrinogen

Low Level
Thrombin Generation

Prothrombin
Fragment 1 + 2
(F1 + 2)

Soluble Fibrin (SF)
(Soluble Fibrin Protofibrils)

Fibrin
Deposition

Factor XIII ⟶ XIIIa

Crossed-Linked Fibrin
Stable Clot

Thrombin Burst
needed to
form a clot

BLUE = Precursor proteins   RED = ACTIVE ENZYMES
GREEN = CoFactors

©2009
Az Coag Cons, Inc
azcoag.com

Figure 6-20 Diagram of in vivo coagulation activation. (Courtesy of Arizona Coagulation Consultants, Inc., azcoag.com)

hemostatic plug; and (4) **fibrinolysis**, the dissolving of the clot after the site has healed. (See Fig. 6-21 for a description of the hemostatic process.)

> **Key Point** Under normal conditions, clot formation is limited to the site of injury and does not disrupt blood flow. Abnormalities in the hemostatic process are potentially life-threatening, as they can result in excessive bleeding or thrombosis (clot formation within a blood vessel).

> **Test your knowledge of this complicated subject with the questions in the EXAM REVIEW.**

Vasoconstriction

The immediate reaction to blood vessel injury is **vasoconstriction**, a reduction in the diameter of the blood vessel caused by contraction of smooth muscle fibers in the tunica media. This narrows the blood vessel, which decreases the flow of blood past the injured area and limits blood loss. This is also the objective behind applying pressure to a bleeding wound.

Vasoconstriction is limited by the opposite process of vasodilation, an increase in vessel diameter due to relaxation of the muscle fibers. Vasodilation prevents the vessel from becoming too narrow and blocking effective blood flow.

> Vasodilation is caused by nitric oxide, a natural muscle relaxant produced by endothelial cells. The use of nitroglycerin tablets to prevent and treat chest pain (angina pectoris) is the same process, because the breakdown of nitroglycerin releases nitric oxide.

Primary Platelet Plug Formation

The second response, platelet plug formation, involves the adhesion, activation, and aggregation of platelets,

The hemostatic process

Vasoconstriction

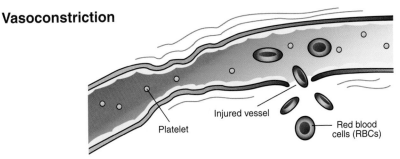

Injured vessel

Platelet

Red blood
cells (RBCs)

Primary platelet plug formation

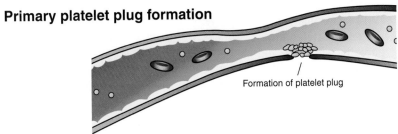

Formation of platelet plug

Secondary hemostatic plug formation

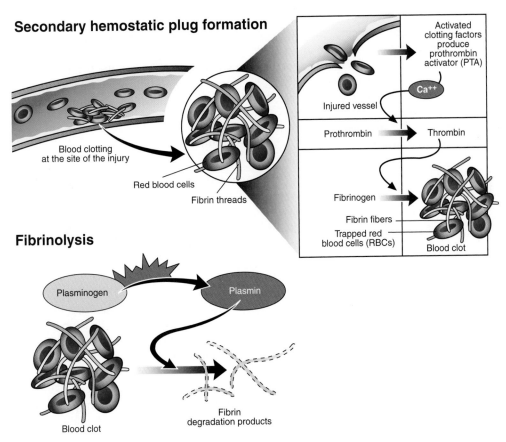

Blood clotting
at the site of the injury

Red blood cells

Fibrin threads

Activated
clotting factors
produce
prothrombin
activator (PTA)

Ca++

Injured vessel

Prothrombin → Thrombin

Fibrinogen

Fibrin fibers
Trapped red
blood cells (RBCs)

Blood clot

Fibrinolysis

Plasminogen → Plasmin

Blood clot

Fibrin
degradation products

Figure 6-21 The hemostatic process.

and the generation of a small amount of fibrin. This response begins with damage to blood vessel endothelial cells caused, for example, by trauma, inflammation, or pathogens. This response has been more recently referred to as the initiation phase of coagulation.

thePoint℠ *View the Platelet Formation animation at http://thepoint.lww.com/McCall6e.*

Initiation

The endothelial cell damage exposes a "glue-like" substance called von Willebrand (vWF) factor that causes platelets to stick to the damaged tissue (**platelet adhesion**). The platelets become partially activated and release clotting factors that begin to produce thrombin from prothrombin, circulating in the blood. The primary role of thrombin is to convert fibrinogen, also present in blood, to soluble fibrin.

> **ⓘ** Under normal circumstances, platelets become activated only at the site of an injured blood vessel, because normal intact blood vessel endothelial cells secrete chemicals that inhibit platelet activation. Aspirin also inhibits platelet activation (and blood clotting in general) and is often prescribed as a "blood *thinner*" or "*antiplatelet agent*" to those at risk of heart attack or stroke.

Blood vessel damage also exposes TF which activates a series of coagulation factors by the extrinsic factor pathway. This leads to the generation of a small amount of thrombin that binds to receptors on the surfaces of the platelets, causing them to change shape, stick to one another (**platelet aggregation**), become activated, and recruit other platelets to the injury site. Some of the thrombin converts fibrinogen to soluble fibrin. The combination of platelet adhesion, aggregation, and fibrin generation results in the formation of the primary platelet plug composed of soluble fibrin and activated platelets.

> **ⓘ** Heparan sulfate is a naturally occurring anticoagulant on the surfaces of blood vessel endothelial cells. It helps prevent clots within vessels (thrombosis) by reducing thrombin generation within normal (noninjured) blood vessels. Heparan sulfate is closely related to the drug heparin. Heparin is derived from certain animal tissues and is used in the treatment of clotting disorders.

The initiation phase (TF activation and formation of the platelet plug as well as a small amount of thrombin) is shut down within 30 seconds by an inhibitor protein secreted by endothelial cells that inactivates several factors critical to the coagulation process. For some very minor injuries, such as a needle puncture of a vein, platelet plug formation and applied pressure are sufficient to seal the site, and coagulation goes no further.

> **🔑 Key Point** Normal platelet plug formation depends on an adequate concentration of platelets (determined by a platelet count), normally functioning platelets (determined by a platelet function assay, PFA), and blood vessel integrity.

Secondary Hemostatic Plug Formation

For injuries with greater tissue damage, the stimulus for coagulation is strong, and the coagulation process continues until the primary platelet plug becomes a stable blood clot called the secondary hemostatic plug. This third hemostatic response is more recently referred to as the amplification and propagation phases of the coagulation process.

Amplification

Much more thrombin is required to create the fibrin needed to reinforce and stabilize the newly formed platelet plug. In the **amplification** phase (see Table 6-7) thrombin enhances its own production by activating a sequence of coagulation factors that ends with a factor complex on the surface of the platelets that begins mass conversion of prothrombin to thrombin.

Propagation

In the **propagation** phase (see Table 6-7), the large amounts of thrombin needed for fibrin formation are produced on the surface of activated platelets as more and more of them are drawn to the site of injury. This ultimately creates a burst of thrombin that triggers the activation of a factor that cross links the fibrin strands into a stable meshwork, forming a net-like structure that traps blood cells and platelets (Fig. 6-22) and produces a dense, stable clot at the injury site in 3 to 5 minutes.

Thrombin production ends with clot formation. A dense clot that activated factors cannot escape, now overlies the site. The trapping of activated factors in the clot and depletion of certain other coagulation factors is thought to be what shuts down thrombin production, terminating the coagulation process and preventing complete clotting of the vessel. Thrombin remaining

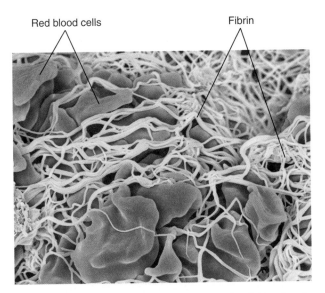

Red blood cells   Fibrin

Figure 6-22 Scanning electron micrograph of blood cells trapped in fibrin. (Reprinted with permission from Mcconnell TH, Hull KH. *Hu man Form, Human Function*. Baltimore, MD: Lippincott Williams & Wilkins; 2011.)

within the clot is still quite active and can make repairs if the clot is disturbed. Activated platelets within the clot release platelet-derived growth factor that begins to repair the vessel.

Key Point Natural inhibitors (Table 6-8) circulate in the plasma along with the coagulation factors. They keep the coagulation process in check and limited to local sites by degrading (breaking down) any activated coagulation factors that escape the injury site or remain within the formed clot.

Table 6-8: Natural Inhibitors of Coagulation

Natural Inhibitor	Function
Antithrombin (AT)	Binds with thrombin to form thrombin/AT complexes that are removed by the liver; inhibits activity of factors IIa, IXa, Xa, XIa, and XIIa.
Heparin cofactor II (HCII)	Thrombin neutralizer activated by substances on arterial endothelial cells.
Proteins C and S	Inactivate cofactors Va and VIIIa. Protein C is activated by a thrombin complex on intact endothelial cell surfaces. Protein S is a binding cofactor for protein C, enhancing its function. Only free circulating protein S can be a protein C cofactor.

Antithrombin, a natural inhibitor, is too large to get into a clot. The drug fondaparinux sodium (Arixtra) was developed to inactivate thrombin inside a clot and prevent clot propagation in individuals with clotting disorders, such as deep venous thrombosis (DVT).

Fibrinolysis

Fibrinolysis (fi'brin-ol'i-sis), the process by which fibrin is dissolved, is an ongoing process responsible for two important activities: (1) It dissolves clots that form within intact vessels (thrombi), thus reopening the vessels, and (2) it removes hemostatic clots from the tissue as healing occurs. The process is possible because activation of the clotting process also activates factors that promote release of plasminogen activators from vessel lining cells and white blood cells. These substances convert plasminogen to plasmin. Plasmin is the enzyme that breaks down fibrin into smaller fragments called **fibrin degradation products (fibrin split products and D-dimers)**, which are then removed by phagocytic cells.

Bleeding may be associated with increased fibrinolytic activity, whereas decreased fibrinolytic activity is associated with thrombosis.

THE ROLE OF THE LIVER IN HEMOSTASIS

The liver plays an important role in the hemostatic process. It is responsible for the synthesis, or manufacture, of many of the coagulation factors, including factors V, VIII, prothrombin, and fibrinogen. It also produces the bile salts needed for the absorption of vitamin K, which is essential to the synthesis of a number of coagulation factors. In addition, mast cells (tissue basophils) in the liver produce heparin, a naturally occurring anticoagulant. When the liver is diseased, the synthesis of coagulation factors is impaired and bleeding may result.

Key Point Because vitamin K is essential to the synthesis of a number of clotting factors, vitamin K deficiency can result in the production of defective clotting factors and lead to an elevated prothrombin time and activated partial thromboplastin time as well as potential bleeding. Coumarins (including Coumadin and other warfarin trade names) are used to treat clotting disorders by inhibiting the proper synthesis of the vitamin K-dependent factors.

HEMOSTATIC DISORDERS AND DIAGNOSTIC TESTS

Examples of disorders and diagnostic tests associated with the hemostatic process are listed in Box 6-6.

ⓘ The first coagulation disorder to be recognized historically was hemophilia, having been described during the second century.

The Lymphatic System

FUNCTIONS

The **lymphatic system** (Fig. 6-23) returns tissue fluid to the bloodstream, protects the body by removing microorganisms and impurities, processes lymphocytes, and delivers fats absorbed from the small intestine to the bloodstream. Lymph vessels extend throughout the entire body, much like blood vessels.

STRUCTURES

The lymphatic system contains fluid called **lymph** and is made up of lymphatic vessels, ducts, and **nodes** (masses of lymph tissue) through which the lymph flows.

LYMPH FLOW

Body cells are bathed in tissue fluid acquired from the bloodstream. Water, oxygen, and nutrients continually diffuse through the capillary walls into the tissue spaces. Much of the fluid diffuses back into the capillaries along with waste products of metabolism. Excess tissue fluid filters into lymphatic capillaries, where it is called lymph. Lymph fluid is similar to plasma but is 95% water.

Lymphatic capillaries join with larger and larger lymphatic vessels until they empty into one of two terminal vessels, either the right lymphatic duct or the thoracic duct. These ducts then empty into large veins in the upper body. Lymph moves through the vessels primarily owing to skeletal muscle contraction, much as blood moves through the veins. Like veins, lymphatic vessels have valves to keep the lymph flowing in the right direction.

Before reaching the ducts, the lymph passes through a series of structures called **lymph nodes**. Lymphoid tissue, of which nodes are composed, is a special kind of tissue with the ability to remove impurities and process lymphocytes. Thus, lymph nodes are able to trap and destroy bacteria and foreign matter and produce lymphocytes. The tonsils, thymus, gastrointestinal tract, and spleen also contain lymphoid tissue.

Box 6-6

Examples of Disorders and Diagnostic Tests of the Hemostatic Process

Hemostatic Disorders

Deep venous thrombosis (DVT): a blood clot that forms in a large vein in the leg.

Disseminated intravascular coagulation (DIC): pathological, widespread clotting and fibrinolysis at the same time, in which coagulation factors are consumed to such an extent that bleeding occurs.

Hemophilia (he'mo-fil'e-a): a hereditary condition characterized by bleeding due to increased coagulation time. The common type of hemophilia is due to factor VIII deficiency along with factor IX (Christmas factor).

Thrombocytopenia (throm'bo-si'to-pe'ne-a): an abnormal decrease in platelets.

Tests of the Hemostatic Process

- D-dimer
- Factor assays
- Fibrin degradation products (FDP)
- Platelet function assay (PFA)
- Prothrombin time (PT)
- Partial thromboplastin time (PTT or APTT)

⚠ **CAUTION** Axillary lymph nodes (nodes in the armpit) are often removed as part of breast cancer surgery. Their removal can impair lymph drainage and interfere with the destruction of bacteria and foreign matter in the affected arm. This is cause for concern in phlebotomy and the reason why an arm on the same side as a mastectomy is not suitable for venipuncture.

🔑 **Key Point** Inflamed lymph nodes may not be able to filter pathogens from the lymph before it returns to the bloodstream. This can lead to septicemia (sep-ti-se'me-ah), the presence of pathogenic microorganisms in the blood.

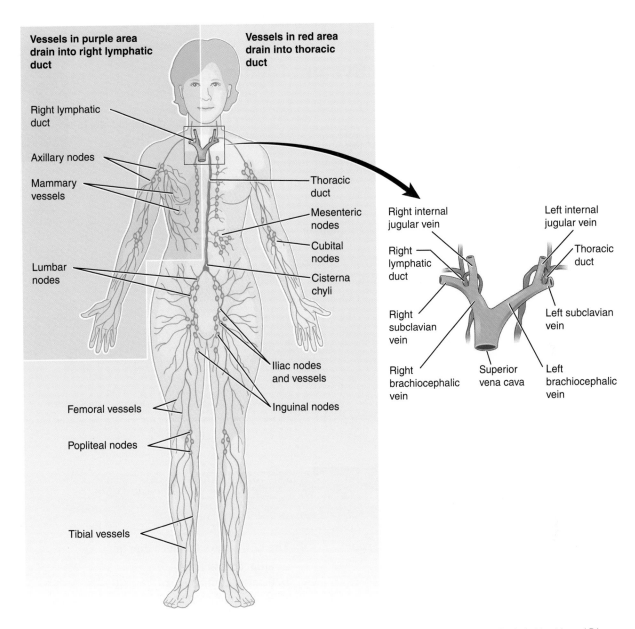

Figure 6-23 Lymphatic system. (Reprinted with permission from Cohen BJ. *Memmler's the Human Body in Health and Disease.* 12th ed. Philadelphia, PA: Lippincott Williams & Wilkins; 2013:366.)

LYMPHATIC SYSTEM DISORDERS AND DIAGNOSTIC TESTS

Examples of disorders and diagnostic tests associated with the lymphatic system are listed in Box 6-7.

Time for some fun. It's good for your heart. Check out the crossword puzzle in Chapter 6 of the WORKBOOK.

Box 6-7

Examples of Lymphatic System Disorders and Diagnostic Tests

Lymphatic System Disorders

Lymphangitis (lim-fan-ji′tis): inflammation of the lymph vessels

Lymphadenitis (lim-fad′e-ni-tis): inflammation of lymph nodes

Lymphadenopathy (lim-fad′e-nop′ah-the): disease of the lymph nodes, often associated with node enlargement such as seen in mononucleosis

Splenomegaly (splen′no-meg′ah-le): spleen enlargement

Hodgkin disease: a chronic, malignant disorder, common in males, characterized by lymph node enlargement

Lymphosarcoma (lim-fo-sar-ko′mah): a malignant lymphoid tumor

Lymphoma: the term for any lymphoid tumor, benign or malignant

Tests for Lymphatic System Disorders

- Bone marrow biopsy
- Complete blood count (CBC)
- Culture and sensitivity (C&S)
- Lymph node biopsy
- Mononucleosis (mono) test

Study and Review Questions

See the EXAM REVIEW for more study questions.

1. **Which of the following is described as an anuclear, biconcave disk?**

   a. Erythrocyte
   b. Granulocyte
   c. Leukocyte
   d. Thrombocyte

2. **The chamber of the heart that receives blood from the systemic circulation is the**

   a. left atrium.
   b. left ventricle.
   c. right atrium.
   d. right ventricle.

3. **The thick muscle layer of the heart is called the**

   a. endocardium.
   b. epicardium.
   c. myocardium.
   d. pericardium.

4. **The ECG shows P waves due to**

   a. atrial contractions.
   b. delayed contractions.
   c. electrical charge revival.
   d. ventricular contraction.

5. **When taking a blood pressure, the systolic pressure is the pressure reading when the**

   a. artery is compressed and blood flow is cut off.
   b. cuff has already been completely deflated.
   c. first heart sounds are heard as the cuff is deflated.
   d. muffled sound is heard as the cuff is deflated.

6. **The purpose of the pulmonary system is to**

   a. carry blood to and from the lungs.
   b. carry nutrients to the cells.
   c. deliver blood to the systemic system.
   d. remove impurities from the blood.

7. **Which of the following blood vessels are listed in the proper order of blood flow?**

    a. Aorta, superior vena cava, vein
    b. Arteriole, venule, capillary
    c. Capillary, venule, vein
    d. Vein, venule, capillary

8. **The internal space of a blood vessel is called the**

    a. atrium.
    b. lumen.
    c. septum.
    d. valve.

9. **The longest vein and the largest artery in the body in that order are**

    a. cephalic and femoral.
    b. great saphenous and aorta.
    c. inferior vena cava and brachial.
    d. pulmonary and femoral.

10. **The preferred vein for venipuncture in the "H" pattern is the**

    a. accessory cephalic.
    b. basilic.
    c. cephalic.
    d. median cubital.

11. **The major difference between plasma and serum is that plasma**

    a. contains fibrinogen, serum does not.
    b. contains nutrients, serum does not.
    c. looks clear, serum looks cloudy.
    d. looks amber, serum looks pale yellow.

12. **An individual's blood type (A, B, AB, or O) is determined by the presence or absence of which of the following on the red blood cells?**

    a. Antigens
    b. Antibodies
    c. Chemicals
    d. Hormones

13. **Which is the correct sequence of events after blood vessel injury?**

    a. Fibrinolysis, platelet adhesion, vasoconstriction
    b. Platelet aggregation, vasoconstriction, fibrin clot formation
    c. Vasoconstriction, platelet aggregation, fibrin clot formation
    d. Vasodilation, platelet adhesion, fibrin clot formation

14. **Lymph originates from**

    a. joint fluid.
    b. plasma.
    c. serum.
    d. tissue fluid.

15. **A heart disorder characterized by fluid buildup in the lungs is called**

    a. aortic stenosis.
    b. bacterial endocarditis.
    c. congestive heart failure.
    d. myocardial infarction.

Case Studies

 See the WORKBOOK for more case studies.

Case Study 6-1: M-Shaped Antecubital Veins

A phlebotomist is examining a patient's arm in search of a suitable vein for a venipuncture. The major visible veins are arranged in the M-shaped pattern.

QUESTIONS

1. Which vein in this pattern is the first choice for venipuncture?

2. Which vein in this pattern is the second choice for venipuncture?

3. Which vein is the last choice for venipuncture?

4. Why is the vein identified in question 3 the last choice for venipuncture?

Case Study 6-2: Blood Specimens

A specimen processor receives a stat chemistry specimen on a patient in the ED at 09:00 hours. The specimen was collected at 08:55 hours. She immediately spins it in the centrifuge, causing the cells to go to the bottom of the tube and leaving clear liquid at the top. She then transfers the clear liquid to another tube that is labeled with the patient's information before delivering the tube to a technician in the chemistry department.

QUESTIONS

1. Was the specimen whole blood or clotted blood before it was centrifuged?

2. What is the term for the part of the specimen that will be used for testing?

3. What clues tell you the type of specimen it is?

Bibliography and Suggested Readings

Blaney KD, Howard PR. *Basic and Applied Concepts of Blood Banking and Transfusion Practices.* 3rd ed. Philadelphia, PA: Mosby/Elsevier; 2013.

Cohen BJ. *Memmler's the Human Body in Health and Disease.* 12th ed. Philadelphia, PA: Lippincott Williams & Wilkins; 2013.

Federated International Programme Anatomical Terminology (FIPAT). *Terminologica Anatomica: International Anatomical Terminology.* New York, NY: Thieme; 2011.

Fischbach FT, Dunning MB. *Laboratory Diagnostic Tests.* 9th ed. Philadelphia, PA: Lippincott Williams & Wilkins; 2014.

Herlihy B. *The Human Body in Health and Illness.* 4th ed. St. Louis, MO: Elsevier/Saunders; 2011.

Moore KL, Agur AM, Dalley AF. *Clincally Oriented Anatomy.* 7th ed. Philadelphia, PA: Lippincott Williams & Wilkins; 2014.

Netter FP. *Atlas of Human Anatomy.* 5th ed. Philadelphia, PA: Saunders/Elsevier; 2011.

Rodak BF, Fritsma GA, Keohane E. *Hematology: Clinical Principles and Applications.* 4th ed. St. Louis, MO: Elsevier/Saunders; 2013.

Stedman's Medical Dictionary. 28th ed. Philadelphia, PA: Lippincott Williams & Wilkins; 2013.

Venes MD. *Taber's Cyclopedic Medical Dictionary.* 22nd ed. Philadelphia, PA: FA Davis; 2013.

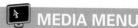

MEDIA MENU

Online Ancillaries (at http://thepoint.lww.com/McCall6e)
- Animations:
  - Cardiac cycle
  - Gas exchange in alveoli
  - Oxygen transport
  - Platelet plug formation
  - Venous valve action
- Interactive exercises and games, including Look and Label, Word Building, Body Building, Roboterms, Crossword Puzzles, Quiz Show, and Concentration
- Audio flash cards and flash card generator
- Audio glossary

Internet Resources
- American Heart Association: http://www.heart.org/HEARTORG/
- American Heart Association Learn and Live Interactive Cardiovascular Library: http://watchlearnlive.heart.org/CVML_Player.php
- Anatomy Arcade, WACK-A-BONE: http://www.anatomyarcade.com/games/WAB/WAB.html

Other Resources
- McCall R, Tankersley C. *Student Workbook for Phlebotomy Essentials.* 6th ed. (Available for separate purchase.)
- McCall R, Tankersley C. *Phlebotomy Exam Review.* 6th ed. (Available for separate purchase.)

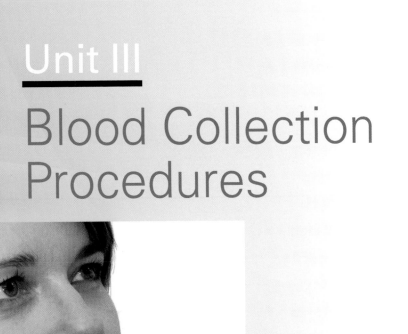

Unit III

Blood Collection Procedures

Chapter 7

Blood Collection Equipment, Additives, and Order of Draw

NAACLS Entry Level Competencies

5.00 Demonstrate knowledge of collection equipment, various types of additives used, special precautions necessary and substances that can interfere in clinical analysis of blood constituents.

5.1 Identify the various types of additives used in blood collection, and explain the reasons for their use.

5.2 Identify the evacuated tube color codes associated with the additives.

5.3 Describe the proper order of draw for specimen collections.

5.4 Describe substances that can interfere in clinical analysis of blood constituents and ways in which the phlebotomist can help to avoid these occurrences.

5.5 List and select the types of equipment needed to collect blood by venipuncture and capillary (dermal) puncture.

5.6 Identify special precautions necessary during blood collections by venipuncture and capillary (dermal) puncture.

Key Terms

Do Matching Exercise 7-1 in the WORKBOOK to gain familiarity with these terms.

ACD
additive
anticoagulant
antiglycolytic
  agent
antiseptic
bevel
butterfly needle
clot activator
disinfectant

EDTA
ETS
evacuated tube
gauge
glycolysis
heparin
hub
hypodermic
  needle
lumen

multisample
  needle
order of draw
potassium
  oxalate
PST
RST
shaft
sharps
  container

silica
sodium citrate
sodium
  fluoride
SPS
SST
thixotropic gel
winged infusion
  set

Objectives

Upon successful completion of this chapter, the reader should be able to:

1 List, describe, and explain the purpose of the equipment and supplies needed to collect blood specimens by venipuncture, and define associated terms and abbreviations.

2 List and describe evacuated tube system (ETS) and syringe system components, explain how each system works, and tell how to determine which system and components to use.

3 Demonstrate knowledge of the types of blood collection additives, identify the chemical composition of the specific additives within each type, and describe how each additive works.

4 Describe ETS tube stopper color coding used to identify the presence or absence of an additive, connect additives and stopper colors with laboratory departments and tests, and list the order of draw and explain its importance.

The primary duty of the phlebotomist is to collect blood specimens for laboratory testing. Blood is collected by several methods, including arterial puncture, capillary puncture, and venipuncture. This chapter describes general blood collection equipment and supplies commonly needed regardless of the method of collection, equipment specific to venipuncture, additives used in blood collection, and the order of draw for collecting or filling blood specimen tubes. A phlebotomist must be familiar with all the types of equipment in order to select appropriate collection devices for the type and condition of the patient's vein and the type and amount of specimen required for the test. Choosing the appropriate tools and using them correctly helps assure the safe collection of high-quality blood specimens. (Equipment specific to capillary puncture and arterial puncture is described in Chapters 10 and 14, respectively.)

General Blood Collection Equipment and Supplies

The following paragraphs describe the equipment and supplies commonly needed for all methods of collecting blood specimens.

BLOOD-DRAWING STATION

A blood-drawing station is a dedicated area of a medical laboratory or clinic equipped for performing phlebotomy procedures on patients, primarily outpatients sent by their physicians for laboratory testing. A typical blood-drawing station includes a table for supplies, a special chair where the patient sits during the blood collection procedure, and a bed or reclining chair for patients with a history of fainting, persons donating blood, and other special situations. A bed or padded table is also needed

if heelsticks or other procedures will be performed on infants and small children.

PHLEBOTOMY CHAIRS

A phlebotomy chair should be comfortable for the patient and have adjustable armrests to achieve proper positioning of either arm. Special phlebotomy chairs (Fig. 7-1) are available from a number of manufacturers. Most have adjustable armrests that lock in place to prevent the patient from falling should fainting occur.

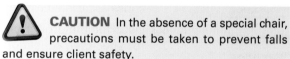

CAUTION In the absence of a special chair, precautions must be taken to prevent falls and ensure client safety.

EQUIPMENT CARRIERS

Equipment carriers make blood collection equipment portable. This is especially important in a hospital setting and other instances in which the patient cannot come to the laboratory.

Handheld Carriers

Handheld phlebotomy equipment carriers or trays (Fig. 7-2) come in a variety of styles and sizes designed to be easily carried by the phlebotomist and to contain enough equipment for numerous blood draws. They are convenient for "stat" or emergency situations or when relatively few patients need blood work.

Phlebotomy Carts

Phlebotomy carts (Fig. 7-3) are typically made of stainless steel or strong synthetic material. They have swivel wheels, which glide the carts smoothly and quietly down hospital hallways and in and out of elevators. They normally have several shelves to carry adequate supplies

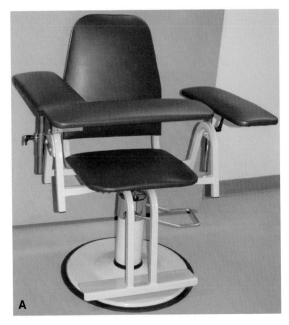

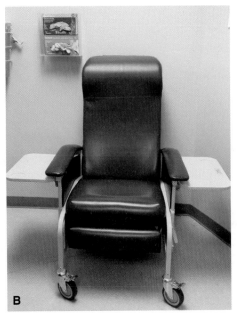

Figure 7-1 Two styles of phlebotomy chairs. **A:** Chair with adjustable arms and hydraulic height adjustment. **B:** Reclinable chair.

for obtaining blood specimens from many patients. Carts are commonly used for early-morning hospital phlebotomy rounds, when many patients need lab work, and for scheduled "sweeps" (rounds that occur at regular intervals throughout the day). Carts are bulky and a potential source of nosocomial infection; they are not normally brought into patients' rooms. Instead, they are parked outside in the hallway. A tray of supplies to be taken into the room is often carried on the cart.

Key Point Keeping carts and trays adequately stocked with supplies is an important duty of the phlebotomist.

GLOVES AND GLOVE LINERS

The Centers for Disease Control/Healthcare Infection Control Practices Advisory Committee (CDC/HICPAC) standard precautions and the Occupational Safety and

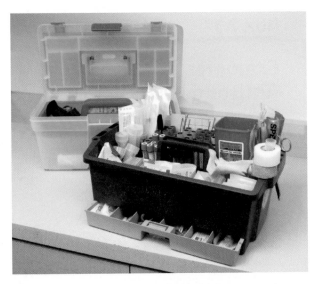

Figure 7-2 Two types of handheld phlebotomy equipment carriers.

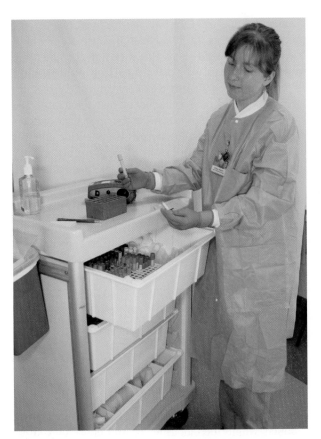

Figure 7-3 A phlebotomist with a phlebotomy cart.

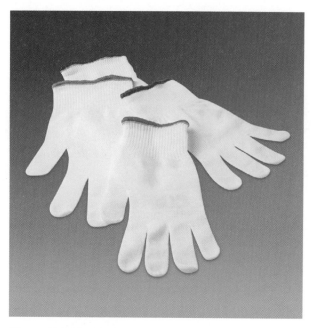

Figure 7-4 UltraFIT glove liners. (Courtesy of Erie Scientific Co., Portsmouth, NH.)

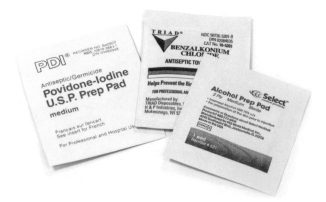

Figure 7-5 Examples of antiseptic prep pads.

Health Administration (OSHA) Bloodborne Pathogen Standard require the wearing of gloves when performing phlebotomy. A new pair must be used for each patient and removed when the procedure is completed. Nonsterile, disposable nitrile, neoprene, polyethylene, and vinyl examination gloves are acceptable for most phlebotomy procedures. A good fit is essential. Because of the prevalence of latex allergies, latex gloves are not recommended. In addition, gloves with powder are not recommended, as the powder can be a source of contamination for some tests (especially those collected by skin puncture) and can also cause allergies in some users. Special glove liners (Fig. 7-4) are available for persons who develop allergies or dermatitis from wearing gloves. Barrier hand creams that help prevent skin irritation and are compatible with most gloves are also available. The U.S. Food and Drug Administration (FDA) regulates glove quality.

 Key Point Decontamination of hands after glove removal is essential. Any type of glove may contain defects, and some studies suggest that vinyl gloves may not provide an adequate barrier to viruses.

ANTISEPTICS

Antiseptics (from Greek *anti*, "against" and *septikos*, "putrefactive") are substances used to prevent sepsis, which is the presence of microorganisms or their toxic products within the bloodstream. Antiseptics prevent or inhibit the growth and development of microorganisms

but do not necessarily kill them. They are considered safe to use on human skin and are used to clean the site prior to blood collection. The antiseptic most commonly used for routine blood collection is 70% isopropyl alcohol (isopropanol) in individually wrapped prep pads (Fig. 7-5). For a higher degree of antisepsis, the traditional antiseptic has been povidone–iodine in the form of swab sticks or sponge pads for blood culture collection and prep pads for blood gas collection. However, the use of alcohol-based preparations for these procedures is increasing because many patients are allergic to povidone–iodine. A list of antiseptics used in blood collection is shown in Box 7-1.

Key Point Cleaning with an antiseptic reduces the number of microorganisms but does not sterilize the site. (Sterilization kills or removes all living organisms and spores from an object; for example, using heat, radiation, or chemical means, and the items are sealed in sterile packages that remain sterile until the seal is broken.)

Box 7-1

Examples of Antiseptics Used in Blood Collection

- 70% Ethyl alcohol
- 70% Isopropyl alcohol (isopropanol)
- Benzalkonium chloride (e.g., Zephiran chloride)
- Chlorhexidine gluconate
- Hydrogen peroxide
- Povidone–iodine (0.1% to 1% available iodine)
- Tincture of iodine

DISINFECTANTS

Disinfectants are chemical substances or solutions regulated by the Environmental Protection Agency (EPA) that are used to remove or kill microorganisms on surfaces and instruments. They are stronger, more toxic, and typically more corrosive than antiseptics and are not safe to use on human skin. (Disinfectants do not kill bacterial spores, so reusable medical equipment must be sterilized before reuse.) According to the CDC and HICPAC *Guidelines for Environmental Infection Control in Healthcare Facilities,* use of EPA-registered sodium hypochlorite products is preferred, but solutions made from generic 5.25% sodium hypochlorite (household bleach) may be used. A 1:100 dilution is recommended for decontaminating nonporous surfaces after cleaning up blood or other body fluid spills in patient-care settings. When spills involve large amounts of blood or other body fluids or occur in the laboratory, a 1:10 dilution is applied prior to cleanup. At least 10 minutes of contact time is required for bleach-based and some other disinfectants to be effective. Consult manufacturer instructions.

 CAUTION Fresh bleach solutions should be made daily or as needed.

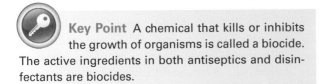 **Key Point** A chemical that kills or inhibits the growth of organisms is called a biocide. The active ingredients in both antiseptics and disinfectants are biocides.

HAND SANITIZERS

The CDC *Guideline for Hand Hygiene in Health Care Settings* recommends the use of alcohol-based hand sanitizers for routine decontamination of hands as a substitute for handwashing provided that the hands are not visibly soiled. If hands are heavily contaminated with organic material and handwashing facilities are not available, it is recommended that hands be cleaned with detergent-containing wipes followed by the use of an alcohol-based hand cleanser. Alcohol-based hand cleansers are available in rinses, gels, and foams and come in various types of containers including personal-size bottles and wall-mounted dispensers (Fig. 7-6). Wall-mounted dispensers are often located just inside the doors to patient rooms and next to handwashing facilities. Phlebotomists typically carry small bottles of sanitizer in their equipment carriers.

GAUZE PADS

Clean 2-by-2–inch gauze pads folded in fourths are used to hold pressure over the site following blood collection procedures. Special gauze pads with fluidproof backing are also available to help prevent contamination of gloves from blood at the site. Use of cotton balls to hold pressure is not recommended because the cotton fibers tend to stick to the site. Consequently, when the cotton ball is removed the platelet plug that is forming to seal the site can be disrupted and bleeding reinitiated.

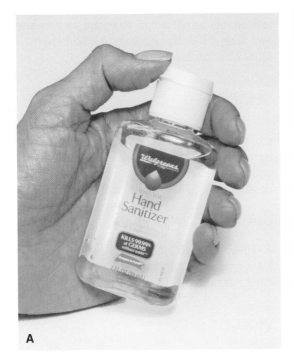

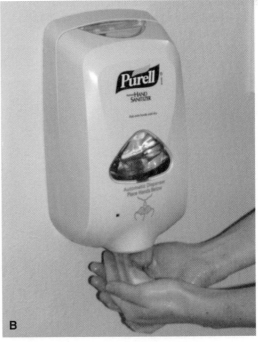

Figure 7-6 A: A personal-size bottle of hand sanitizer. **B:** A wall-mounted hand sanitizer dispenser.

BANDAGES

Adhesive bandages are used to cover a blood collection site after the bleeding has stopped. Paper, cloth, or knitted tape placed over a folded gauze square can also be used. Self-adhesive gauze placed over the gauze pad or cotton ball and wrapped around the arm is being used increasingly, especially for patients who are allergic to adhesive bandages. It is also used to form a pressure bandage following arterial puncture or venipuncture in patients with bleeding problems. Latex-free bandages are available for those with latex allergies.

> ⚠️ **CAUTION** Adhesive bandages should not be used on babies younger than 2 years of age because of the danger of aspiration and suffocation.

NEEDLE AND SHARPS DISPOSAL CONTAINERS

Used needles, lancets, and other sharp objects must be disposed of immediately in special containers referred to as **"sharps" containers** (Fig. 7-7), even if such objects contain safety features. A variety of styles and sizes of sharp containers are available. Most are red, for easy identification, but some are clear or opaque to make it easier to tell when they are full. All must be clearly marked with a biohazard symbol and be rigid, puncture resistant, leakproof, and disposable and have locking lids to seal the contents when filled to the appropriate volume, after which they must be properly disposed of as biohazardous waste.

> ⚠️ **CAUTION** Sharps containers should not be overfilled because this creates a danger of sharps injury or other biohazard exposure (e.g., contact with infectious substances) to subsequent users.

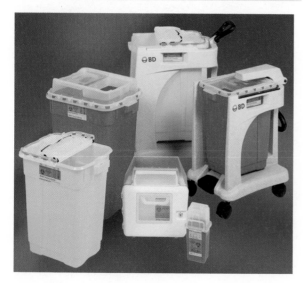

Figure 7-7 Several styles of sharps containers. (Courtesy of Becton Dickinson, Franklin Lakes, NJ.)

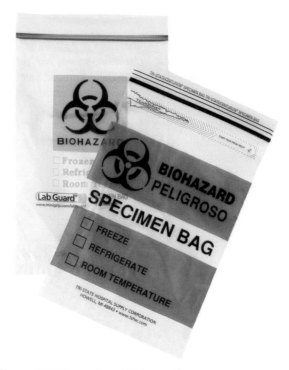

Figure 7-8 Two styles of biohazard bags.

BIOHAZARD BAGS

Biohazard bags (Fig. 7-8) are leakproof plastic bags that are commonly used to transport blood and other specimens from the collection site to the laboratory. The bags are marked with a biohazard label and often have an outside pocket in which requisitions or other forms can be placed. The bags help protect the collector and others from biohazard contamination. They will also contain a leak should a spill occur. There are various other styles and sizes of biohazard bags for biohazard trash and other biohazardous waste.

SLIDES

Precleaned 25-by-75–mm (1-by-3–inch) glass microscope slides are used to make blood films for hematology determinations. Slides are available either plain or with a frosted area at one end where the patient's name or other information can be written in pencil.

PEN

A phlebotomist should always carry a pen with indelible (permanent) nonsmear ink to label tubes and record other patient information.

WATCH

A watch, preferably with a sweep second hand or timer, is needed to accurately determine specimen collection times and time certain tests.

PATIENT IDENTIFICATION EQUIPMENT

Many healthcare facilities use barcode technology to identify patients. The barcode is on the ID band and phlebotomists carry barcode readers to identify patients and generate labels for the specimen tubes. Radio frequency identification (RFID) systems (see Chapter 11) are also gaining acceptance. See Chapter 11.

Venipuncture Equipment

Don't forget that you can test your equipment knowledge with the questions in the EXAM REVIEW.

The following equipment is used for venipuncture procedures in addition to the general blood collection supplies and equipment previously described.

VEIN-LOCATING DEVICES

There are a number of optional but useful portable transillumination devices on the market that make it easier to locate veins that are difficult to see or feel. Transillumination means to inspect an organ by passing light through its walls. These devices typically shine high-intensity LED or infrared red light through the patient's subcutaneous tissue to highlight veins. The hemoglobin in the blood within the veins absorbs the light, causing the veins to stand out as dark lines. Most devices can be used in patients of all ages. Examples include the Venoscope II (Fig. 7-9A,B) and Neonatal Transilluminator (Venoscope, L.L.C., Lafayette, LA), and the AccuVein AV300 (Fig. 7-9C) (AccuVein LLC, Huntington, NY).

TOURNIQUET

A **tourniquet** is a device that is applied or tied around a patient's arm prior to venipuncture to compress the veins and restrict blood flow. A properly applied tourniquet

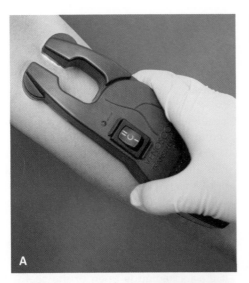

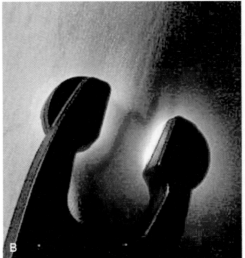

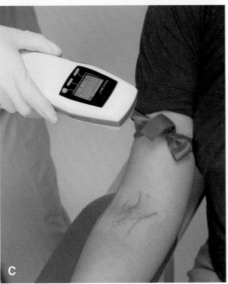

Figure 7-9 A: A Venoscope II transilluminator device. **B:** A vein appears as a dark line between the light-emitting arms of the Venoscope II. (Venoscope II, LLC, Lafayette, LA.) **C:** AccuVein AV300 being used to locate veins on a patient's arm. (AccuVein LLC, Huntington, NY.)

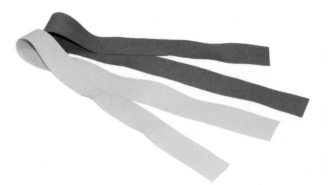

Figure 7-10 Stretchable strap tourniquets.

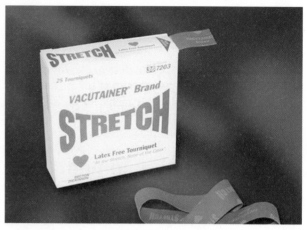

Figure 7-11 Single-use latex-free tourniquets.

is tight enough to restrict venous flow out of the area but not so tight as to restrict arterial flow into the area. Restriction of venous flow distends or inflates the veins, making them larger and easier to find, and stretches the vein walls so they are thinner and easier to pierce with a needle. Restriction of blood flow can change blood components if the tourniquet is left in place for more than 1 minute, so a tourniquet must fasten in a way that is easy to release with one hand during blood collection procedures or in emergency situations, such as when a patient starts to faint or the needle accidentally backs out of the arm during venipuncture.

There are a number of different types of tourniquets, and most are available in both adult and pediatric sizes. The most common type, a strap tourniquet (Fig. 7-10), is a flat strip of stretchable material that is fairly inexpensive and disposable. Although tourniquets at one time were commonly made of latex, nonlatex tourniquets (e.g., nitrile or vinyl) are now readily available.

> **Key Point** A blood pressure cuff may be used in place of a tourniquet. The patient's blood pressure is taken and the pressure is then maintained below the patient's diastolic pressure, or no greater than 40 mm Hg. Disposable blood pressure cuffs are now commonly available.

Although at present there is no regulatory requirement to dispose of tourniquets after a single use, a number of studies have shown that reusable tourniquets have the potential to transmit bacteria, including methicillin-resistant *Staphylococcus aureus* (MRSA). Consequently, CLSI now recommends single-use tourniquets (Fig. 7-11) to prevent HAIs. Reusable tourniquets are still in use at some facilities, however. If disposable tourniquets are reused they must be discarded if dropped or contaminated with blood or other visible contaminants. Nondisposable tourniquets must be disinfected on a regular basis and whenever visibly soiled or contaminated with blood.

Studies have shown that tourniquet contamination often comes from phlebotomists' hands rather than patients' skin, suggesting a need for better hand-hygiene habits by phlebotomists. Although proper hand hygiene is important regardless of the type of tourniquet used, for those who reuse tourniquets, meticulous hand hygiene is crucial.

NEEDLES

Phlebotomy needles are sterile, disposable, and designed for a single use only. They include **multisample needles** (see "Evacuated Tube System," below), **hypodermic needles** (see "Syringe System"), and **winged infusion (butterfly) needle sets** used with both the evacuated tube system (ETS) and the syringe system. Multisample needles are commonly enclosed in sealed twist-off shields or covers. Hypodermic needles and butterfly needles are typically sealed in sterile pull-apart packages.

> **CAUTION** It is important to examine the packaging or seal of a needle before use. If the packaging is open or the seal is broken, the needle is no longer sterile and should not be used.

> **Key Point** It important to visually inspect a needle prior to venipuncture. Needles are mass produced and on rare occasions contain defects such as blocked, blunt, or bent tips or rough bevels or shafts that could injure a patient's vein, cause unnecessary pain, or result in venipuncture failure.

Specific terminology is used to refer to the parts of a needle. The end that pierces the vein is called the **bevel** because it is "beveled," or cut on a slant. The bevel allows the needle to easily slip into the skin and vein without coring (removing a portion of the skin or vein).

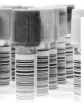

Table 7-1: Common Venipuncture Needle Gauges with Needle Type and Typical Use

Gauge	Needle Type	Typical Use
15–17	Special needle attached to collection bag	Collection of donor units, autologous blood donation, and therapeutic phlebotomy
20 20	Multisample Hypodermic	Sometimes used when large-volume tubes are collected or large-volume syringes are used on patients with normal-size veins
21 21	Multisample Hypodermic	Considered the standard venipuncture needle for routine venipuncture on patients with normal veins or for syringe blood culture collection
22 22	Multisample Hypodermic	Used on older children and adult patients with small veins or for syringe draws on difficult veins
23	Butterfly	Used on the veins of infants and children and on difficult or hand veins of adults

The long cylindrical portion is called the **shaft**. The end that attaches to the blood collection device is called the **hub**, and the internal space of the needle is called the **lumen**. Needles are available in various sizes, indicated by gauge and length.

Gauge

> Have fun finding the word "gauge" in the scrambled words drill in the WORKBOOK.

Needle **gauge** is indicated by a number that is related to the diameter of the lumen. A needle's diameter and gauge have an inverse (opposite) relationship; that is, the higher the gauge number, the smaller the actual diameter of the needle.

Although blood typically flows more quickly through large-diameter needles, needle gauge is selected according to the size and condition of the patient's vein, the type of procedure, the volume of blood to be drawn, and the equipment being used. Appropriate needles for the collection of most blood specimens for laboratory testing include gauges 20 through 23; however, a 21-gauge needle is considered the standard for most routine adult antecubital venipunctures. Common venipuncture needle gauges with needle type and typical use are shown in Table 7-1.

> **Key Point** It is important to select the appropriate needle for the situation. A needle that is too large may damage a vein needlessly, and a needle that is too small may hemolyze the specimen.

Manufacturers typically color code needles by gauge for easy identification. Generally, multisample needles have color-coded caps and hubs, and syringe needles have color-coded hubs. Butterfly needles often have color-coded "wings." Syringe and butterfly needle packaging may also contain color coding. Needle color codes vary among manufacturers; however, several large manufacturers use yellow for 20-gauge, green for 21-gauge, and black for 22-gauge needles (Fig. 7-12).

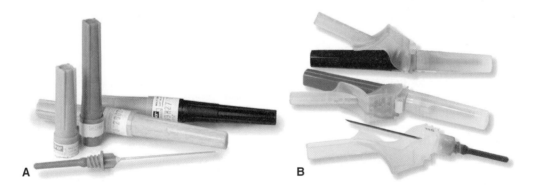

Figure 7-12 Multisample needles with color-coded caps. **A:** Traditional style needles: yellow 20 gauge, green 21 gauge, and black 22 gauge. (Courtesy of Greiner Bio-One International AG, Kremsmünster, Austria.) **B:** BD Eclipse safety needles, black 22 gauge, green 21 gauge. (Becton Dickinson, Franklin Lakes, NJ.)

Box 7-2

Desirable Characteristics of Safety Features

- The safety feature is a fixed safety feature that provides a barrier between the hands and the needle after use; the safety feature should allow or require the worker's hands to remain behind the needle at all times.
- The safety feature is an integral part of the device and not an accessory.
- The safety feature is in effect before disassembly and remains in effect after disposal to protect users and trash handlers and for environmental safety.
- The safety feature is as simple as possible, requiring little or no training to use effectively.

Length

Most multisample needles come in 1- or 1.5-inch lengths. Syringe needles come in many lengths; however 1- and 1.5-inch ones are most commonly used for venipuncture. Butterfly needles are typically ½ to ¾ inch long. Some of the new safety needles come in slightly longer lengths to accommodate resheathing features. Length selection depends primarily upon user preference and the depth of the vein. Many phlebotomists prefer to use 1-inch needles in routine situations because it is less intimidating to the patient. Others, especially those with larger hands, feel that the 1.5-inch needle makes it easier to achieve the proper angle for entering the vein.

Safety Features

Needles are available with or without safety features. Safety features must provide immediate permanent containment and be activated using one hand, which must stay behind the needle at all times. Safety features include **resheathing devices**, such as shields that cover the needle after use; blunting devices; and equipment with devices that retract the needle after use. The FDA is responsible for clearing medical devices for marketing. Box 7-2 lists desirable characteristics of safety features that the FDA considers important in preventing percutaneous injury.

Key Point According to OSHA regulations, if the needle does not have a safety feature, the equipment it is used with (such as tube holder or syringe) must have a safety feature to minimize the chance of an accidental needlestick.

EVACUATED TUBE SYSTEM

The most common and efficient system and that preferred by the CLSI for collecting blood samples is the **evacuated tube system (ETS)** (Fig. 7-13). It is a closed system in which the patient's blood flows through a needle inserted into a vein and then directly into a collection tube without being exposed to the air or outside contaminants. The system allows numerous tubes to be collected with a single venipuncture. ETSs are available from several manufacturers. Although the design of individual elements may vary slightly by manufacturer, all ETS systems have three basic components: a special blood-drawing needle, a tube holder, and various types of evacuated tubes.

Key Point Unless components are specifically designed for use with multiple systems, it is recommended that all ETS components come from the same manufacturer. Mixing components from different manufacturers can lead to problems such as needles coming unscrewed and tubes popping off the needle during venipuncture.

Multisample Needles

ETS needles are called *multisample needles* because they allow multiple tubes of blood to be collected during a single venipuncture. They are threaded in the middle and have a beveled point on each end. The threaded portion screws into a tube holder. The end of the needle that pierces the vein is longer and has a longer bevel. The shorter end penetrates the tube stopper during specimen collection. It is covered by a sleeve that retracts as the needle goes through the tube stopper so that blood can flow into the tube. When the tube is removed, the sleeve slides back over the needle to prevent leakage of blood. ETS needles are available with or without safety features. The color-coded needles shown in Figure 7-12A are traditional-style multiple-sample needles without safety features. The needles shown in Figure 7-12B have safety devices used to resheath the needles after use.

CAUTION ETS needles that lack safety features must be used with tube holders that have safety features.

A welcome innovation in multisample needles is the Greiner Bio-One VACUETTE® VISIO PLUS Needle (Fig. 7-14). This needle has a transparent hub where blood can be seen if the venipuncture is successful. With most other multisample needles, blood flow is not evident until the tube is advanced onto the needle in the tube holder.

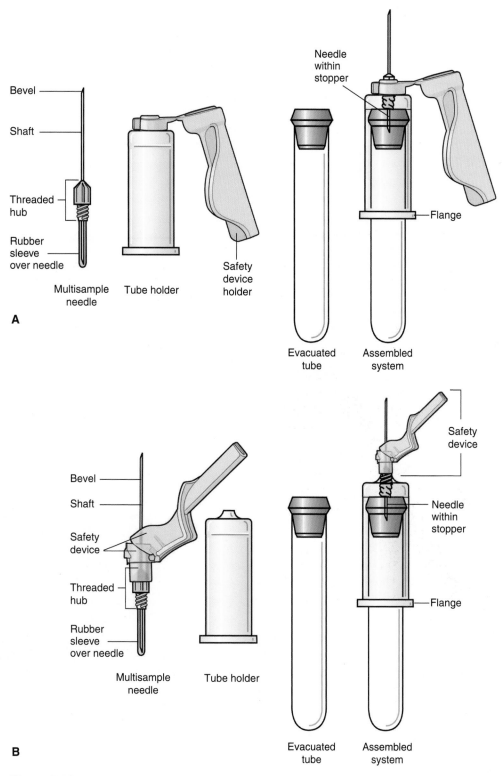

Figure 7-13 Evacuated tube system (ETS) components. **A:** Traditional needle and safety tube holder. **B:** Safety needle and traditional tube holder.

Tube Holders

A **tube holder** is a clear, plastic, disposable cylinder with a small threaded opening at one end (often also called a hub) where the needle is screwed into it and a large opening at the other end where the collection tube is placed. The large end has flanges or extensions on the sides that aid in tube placement and removal.

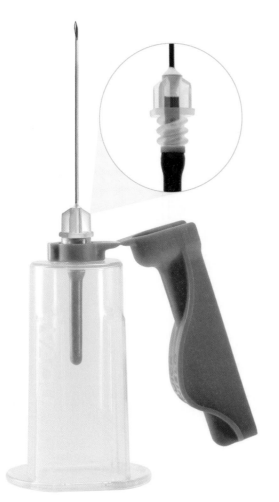

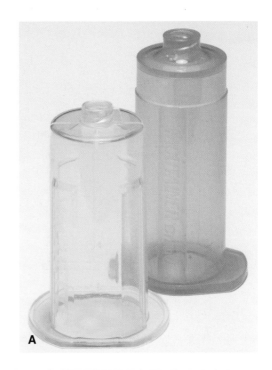

Figure 7-14 VACUETTE® VISIO PLUS needle with see-through hub attached to a safety tube holder. (Courtesy of Greiner Bio-One International AG, Kremsmünster, Austria.)

Key Point OSHA regulations require that the tube holder with needle attached be disposed of as a unit after use and never be removed from the needle and reused.

Holders are typically available in several sizes to accommodate different-sized tubes, including special sizes for large-diameter blood culture bottles, some of which have adapter inserts to narrow the diameter of the holder and allow for the collection of evacuated tubes after the blood culture specimens. Adapter inserts are also available so that small-diameter tubes can be collected in regular-size tube holders. Holders are available with and without safety features (Fig. 7-15).

CAUTION If the tube holder does not have a safety feature, the needle used with it must have a safety feature.

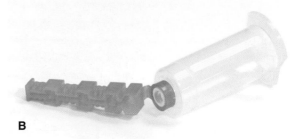

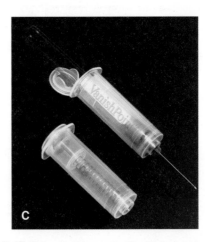

Figure 7-15 Tube holders. **A:** Traditional tube holders. **B:** JELCO Venipuncture Needle-Pro® safety tube holder with resheathing device. (Image courtesy of Smiths Medical North America. JELCO, Needle-Pro is a trademark of Smiths Medical Family of Companies. All Rights Reserved.) **C:** Vanishpoint® safety tube holder with needle-retracting device attached to a traditional nonsafety needle. (Courtesy of Retractable Technologies, Little Elm, TX.)

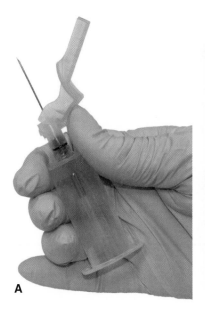
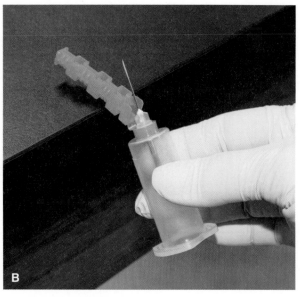

Figure 7-16 Tube holders with needles attached. **A:** Traditional tube holder with safety needle attached. **B:** Venipuncture Needle-Pro safety tube holder with needle resheathing device attached to a traditional nonsafety needle.

Safety features include shields that cover the needle and devices that manually or automatically retract the needle into the holder either before or after it is removed from the vein. Two types of holders (traditional and safety) with needles attached are shown in Figure 7-16.

(i) A needle or tube holder that has a safety device is an example of a SESIP, which is the OSHA acronym for a sharp with engineered sharps injury protection.

Needle and Holder Units

Needle and tube-holder devices are available permanently attached as a single unit or as both devices preassembled. Preassembled devices are often sealed in sterile packaging for use in sterile applications. An example of a single unit is the BD Vacutainer® Passive Shielding Blood Collection Needle (Fig. 7-17). The needle has a shield that releases automatically when the first tube is inserted in the holder. Upon activation, the shield rests against the patient's arm and immediately covers the needle when it is withdrawn from the patient. This safety feature cannot be bypassed by the user, ensuring 100% compliance.

Evacuated Tubes

Evacuated tubes (Fig. 7-18) are used with both the ETS and the syringe method of obtaining blood specimens. (With the syringe method, blood is collected in a syringe and must be immediately transferred into the tubes.) Evacuated tubes are available from a number of different

manufacturers and come in various sizes and volumes ranging from 1.8 to 15 mL. Tube selection is based on the age of the patient, the amount of blood needed for the test, and the size and condition of the patient's vein. Most laboratories stock several sizes of each type of tube to accommodate various needs. Although ETS tubes at one time were made of glass, most are now made of plastic for safety reasons. A few tubes are still available in glass.

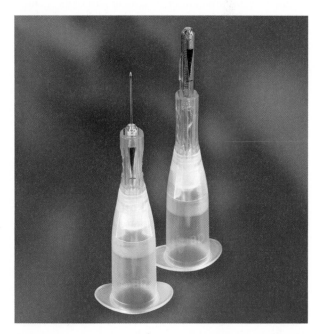

Figure 7-17 BD Vacutainer® Passive Shielding Blood Collection Needle. (Courtesy of Becton Dickinson, Franklin Lakes, New Jersey.)

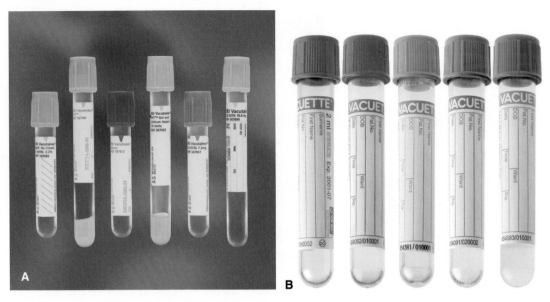

Figure 7-18 Evacuated tubes. **A:** Vacutainer® Plus Plastic brand evacuated tubes. (Courtesy of Becton Dickinson, Franklin Lakes, NJ.) **B:** Vacuette® evacuated tubes. (Greiner Bio-One International AG, Kremsmünster, Austria.)

Vacuum

Evacuated tubes fill with blood automatically because there is a **vacuum** (negative pressure) in them. The vacuum is artificially created during manufacture by pulling air from the tube. The amount of vacuum (i.e., the amount of air removed and negative pressure created) is measured precisely by the manufacturer so that the tube will draw the exact volume of blood indicated on the label. To reach its stated volume, a tube must be allowed to fill with blood until the normal vacuum is exhausted. A tube that has prematurely lost all or part of its vacuum will fail to properly fill with blood.

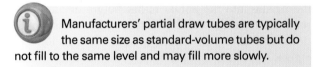

Key Point Tubes do not fill with blood all the way to the stopper. When a tube is filled properly, there is always a consistent amount of head space (air) between the level of blood in the tube and the tube stopper.

Premature loss of vacuum can occur from improper storage, opening the tube, dropping the tube, advancing the tube too far onto the needle before venipuncture, or if the needle bevel becomes partially out of the skin during venipuncture. Premature loss of vacuum, removing the tube before the vacuum is exhausted, or stoppage of blood flow during the blood draw can result in an underfilled tube called a partial draw or **"short draw."** Test results may be compromised in partially filled tubes that contain additives because the ratio of blood-to-additive has been altered. Consequently some manufacturers offer special "short draw" tubes (Fig. 7-19) designed to partially fill without compromising test results. These

tubes are used in situations in which it is difficult or inadvisable to draw larger quantities of blood.

Manufacturers' partial draw tubes are typically the same size as standard-volume tubes but do not fill to the same level and may fill more slowly.

Additive Tubes

Most ETS tubes contain some type of **additive**. An additive is any substance placed within a tube other than the tube stopper or silicone coating, if any. Additives have one or more specific functions, such as preventing clotting or preserving certain blood components. Blood collected in additive tubes may or may not clot,

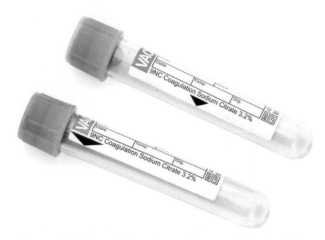

Figure 7-19 Coagulation tubes with arrows indicating fill levels; a regular draw tube **(bottom)** and a short draw tube **(top)**.

depending on the additive type. For example, if the additive prevents clotting, the result is a whole-blood specimen. Some whole-blood specimens are used directly for testing; others are centrifuged to separate the cells from the fluid portion called plasma, which is used for testing. If the additive is a clot activator, the blood will clot and the specimen must be centrifuged to obtain the fluid portion called serum. (See Chapter 6 for a discussion of serum, plasma, and whole blood.)

Key Point Plastic tubes are so smooth inside that platelet aggregation and adhesion are inhibited, resulting in delayed or incomplete clotting. Consequently, clot activators are added to plastic serum tubes. This is not a problem with glass tubes, because glass has a rougher surface.

The amount of additive in a tube has been calibrated by the manufacturer to function optimally and produce accurate results with the amount of blood it takes to fill the tube to the capacity or volume indicated. Specimen quality can be compromised and lead to inaccurate results if the tube is underfilled, so it is important to allow additive tubes to fill with blood until the normal vacuum is exhausted.

CAUTION An underfilled additive tube will have an incorrect blood-to-additive ratio, which can cause inaccurate test results.

Nonadditive Tubes

Very few tubes are additive free. (Even serum tubes need an additive to promote clotting if they are plastic.) Most nonadditive plastic tubes (Fig. 7-20) that do exist are used for clearing or discarding purposes and limited other uses. Examples are the Vacuette® gray top, and the BD clear top. A few glass nonadditive red-top tubes are still in existence (e.g., BD still makes a glass red top primarily used for serum chemistry and blood donor screening), but most have been discontinued for safety

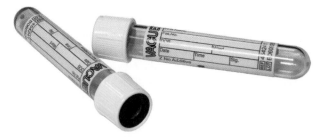

Figure 7-20 Nonadditive tube used as a discard or "clear" tube.

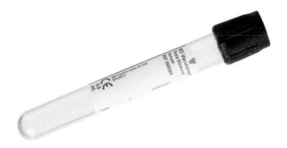

Figure 7-21 Royal-blue–top tube. The red stripe down the left side of the label indicates that it is a serum tube.

reasons. Blood collected in a tube will clot when there is nothing in the tube to prevent it. Consequently, nonadditive tubes yield serum samples.

Stoppers

Tube stoppers (caps, tops, or closures) are typically made of rubber. Some tubes have a rubber stopper covered by a plastic shield designed to protect lab personnel from blood drops remaining on the stopper after the tube is removed from the needle and from aerosols (mists) and sprays of specimen when the stopper is removed from the tube. The rigidity of the plastic also prevents removal of the stopper using a "thumb roll," a technique that has been shown to cause aerosol formation.

Color Coding

Tube stoppers are color coded. Consequently, it is not unusual for evacuated tubes to be referred to as red tops, green tops, and so forth. For most tubes, the stopper color identifies a type of additive placed in the tube by the manufacturer for a specific purpose. However, for some tubes, the stopper color indicates a special property of the tube. For example, a royal-blue stopper (Fig. 7-21) indicates a tube that is as free of trace element contamination as possible. Royal-blue tops either contain no additive, or depending on the manufacturer, heparin or EDTA. The BD tan stopper tube contains EDTA and is used for lead tests because it is certified to contain less than 0.01 µg/mL (ppm) lead.

Key Point If a royal-blue top has an additive, the color code for the additive is often displayed on the label. If not, the proper tube must be selected according to the additive listed on the label.

Occasionally, there is more than one stopper color for the same additive. In addition, although color coding is generally universal, it may vary slightly by manufacturer. Common stopper colors, what they indicate, and what departments use them are shown in Table 7-2. For reference, two manufacturers' tube guides are shown in Appendix F.

Table 7-2: Common Stopper Colors, Additives, and Departments

Stopper Color(s)	Additive	Department(s)
Light blue	Sodium citrate	Coagulation
Red (glass)	None	Chemistry, Blood Bank, Serology/ Immunology
Red (plastic)	Clot activator	Chemistry
Red/light gray Clear	None	NA (discard tube only)
Red/black (tiger) Gold	Clot activator and gel separator	Chemistry
Green/gray Light green	Lithium heparin and gel separator	Chemistry
Green	Lithium heparin Sodium heparin	Chemistry
Lavender (purple)	EDTA	Hematology
Pink	EDTA	Blood Bank
Gray	Sodium fluoride and potassium oxalate Sodium fluoride and EDTA Sodium fluoride	Chemistry
Orange Gray/yellow	Thrombin	Chemistry
Royal blue	None EDTA Sodium heparin	Chemistry
Tan	EDTA	Chemistry
Yellow	Sodium polyanethol sulfonate (SPS)	Microbiology
Yellow	Acid citrate dextrose (ACD)	Blood Bank/Immunohematology

Expiration Dates

Manufacturers guarantee reliability of additives and tube vacuum until an expiration date printed on the label (Fig. 7-22), provided the tubes are handled properly and stored between 4°C and 25°C. Improper handling or storage can affect additive integrity and tube vacuum, which can lead to compromised test results or improper filling, respectively.

Key Point Always check the expiration date on a tube before using it, and never use a tube that has expired or has been dropped. Discard it instead.

SYRINGE SYSTEM

Although the ETS is the preferred method of blood collection, a **syringe system** (Fig. 7-23) is sometimes used for patients with small or difficult veins. This system consists of a sterile syringe needle called a *hypodermic needle* and a sterile plastic syringe with a Luer-lock tip (a special tip that allows the needle to attach more securely than a slip tip).

Syringe Needles

Syringe needles come in a wide range of gauges and lengths for many different uses. Those appropriate for

Figure 7-22 A closeup of the expiration date on a blood specimen tube. (Expiration date has been circled in red.)

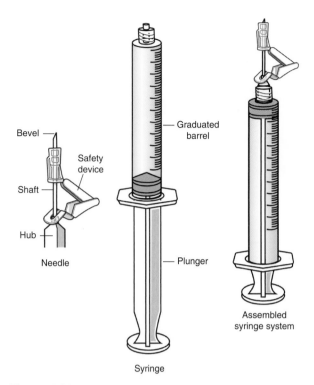

Figure 7-23 Syringe system components.

phlebotomy procedures are generally gauges 21 to 23, in 1- or 1.5-inch lengths. When used to draw blood, a syringe needle must have a resheathing feature to allow it to be safely covered and removed so that a transfer device can be attached to the syringe to fill the evacuated tubes. An example of a safety needle attached to a syringe is shown in Figure 7-24A. A syringe that has a built-in safety device to cover the needle is shown in Figure 7-24B.

⚠️ **CAUTION** Syringe needles used for phlebotomy must have resheathing devices to minimize the chance of accidental needlesticks. Needles used for intradermal skin tests must have resheathing devices or be used with syringes that have devices that cover or retract the needle after use.

Syringes

Syringes typically come in sterile pull-apart packages and are available in various sizes or volumes. The most common volumes used for phlebotomy are 2, 5, and 10 mL. Syringe volume is selected according to the size and condition of the patient's vein and the amount of blood to be collected.

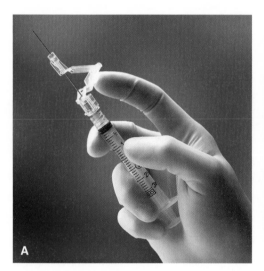

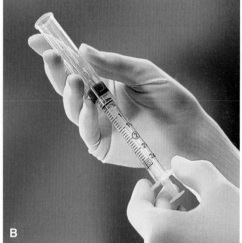

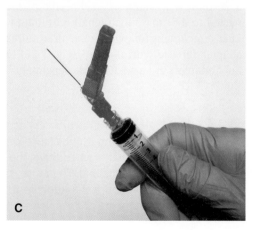

Figure 7-24 Syringe safety devices. **A:** Syringe with BD SAFETYGLIDE™ hypodermic needle attached. **B:** BD SAFETY-LOK™ syringe. (Courtesy of Becton Dickinson, Franklin Lakes, NJ.) **C:** JELCO Hypodermic Needle-Pro® safety needle attached to a syringe. (Smiths Medical North America.)

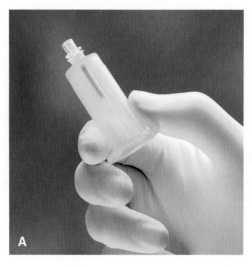

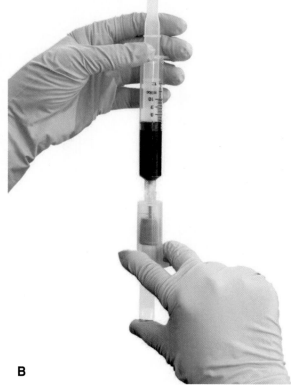

Figure 7-25 Syringe transfer devices. **A:** BD transfer device. (Courtesy of Becton Dickinson, Franklin Lakes, NJ.) **B:** Greiner transfer device attached to a syringe.

Syringes have two parts: a **barrel**, which is a cylinder with graduated markings in either milliliters (mL) or cubic centimeters (cc), and a **plunger**, a rod-like device that fits tightly into the barrel (Fig. 7-23). When drawing venous blood by syringe, the phlebotomist slowly pulls back the plunger, creating a vacuum that causes the barrel to fill with blood.

Syringe Transfer Device

Blood collected in a syringe must be transferred into ETS tubes. In the past blood was transferred by poking the syringe needle through the tube stopper or by removing the tube stopper and ejecting blood from the syringe into the tube. Both practices are now considered unsafe and violate OSHA safety regulations. A **syringe transfer device** (Fig. 7-25A) allows the safe transfer of blood into the tubes without using the syringe needle or removing the tube stopper. The device is similar to an ETS tube holder but has a permanently attached needle inside. After a syringe draw is completed, the needle safety device is activated and the needle is removed and discarded into a sharps container. The transfer device is then attached to the hub of the syringe. An ETS tube is placed inside it and advanced onto the needle until blood flows into the tube (Fig. 7-25B). Additional tubes can be filled as long as there is enough blood in the syringe. The transfer device greatly reduces the chance of accidental needlesticks and confines any aerosol or spraying of the specimen that may be generated as tubes are removed from it.

Key Point A transfer device must be held vertical when tubes are being filled in order to prevent blood in the tube from touching the needle in the transfer device. If blood mixed with additive gets on or in the needle, it could be transferred into the next tube that is filled and contaminate it.

WINGED INFUSION SET

A **winged infusion blood collection set**, or **butterfly**, is an indispensable tool for collecting blood from small or difficult veins such as hand veins and veins of elderly and pediatric patients as it allows much more flexibility and precision than a needle and syringe. It consists of a ½- to ¾-inch stainless steel needle permanently connected to a 5- to 12-inch length of tubing with either a Luer attachment for syringe use or a multisample Luer adapter for use with the ETS (Fig. 7-26). Multisample Luer adapters are also available separately.

Key Point The first tube collected with a butterfly will underfill because of air in the tubing. If the tube contains an additive, the blood-to-additive ratio will be affected. Therefore, to remove air from the tubing before the additive tube is collected, it is important to draw a few milliliters of

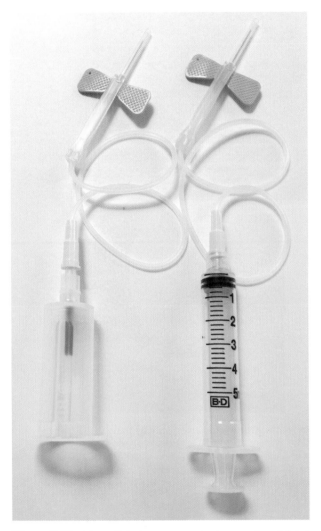

Figure 7-26 Winged infusion sets attached to a syringe **(right)** and an evacuated tube holder by means of a Luer adapter **(left)**.

blood into a nonadditive tube or another additive tube of the same type and discard. Consequently, this is referred to as collecting a "clear" or discard tube and it is especially critical that it be done when a coagulation tube is collected using a butterfly.

Plastic extensions that resemble butterfly wings (thus the name *butterfly*) are attached to the needle where it is joined to the tubing. During use, the needle may be held from above by gripping the "wings" together between the thumb and index finger, thus allowing the user to achieve the shallow angle of needle insertion required to access small veins.

Butterfly needles come in various gauges, although a 23-gauge needle is most commonly used for phlebotomy. In rare situations a 25-gauge needle is used by specially trained personnel to collect blood from scalp or other tiny veins of premature infants and other neonates.

⚠ **CAUTION** It is best to use small-volume tubes when drawing with a butterfly to reduce the chance of specimen hemolysis. Using a needle smaller than 23 gauge increases the chance of hemolysis even when using small-volume tubes.

As with other blood collection needles, butterfly needles are required to have safety devices to reduce the possibility of accidental needlesticks. Butterfly safety devices include locking shields that slide over the needle, blunting devices, and needle-retracting devices. See Figure 7-27 for examples of safety-winged infusion sets (butterflies).

COMBINATION SYSTEMS

The S-Monovette® Blood Collection System (Sarstedt, Inc., Newton, NC) shown in Figure 7-28 is a complete, multisampling venous blood collection system that can be manipulated by the user to perform either vacuum and/or gentle aspiration blood collection based on the condition of the patient's vein. No sample transfers are required with either technique. The tubes are available with a full range of additives and in various sizes and volumes from 1.1 to 9 mL. Tubes connect securely to one-piece safety needles. A fixed needle protector covers the front needle after use, and a small integral holder protects the user from the back end of the needle as well. Safety-Multifly® winged collection needles and adapters for connection to catheters are also available.

Blood Collection Additives

 WORKBOOK Matching 7-2 can help you learn the additives and their functions.

Blood collection tubes and other collection devices often contain one or more additives. There are a number of different types of additives, and each has a specific function. The type of additive required for blood collection generally depends upon the test that has been ordered. No substitution or combining of tubes with different additives is allowed.

⚠ **CAUTION** *Never* transfer blood collected in an additive tube into another additive tube, even if the additives are the same. Different additives may interfere with each other or the testing process. If the additives are the same, an excess of the additive is created, which can negatively affect testing.

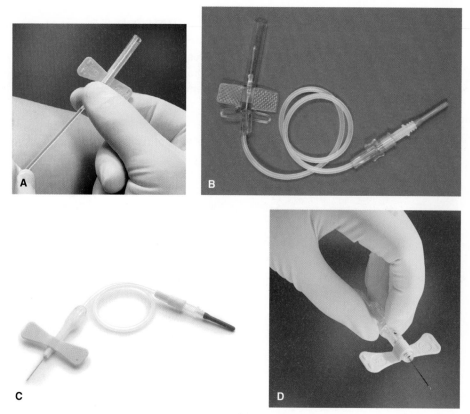

Figure 7-27 Examples of safety-winged infusion sets. **A:** BD Vacutainer® SAFETY-LOK™ Blood Collection Set for use with the evacuated tube system. (Courtesy of Becton Dickinson Vacutainer Systems, Franklin Lakes, NJ.) **B:** Monoject Angel Wing blood collection set. (Kendall CO, LP, Mansfield, MA.) **C:** Vacuette® safety butterfly blood collection system (Greiner Bio-One, Kremsmünster, Austria.) **D:** Vacutainer® push button blood collection set. (Courtesy of Becton Dickinson, Franklin Lakes, NJ.)

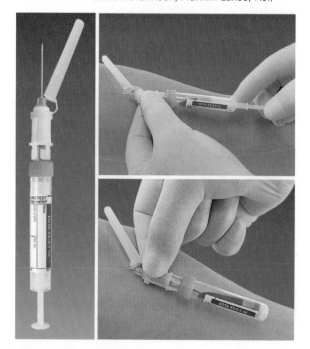

Figure 7-28 Sarstedt S-Monovette® venous blood collection system. **Left:** System with needle attached. **Upper right:** System used as a syringe. **Lower right:** System used as ETS. (Courtesy of Sarstedt, Inc., Newton, NC.)

Additives are available in liquid, spray-dried, and powder forms. A tube with a powdered additive should be lightly tapped prior to use to settle the additive to the bottom of the tube. An additive tube must be gently inverted 3 to 10 times, depending on the type of additive and the manufacturer, immediately after collection to adequately mix the additive with the specimen. (See the tube guides in Appendix F for tube inversion information from two major tube manufacturers.)

Key Point According to tube manufacturer Becton Dickinson (BD), each inversion requires turning the wrist 180 degrees and back again (Fig. 7-29).

CAUTION *Never* shake or otherwise vigorously mix a specimen, as this can cause hemolysis, which makes most specimens unsuitable for testing.

ANTICOAGULANTS

The most common reason for using an additive is to prevent clotting of the specimen. **Anticoagulants** are substances that prevent blood from clotting (coagulating) by either of two methods: by chelating (binding) or precipitating calcium so it is unavailable to the coagulation process or by inhibiting the formation of thrombin needed to convert fibrinogen to fibrin in the coagulation process. If a test requires whole blood or plasma, the specimen must be collected in a tube that contains an anticoagulant. Anticoagulant specimens must be mixed immediately after collection to prevent microclot formation. Gentle mixing is essential to prevent hemolysis. The recommended number of inversions required to sufficiently mix the anticoagulant with the blood may vary by manufacturer. Consult manufacturer instructions.

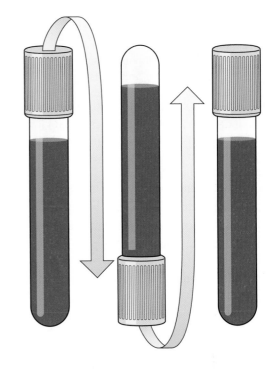

= One inversion

Figure 7-29 Illustration showing one complete tube inversion.

Key Point Because the cells are free flowing and not clotted, a specimen collected in anticoagulant can separate through settling or centrifugation and can be resuspended by intentional or inadvertent mixing of the specimen. (Specimens collected in gel-barrier tubes are protected from resuspension after they are centrifuged.) It is necessary to resuspend whole-blood hematology specimens that have settled before testing. Consult laboratory protocol before recentrifuging a plasma specimen that was inadvertently resuspended with the cells.

There are different types of anticoagulants, each designed for use in certain types of testing. It is important to use the correct anticoagulant for the type of test collected. The most common anticoagulants are **ethylenediaminetetraacetic acid (EDTA), citrates, heparin**, and **oxalates**. Memory joggers to help you learn the most common anticoagulants are found in Table 7-3.

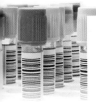

Table 7-3: Memory Joggers for Anticoagulants

Acronym, Mnemonic, or Acrostic	An Easy Way to Remember
ECHO	The most common anticoagulants. E (EDTA) C (citrate) H (heparin) O (oxalate).
phEDTA (*pronounced like fajita*)	Purple tubes go to hematology and contain EDTA. P (purple) h (hematology) EDTA.
Spring Creates Colorful Light-Blue Pansies	Sodium citrate tubes go to coagulation, have light-blue stoppers, and yield plasma. S (sodium) C (citrate) C (coagulation) L (light) B (blue) P (plasma).
HH: Heparin inhibits In-in: Heparin inhibits	Heparin inhibits thrombin formation; "H" in heparin and "H" in inhibits. Heparin ends with "in," and inhibits starts with "in."
Greenhouses Have Colorful Plants	Green tubes contain heparin for chemistry tests on plasma. G (green) H (heparin) C (chemistry) P (plasma).
GO (gray oxalate) or Gray ox (gray oxalate)	Gray tubes typically contain oxalate. G (gray) O (oxalate) Gray (gray); ox (oxalate)
LL (lavender last except for gray)	Lavender is drawn last unless a gray top is ordered. Gray tops are rarely ordered, so lavender is often last.

EDTA

EDTA is commonly available as a spray-coated di-potassium (K_2EDTA), or tri-potassium (K_3EDTA) salt or as liquid K_3EDTA. Salts are preferable due to their high solubility (ability to dissolve). Liquid EDTA can cause a dilution of the blood. Both types of EDTA remove calcium from the blood by binding (or chelating) it to form an insoluble salt. This makes calcium ions unavailable for the coagulation process so the blood in the tube is prevented from clotting.

EDTA is the additive in

- Lavender (or purple)-top tubes (Fig. 7-18).
- Microcollection containers with lavender tops.
- Pink plastic-top tubes with a special blood bank patient ID label.
- Royal-blue–top tubes with lavender color coding on the label.
- White/pearl-top tubes with thixotropic gel separator.

Although EDTA can also be used for blood bank tests, it is primarily used to provide whole-blood specimens for hematology tests (e.g., CBCs) because it preserves cell morphology (shape and structure) and inhibits platelet aggregation better than any other anticoagulant. EDTA specimens must be mixed immediately after collection to prevent platelet clumping and microclot formation, which can negatively affect test results. Eight to ten inversions are normally required for proper mixing.

> **CAUTION** If microclots are detected in a hematology specimen, it cannot be used for testing and must be recollected.

Spray-dried EDTA is used for most hematology tests because liquid EDTA dilutes the specimen and results in lower hemoglobin values, RBC and WBC counts, platelet counts, and packed-cell volumes. The dilutional effect is even more pronounced if the tubes are not completely filled. Therefore, it is important to fill tubes until their normal vacuum is exhausted. Either type of EDTA tube should be filled to its stated volume to maintain the correct blood-to-anticoagulant ratio.

> **Key Point** Excess EDTA, which results when tubes are underfilled, can cause RBCs to shrink and thus change CBC results.

Citrates

Citrates also prevent coagulation by binding or chelating calcium. The most common citrate is **sodium citrate**, which is used for coagulation tests (e.g., PT and aPTT) because it does the best job of preserving the coagulation factors. Sodium citrate tubes have light-blue stoppers (Fig. 7-18).

> **ⓘ** Sodium citrate is also the additive in special erythrocyte sedimentation rate (ESR) tubes with black stoppers.

Coagulation specimens require immediate mixing after collection to prevent activation of the coagulation process and microclot formation, which invalidates test results. Three to four gentle inversions are required for adequate mixing.

> **CAUTION** Vigorous mixing or an excessive number of inversions can activate platelets and shorten clotting times.

Light-blue–top tubes contain a 9:1 ratio of blood to anticoagulant when filled to the stated volume and must be filled to within 90% of that volume for accurate coagulation results. Exact fill volume is hard to tell on most tubes; however, Vacuette® sodium citrate tubes have arrows that are used to identify correct fill volume. A guide provided by the manufacturer also helps phlebotomists or specimen processors determine whether a tube is adequately filled (Fig. 7-30).

> **CAUTION** The 9:1 ratio of blood to anticoagulant in light-blue–sodium citrate tubes is critical; therefore, it is extremely important to fill them to the stated volume. Underfilled tubes can cause artificially prolonged clotting times and visibly underfilled tubes will not be accepted for testing by most laboratories.

Coagulation tests are performed on plasma, so specimens must first be centrifuged to separate the plasma from the cells. Because sodium citrate binds calcium, calcium is added back to the specimen during the testing process so that clotting can be initiated and timed.

Heparin

Heparin prevents clotting by inhibiting **thrombin** (an enzyme needed to convert fibrinogen into the fibrin necessary for clot formation.) and Factor X. Heparinized plasma has traditionally been used for some chemistry tests (e.g., ammonia and plasma hemoglobin). It is now commonly used for stat tests (e.g., electrolytes) and in other rapid-response situations when a fast turnaround time (TAT) for chemistry tests is needed. Faster TAT is possible because tests performed on heparinized whole blood can be performed right away. Specimens for tests

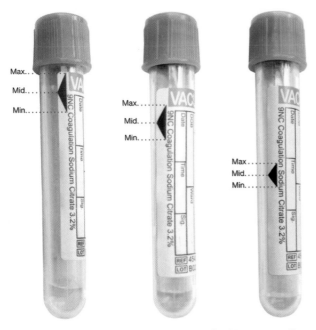

Figure 7-30 Guide showing fill levels for Vacuette sodium citrate tubes. (Courtesy of Greiner Bio-One International AG, Kremsmünster, Austria.)

that are performed on heparinized plasma can be centrifuged right away. This saves the time that would normally be required for a serum specimen to clot before being centrifuged to obtain serum for testing.

Key Point Heparinized plasma is preferred over serum for potassium tests because when blood clots, potassium is released from cells into the serum and can falsely elevate results.

Check out WORKBOOK Knowledge Drill 7-1 to see how well you know this and other cautions and key points.

Heparin is the additive in
- Green-top tubes
- Green-top and light-green–top gel tubes (Fig. 7-18)
- Mottled-green and gray-top tubes
- Royal-blue–top tubes with green color coding on the label
- Green-top and light-green–top microtubes
- Red-banded and green-banded microhematocrit tubes

There are three heparin formulations: ammonium, lithium, and sodium heparin. Lithium heparin causes the least interference in chemistry testing and is the most widely used anticoagulant for both plasma and whole-blood chemistry tests.

CAUTION It is essential to choose the right heparin formulation for the type of test. Lithium heparin must not be used to collect lithium levels. Sodium heparin must not be used to collect sodium specimens or electrolyte panels because sodium is part of the panel.

Heparinized specimens must be mixed immediately upon collection to prevent clot formation and fibrin generation. From five to ten inversions, depending on the manufacturer, are required for proper mixing. Gentle mixing is essential to prevent hemolysis. Hemolyzed specimens are unsuitable for many chemistry tests.

Oxalates

Oxalates remove calcium and prevent clotting by binding and precipitating calcium in the form of an insoluble salt. **Potassium oxalate** is the most widely used. It is commonly added to tubes containing glucose preservatives (see "Antiglycolytic Agents," below) to provide plasma for glucose testing. Potassium oxalate is most commonly found in evacuated tubes and microcollection containers with gray stoppers. Oxalate specimens must be mixed immediately upon collection to prevent clot formation and fibrin generation. Eight to ten inversions are required for proper mixing.

CAUTION It is essential to fill oxalate tubes to the volume stated on the tube because excess oxalate causes hemolysis (destruction of red blood cells, or RBCs) and release of hemoglobin into the plasma.

SPECIAL-USE ANTICOAGULANTS

The following anticoagulants are combined with other additives and have additional properties for special-use situations.

Acid Citrate Dextrose

Acid citrate dextrose **(ACD)** solution is available in two formulations (solution A and solution B) for immunohematology tests such as DNA testing and human leukocyte antigen (HLA) phenotyping, which is used in paternity evaluation and to determine transplant compatibility. The acid citrate prevents coagulation by binding calcium, with little effect on cells and platelets. Dextrose acts as an RBC nutrient and preservative by maintaining RBC viability. ACD tubes have yellow tops and require eight inversions immediately after collection to prevent clotting.

Citrate Phosphate Dextrose

Citrate phosphate dextrose (**CPD**) is used in collecting units of blood for transfusion. Citrate prevents clotting by chelating calcium, phosphate stabilizes pH, and dextrose provides cells with energy and helps keep them alive.

Sodium Polyanethol Sulfonate

Sodium polyanethol sulfonate (**SPS**) prevents coagulation by binding calcium. It is used for blood culture collection because, in addition to being an anticoagulant, it reduces the action of a protein called *complement*, which destroys bacteria. It also slows down phagocytosis (ingestion of bacteria by leukocytes), and reduces the activity of certain antibiotics. SPS tubes have yellow stoppers and require eight inversions to prevent clotting.

ANTIGLYCOLYTIC AGENTS

An **antiglycolytic agent** is a substance that prevents **glycolysis**, the breakdown or metabolism of glucose (blood sugar) by blood cells. If glycolysis is not prevented, the glucose concentration in a blood specimen decreases at a rate of 10 mg/dL per hour.

> **Key Point** Glycolysis occurs faster in newborns because their metabolism is increased, and in patients with leukemia because of high metabolic activity of WBCs.

The most common antiglycolytic agent is **sodium fluoride**. It preserves glucose and also inhibits the growth of bacteria. Sodium fluoride by itself will clot the blood and can be used when a serum specimen is required. Sodium fluoride is commonly used in combination with the anticoagulant potassium oxalate or EDTA to provide plasma specimens, especially for rapid-response situations. Sodium fluoride tubes have gray stoppers and require between five and ten inversions, depending on the manufacturer, for proper mixing, whether or not they also contain an anticoagulant.

> **Key Point** Sodium fluoride tubes are used to collect ethanol specimens to prevent either a decrease in alcohol concentration due to glycolysis or an increase due to fermentation by bacteria.

CLOT ACTIVATORS

A **clot activator** is a substance that enhances coagulation in tubes used to collect serum specimens. Clot activators include substances that provide more surface for platelet activation, such as glass (**silica**) particles and clotting factors such as **thrombin.** Silica particles are the clot activators

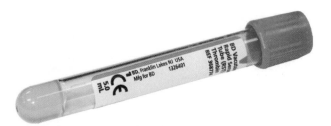

Figure 7-31 BD Vacutainer® Rapid Serum Tube (RST). (Courtesy of Becton Dickinson, Franklin Lakes, NJ.)

in serum-separator tubes (SSTs) and plastic red-top tubes. Silica particles cause the blood to clot within 15 to 30 minutes. Blood collected in thrombin tubes such as the Becton Dickinson (BD) **Rapid Serum Tube™ (RST)** (Fig. 7-31) normally clots within 5 minutes. RST tubes have an orange stopper. Tubes containing clot activators require five to ten gentle inversions depending on the manufacturer, for complete and rapid clotting to occur.

> **Key Point** Blood in an SST tube will eventually clot without mixing; however, when it is not mixed, glass particles may become suspended in the serum and could interfere in the testing process, as glass particles have been known to plug the small diameter tubing in some analyzers.

THIXOTROPIC GEL SEPARATOR

Thixotropic gel is an inert (nonreacting) synthetic substance initially contained in or near the bottom of certain blood collection tubes. The density of the gel is between that of the cells and the serum or plasma. When a specimen in a gel tube is centrifuged, the gel undergoes a change in viscosity (thickness) and moves to a position between the cells and the serum or plasma, forming a physical barrier between them. This physical separation prevents the cells from continuing to metabolize substances such as glucose in the serum or plasma. Serum gel-barrier tubes include BD tubes with gold plastic (Fig. 7-18) stoppers and tubes with mottled red/gray-rubber stoppers called **serum-separator tubes (SSTs)**; some orange stopper RST tubes, and Kendall tubes with mottled red/gray-rubber stoppers (sometimes called tiger tops) called Monoject **Corvac tubes**; and Greiner Bio-One Vacuette serum tubes with yellow plastic over red-rubber stoppers. Heparinized plasma gel-barrier tubes include BD tubes with light-green plastic or mottled gray/green-rubber stoppers called **plasma-separator tubes (PSTs)** and Vacuette tubes with green plastic stoppers and yellow tops. In addition, BD has EDTA gel-barrier tubes with white/pearl-colored stoppers called **plasma-preparation tubes (PPTs)**.

TRACE ELEMENT–FREE TUBES

Although stopper colors normally indicate a type of additive in a tube, royal-blue stoppers indicate **trace element–free tubes**. These tubes are made of materials that are as free of trace element contamination as possible; they are used for trace element tests, toxicology studies, and nutrient determinations. These tests measure substances present in such small quantities that trace element contamination commonly found in the glass, plastic, or stopper material of other tubes may leach into the specimen and falsely elevate test results. Royal-blue–top tubes (Fig. 7-21) contain EDTA, heparin, or no additive to meet various test requirements. Tube labels may be color coded to indicate the type of additive, if any, in the tube.

Order of Draw

![open book icon] **Grab some colored pencils and have some fun with the order of draw with WORKBOOK Labeling Exercise 7-2.**

Order of draw refers to the order in which tubes are collected during a multiple-tube draw or are filled from a syringe. CLSI recommends the following order of draw for both ETS collection and in filling tubes from a syringe.

1. Blood culture tube
2. Sodium citrate tube (e.g., light-blue–top coagulation tube)
3. Serum tube with or without clot activator, with or without gel (e.g., red, red/gray-mottled, or gold stopper)
4. Heparin tube with or without gel plasma separator (e.g., green top)
5. EDTA tube with or without gel separator (e.g., lavender, purple, or white/pearl top)
6. Sodium fluoride/potassium oxalate glycolytic inhibitor (e.g., gray top)

Note: According to CLSI, the order of draw for tubes not listed above should take into consideration the additive and the potential for the specimen collected in it to alter or be altered by carryover. Follow facility policy.

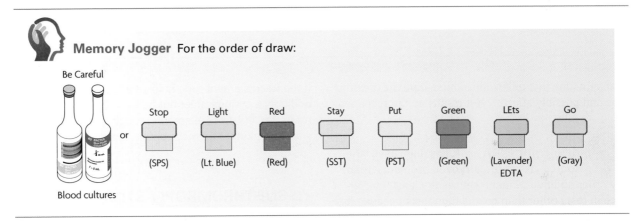

Memory Jogger For the order of draw:

Be Careful — Blood cultures

| Stop | Light | Red | Stay | Put | Green | LEts | Go |
| (SPS) | (Lt. Blue) | (Red) | (SST) | (PST) | (Green) | (Lavender) EDTA | (Gray) |

![info icon] The memory jogger for the order of draw places the red top before the SST and places the PST before the green top for convenience in memorization.

Filling tubes in the wrong order can lead to interference in testing from cross-contamination of the specimen by additive carryover, tissue thromboplastin, or microorganisms. The special sequence of tube collection (order of draw) is intended to minimize these problems. The CLSI order of draw including stopper colors and rationale for collection order, is summarized in Table 7-4.

If during a multiple-tube draw you realize that a tube has just been drawn in the wrong order, draw a second one of that tube, discard the first one, draw a few mL of blood into a discard tube, and resume the order of draw for any subsequent tubes.

![key icon] **Key Point** Carryover from an underfilled additive tube has a greater potential to negatively affect test results in a subsequent tube.

![info icon] Order of draw may vary slightly among institutions. Consult institutional protocol before using a specific order of draw.

CARRYOVER/CROSS-CONTAMINATION

Carryover or cross-contamination is the transfer of additive from one tube to the next. It can occur when blood in an additive tube touches the needle during ETS blood collection or when blood is transferred from a syringe into ETS tubes. Blood remaining on or within the needle can be transferred to the next tube drawn or filled,

Table 7-4: Order of Draw, Stopper Colors, and Rationale for Collection Order

Order of Draw	Tube Stopper Color	Rationale for Collection Order
Blood cultures (sterile collections)	Yellow SPS Sterile media bottles	Minimizes chance of microbial contamination.
Coagulation tubes	Light blue	The first additive tube in the order because all other additive tubes affect coagulation tests.
Glass nonadditive tubes	Red	Prevents contamination by additives in other tubes.
Plastic clot activator tubes Serum-separator tubes (SSTs)	Red Red and gray rubber gold plastic	Filled after coagulation tests because silica particles activate clotting and affect coagulation tests (carryover of silica into subsequent tubes can be overridden by anticoagulant in them).
Heparin tubes with gel/ Plasma-separator tubes (PSTs) Heparin tubes	Green and gray rubber Light-green plastic Green	Heparin affects coagulation tests and interferes in collection of serum specimens; it causes the least interference in tests other than coagulation tests.
EDTA tubes	Lavender, pink, purple	Responsible for more carryover problems than any other additive: elevates Na and K levels, chelates and decreases calcium and iron levels, elevates PT and PTT results.
EDTA tubes with gel/Plasma-preparation tubes (PPTs)	Pearl/white top	
Oxalate/fluoride tubes	Gray	Sodium fluoride and potassium oxalate affect sodium and potassium levels, respectively. Filled after hematology tubes because oxalate damages cell membranes and causes abnormal RBC morphology. Oxalate interferes in enzyme reactions.

contaminating that tube with additive from the previous tube and possibly affecting test results on the specimen.

Key Point EDTA in tubes has been the source of more carryover problems than any other additive. Heparin causes the least interference in tests other than coagulation tests because it also occurs in blood naturally.

Remembering which tests the various additives affect can be difficult. Order of draw eliminates confusion by presenting a sequence of collection that results in the least amount of interference should carryover occur. The chance of carryover can be minimized by making certain that specimen tubes fill from the bottom up during collection and that the contents of the tube do not come in contact with the needle during the draw or in transferring blood into tubes from a syringe.

Key Point According to the Center for Phlebotomy Education (www.phlebotomy. com), when using the ETS, royal-blue tops for trace element studies should be collected separately to avoid even the smallest amount of carryover. If a syringe is used, the transfer device should be changed

if the trace element tube is filled after other tubes. In addition, a syringe must not be used to collect specimens for the trace elements cobalt and chromium since the plunger tip may contain these elements.

TISSUE THROMBOPLASTIN CONTAMINATION

Tissue thromboplastin, a substance present in tissue fluid, activates the extrinsic coagulation pathway and can interfere with coagulation tests. It is picked up by the needle during venipuncture and flushed into the first tube filled during ETS collection, or it is mixed with blood collected in a syringe. Although tissue thromboplastin is no longer thought to pose a clinically significant problem for prothrombin time (PT/INR), partial thromboplastin time (PTT or aPTT), and some special coagulation tests unless the draw is difficult and involves a lot of needle manipulation, it may compromise results of other coagulation tests. Therefore unless there is documented evidence to show the test to be unaffected by tissue thromboplastin any time a coagulation test other than a PT/INR or PTT/aPTT is the first or only tube collected, a few milliliters of blood should be drawn into a nonadditive tube or another coagulation tube before it is collected. The extra tube is called a "clear" or "discard" tube because it is used to remove (or clear) tissue fluid from the needle and is then thrown away.

⚠️ **CAUTION** A discard tube must be drawn to protect the critical 9:1 blood-to-additive ratio of a coagulation tube that is the first or only tube collected using a butterfly because air in the tubing displaces (takes the place of) blood in the tube.

MICROBIAL CONTAMINATION

Blood cultures detect microorganisms in the blood and require special site-cleaning measures prior to collection to prevent contamination of the specimen by microorganisms that are normally found on the skin. Blood culture tubes or bottles are sterile and are collected first in the order of draw to ensure that they are collected when sterility of the site is optimal and to prevent microbial contamination of the needle from the unsterile tops of tubes used to collect other tests. Blood cultures do not often factor into the sequence of collection because they are typically drawn separately.

🔑 **Key Point** Contamination of blood culture bottles can lead to false-positive results and inappropriate or delayed care for the patient.

Study and Review Questions

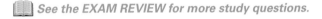

📖 *See the EXAM REVIEW for more study questions.*

1. **Which additive prevents glycolysis?**
   a. EDTA
   b. Heparin
   c. Potassium oxalate
   d. Sodium fluoride

2. **The following supplies were gathered for a routine venipuncture. Which item is incorrect?**
   a. ETS tubes
   b. Iodine swab
   c. Safety needle
   d. Tourniquet

3. **Which of the following tubes can be used to collect a serum specimen?**
   a. Light-blue top
   b. Green top
   c. PST
   d. Red top

4. **A tourniquet is used in venipuncture to**
   a. concentrate the blood specimen.
   b. find and enter veins more easily.
   c. keep the vein from collapsing.
   d. all of the above.

5. **You are about to perform routine venipuncture on a patient with no known allergy to antiseptics. Which of the following substances would you use to clean the site?**
   a. 5.25% sodium hypochlorite
   b. 70% isopropyl alcohol
   c. Antibacterial soap and water
   d. Povidone–iodine

6. **Which of the following needles has the largest diameter?**
   a. 18 gauge
   b. 20 gauge
   c. 21 gauge
   d. 23 gauge

7. **What causes evacuated tubes to fill with blood automatically?**
   a. Arterial blood pressure
   b. Fist pumping by the patient
   c. Pressure from the tourniquet
   d. Premeasured tube vacuum

8. **Lavender-top tubes are most commonly used to collect**
   a. chemistry tests.
   b. coagulation specimens.
   c. hematology tests.
   d. immunology tests.

9. **Of the following tubes or containers, which is filled last in the recommended order of draw?**
   a. Blood culture bottle
   b. Lavender top
   c. Light-blue top
   d. Red top

10. **A butterfly is typically used for**
    a. coagulation specimens.
    b. difficult and hand veins.
    c. draws from a basilic vein.
    d. all of the above.

11. **EDTA can be found in**
    a. lavender-top tubes.
    b. purple-top tubes.
    c. white-top tubes.
    d. all of the above.

12. **Blood in this tube normally clots within 5 minutes.**
    a. PST
    b. RST
    c. SPS
    d. SST

13. **Which of the following is a biocide?**
    a. 70% isopropanol
    b. Hydrogen peroxide
    c. Povidone–iodine
    d. All of the above

14. **Mixing an additive correctly involves turning the wrist this many degrees and back again.**
    a. 45
    b. 90
    c. 120
    d. 180

15. **If a CBC, PT, plasma potassium, and glucose (with glycolysis inhibitor) are all to be collected during a multiple-tube draw on a patient, which of the following choices shows the correct stopper colors to use in the correct order of draw?**
    a. Lavender, light blue, gold, green
    b. Light blue, green, lavender, gray
    c. Red, royal blue, green, lavender
    d. Yellow, orange, lavender, gray

Case Studies

 See the WORKBOOK for more case studies.

Case Study 7-1: Proper Handling of Anticoagulant Tubes

A mobile blood collector named Chi is collecting an SST and two lavender tops (one for a glycohemoglobin and one for a CBC) on a client named Louise Jones. He fills the SST, lays it down while he places the first lavender top in the tube holder, then picks it up and mixes it as the lavender top is filling. When the lavender top is full, he lays it down while he places the second lavender top in the tube holder. The second lavender top fails to fill with blood, so he makes several needle adjustments to try to establish blood flow. Nothing works, so he decides to try a new tube. The new tube works fine. While it is filling, he picks up the first lavender top and mixes it. After completing the draw he labels his tubes, putting the hematology label on the lavender top he collected first. He finishes up with the client, delivers the specimens to the laboratory, and goes to lunch. When he returns from break his supervisor tells him to recollect the CBC on Louise Jones because the specimen had a clot in it.

QUESTIONS

1. What can cause clots in EDTA specimens?
2. What most likely caused the clot in this specimen?
3. Did the problem with the second lavender top contribute to the problem?
4. Would the problem with the second lavender top have been an issue if Chi had handled the first lavender top properly? Explain your answer.
5. What can Chi do to prevent this type of thing from happening in the future?

Case Study 7-2: Order of Draw

Jake, a phlebotomist, is sent to the ER to collect an EDTA specimen for a stat type and crossmatch on an accident victim. He properly identifies the patient and is in the process of filling the lavender-top tube when an ER nurse tells him that the patient's physician wants to add a stat set of electrolytes to the test order. Jake acknowledges her request. He finishes filling the lavender top and grabs a green top. After completing the draw, he takes the specimens straight to the laboratory to be processed immediately.

QUESTIONS

1. One of the specimens that Jake drew is compromised. Which one is it?
2. Why is the specimen compromised and how may test results be affected?
3. How could Jake have avoided the problem without drawing blood from the patient twice?

Bibliography and Suggested Readings

Bishop M, Fody E, Schoeff L. *Clinical Chemistry, Principles, Procedures, Correlations.* 7th ed. Philadelphia, PA: Lippincott Williams & Wilkins; 2013.

Burtis C, Ashwood E. *Tietz Fundamentals of Clinical Chemistry.* 7th ed. Philadelphia, PA: Saunders; 2015.

CDC. Guideline for hand hygiene in health care settings. *Morbidity and Mortality Weekly Report (MMWR).* October 25, 2002;51 (RR-16). Complete report available at http://www.cdc.gov

CDC/HICPAC. Guideline for environmental infection control in health-care facilities. Recommendations of CDC and the Healthcare Infection Control Practices Advisory Committee (HICPAC). *Morbidity and Mortality Weekly Report (MMWR).* June 2003;52 (RR-10).

Clinical and Laboratory Standards Institute, GP34-A. *Validation and Verification of Tubes for Venous and Capillary Blood Specimen Collection: Approved Guideline.* Wayne, PA: CLSI; 2010.

Clinical and Laboratory Standards Institute, GP39-A6. *Tubes and Additives for Blood Specimen Collection: Approved Standard.* 6th ed. Wayne, PA: CLSI; 2010.

Clinical and Laboratory Standards Institute, GP41-A6. *Procedures for the Collection of Diagnostic Blood Specimens by Venipuncture: Approved Standard.* 6th ed. Wayne, PA: CLSI; 2007.

Clinical Laboratory Standards Institute, M29-A4. *Protection of Laboratory Workers from Occupationally Acquired Infections; Approved Guideline.* 3rd ed. Wayne, PA: CLSI; 2014.

College of American Pathologists (CAP). *So You're Going to Collect a Blood Specimen.* 14th ed. Northfield, IL: CAP; 2013.

Ernst DJ. *Applied Phlebotomy.* Baltimore, MD: Lippincott Williams & Wilkins; 2005.

Gottfried EL, Adachi MM. Prothrombin time (PT) and activated partial thromboplastin time (APTT) can be performed on the first tube. *Am J Clin Pathol.* 1997;107:681–683.

Leitch A, McCormick I, Gunn I, Gillespie T. Reducing the potential for phlebotomy tourniquets to act as a reservoir for methicillin-resistant Staphylococcus aureus. *J Hosp Infect.* 2007;65(2):173–175.

OSHA. Disposal of contaminated needles and blood tube holders used for phlebotomy. *Safety and Health Information Bulletin.* http://www.osha.gov/dts/shib/shib101503.html. October 15, 2003.

Roark C, Bates C, Read R. Poor hospital infection control practice in venipuncture and use of tourniquets. *J Hosp Infect.* 2002: 49(1):59–61.

Siegel JD, Rhinehart E, Jackson M, Chiarello L; the Healthcare Infection Control Practices Advisory Committee (HICPAC). *Guideline for Isolation Precautions: Preventing Transmission of Infectious Agents in Healthcare Settings.* Atlanta, GA: CDC/HICPAC; 2007.

Turgeon ML. *Clinical Hematology.* 5th ed. Baltimore, MD: Lippincott Williams & Wilkins; 2012.

 MEDIA MENU

Online Ancillaries (at http://thepoint.lww.com/McCall6e)
- Interactive exercises and games, including Look and Label, Word Building, Body Building, Roboterms, Crossword Puzzles, Quiz Show, and Concentration
- Audio flash cards and flash card generator
- Audio glossary

Internet Resources
- Accuvein vein locator demo: http://accuvein.com/
- Becton Dickinson (BD) Lab notes Volume 19, No. 1, 2009: The evolution of evacuated blood collection tubes: http://www.bd.com/vacutainer/labnotes
- Center for Phlebotomy Education: http://www.phlebotomy.com/
- Clinical Laboratory Science Internet Resources Website: www.tarleton.edu/library/inetlinks/cls_il.html
- LabCorp (Laboratory Corporation of America): https://www.labcorp.com/wps/portal/provider/testmenu/
- Quia Corp; online education support: http://www.quia.com/fc/71443.html

Other Resources
- McCall R, Tankersley C. *Student Workbook for Phlebotomy Essentials.* 6th ed. (Available for separate purchase.)
- McCall R, Tankersley C. *Phlebotomy Exam Review.* 6th ed. (Available for separate purchase.)

Chapter 8

Venipuncture Procedures

NAACLS Entry Level Competencies

6.00 Follow standard operating procedures to collect specimens.

6.3 Describe and demonstrate the steps in the preparation of a puncture site.

6.5 Recognize proper needle insertion and withdrawal techniques, including direction, angle, depth and aspiration, for venipuncture.

6.9 Describe signs and symptoms of physical problems that may occur during blood collection.

6.10 List the steps necessary to perform a venipuncture and a capillary (dermal) puncture in order.

6.11 Demonstrate a successful venipuncture following standard operating procedures.

7.00 Demonstrate understanding of requisitioning, specimen transport, and specimen processing.

7.1 Describe the process by which a request for a laboratory test is generated.

9.00 Communicate (verbally and nonverbally) effectively and appropriately in the workplace.

9.1 Maintain confidentiality of privileged information on individuals, according to federal regulations (e.g., HIPAA).

9.3 Interact appropriately and professionally.

Key Terms

Do Matching Exercise 8-1 in the WORKBOOK to gain familiarity with these terms.

accession	belonephobia	ID card	patency
anchor	DNR/DNAR	MR number	patient ID
arm/wrist band	EMLA	needle phobia	preop/postop
ASAP	fasting	needle sheath	reflux
bar code	hospice	NPO	requisition
bedside manner	ID band/bracelet	palpate	stat

Objectives

Upon successful completion of this chapter, the reader should be able to:

1 Demonstrate knowledge of each venipuncture step from the time the test request is received until the specimen is delivered to the lab, and define associated terminology.

2 Describe how to perform a venipuncture using ETS, syringe, or butterfly, list required patient and specimen identification information, describe how to handle patient ID discrepancies, and state the acceptable reasons for inability to collect a specimen.

3 Identify challenges and unique aspects associated with collecting specimens from pediatric and geriatric patients.

4 Describe why a patient would require dialysis and how it is performed, and exhibit an awareness of the type of care provided for long-term care, home care, and hospice patients.

Venipuncture is the process of collecting or "drawing" blood from a vein and the most common way to collect blood specimens for laboratory testing. It is the most frequent procedure performed by a phlebotomist and the most important step in this procedure is patient identification. This chapter addresses how to correctly identify all types of patients and how to safely obtain high-quality blood specimens from them. Venipuncture techniques covered in this chapter include ETS, butterfly, and syringe procedures on arm and hand veins. This chapter also addresses challenges and unique issues associated with pediatric, geriatric, dialysis, long-term care, home care, and hospice patients. Venipuncture procedures in this chapter conform to CLSI standards.

 Key Point In the interest of achieving global harmonization (worldwide uniformity) and to align the use of terminology with that of the International Standards Organization (ISO), the CLSI has begun using the terms *pre-examination, examination, and postexamination* in place of *pre-analytical, analytical, and postanalytical* in recent guidelines.

The Test Requisition

The form on which test orders are entered is called a **requisition**. Test requisitions become part of a patient's medical record and require specific information to ensure that the right patient is tested, the physician's

Venipuncture Steps

STEP 1: REVIEW AND ACCESSION TEST REQUEST

 WORKBOOK Skills Drill 8-3 can help you commit these steps to memory.

Blood-collection procedures legally begin with the test request. This is the first step for the laboratory in the preanalytical (before analysis) or pre-examination phase of the testing process. Typically, a physician or other qualified healthcare professional requests laboratory testing; the exceptions are certain rapid tests that can be purchased and performed at home by consumers and blood specimens requested by law enforcement officials that are used for evidence. Some states have legalized "Direct Access Testing" (DAT), in which patients are allowed to order some of their own blood tests.

Box 8-1

Required Requisition Information

- Ordering physician's name
- Patient's first and last names and middle initial
- Patient's medical record number (if inpatient)
- Patient's date of birth or age
- Room number and bed (if inpatient)
- Type of test to be performed
- Date test is to be performed
- Billing information and ICD-9 codes (if outpatient)
- Test status (e.g., timed, fasting, priority)
- Special precautions (e.g., latex sensitivity)

orders are met, the correct tests are performed at the proper time under the required conditions, and the patient is billed properly. Required requisition information is listed in Box 8-1. Requisitions come in manual and computer-generated forms.

Key Point Verbal test requests are sometimes used in emergencies; however, the request is usually documented on standard request forms or entered in the computer by the time the phlebotomist arrives to collect the specimen.

Manual Requisitions

Manual requisitions come in a number of different styles and types as simple as a test request written on a prescription pad by a physician, or a special form (Fig. 8-1) issued by a reference laboratory. With increased use of computer systems, the use of manual requisitions is declining. However, they are typically used as a backup when computer systems fail.

Computer Requisitions

Computer requisitions (Fig. 8-2) normally contain the actual labels that are placed on the specimen tubes immediately after collection. In addition to patient

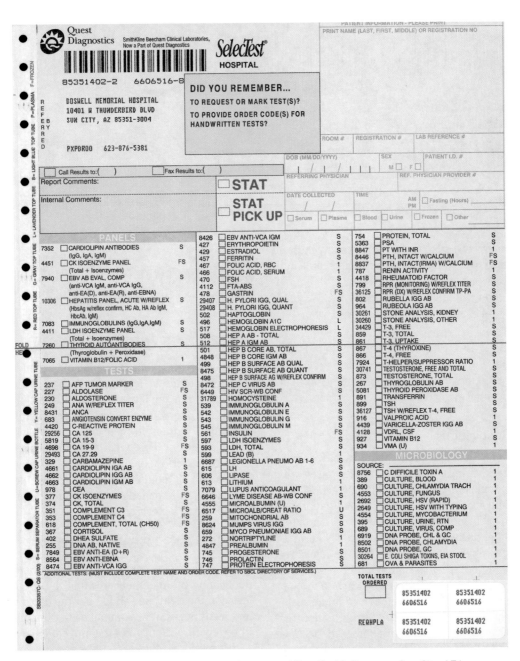

Figure 8-1 A manual requisition. (Courtesy of Sun Health Systems, Sun City, AZ.)

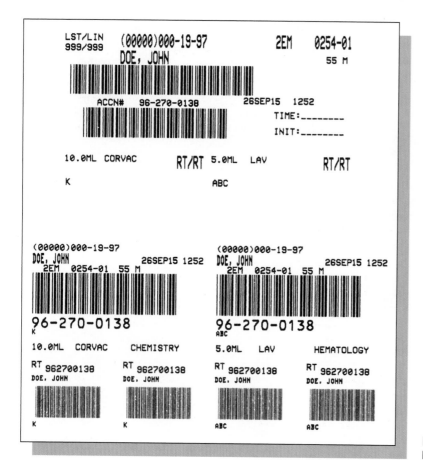

Figure 8-2 A computer requisition with bar code.

identification and test status information, many indicate the type of tube needed for the specimen and some indicate additional patient information such as "potential bleeder" or "no venipuncture right arm."

> **Key Point** When a computer-generated label is used, the phlebotomist is typically required to write the time of collection and his or her initials on the label after collecting the specimen.

Bar-Code Requisitions

Either type of requisition may contain a **bar code**, a series of black stripes and white spaces of varying widths that correspond to letters and numbers (Fig. 8-2). The stripes and spaces are grouped together to represent patient names, identification numbers, or laboratory tests. Manual requisitions that have bar codes normally contain copies of the bar code that can be peeled off and placed on the specimens. Computer requisitions typically have the bar code printed on each label. Bar-code information can be scanned into a computer using a special light or laser to identify the information represented. Bar-code systems allow for fast, accurate processing, and their use has been shown to decrease laboratory errors associated with clerical mistakes.

> **Key Point** With any type of requisition it is essential for the information to be transcribed or entered correctly.

RECEIPT OF THE TEST REQUEST

Computer requisitions for inpatients usually print out at a special computer terminal (Fig. 8-3) at the phlebotomist station in the laboratory. Typically, outpatients are given laboratory requisitions or prescription slips with test orders written on them by their physicians and are responsible for taking them to a blood-collection site. It is up to personnel of the blood-collection site to make certain that all required information is on the requisition provided by the patient or to fill out a requisition from the physician's prescription slip.

REVIEWING THE REQUISITION

A thorough review of the test requisition helps to avoid duplication of orders, ensures that the specimen is collected at the right time and under the proper conditions, and identifies special equipment that may be required. In reviewing a requisition the phlebotomist must:

- Check to see that all required information is present and complete.

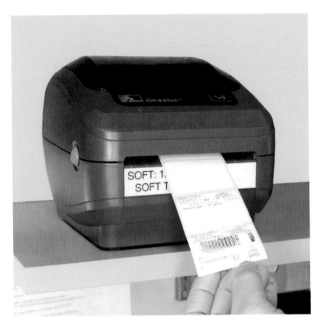

Figure 8-3 Computer requisitions printing at a terminal in the laboratory.

- Verify the tests to be collected and time and date of collection.
- Identify diet restrictions or other special circumstances that must be met prior to collection.
- Determine test status or collection priority (Table 8-1).

Accessioning the Test Request

The definition of **accession** is "the process of recording in the order received." To accession a specimen means to take steps to unmistakably connect the specimen and the accompanying paperwork with a specific individual. When a test request is accessioned it is assigned a unique number used to identify the specimen and all associated processes and paperwork and connect them to the patient. This helps to ensure prompt and accurate processing from receipt of the order to reporting of test results.

STEP 2: APPROACH, IDENTIFY, AND PREPARE PATIENT

Approaching the Patient

Being organized and efficient plays a role in a positive and productive collection experience. Before collecting the specimens, the phlebotomist should arrange the requisitions according to priority and review them to see that needed equipment is on the blood-collecting tray or cart before proceeding to the patient's room. Outpatients are typically summoned into the drawing area from the waiting room in order of arrival and check-in. As with inpatients, stat requests take priority over all others.

Looking for Signs

Looking for signs containing information concerning the patient is an important part of the approach to an inpatient. Signs are typically posted on the door to the patient's room or on the wall beside or behind the head of the patient's bed. Of particular importance to phlebotomists are signs indicating that infection-control precautions are to be followed on entering the room and signs that prohibit the taking of blood pressures or blood draws (Fig. 8-4A) from a particular arm. Other commonly encountered signs may identify limits to the number of visitors allowed in the room at one time, indicate that "fall" precautions are to be observed for the patient, or warn that the patient has a severe allergy (e.g., to latex or flowers). A sign with the letters **DNR** (do not resuscitate) or **DNAR** (do not attempt resuscitation) means that there is an order (also called a no code order) stating that the patient should not be revived if he or she stops breathing. A physician—at the request of the patient or the patient's guardian—typically writes the order.

> (i) A code is a way to transmit a message, normally understood by healthcare personnel only, over the facility's public address system. A code uses numbers or words to convey information needed by healthcare personnel to respond to certain situations.

Pictures are sometimes used in place of written warnings. For example, a sign with a picture of fall leaves (Fig. 8-4B) is sometimes used to indicate that the patient is at risk of falling. A picture of a fallen leaf with a teardrop on it (Fig. 8-4C) is sometimes used on obstetric wards to indicate that a patient has lost a baby.

Entering a Patient's Room

Doors to patients' rooms are usually open. If the door is closed, knock lightly, open the door slowly, and say something like "good morning" before proceeding into the room. Even if the door is open, it is a good idea to knock lightly to make occupants aware that you are about to enter. Curtains are often pulled closed when nurses are working with patients or when patients are using bedpans or urinals. Make your presence known before proceeding or opening the curtain so as to protect the patient's privacy and avoid embarrassment.

Physicians and Clergy

If a physician or a member of the clergy is with the patient, don't interrupt. The patient's time with these individuals is private and limited. If the draw is not stat, timed or other urgent priority, go draw another patient and check back after that. If that is the only patient,

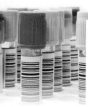

Table 8-1: Common Test Status Designations

Status	Meaning	When Used	Collection Conditions	Test Examples	Priority
Stat	Immediately (from Latin *statim*)	Test results are urgently needed on critical patients	Immediately collect, test, and report results. Alert lab staff when delivered. ER stats typically have priority over other stats	Glucose H&H Electrolytes Cardiac enzymes	First
Med Emerg	Medical emergency (replaces stat)	Same as stat	Same as stat	Same as stat	Same as stat
Timed	Collect at a specific time	Tests for which timing is critical for accurate results	Collect as close as possible to requested time. Record actual time collected	2-hour PP GTT, Cortisol Cardiac enzymes TDM Blood cultures	Second
ASAP	As soon as possible	Test results are needed soon to respond to a serious situation, but patient is not critical	Follow hospital protocol for type of test	Electrolytes Glucose H&H	Second or third depending on test
Fasting	No food or drink except water for 8–12 hours prior to specimen collection	To eliminate diet effects on test results	Verify patient has fasted. If patient has not fasted, check to see if specimen should still be collected	Glucose Cholesterol Triglycerides	Fourth
NPO	Nothing by mouth (from Latin *nil per os*)	Prior to surgery or other anesthesia procedures	Do not give patient food or water. Refer requests to physician or nurse	N/A	N/A
Preop	Before an operation	To determine patient eligibility for surgery	Collect before the patient goes to surgery	CBC PTT Platelet function studies	Same as ASAP
Postop	After an operation	Assess patient condition after surgery	Collect when patient is out of surgery	H&H	Same as ASAP
Routine	Relating to established procedure	Used to establish a diagnosis or monitor a patient's progress	Collect in a timely manner but no urgency involved. Typically collected on morning sweeps or the next scheduled sweep	CBC Chem profile	None

wait outside the room for a few minutes or go back to the lab and draw the specimen on the next sweep. (In any case, always make certain your actions follow facility policy.) If the request is stat, timed, or other urgent priority, excuse yourself, explain why you are there, and ask permission to proceed.

Family and Visitors

Often there are family members or visitors with the patient. It is best to ask them to step outside the room until you are finished. Most will prefer to do so; however, some family members will insist on staying in the room. It is generally acceptable to let a willing family member help steady the arm or hold pressure over the site while you label tubes.

Unavailable Patient

If the patient cannot be located, is unavailable, or you are unable to obtain the specimen for any other reason, it is the policy of most laboratories that you fill out a form stating that you were unable to obtain the specimen at the requested time and the reason why. The original copy of this form is left at the nurses' station and a copy goes to the lab.

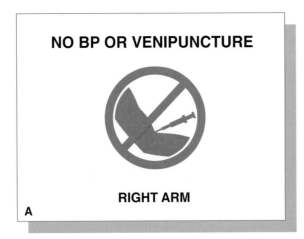

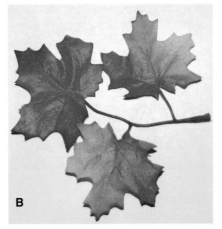

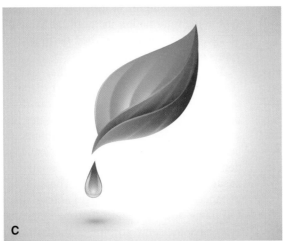

Figure 8-4 Three examples of warning signs. **A:** No blood pressures or venipuncture in right arm. (Courtesy of Brevis Corp, Salt Lake City, UT.) **B:** Fall-colored leaves symbolizing fall precautions. **C:** Falling leaf with a teardrop symbolizing the loss of a newborn.

Identifying Yourself

Identify yourself to the patient by stating your name, your title, and why you are there (e.g., "Good morning. I am Joe Smith, from the lab. I'm here to collect a blood specimen if it is all right with you."). If you are a student, let the patient know this and ask permission to do the blood draw. This is a part of informed consent and patient rights. The patient has a right to refuse to have blood drawn by a student or anyone else.

Obtaining Consent

The patient's consent must be obtained before starting the venipuncture. Always ask a patient for permission to collect the specimen (see "Identifying Yourself," above). This is not only courteous but also legally required. Consent does not always have to be stated verbally, however. It can be implied by actions—for example, if the patient extends an arm when you explain why you are there. A phlebotomist must never collect a blood specimen without permission or against a patient's will. Objections should be reported to the appropriate personnel. (See "Patient Consent" in Chapter 2.)

CAUTION Be aware of conflicting permission statements. This often happens with student phlebotomists. For example, when a student asks permission to collect the specimen, a patient may say "Yes, but I would rather not." The patient has given permission and taken back that permission in the same statement. In this case it is best if the student's instructor or another phlebotomist employed by the facility collects the specimen.

Bedside Manner

The behavior of a healthcare provider toward, or as perceived by, a patient is called **bedside manner**. Approaching a patient is more than simply calling an outpatient into the blood-drawing room or finding an inpatient's room and proceeding to collect the specimen. The manner in which you approach and interact with the patient sets the stage for whether or not the patient perceives you as a professional. Gaining the patient's trust and confidence and putting the patient at ease are important aspects of a successful encounter and an important part of professional bedside manner. A phlebotomist with a professional bedside manner and appearance will more easily gain a patient's trust. A confident phlebotomist will convey that confidence to patients and help them feel at ease.

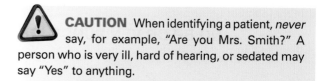

Key Point A cheerful, pleasant manner and an exchange of small talk will help to put a patient at ease as well as divert attention from any discomfort associated with the procedure.

Patient Identification

Patient Identification (ID) Importance

thePoint. *View the Introductory and Identification Processes Required Prior to Blood Specimen Collection video at http://thepoint.lww.com/McCall6e.*

Patient ID, the process of verifying a patient's identity, is the most important step in specimen collection. Obtaining a specimen from the wrong patient can have serious, even fatal, consequences, especially specimens for type and cross-match prior to blood transfusion. Misidentifying a patient or specimen can be grounds for dismissal of the person responsible and can even lead to a malpractice lawsuit against that person.

Verifying Name and Date of Birth

The patient must be actively involved in the identification process. When identifying a patient, ask the patient to state his or her full name and date of birth. In addition, the CLSI guideline GP33-A (*Accuracy in Patient and Sample Identification*) recommends having the patient spell the last name. This also serves as a memory jogger to help the phlebotomist remember that the patient's ID was verified. The patient's response must match the information on the requisition and/or computer-generated specimen labels. Any errors or differences must be resolved before a sample is collected.

CAUTION When identifying a patient, *never* say, for example, "Are you Mrs. Smith?" A person who is very ill, hard of hearing, or sedated may say "Yes" to anything.

Checking Identification Bracelets

If the patient's response matches the information on the requisition, proceed to check the patient's **ID band** or **bracelet** (Fig. 8-5A) (also called an **arm band** or **wrist band**) if applicable. Inpatients are normally required to wear an ID band, usually on the wrist. The typical ID band (Fig. 8-5B) lists the patient's name and hospital identification number or **medical record (MR) number**. Additional information includes the patient's birth date or age, room number and bed designation, and physician's name.

The patient's name, MR number, and date of birth (DOB) or age on the ID band must match the information on the requisition *exactly*. It is not unusual to have patients with the same or similar names in the hospital at the same time. (Examples are patients with common last names, fathers and sons who have been in accidents, multiple-birth babies, and relatives involved in tissue transplant procedures.) There have even been instances when two unrelated patients shared the same full name and birth date. Two patients will not, however, have the same hospital or medical record number, although they may be similar.

Identification protocol may vary slightly from one healthcare institution to another. Generally, ID information such as room number, bed number, and physician name are allowed to differ. For instance, occasionally a room number will differ because the patient has been moved. The name of the ordering physician may be different, since it is not unusual for a patient to be under the care of several different physicians at the same time.

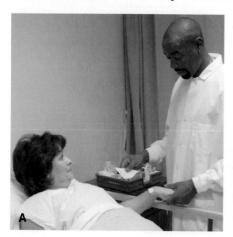
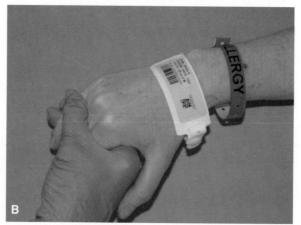

Figure 8-5 A: A phlebotomist at bedside checking patient identification band. **B:** Closeup of a typical identification bracelet.

Three-Way ID

To avoid identification and mislabeling errors, some inpatient facilities require what is referred to as three-way ID, in which the patient is identified by three means: the patient's verbal ID statement, a check of the ID band, and a visual comparison of the labeled specimen with the patient's ID band before leaving the bedside. Some facilities are now also showing the labeled specimen to the patient and asking for verification that the correct name is on the label.

ID Discrepancies

If there is a discrepancy between the name, MR number, or date of birth on the ID band and the information on the requisition, the patient's nurse should be notified. The specimen must not be obtained until the discrepancy is addressed and the patient's identity has been verified.

Missing ID

If there is no ID band on either of an inpatient's wrists, ask the patient if you can check to see if it is on an ankle. Intravenous (IV) lines in patient's arms often infiltrate the surrounding tissues and cause swelling, which necessitates removal of the ID band. When this occurs, especially on a patient with IV lines in both arms, nursing personnel sometimes place the ID band around an ankle. (The patient is not always aware that this has been done.) In some instances, an ID band is removed from an IV-infiltrated arm or while other procedures are being performed on the patient and placed on an IV pole or the night table by the patient's bed. An ID band on an IV pole or night table could belong to a patient who previously occupied that bed and should not be used for identification purposes. It is also not unusual for a new patient to occupy a bed before the nursing staff has had a chance to attach his or her ID band.

> **⚠ CAUTION** *Never* verify information from an ID band that is not attached to the patient or collect a specimen from an inpatient who is not wearing an ID band.

In rare cases, such as a patient with severe burns, the ID is left off intentionally. In such cases follow facility protocol, which typically involves a verbal statement of ID by the patient and confirmation of ID by a nurse or relative with documentation of that person's name.

If an ID band is required and the patient is not wearing one, it is usually acceptable to ask the patient's nurse to attach an ID band before collecting the specimen. Some sites require the phlebotomist to refrain from collecting the specimen and fill out a special form stating that the specimen was not collected because the patient did not have an ID band. The form is left at the nurse's station. It is then up to the patient's nurse to attach an ID band and inform the lab when it has been done so that the specimen can be collected. In rare emergency situations in which there is no time to wait for the attachment of an ID band, the patient's nurse is allowed to verify the patient's ID. In such cases the nurse must sign or initial the requisition. Follow institution protocol.

Sleeping Patients

Obviously, proper identification and informed consent cannot occur if the patient is asleep. If you encounter a sleeping patient, as is often the case in hospitals and nursing homes, wake the person gently. Try not to startle the patient, as this can affect test results. Speak softly but distinctly. If the room is darkened, avoid turning on bright overhead lighting, at least until the patient's eyes have adjusted to being open, and warn the patient first.

> **⚠ CAUTION** *Never* attempt to collect a blood specimen from a sleeping patient. Such an attempt may startle the patient and cause injury to the patient or the phlebotomist.

Unconscious Patients

Unconscious patients are often encountered in emergency rooms and intensive care units. Ask a relative or the patient's nurse or physician to identify the patient and record the name of that person. Speak to the patient as you would to someone who is alert. Identify yourself and inform the patient of your intent. Unconscious patients can often hear what is going on around them even though they are unresponsive.

> **⚠ CAUTION** An unconscious patient may be able to feel pain and move when you insert the needle, so it may be necessary to have someone assist you by holding the arm during the blood draw.

Emergency Room ID Procedures

It is not uncommon for an emergency room (ER), or emergency department (ED), to receive an unconscious patient with no identification. Clear guidelines for this situation, provided by the American Association of Blood Banks (AABB), include the following:

- Assign a temporary number to the patient and record it on the test request forms.
- Fill out labels by hand or computer and apply them to the test request and specimens after collection. (Some tubes have bar codes and bar-code labels that can be peeled off and placed on the test request form.)

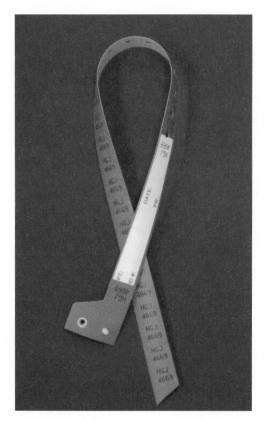

Figure 8-6 An example of a special three-part ID band used for unidentified ER patients.

- When a permanent number is issued, it must be cross-referenced to the temporary number.
- Attach an ID band or device to the patient that has the name and temporary number on it. In many institutions, the phlebotomist is allowed to attach a special three-part identification band (Fig. 8-6) such as a Typenex Blood Recipient ID band (Typenex Medical LLC, Chicago, IL) to an unidentified ER patient's wrist. All three parts contain the same number. The first part becomes the patient's ID band. The second part is attached to the specimen. The third part is used if the patient needs a transfusion, and it is attached to the unit of blood. Follow your institution's protocol for unidentified patients.

> ⚠️ **CAUTION** *Never* collect a specimen without some way to positively connect that specimen to the patient.

Identification of Young, Mentally Incompetent, or Non–English-Speaking Patients

If the patient is young, mentally incompetent, or non–English-speaking, ask the patient's nurse, attendant, relative, or friend to identify the patient by name, address, and identification number or birth date. This information

must match the information on the test requisition and the patient's ID band if applicable.

Neonates and Other Infants

ID bands may be placed on the lower leg instead of the arm of inpatient newborns or babies under 2 years of age. (In some facilities, newborns may also have another ID with the mother's information.) In addition, there is usually a card on the isolette with the baby's information on it. It can be used to locate the infant; however, it must not be used for final identification purposes. The child may be identified by a nurse, relative, or guardian. The name and relationship of a relative or guardian or the name and title of a nurse who identifies the child should be recorded on the requisition. Information that must be confirmed on a baby includes the following:

- Name (if available) and date of birth
- Gender
- Medical record number or other unique identifier
- Mother's last name or name of person provided at registration

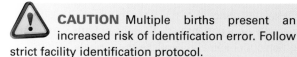

> ⚠️ **CAUTION** Multiple births present an increased risk of identification error. Follow strict facility identification protocol.

Outpatient ID

Typically, the outpatient collection site's receptionist verifies the patient's identity and fills out the proper lab requisition or generates one via computer. Some labs supply requisition forms to physicians who use their services, so some outpatients arrive at the collection site with lab requisitions that are already filled out. Information must still be verified, and patients may be required to show proof of identification such as a driver's license or other picture ID. Outpatients do not normally have ID bands. However, they may have a clinic-issued **ID card** that contains their name and other information identifying them as clinic patients. ID cards are sometimes used to imprint requisitions or labels using an addressograph type of machine. Even if a receptionist has identified the patient, a phlebotomist must still personally verify the patient's ID after calling him or her into the blood-drawing area from the waiting room. Simply calling a person's name and having someone respond is not verification enough. An anxious or hard-of-hearing patient may think that his or her name has been called when in fact a similar name was called. Always ask an outpatient to state his or her name and date of birth and spell the last name. Make certain that the patient's response matches the requisition information before obtaining the specimen.

Preparing the Patient

Explaining the Procedure

Most patients have had a blood test before. A statement of your intent to collect a specimen for a blood test is usually sufficient for them to understand what is about to occur. A patient who has never had a blood test may require a more detailed explanation. Special procedures may require additional information. If a patient does not speak or understand English, you may have to use sign language or other nonverbal means to demonstrate what is to occur. If this fails, an interpreter must be located. Speaking slowly and distinctly, using sign language, or writing down information may be necessary for patients with hearing problems.

Key Point Regardless of the difficulties involved, you must always determine that the patient understands what is about to take place and obtain permission before proceeding. This is part of informed consent.

Addressing Patient Inquiries

Some healthcare facilities will allow the phlebotomist to tell the patient the name of the test or tests to be performed. Others prefer that all inquiries be directed to the patient's physician. Never attempt to explain the purpose of a test to a patient. Because a particular test can be ordered to rule out a number of different problems, any attempt to explain its purpose could mislead or unduly alarm the patient. Handle such inquiries by stating that it is best to have the doctor or nurse explain the tests to them.

When bedside testing is being performed (such as glucose monitoring), the patient is often aware of the type of test being performed and may ask about results. Follow facility protocol for addressing such requests or check with the patient's nurse or physician to see if it is acceptable to tell the patient the results at this time.

Handling Patient Objections

Although most patients understand that blood tests are needed in the course of treatment, occasionally a patient will object to the procedure. Outpatients rarely object because typically they have been personally directed by their physician to obtain testing and in most cases have been given a test requisition. Inpatients, on the other hand, may not be aware of all the tests that have been ordered or the frequency with which some tests must be repeated. Some may have difficult veins and just get tired of the ordeal. A reminder that the doctor ordered the test and needs the results to provide proper care will sometimes convince the patient to cooperate.

Key Point Do not attempt to badger the patient into cooperating or to restrain a conscious, mentally alert adult patient to obtain a specimen. Remember, a patient has the right to refuse testing.

Sometimes a patient objects at first but is not really serious. However, if a patient truly objects and refuses to let you collect the specimen, write on the requisition that the patient has refused to have blood drawn and notify the appropriate personnel that the specimen was not obtained because of patient refusal. Depending upon institution policy, you may be required to fill out a special form stating why you were unable to collect the specimen.

Handling Difficult Patients

The patient may not echo your cheerful, pleasant manner. Hospitalization or illness is typically a stressful situation. The patient may be lonely, scared, fearful, or just plain disagreeable and may react in a negative manner toward you. It is important to remain calm and professional and treat the patient in a caring manner under all circumstances.

Cognitively Impaired or Combative Patients

Some patients may display unpredictable or sudden movements and behaviors that could pose a danger to themselves, the phlebotomist or others nearby. If a patient exhibits such behaviors it is essential for an additional person or employee to be enlisted to assist if necessary. In addition, make certain you have an unobstructed exit route in case it is needed. Also be mindful of where you place equipment, being certain to keep it out of the reach of the patient. As with venipuncture on every patient, always have a gauze pad ready and be prepared to release the tourniquet quickly in case the patient pulls the needle out, or suddenly jerks causing the needle to either come out or go deep into the arm. Should the needle penetrate deep into the arm the patient's nurse or healthcare provider must be informed and the incident documented according to facility policy.

 CAUTION Never position a potentially combative patient between yourself and the only exit.

Patients in Altered Mental States

An altered mental state (also called altered state of consciousness or state of mind) is state that is significantly different from the normal waking state of a conscious person. It is characterized by changes in brain function such as confusion, disorientation, memory loss, disruptions in perception and abnormal behaviors such as emotional outbursts. Examples of patients who may undergo a change in mental status include transplant patients, patients with liver failure, and those suffering from post-traumatic stress syndrome. Alcohol abuse, illegal drugs, marijuana, and even prescription drugs can also be associated with mental problems in patients. Such conditions can cause problems with blood collection including verifying patient identification, obtaining informed consent for procedures, and trying to safely obtain specimens if the patient is combative or unaware of what is happening. Drug addicted patients can have scaring of the skin and veins that makes finding and palpating veins difficult. Assistance with patients who are in an altered state of consciousness is required for the safety of everyone involved and others nearby. In addition certain liabilities may be associated with dealing with these patients. Consult facility protocol for guidance.

Addressing Needle Phobia

An admission of **needle phobia** (intense fear of needles) by a patient or signs that suggest it, such as extreme fear or apprehension in advance of venipuncture, should not be taken lightly. Needle-phobic individuals typically have a heightened sensitivity to pain and can experience a shock type reaction during or immediately following venipuncture. Symptoms include pallor (paleness), profuse sweating, light-headedness, nausea, and fainting. In severe cases, patients have been known to suffer arrhythmia and even cardiac arrest. Needle phobia is estimated to affect more than 10% of the population to such a degree that they avoid medical care. It is important that those who do have the courage to submit to blood tests are treated with empathy and special attention and that steps be taken to minimize any trauma associated with the venipuncture. Basic steps that can be taken include the following:

- Have only the most experienced and skilled phlebotomist perform the venipuncture.
- Have the patient lie down during the procedure, with legs elevated.
- Apply an ice pack to the site for 10 to 15 minutes to numb it before venipuncture.

It is recommended that anyone who has suffered a severe reaction as a result of needle phobia have future procedures involving needles performed at sites where personnel are trained in CPR and a defibrillator is readily accessible.

> **(i)** A persistent irrational fear of pins and needles is called **belonephobia**. It is derived from the Greek word "belone," meaning *needle,* and "phobos," which means *fear.*

Addressing Objects in the Patient's Mouth

Do not allow a patient to eat, drink, chew gum, or have a thermometer, toothpick, or any other foreign object in the mouth during blood collection. Objects in the mouth can cause choking. A bite reflex could break a thermometer and injure a patient. Politely ask patients to stop eating or drinking and remove objects from their mouths until you are finished with the venipuncture.

STEP 3: VERIFY DIET RESTRICTIONS AND LATEX SENSITIVITY

Diet Restrictions

It is important to verify that any special diet instructions or restrictions have been followed. The most common diet requirement is for the patient to fast (refrain from eating) for a certain period of time, typically overnight, such as after the last meal of the day or after midnight in some cases (e.g., outpatients if they will not have the specimen drawn until after 8 AM) until the specimen is collected the following morning. The total time required is usually 8 to 12 hours. If no other restrictions are required, the patient may have water during the fasting period. Drinking water is important so that the patient does not become dehydrated, which can affect test results and make it harder to collect a blood specimen.

Eating can alter blood composition considerably. Consequently, if the patient did not fast or follow other diet instructions, it is important to notify and consult with the patient's physician or nurse so that a decision can be made as to whether or not to proceed with the test.

> **Key Point** If the patient has eaten and you are told to proceed with specimen collection, it is important to write "nonfasting" on the requisition and the specimen label.

Latex Sensitivity

Exposure to latex can trigger life-threatening reactions in those allergic to it. If a patient is allergic to latex, it is extremely important to verify that all equipment used on that individual is latex-free and that no latex items are brought into the room, even if they are for use on another patient in the same room.

STEP 4: SANITIZE HANDS AND PUT ON GLOVES

thePoint *View a video of Hand Washing/Hand Antisepsis at http://thepoint.lww.com/McCall6e.*

Proper hand hygiene plays a major role in preventing the spread of infection by protecting the phlebotomist, patient, and others from contamination. It

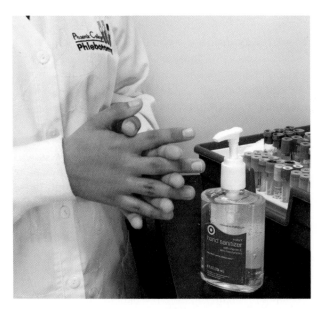

Figure 8-7 A phlebotomist applying hand sanitizer.

is an important step in the venipuncture procedure that should not be forgotten or performed poorly. Depending on the degree of contamination, hands can be decontaminated by washing or use of alcohol-based hand sanitizers (Fig. 8-7), which are normally available in the form of gels or foams. In using hand sanitizers it is important to use a generous amount and allow the alcohol to evaporate to achieve proper antisepsis. If hands are visibly dirty or contaminated with blood or other body fluids, they must be washed with soap and water. If hand-washing facilities are not available, visibly contaminated hands should be cleaned with detergent-containing wipes followed by the use of an alcohol-based hand cleaner. Hands must be sanitized in view of the patient, immediately before contact with the patient.

Wearing gloves is required by OSHA to protect the phlebotomist from potential exposure to bloodborne pathogens. Due to infection-control issues, most healthcare facilities require phlebotomists to put on gloves immediately after hand sanitization, before touching the patient. Follow facility protocol.

> (i) In absence of facility protocol, some phlebotomists prefer to wait until after vein selection to don gloves because they find it easier to feel veins without gloves on.

> ⚠ **CAUTION** Gloves must remain intact throughout the procedure (e.g., do not remove the fingertips).

STEP 5: POSITION PATIENT, APPLY TOURNIQUET, AND ASK PATIENT TO MAKE A FIST

Positioning the Patient

Inpatients normally have blood drawn while lying down in their beds. Outpatients at most facilities are drawn while sitting up in special blood-drawing chairs (Fig. 8-8A). If a special phlebotomy chair is not available (e.g., home draws), the patient should be seated in one that is sturdy and comfortable and has armrests in case the patient faints. If a suitable chair is not available or an outpatient is in a weakened condition or known to have fainting tendencies, the blood can be drawn with the patient in a reclining chair (Fig. 8-8B) or lying on a sofa or bed. With all blood draws, be prepared to react in case the patient feels faint or loses consciousness.

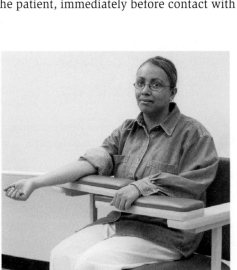
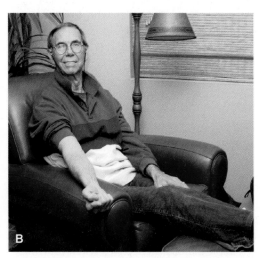

Figure 8-8 A: A patient seated in a special blood-drawing chair. **B:** A home-draw patient seated in a reclining chair.

CAUTION Because of the possibility of fainting, a patient should *never* be standing or seated in a chair without arms or on a high or backless stool during blood collection.

When venipuncture is performed on a hand or wrist vein, the patient's hand must be well supported on a bed, rolled towel, or armrest. For venipuncture in the antecubital (AC) area, the patient's arm should extend downward in a straight line from shoulder to wrist and *not* be bent at the elbow. (In some cases a slight bend may be necessary to avoid hyperextension of the elbow.) This position helps "fix" the veins so they are less apt to roll and makes them easier to locate because gravity causes them to enlarge and become more prominent. In addition, a downward position is necessary to ensure that blood-collection tubes fill from the bottom up. This prevents reflux or backflow of tube contents into the patient's vein (see Chapter 9) as well as additive carryover between tubes if multiple tubes are collected.

Proper positioning is somewhat harder to achieve with patients who are lying down, especially if the head of the bed cannot be raised. If necessary, a pillow or rolled towel can be used to support and position the arm so that at least the hand is lower than the elbow. Bed rails may be let down, but be careful not to catch IV lines, catheter bags and tubing, or other patient apparatus. Bed rails *must* be raised again when the procedure is finished. Many phlebotomists have learned to draw blood specimens with bed rails in place, so they don't have to worry about forgetting to put them back up when they are finished.

CAUTION A phlebotomist who lowers a bed rail and forgets to raise it can be held liable if the patient falls out of bed and is injured.

Tourniquet Application and Fist Clenching

thePoint *View the Proper Tourniquet Application for Venipuncture video at http://thepoint.lww.com/McCall6e.*

A tourniquet is applied 3 to 4 inches above the intended venipuncture site to restrict venous blood flow and make the veins more prominent. If it is closer to the site, the vein may collapse as blood is removed. If it is too far above the site, it may be ineffective. When drawing blood from a hand vein, the tourniquet is applied proximal to the wrist bone.

Key Point If a patient has prominent, visible veins that can be palpated and determined to be patent without it, tourniquet application can wait until after the site has been cleaned and you are ready to insert the needle.

The tourniquet should be tight enough to slow venous flow without affecting arterial flow. This allows more blood to flow into the area than out. As a result, blood backs up in the veins, enlarging them so they are easier to see and distending or stretching them so the walls are thinner and easier to pierce with a needle. A tourniquet that is too tight may prevent arterial blood flow into the area and result in failure to obtain blood. A tourniquet that is too loose will be useless. The tourniquet should feel snug or slightly tight to the patient, but not uncomfortable. It should lie flat around the circumference of the arm and not be rolled, twisted, or so tight that it pinches, hurts, or causes the arm to turn red or purple.

 A tourniquet has a greater tendency to roll or twist on the arms of obese patients. Bariatric tourniquets are available from manufacturers. However, if one is not available, two tourniquets placed on top of each other and used together will sometimes be sturdy enough to prevent this problem.

For patient comfort or if a patient has sensitive skin or dermatitis, apply the tourniquet over clothing or the sleeve of a hospital gown to prevent pinching the skin. An alternative is to use a clean washcloth or unfolded 4 × 4 gauze wrapped around the arm. Ask patients for permission before applying the tourniquet over street clothing however, as some may object. Instructions for tying a strap tourniquet are shown in Procedure 8-1.

CAUTION *Never* apply a tourniquet over an open sore. Choose another site.

When the tourniquet is in place, ask the patient to clench or make a fist. When a patient makes a fist, the veins in that arm become more prominent, making them easier to locate and enter with a needle. Pumping (repeatedly opening and closing) the fist should be prohibited, as it causes muscle movement that can make vein location more difficult; it can also cause changes in blood components that could negatively affect test results.

Procedure 8-1: Tourniquet Application

PURPOSE: Properly apply a tourniquet to a patient's arm as an aid to venipuncture

EQUIPMENT: Nonlatex strap tourniquet

NOTE: Steps listed are for a right-handed individual. If you are left handed, substitute dominant and nondominant, respectively, for right and left references.

Step	Explanation/Rationale
1. Place the tourniquet around the arm 3–4 inches above the intended venipuncture site.	If closer to the site, the vein may collapse as blood is withdrawn. If too far above the site, it may be ineffective.

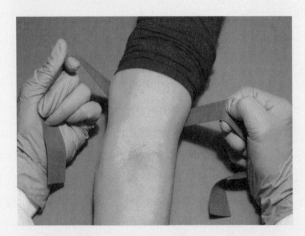

Step	Explanation/Rationale
2. Grasp one side of the tourniquet in each hand a few inches from the end.	Allows sufficient length for fastening the tourniquet and creating the loop in step 7.
3. Apply a small amount of tension and maintain it throughout the process.	Tension is needed so the tourniquet will be snug when tied. If too much tension is applied, it will be too tight and will roll up on itself or twist and cause discomfort.
4. Bring the two sides together and grasp them both between the thumb and forefinger of the right hand.	This is preparation for crossing the sides over each other.

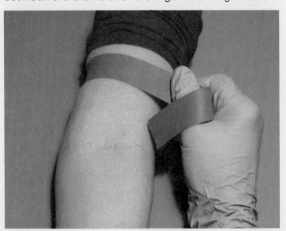

Step	Explanation/Rationale
5. Reach over the right hand and grasp the right side of the tourniquet between the thumb and forefinger of the left hand and release it from the grip of the right hand.	The tourniquet ends will now be held in opposite hands, with the sides crossed over each other.

Procedure 8-1: Tourniquet Application (Continued)

Step	Explanation/Rationale
6. Cross the left end over the right end near the left index finger, grasping both sides together between the thumb and forefinger of the left hand, close to the patient's arm.	If there is too much space between the left index finger and the patient's arm, the tourniquet will be too loose.

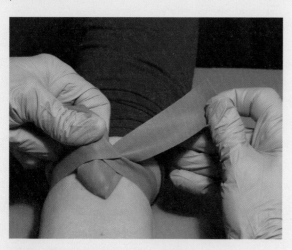

Step	Explanation/Rationale
7. While securely grasping both sides, use either the left middle finger or the right index finger to tuck a portion of the left side under the right side and pull it into a loop.	The loop allows the tourniquet to be released quickly by a slight tug on the end that forms it.

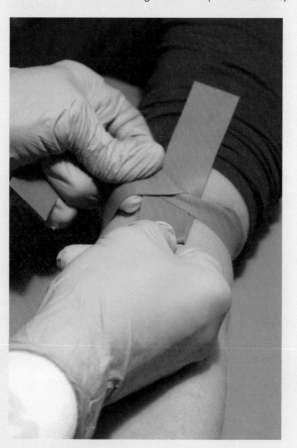

Procedure 8-1: Tourniquet Application (Continued)

Step	Explanation/Rationale
8. A properly tied tourniquet with the ends pointing toward the shoulder.	The tourniquet ends should point toward the shoulder to prevent them from contaminating the blood-collection site.

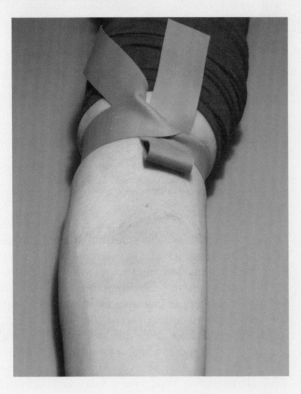

 Key Point Fist pumping most notably affects levels of potassium and ionized calcium.

STEP 6: SELECT VEIN, RELEASE TOURNIQUET, AND ASK PATIENT TO OPEN FIST

The preferred venipuncture site is the AC area of the arm, where a number of veins lie fairly close to the surface. Typically, the most prominent of these are the median cubital, cephalic, and basilic veins in the "H" pattern and the median, median cephalic, and median basilic veins in the "M" pattern (see Chapter 6). The median cubital and median veins are normally closer to the surface, more stationary, and in an area where nerve injury is least likely. Consequently, they are the first choices for venipuncture, followed by the cephalic and median cephalic veins. The basilic and median basilic veins are the last-choice veins because they are near the median nerve and brachial artery, which could be punctured accidentally.

CAUTION According to CLSI Standards, an attempt must be made to locate the veins in the median aspect (center of the arm) on both arms before considering an alternate vein. Because of the possibility of nerve injury and damage to the brachial artery, the basilic vein or other veins in the medial aspect (inside of the arm) should not be chosen unless it appears that no other vein can be safely or successfully accessed.

A patient will generally have the most prominent veins in the dominant arm. It should be examined first unless there is a reason that it should not be used. However, if the nondominant arm has an equally suitable vein, it may be a good idea to draw that arm since the patient is less likely to use it after the draw and disturb healing at the site that could result in bruising. Some veins may be easily visible (Fig. 8-9); others will have to be located entirely by feel. To locate a vein, **palpate** (examine by touch or feel) the area by pushing down on the skin with the tip of the index finger (Fig. 8-10). In addition to

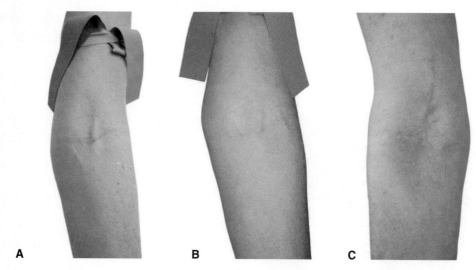

A   **B**   **C**

Figure 8-9 Three examples of antecubital vein patterns. **A:** H-pattern. **B:** M-pattern. **C:** Atypical pattern.

locating veins, palpating helps determine their **patency** (state of being freely open), size and depth, and the direction or the path they follow. Consequently, even visible veins must be palpated to judge their suitability for venipuncture.

Have fun unscrambling patency and other words with the Scrambled Words activity in the WORKBOOK.

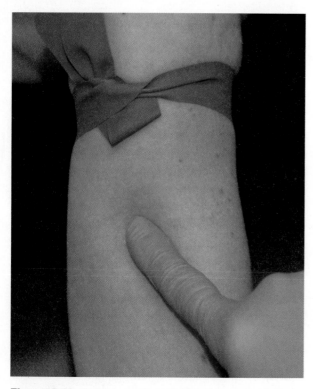

Figure 8-10 A phlebotomist palpating the antecubital area for a vein.

When you have found a vein, roll your finger from one side to the other while pressing against it to help judge its size. Trace its path to determine a proper entry point by palpating above and below where you first feel it. Press and release it several times to determine depth and patency. Depth is indicated by the degree of pressure required to feel it. A **patent** (freely open) vein is turgid (distended from being filled with blood), giving it a bounce or resilience, and has a tube-like feel. An artery has a pulse and must be avoided. (Do not use your thumb to palpate as it has a pulse that could lead you to think that a vein is an artery.)

CAUTION To avoid inadvertently puncturing an artery, *never* select a vein that overlies or is close to where you feel a pulse.

Do not select a vein that feels hard and cord-like or lacks resilience, as it is probably sclerosed or thrombosed (see Chapter 9). Such veins roll easily, are hard to penetrate, and may not have adequate blood flow to yield a representative blood sample. Tendons are also hard and lack resilience. Rotating the patient's arm slightly helps to locate veins and differentiate them from other structures. Dimming the lights and using a transilluminator device or halogen flashlight can help locate veins, especially in infants and children. Wiping the site with alcohol often makes surface veins such as hand veins appear more visible. (This step *does not* take the place of cleaning after vein selection.) If no suitable AC vein can be found, check the other arm. If no suitable AC vein can be found in either arm, check for veins on the back of the hand or wrist.

If a suitable vein still cannot be found, massage the arm from wrist to elbow to force blood into the area or wrap a warm, wet towel around the arm or hand for a few minutes. Warming the site increases blood flow and makes veins easier to feel. The site should not be manipulated excessively, however, as this may change the composition of blood in the area and cause erroneous test results. In the absence of a suitable vein, a capillary puncture may have to be considered if the test can be performed on capillary blood.

After you have selected a suitable vein, mentally visualize its location if it is not obvious. Making a mental note of the position of the vein in reference to landmarks such as a freckle, mole, hair, skin crease, superficial surface vein, or imperfection makes relocation easier after the delay while the site is cleaned. Do not mark the site with a pen. This contaminates the site and the pen. The pen can become a source of infection transmission if it is used on other patients. An acceptable way to mark the site using an alcohol pad is shown in Figure 8-11. This,

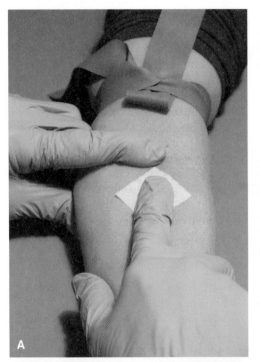

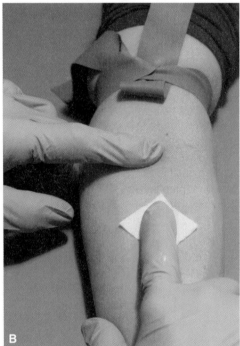

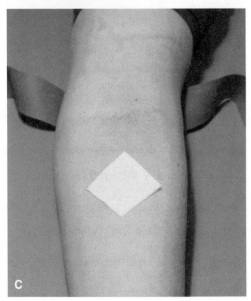

Figure 8-11 Marking the site with an alcohol pad before cleaning the site. **A:** Align the corner of a clean alcohol pad with the vein located by the index finger. **B:** Slide the pad away from the site, paralleling the direction of the vein and keeping the corner of the pad pointing in the direction of the vein. **C:** Alcohol pad pointing in the direction of the vein.

of course, is done before the site is cleaned, so the pad must be placed far enough away from the site so it is not disturbed in the cleaning process.

If the tourniquet was applied during vein selection, release it and ask the patient to open the fist. This allows the vein to return to normal and minimizes the effects of stasis from blockage of blood flow on specimen composition.

 Key Point According to the CLSI, when a tourniquet has been in place for longer than one minute, it should be released and reapplied after 2 minutes.

STEP 7: CLEAN AND AIR-DRY THE SITE

The venipuncture site must be cleaned with an antiseptic prior to venipuncture. Otherwise, microorganisms from the skin could be picked up by the needle and carried into the vein, creating the possibility of infection, or flushed into the collection tube on blood flow, contaminating the specimen. The recommended antiseptic for cleaning a venipuncture site is 70% isopropyl alcohol, which is typically available in sterile, prepackaged pads referred to as alcohol prep pads.

An antiseptic does not sterilize the site; however, it does inhibit microbial growth.

Clean the site with a gauze pad soaked with 70% isopropyl alcohol or a commercially prepared alcohol prep pad. Use friction to clean an area 2 to 3 inches in diameter around the selected site of needle entry. Although previous CLSI standards recommended using a circular motion, starting at the point of expected needle entry, and moving outward in ever-widening **concentric circles** (circles with a common center), this is no longer considered necessary. Use sufficient pressure to remove surface dirt and debris but do not rub so vigorously that you abrade the skin, especially on infants and elderly patients whose skin is thin and more delicate. If the site is especially dirty, clean it again using a new alcohol soaked gauze or alcohol prep pad. Allow the area to dry naturally for 30 seconds to 1 minute.

Key Point The evaporation and drying process helps destroy microbes, and avoids a burning or stinging sensation when the needle is inserted.

To prevent contamination of the site,

- *Do not* dry the alcohol with unsterile gauze.
- *Do not* fan the site with your hand or blow on it to hasten drying time.
- *Do not* touch the site after cleaning it.

Key Point If it is necessary to repalpate the vein after the site has been cleaned, the site must be cleaned again.

STEP 8: PREPARE EQUIPMENT

Assemble the components of the blood-collection system and supplies if you have not already done so. Choose the collection system, needle size, and tube volume according to the age of the patient, size and location of the vein, and amount of blood to be collected. Select tubes according to the tests that have been ordered. Select and attach the needle to the collection device but *do not* remove the **needle sheath** (cap or cover) at this time. Put on a clean pair of gloves if you have not already done so.

CAUTION Either the needle, tube holder, or syringe selected must have an OSHA-required safety feature to help protect the user from accidental needlesticks.

ETS Equipment Preparation

Select the appropriate ETS tubes. Check the expiration date on each one to make certain that it has not expired. (Discard any tube that is beyond its expiration date.) Tap additive tubes lightly to dislodge any additive that may be adhering to the tube stopper. Inspect the seal of the needle. If it is broken, discard it and select a new one. Twist the needle cover apart to expose the short or back end of the needle, which is covered by a retractable sleeve. Screw this end of the needle into the threaded hub of an ETS tube holder. Place the first tube in the holder and use a slight clockwise twist to push it onto the needle just far enough to secure it and keep it from falling out but not far enough to release the tube vacuum. It is acceptable to delay positioning the tube in the holder until the needle is inserted in the patient's vein.

Preparation of a Winged Infusion Set (Butterfly)

Although they are available in various gauges, a 23-gauge butterfly is most commonly used for small and difficult veins. Butterfly needles are also available in two basic types. One type has a hub that can be attached to a syringe. The second type has a hub with a multisample Luer adapter that can be threaded onto an ETS tube holder. The adapter can typically be removed to also allow the needle to be used with a syringe. Select the type according to the system (ETS or syringe) you have chosen to collect the specimen. The system to use typically depends on the size, condition, and location of the vein as well as the skill and personal preference of the user. In some cases a syringe and butterfly are used after a failed attempt at blood collection using a butterfly and ETS holder. For either method, the butterfly needle typically contains the safety feature.

Verify sterility of the butterfly packaging (i.e., package is sealed and intact) before aseptically opening it and removing the butterfly. To help preserve needle sterility (a butterfly needle cover is typically an open-ended tubular sheath), it is a good idea to retain the package so you can put the needle back in it temporarily while retying the tourniquet. Attach the butterfly to the evacuated tube holder or syringe. Butterfly tubing may be coiled somewhat because it was coiled in the package. To help straighten it and keep it from coiling back up, use the thumb and index finger of one hand to grasp the tubing just beyond the point where it attaches to the needle. Gently grasp the tubing a little below this point with the thumb and index finger of the opposite hand and slide these fingers down the length of the tubing while stretching it slightly, until you are just above the point where it attaches to the tube holder. Be extremely careful not to loosen the tubing from the needle or the holder. Select the appropriate small-volume tubes for the tests ordered. (The vacuum draw of large-volume tubes may collapse the vein or hemolyze the specimen.)

Preparation of Syringe Equipment

Select a syringe and needle size compatible with the size and condition of the patient's veins and the amount of blood to be collected. To comply with OSHA regulations, you must select a needle-locking syringe (e.g., Luer lock) to use for the draw and a syringe transfer device to transfer blood from the syringe to the ETS tubes. Syringes and syringe needles designed for blood collection are normally available in sterile pull-apart packages. The syringe plunger is typically already pulled back slightly. To ensure that it moves freely but still maintain syringe sterility, move the plunger back and forth slightly a few times and advance it to the end of the syringe before opening the sterile package. Open the needle packages in an aseptic manner and securely attach the needle to the syringe. A blood specimen collected in a syringe will have to be transferred to ETS tubes. Small-volume tubes are typically chosen because the amount of blood that can be collected in a syringe is limited. Partially open the package containing the transfer device to make removal easy when it comes time to use it.

Positioning Equipment for Use

Place collection equipment and other supplies, such as gauze and alcohol pads, within easy reach, typically on the same side of the patient's arm as your free hand during venipuncture. Make certain that extra supplies, ETS tubes for example, are within easy reach. If you are using a phlebotomy tray, place it within easy reach.

> **⚠ CAUTION** *Do not* place the phlebotomy tray on a patient's bed or any other place that could be contaminated by it. If you set it on the patient's bedside table, place it on a clean paper towel.

STEP 9: REAPPLY TOURNIQUET, UNCAP AND INSPECT NEEDLE

Reapply the tourniquet, being careful not to touch the cleaned area. Be aware that there are a few tests (i.e., lactic acid) that must be collected without using a tourniquet.

Pick up collection equipment with your dominant hand. Both an ETS tube holder and a syringe are held close to the needle hub with the thumb on top and two or three fingers underneath and slightly to the side. Turn your wrist upward slightly so the opening of the tube holder remains accessible. Hold the wing portion of the butterfly between your thumb and index finger or fold the wings upright and grasp them together. Cradle the butterfly tubing and holder or syringe in the palm of your dominant hand or lay it next to the patient's hand.

Remove the needle cover and visually inspect the needle. Although rare, a needle can have obstructions that could impair blood flow or imperfections such as roughness or barbs that could hurt the patient or damage the vein. If any are noted, discard the needle and select a new one.

> **⚠ CAUTION** Once the cap is removed, *do not* let the needle touch anything prior to venipuncture. If it does, remove it and replace it with a new one.

STEP 10: ASK PATIENT TO MAKE A FIST, ANCHOR VEIN, AND INSERT NEEDLE

At this time the patient is asked to again make a fist. The nondominant hand is used to **anchor** (secure firmly) the vein while the collection equipment is held and the needle inserted using the dominant hand.

Anchoring

To anchor AC veins, grasp the patient's arm with your free hand, using your fingers to support the back of the arm just below the elbow. Place your thumb a minimum of 1 to 2 inches below and slightly to the side of the intended venipuncture site and pull the skin toward the wrist (Fig. 8-12). This stretches the skin taut (pulled tight or without slack), anchoring the vein and helping

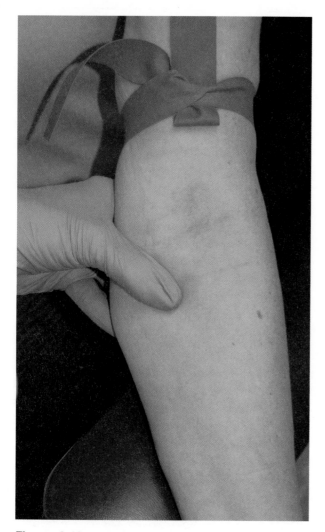

Figure 8-12 Proper placement of thumb and fingers in anchoring a vein.

One way to anchor a hand vein is to use your free hand to hold the patient's hand just below the knuckles and use your thumb to pull the skin taut over the knuckles while bending the patient's fingers. Another way is to have the patient make a tight fist. Encircle the fist with your fingers and use your thumb to pull the skin over the knuckles.

Needle Insertion

Hold the collection device or butterfly needle in your dominant hand as described in step 9. The bevel of the needle should be facing up. Position the needle above the vein so it is lined up with it and paralleling or following its path. Your body should be positioned directly behind the needle so that you are not trying to insert the needle with your arm or hands at an awkward angle. Warn the patient by saying something like "There is going to be a little poke (or stick) now."

> ⚠️ **CAUTION** If the needle touches the skin, but you change your mind and lift it off of the skin, it is no longer sterile and must be replaced.

For AC site venipunctures, insert the needle into the skin at an angle of 30 degrees or less (Fig. 8-13A), depending on the depth of the vein. (A shallow vein may need an angle closer to 15 degrees, while a deeper vein may require an angle closer to 30 degrees.) Use one smooth, steady forward motion to penetrate first the skin and then the vein. Advancing the needle too slowly prolongs any discomfort. A rapid jab can result in missing the vein or going all the way through it.

> 🔑 **Key Point** You have less control over the needle the faster it goes into the arm. In addition to possibly missing the vein or going through it, you impair the ability to immediately stop advancing the needle if it hits a nerve.

to keep it from moving or rolling to the side upon needle entry. (If the vein rolls, the needle may slip beside the vein, not into it.) In addition, a needle passes through taut skin more easily and with less pain. Even so, it is not uncommon for an apprehensive patient to suddenly pull back the arm as the needle is inserted. Because your fingers are wrapped around the arm, the patient is less likely to pull away from your grasp and the needle is more likely to stay in the vein. This is known as the "L" hold technique for anchoring the vein.

> ⚠️ **CAUTION** For safety reasons, *do not* use a two-finger technique (also called the "C" hold) in which the entry point of the vein is straddled by the index finger above and the thumb below. If the patient abruptly pulls the arm back when the needle is inserted, a reflex reaction could cause the needle to recoil as it comes out of the arm and spring back into your index finger.

When the needle enters the vein, you will feel a slight "give" or decrease in resistance. Some phlebotomists describe this as a "pop," although it may be described as a feeling and not a sound. (It is especially important to recognize the decrease in resistance when using an ETS needle and tube holder, because most needles do not provide visual confirmation that the vein has been entered.) When you sense the "pop" or recognize the lessening of resistance signaling that the needle is in the vein, stop advancing it and securely anchor the tube holder or syringe by pressing the back of your fingers or knuckles against the arm. Discontinue anchoring with your thumb and let go of the arm with that hand.

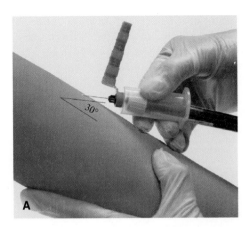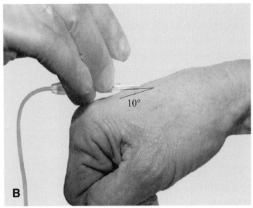

Figure 8-13 A: Illustration of a 30-degree angle of needle insertion. **B:** Illustration of a 10-degree angle of needle insertion.

⚠ **CAUTION** Do not deeply depress the skin by forcefully pushing down on the needle as it is inserted. This causes pain and enlarges the vein opening, increasing the risk of blood leakage at the site.

When using a butterfly needle on a hand vein, insert it into the vein at a shallow angle of approximately 10 degrees or less (Fig. 8-13B), being careful not to push it through the back wall of the vein. You may need to slightly increase the angle of the needle bevel at first to get it to slip into the vein. A "flash" or small amount of blood will usually appear in the tubing when the needle is in the vein. "Seat" the needle by slightly threading it within the lumen (central area of the vein). This helps keep the needle from twisting back out of the vein if you let go of it. If the needle does start to come out of the vein, secure it with the thumb of the opposite hand.

At this point, some phlebotomists switch to holding the blood-collection device in their nondominant hand so that tube changes can be made with the dominant hand. This is accomplished by gently slipping the fingers of the opposite hand under the holder and placing the thumb atop the holder as the other hand lets go. Many phlebotomists, particularly those who are left-handed, do not change hands but continue to steady the holder in the same hand and change tubes with the opposite one. Whatever the method, it is important to hold the blood-collection device steady so there is minimal needle movement.

🔑 **Key Point** If the tube holder or syringe is not securely anchored, the needle can push through the back of the vein or pull out of the vein when tubes are changed or the syringe is filled.

STEP 11: ESTABLISH BLOOD FLOW, RELEASE TOURNIQUET, AND ASK PATIENT TO OPEN FIST

To establish blood flow when using the ETS system, the collection tube must be advanced into the tube holder until the stopper is completely penetrated by the needle. This is accomplished most efficiently by pushing the tube with your thumb while your index and middle fingers straddle and grasp the flanges of the tube holder (Fig. 8-14), pulling back on them slightly to prevent forward motion of the tube holder. If the vein has been successfully entered, blood will begin to flow into the tube. If you are using a syringe, a flash of blood in the syringe hub indicates that the vein has been successfully entered. Blood flow into the syringe is achieved by slowly pulling back on the plunger with your free hand.

Release the tourniquet and ask the patient to release the fist as soon as blood flows freely into the first ETS tube or is established in the syringe. Blood should continue to flow until multiple tubes have been collected or the syringe filled. On elderly patients and others with fragile veins that

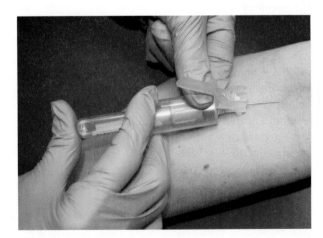

Figure 8-14 Proper placement of fingers and thumb in advancing a tube in an ETS holder.

might collapse or in other difficult-draw situations where release of the tourniquet might cause blood flow to stop, the tourniquet is sometimes left on until the last tube is filled. *Do not,* however, leave the tourniquet on for more than 1 minute, or test results may be affected.

 Typically, several tubes can be filled in less than a minute.

STEP 12: FILL, REMOVE, AND MIX TUBES IN ORDER OF DRAW, OR FILL SYRINGE

Following the order of draw, place ETS tubes in the holder and advance them onto the needle.

ETS tubes fill automatically until the tube vacuum is exhausted or lost. A syringe is filled manually by slowly and steadily pulling back on the plunger until the barrel is filled to the appropriate level.

Key Point According to the CLSI, if a coagulation tube is the first tube to be drawn when using a butterfly, a discard tube should be drawn first to fill the tubing dead space and ensure a correct blood-to-anticoagulant ratio when the coagulation tube is filled. The discard tube can be a nonadditive tube or another coagulation tube and does not have to be filled completely.

Maintain needle position while the tubes or syringe are filling. Try not to pull up, press down, or move the needle back and forth or sideways in the vein. These actions can be painful to the patient and enlarge the hole in the vein, resulting in leakage of blood and hematoma formation.

Keep the arm in a downward position so that blood fills ETS tubes from the bottom up and does not contact the needle in the tube holder. Under certain conditions, **reflux** (flow of blood from the tube back into the vein) and a possible adverse patient reaction from additives can occur if tube blood is in contact with the needle. Additive-containing blood on or in the needle could also contaminate subsequent tubes when multiple tubes are collected. Do not change position of the tube or allow back-and-forth movement of the blood in the tube, as this too can cause reflux. A downward arm position also helps maintain blood flow.

Key Point If the stopper end of the tube fills first, blood in the tube is in contact with the needle and reflux can occur if there is a change in pressure in the patient's vein.

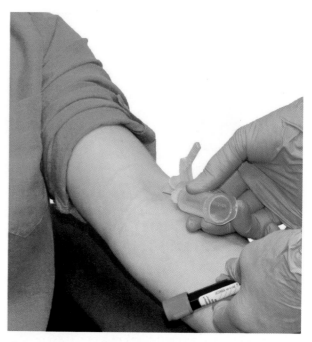

Figure 8-15 A phlebotomist mixing a heparin tube.

To ensure a proper ratio of blood to additive, allow ETS tubes to fill until the normal vacuum is exhausted and blood ceases to flow. Tubes do not fill completely to the top. When blood flow stops, remove the tube, using a reverse twist and pulling motion while bracing the thumb or index finger against the flange of the holder. The rubber sleeve will cover the needle and prevent leakage of blood into the tube holder. If the tube contains an additive, mix it by gently inverting it three to eight times (depending upon the type of additive and manufacturer's recommendations) as soon as it is removed from the tube holder and before putting it down (Fig. 8-15). Remember, each inversion requires turning the wrist 180 degrees and back again. Lack of, delayed, or inadequate mixing can lead to clot formation and necessitate recollection of the specimen. Nonadditive tubes do not require mixing.

See how well you know the key points and cautions in this chapter with WORKBOOK Knowledge Drill 8-1.

CAUTION *Do not* shake or vigorously mix blood specimens, as this can cause hemolysis (breakage of red blood cells and release of hemoglobin into the serum or plasma).

If other ETS tubes are to be drawn, place them in the holder, use a clockwise twist to engage them with the needle, and push them the rest of the way onto the needle until blood flow is established. Steady the tube holder so that the needle does not pull out of or penetrate through the vein as tubes are placed and removed. If the needle backs out of the skin even slightly, the vacuum of the tube will be lost (evidenced by a hissing sound) and the tube will stop filling. Unless the tube already has an adequate amount of blood for the test, a new one will have to be filled. Remember to follow the proper order of draw (see Chapter 7).

When the last ETS tube has been filled, remove it from the holder and mix it, if applicable, before removing the needle from the arm. If the tube is still engaged when the needle is removed from the arm, the needle may drip blood and cause needless contamination.

Key Point The practice of releasing the tube from the needle but leaving it in the holder during needle removal is awkward and increases the chance of needlesticks. It also delays proper mixing of tube contents, which can lead to microclot formation in anticoagulant tubes.

If the tourniquet is still on, release it before removing the needle. If the needle is removed with the tourniquet in place, blood may run down the arm and alarm the patient.

STEP 13: PLACE GAUZE, REMOVE NEEDLE, ACTIVATE SAFETY FEATURE, AND APPLY PRESSURE

After the last tube has been removed from the holder or an adequate amount of blood has been collected (if you are using a syringe), fold a clean gauze square into fourths and place it directly over the site where the needle enters the skin. Hold the gauze lightly in place but do not press down on it until the needle is removed.

CAUTION *Do not* press down on the gauze while the needle is in the vein. It puts pressure on the needle during removal, causing pain, and the needle may slit the vein and skin as it is withdrawn.

If the needle safety feature is designed to function within the vein, activate it according to the manufacturer's instructions. Withdraw the needle from the vein in one smooth motion. If the needle safety feature operates outside the vein, activate it immediately while simultaneously applying pressure to the site with your free hand. Apply pressure to the site for 3 to 5 minutes

or until the bleeding stops. Failure to apply pressure or applying inadequate pressure can result in leakage of blood and hematoma formation. It is acceptable to have the patient hold pressure while you proceed to label tubes (or fill them if a syringe was used) provided that the patient is fully alert and able to so. *Do not* ask the patient to bend the arm up. The arm should be kept extended or even raised.

Key Point Studies show that folding the arm back at the elbow to hold pressure or keep the gauze in place after a blood draw actually increases the chance of bruising by keeping the wound open (especially if it is to the side of the arm) or disrupting the platelet plug when the arm is lowered.

If the sharps container has been moved out of reach (as sometimes happens in emergencies when others are working on the patient at the same time) and the patient is not able to hold pressure, it is generally acceptable to bend the patient's arm up temporarily while locating the sharps container and disposing of the collection device.

STEP 14: DISCARD COLLECTION UNIT, SYRINGE NEEDLE, OR TRANSFER DEVICE

CAUTION OSHA regulations prohibit cutting, bending, breaking, or recapping blood-collection needles or removing them from tube holders after use.

A needle and tube holder must be promptly discarded in a sharps container as a single unit. A syringe safety needle, however, may be removed and discarded separately so that the syringe can be attached to a syringe transfer device and tubes filled at this point. A transfer device is similar to an ETS holder but has a permanently attached needle inside. After the device is attached to the syringe, an ETS tube is placed inside it and advanced onto the needle until blood flows into the tube. Additional tubes can be filled as long as there is enough blood left in the syringe. When the transfer is complete, the syringe and transfer device are discarded in a sharps container as a single unit.

STEP 15: LABEL TUBES

the Point_· *View the Specimen Labeling and Venipuncture Follow-up Procedures video at http://thepoint.lww.com/McCall6e.*

⚠️ **CAUTION** Do not turn your back to the patient after the draw. Face the patient while labeling tubes or finishing paperwork and be prepared to react should the patient have an adverse reaction.

Tubes must be labeled in the presence of the patient immediately after blood collection, never before, and the label must be permanently attached to the tube before leaving an inpatient's bedside or dismissing an outpatient.

If you are using a preprinted computer or bar-code label, you will need to write the date, time, your initials, and other pertinent information on the label immediately before or after attaching it to the tube. If you do not have a preprinted label, you will have to hand print the required information on the tube yourself. Any handwritten labeling must be done with a permanent-ink pen. Labels should include the following information as a minimum:

- Patient's first and last names
- Patient's identification number (inpatient) or date of birth (outpatient)
- Date and time of collection
- Phlebotomist's initials
- Pertinent additional information, such as "fasting"

Before leaving an inpatient, compare the information on each labeled tube with the patient's ID band (Fig. 8-16) and the requisition. Some facilities have the phlebotomist show the labeled tube to the patient and ask the patient to verify that the correct name is on the tube. Both inpatient and outpatient tubes must then be placed upright in a biohazard specimen bag or other suitable container for transport to the laboratory.

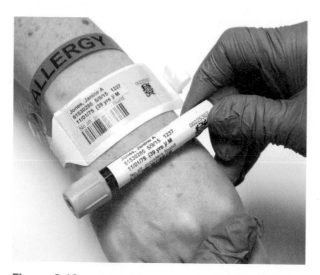

Figure 8-16 A phlebotomist comparing labeled tube with patient's ID band.

STEP 16: OBSERVE SPECIAL HANDLING INSTRUCTIONS

Follow applicable special handling requirements. Place specimens that must be cooled (e.g., ammonia) in crushed ice slurry. Put specimens that must be kept at body temperature (e.g., cold agglutinin) in a 37°C heat block or other suitable warming device. Wrap specimens that require protection from light (e.g., bilirubin) in aluminum foil or other light-blocking material or place them in a light-blocking container.

STEP 17: CHECK PATIENT'S ARM AND APPLY BANDAGE

Examine the venipuncture site to determine if bleeding has stopped. (Bleeding from the vein can continue even though it has stopped at the surface of the skin). If you are certain it has stopped, apply an adhesive bandage (or tape and folded gauze square) over the site. If the patient is allergic to adhesive bandages, apply paper tape over a clean, folded gauze square. If the patient has sensitive skin or is allergic to adhesives, place a folded gauze square over the site and wrap gauze around it, fastening the gauze with paper tape, or wrap the site with a self-adhering gauze-like material such as Coban. Instruct the patient to leave the bandage on for a minimum of 15 minutes, after which it should be removed to avoid irritation. Instruct an outpatient not to carry a purse or other heavy object or lift heavy objects with that arm for a minimum of 1 hour.

⚠️ **CAUTION** If bleeding has not stopped, the phlebotomist must apply pressure until it does. If the patient continues to bleed beyond 5 minutes, the appropriate personnel such as the patient's physician or nurse should be notified.

STEP 18: DISPOSE OF CONTAMINATED MATERIALS

Dispose of contaminated materials in the proper biohazard containers or according to facility protocol; discard other used disposable items in the regular trash. Make sure that any other equipment is returned to its proper place.

STEP 19: THANK PATIENT, REMOVE GLOVES, AND SANITIZE HANDS

Thank the patient for his or her cooperation. This is courteous and lets the patient know that the procedure is complete. Remove gloves aseptically as described in Chapter 3, discard them in the manner required by your institution, and sanitize your hands before leaving the area.

STEP 20: TRANSPORT SPECIMEN TO THE LAB

Transport specimens to the laboratory or designated pickup site in a timely fashion. Prompt delivery to the laboratory protects specimen integrity and is typically achieved by personal delivery, transportation through a pneumatic tube system, or arranged pickup by a courier service. The phlebotomist is typically responsible for verifying and documenting collection by computer entry or manual entry in a logbook.

Don't forget that questions in the EXAM REVIEW can help you see how well you have learned venipuncture procedures.

Routine ETS Venipuncture

Most venipunctures are routine and can be performed on AC veins using an ETS system. This system is preferred because it is direct, efficient, relatively safe for the patient and the blood drawer, and allows multiple tubes to be easily collected. Routine ETS venipuncture is illustrated in Procedure 8-2.

thePoint *View the Collecting a Blood Specimen by Venipuncture Using the Evacuated Tube System Video at http://thepoint.lww.com/McCall6e. For tips on proper ergonomics for this technique, watch the video Poor and Good Workplace Ergonomics for Phlebotomy, found at the same location.*

Procedure 8-2: Routine ETS Venipuncture

PURPOSE: To obtain a blood specimen for patient diagnostic or monitoring purposes from an antecubital vein using the evacuated tube system (ETS)

EQUIPMENT: Tourniquet; gloves; antiseptic prep pad; ETS needle,* tube holder* and tubes; gauze pads; sharps container; permanent ink pen; bandage

*Either the needle or tube holder must have a safety feature to prevent needlesticks.

Step	Explanation/Rationale
1. Review and accession test request.	A test request must be reviewed for completeness, date and time of collection, status, and priority. The accession process records the request and assigns it a unique number used to identify the specimen, related processes, and paperwork.
2. Approach, identify, and prepare patient. 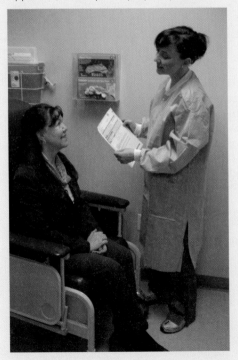	The right approach for a successful patient encounter includes a professional bedside manner, being organized and efficient, and looking for signs that convey important inpatient information or infection-control precautions.
	Correct ID is vital to patient safety and meaningful test results. Name, DOB, and MR number must be verified and matched to the test order and inpatient's ID band. Preparing the patient by explaining procedures and addressing inquiries helps reduce patient anxiety.

Procedure 8-2: Routine ETS Venipuncture (Continued)

Step	Explanation/Rationale

3. Verify diet restrictions and latex sensitivity.

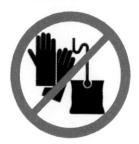

Test results can be meaningless or misinterpreted and patient care compromised if diet requirements have not been met. Exposure to latex can trigger a life-threatening reaction in those allergic to it.

4. Sanitize hands and put on gloves.

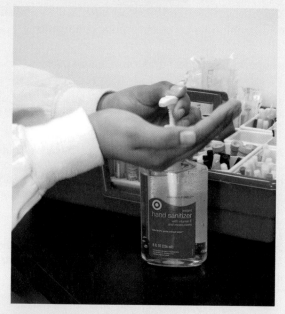

Proper hand hygiene plays a major role in infection control by protecting the phlebotomist, patient, and others from contamination. Gloves are required by OSHA to protect the phlebotomist from potential bloodborne pathogen exposure.

5. Position patient, apply tourniquet, and ask patient to make a fist.

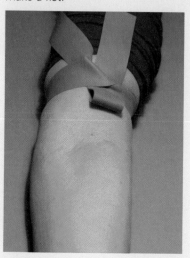

Proper positioning is important to patient comfort and venipuncture success. The patient's arm should be placed downward in a straight line from shoulder to wrist to aid in vein selection and avoid reflux as tubes are filled.

Tourniquet application enlarges veins and makes them easier to see, feel, and enter with a needle.

A clenched fist make the veins easier to see and feel and helps keep them from rolling.

Procedure 8-2: Routine ETS Venipuncture (Continued)

Step	Explanation/Rationale
6. Select vein, release tourniquet, ask patient to open fist. 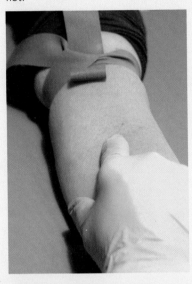	Select a large, well-anchored vein. The median cubital should be the first choice, followed by the cephalic. The basilic should not be chosen unless it appears that no other vein can be safely or successfully accessed. Releasing the tourniquet and opening the fist helps prevent hemoconcentration.
7. Clean and air-dry site. 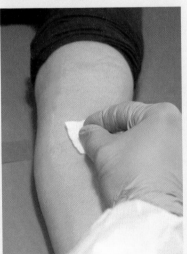	Cleaning the site with an antiseptic helps avoid contaminating the specimen or patient with skin-surface bacteria picked up by the needle during venipuncture. Letting the site dry naturally permits maximum antiseptic action, prevents contamination caused by wiping, and avoids stinging or burning on needle entry.
8. Prepare equipment. 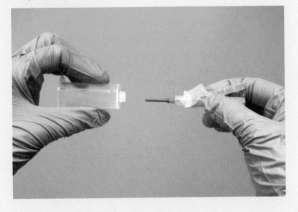	Selecting appropriate equipment for the size, condition, and location of the vein is easier after vein selection. Preparing it while the site is drying saves time. Attach a needle to an ETS holder. Put the first tube in the holder now (see step 10) or wait until after needle entry. Gloves must be put on now if not already on.

Procedure 8-2: Routine ETS Venipuncture (Continued)

Step	Explanation/Rationale
9. Reapply tourniquet, uncap and inspect needle.	The tourniquet aids needle entry. Pick up the tube holder with your dominant hand, placing your thumb on top near the needle end and fingers underneath. Uncap and inspect the needle for defects and discard it if flawed.

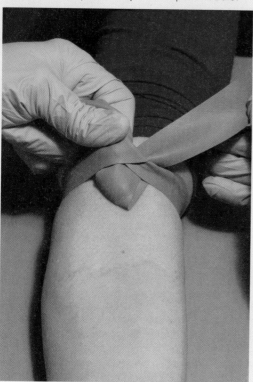

Step	Explanation/Rationale
10. Ask patient to remake a fist, anchor vein, and insert needle.	The fist aids needle entry. Anchoring stretches the skin so the needle enters easily and with less pain, and keeps the vein from rolling. Warn the patient. Line the needle up with the vein and insert it bevel up into the skin using a smooth forward motion. Stop when you feel a decrease in resistance, often described as a "pop," and press your fingers into the arm to anchor the holder.

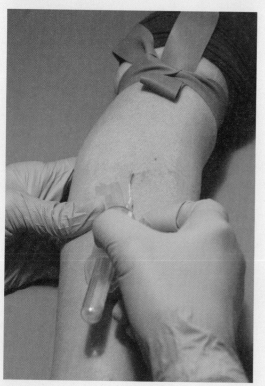

Procedure 8-2: Routine ETS Venipuncture (Continued)

Step	Explanation/Rationale
11. Establish blood flow, release tourniquet, ask patient to open fist. 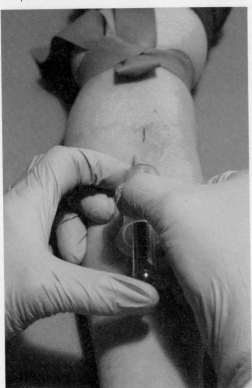 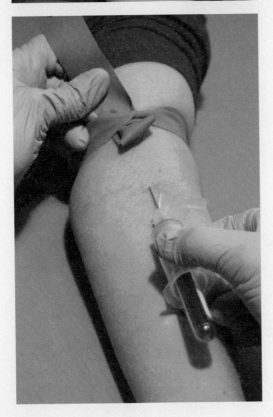	Blood will not flow until the needle pierces the tube stopper. Place a tube in the holder and push it part way onto the needle with a clockwise twist. Grasp the holder's flanges with your middle and index fingers, pulling back slightly to keep the holder from moving, and push the tube onto the needle with your thumb. Releasing the tourniquet and opening the fist allows blood flow to normalize (see step 6). According to CLSI standards, the tourniquet should be released as soon as possible after blood begins to flow and should not be left on longer than 1 minute.

Procedure 8-2: Routine ETS Venipuncture (Continued)

Step	**Explanation/Rationale**
12. Fill, remove, and mix tubes in order of draw. 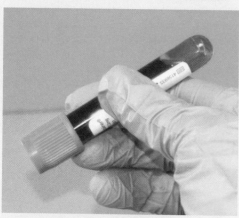	Fill additive tubes until the vacuum is exhausted to ensure correct blood-to-additive ratio and mix them immediately upon removal from the holder using three to eight gentle inversions (depending on type and manufacturer) to prevent clot formation. Follow the CLSI order of draw to prevent additive carryover between tubes.
13. Place gauze, remove needle, activate safety feature, and apply pressure. 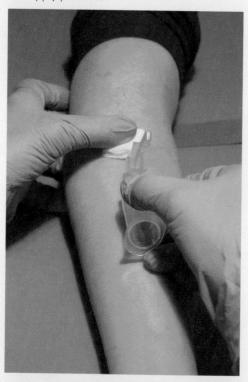 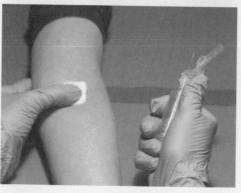 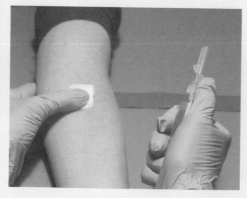	A clean, folded gauze square is placed over the site so pressure can be applied immediately after needle removal. Remove the needle in one smooth motion without lifting up or pressing down on it. Immediately apply pressure to the site with your free hand while simultaneously activating the needle safety feature with the other to prevent the chance of a needlestick.

Procedure 8-2: Routine ETS Venipuncture (Continued)

Step	Explanation/Rationale
14. Discard collection unit. 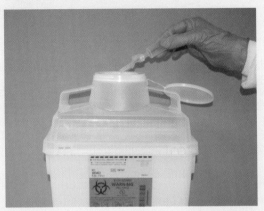	According to OSHA, the needle and the tube holder must go into the sharps container as a unit because removing a needle from the holder exposes the user to sharps injury.
15. Label tubes. 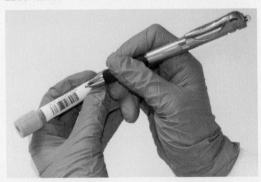	To avoid mislabeling errors, label tubes before leaving the bedside or dismissing the patient.
16. Observe special handling instructions. 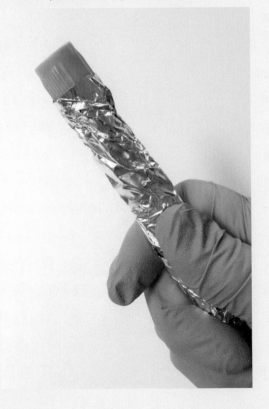	For accurate results, some specimens require special handling such as cooling in crushed ice (e.g., ammonia), transportation at body temperature (e.g., cold agglutinin), or protection from light (e.g., bilirubin).

Procedure 8-2: Routine ETS Venipuncture (Continued)

Step	Explanation/Rationale
17. Check patient's arm and apply bandage.	The patient's arm must be examined to verify that bleeding has stopped. The site must also be checked for signs of bleeding beneath the skin. If bleeding has stopped, apply a bandage and advise the patient to keep it in place for at least 15 minutes. Note: If bleeding persists beyond 5 minutes, notify the patient's nurse or physician.
18. Dispose of used and contaminated materials.	Materials such as needle caps and wrappers are normally discarded in the regular trash. Some facilities require that contaminated items such as blood-soaked gauze be discarded in biohazard containers.
19. Thank patient, remove gloves, and sanitize hands.	Thanking the patient is courteous and professional. Gloves must be removed in an aseptic manner and hands washed or decontaminated with hand sanitizer as an infection-control precaution.

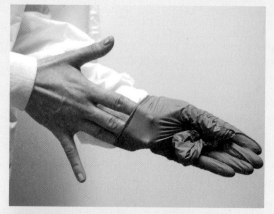

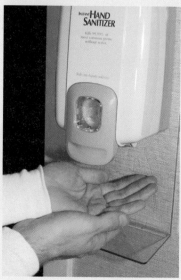

20. Transport specimen to the lab.	Prompt delivery to the lab protects specimen integrity and is typically achieved by personal delivery, transportation via a pneumatic tube system, or by a courier service.

Butterfly Procedure

A phlebotomist may elect to use a winged infusion set (butterfly) in attempting to draw blood from AC veins of infants and small children or from difficult adult veins, such as small AC veins or wrist and hand veins. A butterfly needle (i.e., 23 gauge) is appropriate in these situations because it is less likely to collapse or "blow" (rupture) the vein. A butterfly can be used with an ETS tube holder or a syringe (see "Syringe

Venipuncture Procedure"). Small-volume tubes should be chosen when a butterfly is used with an ETS holder because the vacuum of large tubes may collapse the vein or hemolyze the specimen. Venipuncture of a hand vein using a butterfly and ETS holder is illustrated in Procedure 8-3.

thePoint: *View the video of the Blood Collection from a Hand Vein Using a Butterfly and ETS Holder procedure at http://thepoint.lww.com/McCall6e.*

Procedure 8-3: Venipuncture of a Hand Vein Using a Butterfly and ETS Holder

PURPOSE: To obtain a blood specimen for patient diagnostic or monitoring purposes from a hand vein using a butterfly and ETS holder.

EQUIPMENT: Tourniquet, gloves, antiseptic prep pad, butterfly needle with safety feature, ETS tube holder and tubes, gauze pads, sharps container, permanent ink pen, bandage

Step	Explanation/Rationale
1–4. (Same as routine ETS venipuncture.)	See Procedure 8-2: steps 1–4.
5. Position hand, apply tourniquet, ask patient to close the hand.	Proper arm position is important to the comfort of the patient and the success of venipuncture. Support the hand on the bed or armrest. Have the patient bend the fingers slightly or make a fist. A tourniquet is necessary to increase venous filling and aid in vein selection. Apply it proximal to the wrist bone. A closed hand or clenched fist sometimes makes the veins easier to see and feel.
6. Select vein, release tourniquet, ask patient to relax hand.	Select a vein that has bounce or resilience and can be easily anchored. Wiping the hand with alcohol sometimes makes the veins more visible. Finding a suitable vein can take a while. Releasing the tourniquet and opening the fist allows blood flow to return to normal and minimizes effects of hemoconcentration.
7. Clean and air-dry site.	Same as routine ETS venipuncture (see Procedure 8-2: step 7).
8. Prepare equipment and put on gloves.	It is easier to select appropriate equipment after the vein has been chosen. Preparing it while the site is drying saves time. Attach the butterfly to an ETS holder. Grasp the tubing near the needle end and run your fingers down its length, stretching it slightly to help keep it from coiling back up. Position the first tube in the holder now or wait until after needle entry. According to the OSHA BBP standard, gloves must be worn during phlebotomy procedures.
9. Reapply tourniquet, uncap and inspect needle.	The tourniquet aids needle entry. Hold the wing portion of the butterfly between your thumb and index finger or fold the wings upright and grasp them together. Cradle the tubing and holder in the palm of your dominant hand or lay it next to the patient's hand. Uncap and inspect the needle for defects and discard it if flawed.

Procedure 8-3: Venipuncture of a Hand Vein Using a Butterfly and ETS Holder (Continued)

Step	Explanation/Rationale
10. Anchor vein and insert needle.	Anchoring stretches the skin so the needle enters easily and with less pain, and it keeps the vein from rolling. Insert the needle into the vein at a shallow angle of approximately 10 degrees or less. A "flash" or small amount of blood will appear in the tubing when the needle is in the vein. "Seat" the needle by slightly threading it within the lumen of the vein to keep it from twisting back out of the vein if you let go of it.

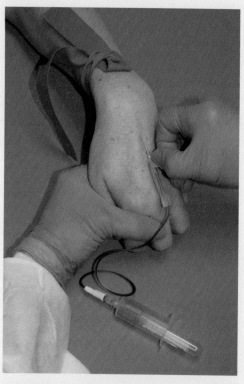

Step	Explanation/Rationale
11. Establish blood flow and release tourniquet.	The flash of blood in the tubing indicates vein entry. Blood will not flow until the needle pierces a tube stopper. Place a tube in the holder and push it part way onto the needle with a clockwise twist. Grasp the holder flanges with your middle and index fingers, pulling back slightly to keep the holder from moving, and push the tube onto the needle with your thumb. Releasing the tourniquet allows blood flow to normalize (see step 6).

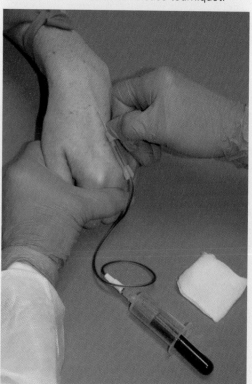

Procedure 8-3: Venipuncture of a Hand Vein Using a Butterfly and ETS Holder (Continued)

Step	Explanation/Rationale
12. Fill, remove, and mix tubes in order of draw.	Maintain tubing and holder below the site, and positioned so that the tubes fill from the bottom up to prevent reflux. Fill additive tubes until the vacuum is exhausted to ensure the correct blood-to-additive ratio and mix them immediately upon removal from the holder, using three to eight gentle inversions (depending on type and manufacturer) to prevent clot formation. Follow the CLSI order of draw to prevent additive carry-over between tubes. If a coagulation tube is the first or only tube collected, draw a discard tube first to remove air in the tubing and assure proper filling of the coagulation tube.
13. Place gauze, remove needle, activate safety device, and apply pressure.	A clean, folded gauze square is placed over the site so pressure can be applied immediately after needle removal. Remove the needle in one smooth motion without lifting it up or pressing down on it. Immediately apply pressure to the site with your free hand while simultaneously activating the needle safety device with the other to prevent the chance of a needlestick.

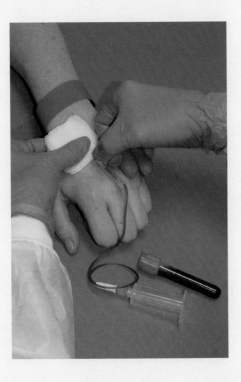

Procedure 8-3: Venipuncture of a Hand Vein Using a Butterfly and ETS Holder (Continued)

Step	Explanation/Rationale

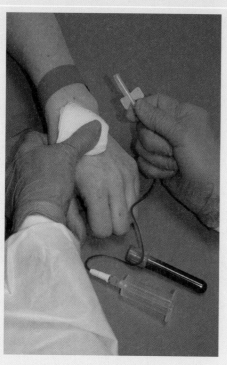

14. Discard collection unit.

According to OSHA, the needle and tube holder must go into the sharps container as a unit because removing a needle from the holder exposes the user to sharps injury.

15–20. (Same as routine ETS venipuncture.)

See Procedure 8-2: steps 15–20.

Syringe Venipuncture Procedure

The preferred method of obtaining venipuncture specimens is the evacuated tube method. In fact, according to CLSI standard GP41 blood collection with a needle and syringe should be avoided for safety reasons. Even so, a needle or butterfly and syringe are sometimes used when the patient has extremely small, fragile, or weak veins. The vacuum pressure of an evacuated tube may be too great for such veins and cause them to collapse easily. This is often the case with elderly patients and newborn infants. When a syringe is used, the amount of pressure can be reduced somewhat over that of a tube by pulling the plunger back slowly. If the syringe fills too slowly, however, there is the possibility that the specimen will begin to clot either before enough blood is collected or before it can be transferred to the appropriate tubes. A special syringe transfer device is required to safely transfer blood from the syringe into the ETS tubes. Venipuncture with a needle and syringe is illustrated in Procedure 8-4. Steps to follow when using a transfer device to fill tubes with blood from a syringe are shown in Procedure 8-5.

Procedure for Inability to Collect Specimen

If you are unable to obtain a specimen on the first try, evaluate the problem and try again below the first site, on the opposite arm, or on a hand or wrist vein. If the patient's veins are small or fragile, it may be necessary to use a butterfly or syringe on the second attempt.

thePoint *View the video of the procedure for Collecting Blood from an Antecubital Vein Using a Needle and Syringe at http://thepoint.lww.com/McCall6e.*

Procedure 8-4: Needle-and-Syringe Venipuncture

PURPOSE: To obtain a blood specimen for patient diagnostic or monitoring purposes from an antecubital vein using a needle and syringe.

EQUIPMENT: Tourniquet, gloves, antiseptic prep pad, syringe needle,* syringe,* ETS tubes, gauze pads, sharps container, permanent ink pen, bandage

*Either the needle or syringe must have a safety feature to prevent needlesticks.

Step	Rationale/Explanation
1–7. (Same as routine ETS venipuncture.)	See Procedure 8-2: steps 1–7.
8. Prepare equipment.	It is easier to select appropriate equipment after the vein has been chosen. Preparing it while the site is drying saves time. Select the syringe needle according to the size and location of the vein and select the syringe and tube size according to the volume of blood required for the tests. Attach the needle to the syringe but do not remove the cap at this time. Hold the syringe as you would an ETS tube holder. Gloves must be put on now if not already on.
9. Reapply tourniquet, uncap and inspect needle.	The tourniquet aids in venipuncture. Hold the syringe in your dominant hand as you would an ETS holder. Place your thumb on top near the needle end and fingers underneath. Uncap and inspect the needle for defects and discard it if flawed. Although it is rare, a needle can have defects.
10. Ask patient to make a fist, anchor vein, and insert needle. 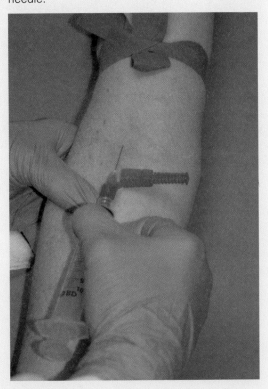	The fist aids needle entry. Anchoring stretches the skin so the needle enters easily and with less pain and keeps the vein from rolling. Anchor by grasping the arm just below the elbow, supporting the back of it with your fingers. Place your thumb 1–2 inches below and slightly beside the vein and pull the skin toward the wrist. Warn the patient. Line the needle up with the vein and insert it into the skin using a smooth forward motion. Stop when you feel a decrease in resistance, often described as a "pop," and press your fingers into the arm to anchor the holder.

Procedure 8-4: Needle-and-Syringe Venipuncture (Continued)

Step	Rationale/Explanation
11. Establish blood flow, release tourniquet, ask patient to open fist.	Establishment of blood flow is normally indicated by blood in the hub of the syringe. In some cases blood will not flow until the syringe plunger is pulled back.
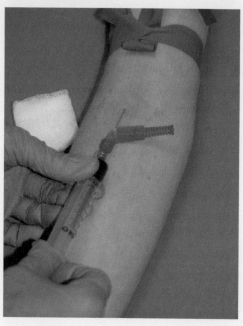	Releasing the tourniquet and opening the fist allows blood flow to return to normal and helps prevent hemo-concentration.
	According to CLSI Standard H3-A5, the tourniquet should be released as soon as possible after blood begins to flow and should not be left on longer than 1 minute.
12. Fill syringe.	Venous blood will not automatically flow into a syringe. It must be filled by slowly pulling back on the plunger with your free hand. Steady the syringe as you would an ETS holder during routine venipuncture.
13. Place gauze, withdraw needle, activate safety device, apply pressure.	A clean, folded gauze square is placed over the site so pressure can be applied immediately after needle removal.
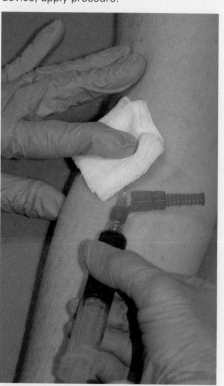	Remove the needle without lifting it up or pressing down on it. Immediately apply pressure to the site with your free hand and simultaneously activate the needle safety device with the other.

Procedure 8-4: Needle-and-Syringe Venipuncture (Continued)

Step	Rationale/Explanation

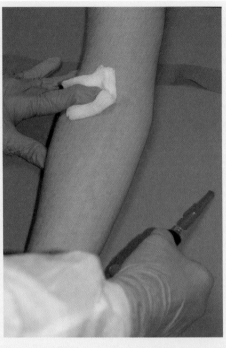

14. Discard needle, fill tubes, discard syringe and transfer device.

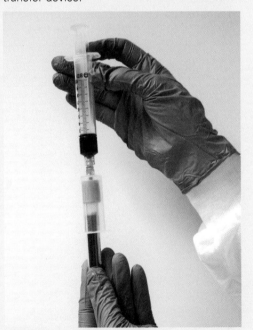

The needle must be removed and discarded in the sharps container so that a transfer device for filling the tubes can be attached to the syringe. A transfer device greatly reduces the chance of accidental needlesticks and confines any aerosol or spraying that may be generated as the tube is removed. An ETS tube is placed in the transfer device in the order of draw and pushed onto the internal needle until the stopper is pierced. Blood from the syringe is then safely drawn into the tube. Several tubes can be filled as long as there is enough blood in the syringe. After use, the syringe and transfer device unit is discarded in the sharps container.

15–20. (Same as routine ETS venipuncture.)

See Procedure 8-2, steps 15–20.

thePoint₊ *View the video Transferring Blood from a Syringe into ETS Tubes at http://thepoint.lww.com/McCall6e.*

Procedure 8-5: Using a Syringe Transfer Device

PURPOSE: To safely transfer blood from a syringe into ETS tubes.

EQUIPMENT: Syringe transfer device

Step	Explanation/Rationale
1. Remove the needle from the syringe and discard it in a sharps container.	The needle must be removed to attach the transfer device.
2. Attach the syringe hub to the transfer device hub, rotating it to ensure secure attachment.	Secure attachment is necessary to prevent blood leakage during transfer.

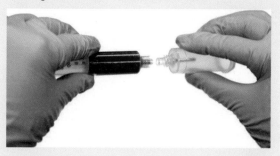

Step	Explanation/Rationale
3. Hold the syringe vertically with the tip down and the transfer device at the bottom.	This ensures vertical placement of tubes to prevent additive carryover.
4. Place an ETS tube in the barrel of the transfer device and push it all the way to the end.	The device has an internal needle that will puncture the stopper and allow blood to flow into the tube.

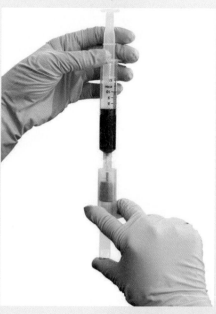

Step	Explanation/Rationale
5. Follow the order of draw if multiple tubes are to be filled.	The order of draw is designed to prevent additive carryover between tubes.
6. Keep the tubes and transfer device vertical.	This ensures that tubes fill from bottom to top, preventing additive contact with the needle and cross-contamination of subsequent tubes.

Procedure 8-5: Using a Syringe Transfer Device (Continued)

Step	Explanation/Rationale
7. Let tubes fill using the vacuum draw of the tube. Do not push on the syringe plunger.	Forcing blood into a tube by pushing the plunger can hemolyze the specimen or cause the tube stopper to pop off, splashing tube contents.

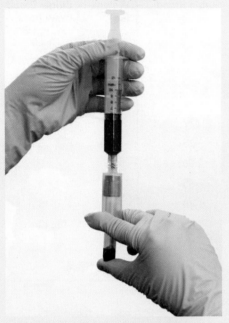

Step	Explanation/Rationale
8. If you must underfill a tube, hold back the plunger to stop blood flow before removing it.	Tubes quickly fill until the vacuum is gone. Holding back the plunger stops the tube from filling.
9. Mix additive tubes as soon as they are removed.	Additive tubes must be mixed immediately for proper function, including preventing clot formation in anticoagulant tubes.
10. When finished, discard the syringe and transfer device unit in a sharps container.	Removing the transfer device from the syringe would expose the user to blood in the hubs of both units. The transfer device must go into the sharps container because of its internal needle.

If the second attempt is unsuccessful, ask another phlebotomist to take over. Unsuccessful venipuncture attempts are frustrating to the patient and the phlebotomist. Should the second phlebotomist be unsuccessful after two attempts, it is a good idea to give the patient a rest if the request is not stat or timed and try again at a later time.

> ⚠️ **CAUTION** According to CLSI, arterial puncture should not be used as an alternative to venipuncture on difficult veins. If it appears to be the only choice, the patient's physician should be consulted first.

There are times when a phlebotomist is not able to collect a specimen from a patient even before attempting venipuncture. Occasionally, a patient will refuse to have blood drawn. Other times, the patient may be unavailable because he or she has gone to surgery or for another test, as in radiology. Whatever the reason, if the specimen cannot be obtained, notify the patient's nurse or physician. You may be required to fill out a form stating that the specimen was not obtained and the reason why. The original form is placed in the patient's chart and the laboratory retains a copy. The following are the most common and generally accepted reasons for inability to obtain a specimen:

- Phlebotomist attempted but was unable to draw blood.
- Patient refused to have blood drawn.
- Patient was unavailable.

Pediatric Venipuncture

Collecting blood by venipuncture from infants and children may be necessary for tests that require large amounts of blood (i.e., cross-matching and blood cultures) and tests that cannot normally be performed by skin puncture (i.e., ammonia levels and most coagulation studies). Venipuncture in children under the age of 2 should be limited to superficial veins and not deep, hard-to-find veins. Normally, the most accessible veins of infants and toddlers are the veins of the AC fossa and forearm. Other potential venipuncture sites include the medial back side of the wrist, the dorsum of the foot, the scalp, and the medial ankle. Venipuncture of these alternate sites, however, requires special training and the permission of the patient's physician.

CHALLENGES

Capillary collection is normally recommended for pediatric patients, especially newborns and infants up to 12 months, because their veins are small and not well developed and there is a considerable risk of permanent damage. There are, however, times when capillary collection is not feasible or possible owing to type or volume requirements of tests ordered; in such instances a venipuncture is necessary. Performing venipuncture on pediatric patients presents special challenges and requires the expertise and skill of an experienced phlebotomist. In addition, every attempt should be made to collect the minimum amount of blood required for testing, because infants and young children have much smaller blood volumes than older children and adults. Removal of large quantities of blood at once or even small quantities on a regular basis, as is often the case when an infant or child is in intensive care, can lead to anemia. Removing more than 10% of an infant's blood volume at one time can lead to shock and cardiac arrest. Consequently, most facilities have limits on the amount of blood that can be removed per draw and for various time periods from 24 hours up to a month. For example, many facilities do not allow more than 3% of a child's blood volume to be collected at any one time and allow no more than 10% in an entire month. See Table 8-2 for recommended blood draw volumes for pediatric patients.

> (i) The CLSI recommends that procedures be in place to monitor amounts of blood drawn from pediatric, geriatric, and other vulnerable patients to avoid phlebotomy-induced anemia.

No one would intentionally put a patient's life at risk by drawing too much blood. However, a phlebotomist who fails to keep track of amounts of blood collected or who is unable to judge how much blood can be collected safely could do just that. Consequently, for safe practice, a competent phlebotomist should be able to calculate blood volume. The formula for calculating blood volume is shown in Appendix B.

Table 8.2: Recommended Blood Draw Volumes for Pediatric Patients

Weight (kg)	Maximum Volume for a Single Blood Draw (mL)	Weight (kg)	Maximum Volume for a Single Blood Draw (mL)
2	4	30	60
4	8	32.5	65
6	12	35	70
8	16	37.5	75
10	20	40	80
12.5	25	42.5	85
15	30	45	90
17.5	35	47.5	95
20	40	50	100
22.5	45	52.5	105
25	50	55	110
27.5	55		

Courtesy of Dr. David Friedman, Children's Hospital of Philadelphia, Philadelphia, PA.
Reprinted with permission from Bishop ML, Fody EP, Schoeff LE. *Clinical Chemistry, Principles, Techniques, and Correlations.* 7th ed. Philadelphia, PA: Lippincott Williams & Wilkins; 2013:722.

DEALING WITH PARENTS OR GUARDIANS

Parents or guardians may give the best prediction of how cooperative the child will be. Anxiety on the part of a parent can negatively influence the child's coping mechanisms. If parents or guardians are present, it is important for the phlebotomist to earn their trust before attempting venipuncture. A phlebotomist who behaves in a warm and friendly manner and displays a calm, confident, and caring attitude will more easily earn that trust and limit his or her own anxiety as well. Ask the parent or guardian about the child's past experiences with blood collection so as to gain insight into how the child may behave and approaches that might work. Give them the option of staying in the room during the procedure or waiting outside until you are finished. Their presence and involvement should be encouraged, however, as studies show that this reduces a child's anxiety and has a positive effect on the child's behavior.

DEALING WITH THE CHILD

Venipuncture in children that results in a traumatic experience can have lasting negative consequences, including increased sensitivity to pain, a decreased capacity to cope with it, and a lifelong fear of needles. The best strategy to reduce the child's anxiety should be employed.

With older children, it is as important as with adults to gain their trust. However, children typically have a wider zone of comfort, which means that you cannot get as close to them as you can to an adult without making them feel threatened. Approach them slowly and determine their degree of anxiety or fear before handling equipment or touching their arms to look for a vein. An adult towering over a child is intimidating. Physically lower yourself to the patient's level. Explain what you are going to do in terms that the child can understand and answer questions honestly.

> **Key Point** *Never* tell a child that it won't hurt. Instead, say that it may hurt just a little bit, but it will be over quickly.

Help the child to understand the importance of remaining still. Give the child a job to do such as holding the gauze or adhesive bandage. Studies have demonstrated that age-appropriate distractions such as videos, movies, games, counting and singing can minimize the stress and anxiety of potentially painful procedures such as venipuncture. Offer the child a reward for being brave. However, *do not* put conditions on receiving the reward, such as "you can have a sticker if you don't cry." Some crying is to be anticipated, and it is important to let the child know that it is all right to cry.

> **Key Point** Calm a crying child as soon as possible, because the stress of crying and struggling can alter blood components and lead to erroneous test results.

PAIN INTERVENTIONS

Interventions to minimize pain transmission or ease the pain of venipuncture include the use of cold or vibration, **EMLA**, a **eutectic** (easily melted) **mixture of local anesthetics** for newborns through adults, and oral sucrose and pacifiers for infants and toddlers.

EMLA is a topical anesthetic–containing lidocaine and prilocaine. It is available in a cream that must be covered with a clear dressing or a patch after application. It takes approximately 1 hour (a major drawback to its use) for it to anesthetize the area to a depth of approximately 5 mm. It cannot be used on patients who are allergic to local anesthetics. It can only be applied to intact skin, and must be applied by a licensed healthcare practitioner following strict dosage, amount of area covered, and application times based on the child's age and weight to prevent toxicity from absorption through the skin. It cannot be used on patients who are allergic

to local anesthetics, infants with a gestational age of less than 37 weeks, or infants under 12 months of age who are receiving treatment with methemoglobin-inducing agents.

Use of a 12% to 24% solution of oral sucrose has been shown to reduce the pain of procedures such as heel puncture and venipuncture in infants up to 6 months of age. A 24% solution of sucrose (prepared by mixing 4 teaspoons of water with 1 teaspoon of sugar) can be administered by dropper, nipple, oral syringe, or on a pacifier provided that it will not interfere with the tests to be collected or diet restrictions. Sucrose nipples or pacifiers are available commercially. The sucrose must be given to the infant 2 minutes before the procedure, and its pain-relieving benefits last for approximately 5 minutes. Studies have shown that infants given sucrose or even a regular pacifier by itself cry for a shorter time and are more alert and less fussy after the procedure.

SELECTING A METHOD OF RESTRAINT

Immobilization of the patient is a critical aspect in obtaining an adequate specimen from infants and children while ensuring their safety. A newborn or young infant can be wrapped in a blanket, but physical restraint is often required for older infants, toddlers, and younger children. Older children may be able to sit by themselves in the blood-drawing chair, but a parent or another phlebotomist should help steady the child's arm.

Toddlers are most easily restrained by having them sit upright on a parent's lap (Fig. 8-17). The arm to be used for venipuncture is extended to the front and downward. The parent places an arm around the toddler and over the arm that is not being used. The other arm supports the venipuncture arm from behind, at the bend of the elbow. This helps steady the child's arm and prevents the child from twisting the arm during the draw. It is also helpful if the parent's legs are wrapped around the toddler's legs to prevent kicking.

If the child is lying down, the parent or another phlebotomist typically leans over the child from the opposite side of the bed. One arm reaches around and holds the venipuncture arm from behind, the other reaches across the child's body, holding the child's other arm secure against his or her torso.

EQUIPMENT SELECTION

Venipuncture of an AC vein is most easily accomplished using a 23-gauge butterfly needle attached to an evacuated tube holder or syringe. The tubing of the butterfly allows flexibility if the child struggles or twists during the draw. Use of an evacuated-tube holder and butterfly needle is preferred because it minimizes chances of producing clotted specimens and inadequately filled tubes. However, the smallest tubes available should be used

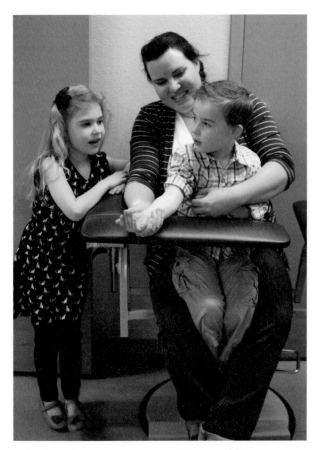

Figure 8-17 A seated adult restraining a toddler.

to reduce the risk of creating too much vacuum draw on the vein and causing it to collapse. In difficult-draw situations, a small amount of blood can be drawn into a syringe and the blood placed in microcollection tubes (microtubes or "bullets") rather than ETS tubes.

⚠ **CAUTION** Laboratory personnel will assume that blood in microtubes is capillary blood. If venous blood is placed in a microtube, it is important to label the specimen as venous blood because reference ranges for some tests differ depending on the source of the specimen.

PROCEDURES

Regardless of the collection method, every attempt should be made to collect the minimum amount of blood required for testing because of the small blood volume of the patient. In addition to reducing the risk of iatrogenic anemia, minimizing the volume of blood drawn shortens the duration of the draw and the time the patient is under stress. Follow strict identification requirements and venipuncture procedures outlined earlier in the chapter. You may be required to wear a mask, gown, and gloves in the newborn nursery or neonatal ICU.

Geriatric Venipuncture

Geriatric means relating to old age. According to the National Institute on Aging (NIA), life expectancy has doubled over the last century, and there are now over 35 million Americans of age 65 or older. This segment of the population is expected to grow by 137% over the next 50 years and to become the major focus of health care. Already a major portion of laboratory testing is performed on the elderly. (See Table 8-3 for a list of tests commonly ordered on geriatric patients.)

📖 **Matching 8-3 in the WORKBOOK tests knowledge of geriatric tests and indications for ordering them.**

Although aging is a normal process, it involves physical, psychological, and social changes leading to conditions, behaviors, and habits that may seem unusual to those unaccustomed to working with elderly patients. To feel comfortable working with them one must understand the aging process and be familiar with the physical limitations, diseases, and illnesses associated with it. It is also important to remember that elderly patients are unique individuals with special needs who deserve as with all patients, to be treated with compassion, kindness, patience, and respect.

CHALLENGES

Physical effects of aging, such as skin changes, hearing and vision problems, mobility issues—often related to arthritis and osteoporosis, diseases such as diabetes, and mental and emotional conditions often present challenges not only to the patient but to a phlebotomist's technical expertise and interpersonal skills as well.

Skin Changes

Skin changes include loss of collagen and subcutaneous fat, resulting in wrinkled, sagging, thin skin with a decreased ability to stay adequately hydrated. Lack of hydration along with impaired peripheral circulation caused by age-related narrowing of blood vessels makes it harder to obtain adequate blood flow, especially during skin puncture. In addition, aging skin cells are replaced more slowly, causing the skin to lose elasticity and increasing the likelihood of injury. Blood vessels also lose elasticity, becoming more fragile and more likely to collapse, resulting in an increased chance of bruising and the failure to obtain blood.

🔑 **Key Point** Skin changes make veins in the elderly easier to see; however, sagging skin combined with loss of muscle tone may make it harder to anchor veins and keep them from rolling.

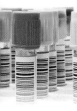

Table 8-3: Tests Commonly Ordered on Geriatric Patients

Test	Typical Indications for Ordering
ANA, RA, or RF	Diagnose lupus and rheumatoid arthritis, which can affect nervous system function
CBC	Determine hemoglobin levels, detect infection, and identify blood disorders
BUN/creatinine	Diagnose kidney function disorders that may be responsible for problems such as confusion, coma, seizures, and tremors
Calcium/magnesium	Identify abnormal levels associated with seizures and muscle problems
Electrolytes	Determine sodium and potassium levels, critical to proper nervous system function
ESR	Detect inflammation; identify collagen vascular (i.e., connective tissue) diseases
Glucose	Detect and monitor diabetes; abnormal levels can cause confusion, seizures, or coma or lead to peripheral neuropathy
PT/PTT	Monitor blood-thinning medications; important in heart conditions, coagulation problems, and stroke management
SPEP, IPEP	Identify protein or immune globulin disorders that lead to nerve damage
VDRL/FTA	Diagnose or rule out syphilis, which can cause nerve damage and dementia

Hearing Impairment

Effects of aging include loss of auditory hair cells, resulting in a hearing loss in upper frequencies and trouble distinguishing sounds such as ch, s, sh, and z. Hearing-impaired patients may strain to hear and have difficulty answering questions and understanding instructions. If you know or have reason to suspect that a patient has a hearing impairment, move closer and face the patient when you speak. Speak clearly and distinctly, but use your normal tone of voice. Never shout; shouting raises the pitch of your voice and makes it harder to understand. Allow the patient enough time to answer questions, and confirm patient responses to avoid misunderstanding. Repeat information if necessary. Watch for nonverbal verification that the patient understands. Be mindful of nonverbal messages you may be sending inadvertently. Use pencil and paper to communicate if necessary. A relative or attendant often accompanies a patient with a hearing impairment or other communication problem. If this person is included in the conversation, do not speak to him or her directly as if the patient were not present.

Key Point Although hearing loss is common in the elderly, never assume that an elderly person is hard of hearing.

Visual Impairment

Effects of aging on the eyes include a diminished ability of the lens to adjust, causing farsightedness; clouding of the lens or cataract formation resulting in dim vision; and other changes that lead to light intolerance and poor night vision. The phlebotomy area should have adequate lighting without glare. Be aware that you may need to guide elderly patients to the drawing chair or escort them to the restroom if a urine specimen is requested. Provide written instructions in large print, avoid using gestures when speaking, and use a normal tone of voice.

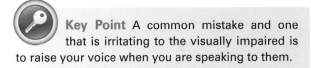

Key Point A common mistake and one that is irritating to the visually impaired is to raise your voice when you are speaking to them.

Mental Impairment

Slower nerve conduction associated with aging leads to slower learning, slower reaction times, and a diminished perception of pain, which, in turn, can lead to an increase in injuries. Reduced cerebral circulation can lead to loss of balance and frequent falls. The effects of some medications can make problems worse. Speak clearly and slowly and give the patient plenty of time to respond. You may need to repeat your statement or question more than once. Be especially careful in obtaining patient identification information and verifying compliance with diet instructions. If a relative or attendant is with the patient, verify information with him or her.

Alzheimer disease and other forms of dementia can render a patient unable to communicate meaningfully, requiring you to communicate through a relative or other caregiver. Some Alzheimer patients will act absolutely normal and others will exhibit anger and hostility, which should not be taken personally. Always approach patients in a calm, professional manner. Use short, simple statements and explain things slowly. You may require assistance to keep the patient's arm in place during the draw.

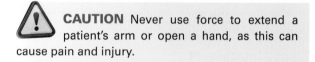

Key Point Although mental confusion and dementia are common in elderly patients, always assume that an elderly person is of sound mind unless you have information to the contrary.

Effects of Disease

Although most elderly persons are generally healthy, many are not. Some of the diseases that affect the elderly and the challenges they present to the patient and the phlebotomist include the following:

Arthritis

The two basic types of arthritis are osteoarthritis and rheumatoid arthritis. Osteoarthritis occurs with aging and also results from joint injury. The hips and knees are most commonly affected; this can cause difficulty getting in and out of a blood-drawing chair. Rheumatoid arthritis affects connective tissue throughout the body and can occur at any age. It primarily affects the joints, but connective tissue in the heart, lungs, eyes, kidneys, and skin may also be affected. Inflammation associated with both types of arthritis may leave joints swollen and painful and cause the patient to restrict movement. It may result in the patient being unable or unwilling to straighten an arm or open a hand. Use the other arm if it is unaffected. If that is not an option, let the patient decide what position is comfortable. A butterfly needle with 12-inch tubing helps provide the flexibility needed to access veins from awkward angles.

CAUTION Never use force to extend a patient's arm or open a hand, as this can cause pain and injury.

Coagulation Problems

Patients who have coagulation disorders or who take blood-thinning medications as a result of heart problems or strokes are at risk of hematoma formation or uncontrolled bleeding at the blood-collection site. Make certain that adequate pressure is held over the site until bleeding is stopped. You must hold pressure if the patient is unable to do so. However, do not hold pressure so tightly that the patient is injured or bruised, and do not apply a pressure bandage in lieu of holding pressure. If bleeding persists, notify the patient's physician or follow your facility's policy.

Diabetes

Many elderly patients have diabetes. Diabetes affects circulation and healing, particularly in the lower extremities, and generally makes venipuncture of leg, ankle, and foot veins off limits. Peripheral circulation problems and scarring from numerous skin punctures to check glucose can make skin puncture collections difficult. Warming the site before blood collection can help encourage blood flow.

Parkinson Disease and Stroke

Stroke and Parkinson disease can affect speech. The frustration this can cause to both the patient and the phlebotomist can present a barrier to effective communication. Allow these patients time to speak and do not try to finish their sentences. Keep in mind that difficulty in speaking does not imply problems in comprehension. Tremors and movement of the hands of Parkinson patients can make blood collection difficult; such patients may require help to hold still.

Pulmonary Function Problems

The effects of colds and influenza are more severe in the elderly. Age-related changes in pulmonary function reduce the elasticity of airway tissues and decrease the effectiveness of respiratory defense systems. Weakened chest muscles reduce the ability to clear secretions and increase the chance of developing pneumonia. If you have a cold, refrain from drawing blood from elderly patients if possible or wear a mask.

Other Problems

Disease and loss of immune function in the elderly increase the chance of infection. Lack of appetite due to disease or a decreased sense of smell and taste can result in emaciation. Poor nutrition can intensify the effects of aging on the skin, affect clotting ability, and contribute to anemia.

SAFETY ISSUES

Although all patients require an unencumbered traffic pattern, geriatric patients may need wider open areas to accommodate wheelchairs and walkers. Some patients tend to shuffle when they walk, so floors should have nonslip surfaces and be free of clutter. Dispose of equipment packaging properly and look out for items inadvertently dropped on the floor. Floor mats should stay snug against the floor so that they do not become a tripping hazard for any patient or employee as well.

PATIENTS IN WHEELCHAIRS

Many geriatric patients are wheelchair-bound or are so weak that they are transported to the laboratory in wheelchairs. Be careful in moving wheelchair patients (Fig. 8-18) from the waiting room to the blood-drawing room. Remember to lock wheels when drawing blood from patients in wheelchairs, assisting them to and from the drawing chair, or after returning them to waiting areas. Never attempt to lift patients to transfer them from a wheelchair to a drawing chair. Attempting to do so can result in injury to the patient, the phlebotomist, or both.

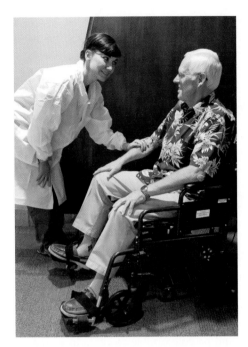

Figure 8-18 An elderly patient in a wheelchair.

Key Point It is generally safest and easiest to draw blood with the patient in the wheelchair, supporting the arm on a pillow or on a special padded board placed across the arms of the chair.

BLOOD-COLLECTION PROCEDURES

Although the venipuncture steps are basically the same for all patients, extra care must be taken in the following areas when drawing from elderly patients.

Patient Identification

Be extra careful in identifying patients with mental or hearing impairments. Never rely on nods of agreement or other nonverbal responses. Verify patient information with a relative or attendant if possible.

Equipment Selection

It is often best to use butterfly needles and pediatric or short-draw tubes for venipuncture on the elderly. Although the veins may appear prominent, they are apt to roll or collapse easily, making blood collection difficult. It is best to select equipment after you have selected the venipuncture site so that you can choose the best equipment for the size, condition, and location of the vein. If the veins are extremely fragile, you may have to collect the specimen by syringe or finger puncture.

Tourniquet Application

Apply the tourniquet snugly but loose enough to avoid damaging the patient's skin. A tourniquet that is too tight can cause the vein to collapse when it is released

or the tube is engaged. It can also distend the vein so much that it "blows" or splits open on needle entry, resulting in hematoma formation. It is acceptable to apply the tourniquet over the patient's sleeve or a clean dry washcloth wrapped around the arm.

Key Point Geriatric patients in their 90s and 100s are seen more often lately, and their veins are very sensitive to tourniquet pressure.

Site Selection

Elderly patients, especially inpatients, often have bruising in the AC area from previous blood draws. Venipuncture in a bruised site should be avoided, as it can be painful to the patient and the hemostatic process occurring in the area can lead to erroneous test results. If both AC areas are bruised, select a needle entry point below the bruising. Be aware that some elderly patients may not be able to make a fist because of muscle weakness.

If no suitable vein can be found, gently massage the arm from wrist to elbow to force blood into the area or wrap a warm, wet towel around the arm or hand for a few minutes to increase blood flow. Avoid heavy manipulation of the arm, as this can cause bruising and affect test results. Have the patient hold the arm down at his or her side for a few minutes to let gravity help back up blood flow. When a suitable vein has been selected, release the tourniquet to allow blood flow to return to normal while you clean the site and ready your equipment.

Cleaning the Site

Clean the site in the same manner as in routine venipuncture, being careful not to rub too vigorously, as that may abrade or otherwise damage the skin. The site may have to be cleaned a second time on some elderly patients who are unable to bathe regularly.

Performing the Venipuncture

Although actually quite fragile, an elderly patient's veins often feel tough and have a tendency to roll. Anchoring them firmly and entering quickly increases the chance of successful venipuncture. If the skin is loose and the vein poorly fixed in the tissue, it sometimes helps to wrap your hand around the arm from behind and pull the skin taut from both sides rather than anchoring with your thumb. Because veins in the elderly tend to be close to the surface of the skin, a shallow angle of needle insertion may be required.

Holding Pressure

As discussed earlier under "Coagulation Problems," it may take longer for bleeding in elderly patients to stop, especially if they are on anticoagulant therapy. Bleeding must have stopped before the bandage is applied. If bleeding is excessively prolonged, the patient's nurse or physician must be notified and laboratory facility procedures followed.

Dialysis Patients

Dialysis is a procedure in which patients whose kidneys do not function adequately have their blood artificially filtered to remove waste products. The most common reason for dialysis is end-stage renal disease (ESRD), a serious condition in which the kidneys have so deteriorated that they fail to function. The most common cause of ESRD is diabetes. The second most common cause is high blood pressure. Patients with ESRD require ongoing dialysis treatments or a kidney transplant.

In one type of dialysis, called hemodialysis, the patient's blood is filtered through a special machine often referred to as an artificial kidney. Access for hemodialysis is commonly provided by permanently fusing an artery and vein in the forearm, creating an arteriovenous (AV) shunt or fistula (see Chapter 9). During dialysis a special needle and tubing set is inserted into the fistula to provide blood flow to the dialysis machine. A typical AV fistula appears as a large bulging vein in the forearm above the wrist and causes a buzzing sensation called a "thrill" when palpated. The fistula arm must not be used to take blood pressures or perform venipuncture.

> **Key Point** A phlebotomist must be able to recognize a fistula to avoid damaging it, as it is the dialysis patient's lifeline.

Long-Term Care Patients

Long-term care includes a variety of healthcare and social services required by certain patients with functional disabilities who cannot care for themselves but do not require hospitalization. Although long-term care serves the needs of patients of all ages, primary recipients are the elderly. Long-term care is delivered in adult daycare facilities, nursing homes, assisted living facilities, rehabilitation facilities (Fig. 8-19), and even private homes.

Home Care Patients

Care for the sick at home plays an important role in today's healthcare delivery system. Many individuals who in the past would have been confined to a healthcare institution are now able to remain at home, where numerous studies show they are happier and get better sooner or survive longer. Home care services are provided through numerous agencies and include professional nursing; home health aid; physical, occupational, and respiratory therapy; and laboratory services. Laboratory services are often provided by mobile phlebotomists who go to

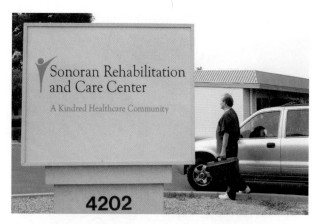

Figure 8-19 A phlebotomist making a visit to a rehabilitation center.

the patient's home to collect specimens and then deliver them to the laboratory for testing. A home care phlebotomist must have exceptional phlebotomy, interpersonal, and organizational skills; be able to function independently; and be comfortable working in varied situations and under unusual circumstances. Mobile phlebotomists must carry with them all necessary phlebotomy supplies including sharps containers and biohazard bags for disposal of contaminated items and containers for properly protecting specimens during transportation, typically in their own vehicles (Fig. 8-20).

Hospice Patients

Hospice is a type of care for patients who are terminally ill. Hospice care allows them to spend their last days in a peaceful, supportive atmosphere that emphasizes pain management to help keep them comfortable. Some individuals are uncomfortable with the subject of death or being around patients who are dying and react with indifference out of ignorance. Phlebotomists who deal with hospice patients must understand the situation and be able to approach them with care, kindness, and respect.

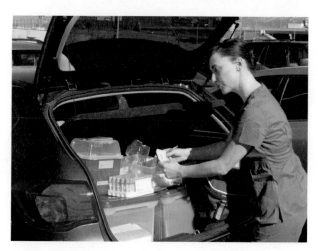

Figure 8-20 A traveling phlebotomist getting supplies from the back of her vehicle.

Study and Review Questions

See the *EXAM REVIEW* for more study questions.

1. **NPO means:**
   a. new patient orders.
   b. needed postoperative.
   c. nothing by mouth.
   d. nutrition postoperative.

2. **Which of the following is required requisition information?**
   a. Ordering physician's name
   b. Patient's first and last names
   c. Type of test to be performed
   d. All of the above

3. **The following test orders for different patients have been received at the same time. Which test would you collect first?**
   a. Fasting glucose
   b. STAT glucose in the ER
   c. STAT hemoglobin in ICU
   d. ASAP CBC in ICU

4. **A member of the clergy is with the patient when you arrive to collect a routine specimen. What should you do?**
   a. Ask the patient's nurse what you should do.
   b. Come back after the clergy person has gone.
   c. Fill out a form saying you were unable to collect the specimen.
   d. Say "Excuse me, I need to collect a specimen from this patient."

5. **You are asked to collect a blood specimen from an inpatient. The patient is not wearing an ID band. What is the best thing to do?**
   a. Ask the patient's name and collect the specimen if it matches the requisition.
   b. Ask the patient's nurse to put an ID band on the patient before you draw the specimen.
   c. Identify the patient by the name card on the door.
   d. Refuse to draw the specimen and cancel the request.

6. **If a patient adamantly refuses to have blood drawn, you should**
   a. convince the patient to be cooperative.
   b. notify the patient's nurse or physician.
   c. restrain the patient and draw the blood.
   d. write a note to the patient's physician.

7. **An inpatient is eating breakfast when you arrive to collect a fasting glucose. What is the best thing to do?**
   a. Consult with the patient's nurse to see if the specimen should be collected.
   b. Draw the specimen quickly before the patient finishes eating.
   c. Draw the specimen and write "nonfasting" on the requisition.
   d. Fill out a form stating the patient had eaten so the specimen was not drawn.

8. **After cleaning the venipuncture site with alcohol, the phlebotomist should**
   a. allow the alcohol to dry completely.
   b. fan the site to help the alcohol dry.
   c. dry the site with a clean gauze pad or cotton ball.
   d. insert the needle quickly before the alcohol dries.

9. **The tourniquet should be released**
   a. as soon as blood flow is established.
   b. before needle removal from the arm.
   c. within 1 minute of its application.
   d. all of the above.

10. **What is the recommended angle of needle insertion when performing venipuncture on an arm vein and on a hand vein, respectively?**
    a. 20 degrees or less, 20 degrees or less.
    b. 25 degrees or less, 15 degrees or less
    c. 30 degrees or less, 10 degrees or less
    d. 45 degrees or less, 20 degrees or less.

11. **After inserting a butterfly needle, the phlebotomist must "seat" it, meaning:**
    a. have the patient make a fist to keep it in place.
    b. keep the skin taut during the entire procedure.
    c. push the bevel against the back wall of the vein.
    d. slightly thread it within the lumen of the vein.

12. **Blood collection tubes are labeled**
    a. as soon as the test order is received.
    b. before the specimen is even collected.
    c. immediately after specimen collection.
    d. whenever it is the most convenient.

13. **What is the best approach to use on an 8-year-old child who needs to have blood drawn?**

    a. Explain the draw in simple terms and ask for the child's cooperation.

    b. Have someone restrain the child and collect the specimen.

    c. Offer the child a treat or a toy if he or she does not cry.

    d. Tell the child it won't hurt and will only take a few seconds.

14. **Which type of patient is most likely to have an arteriovenous fistula or graft?**

    a. Arthritic

    b. Dialysis

    c. Hospice

    d. Wheelchair-bound

15. **Which of the following is proper procedure when dealing with an elderly patient?**

    a. Address your questions to an attendant if the patient has a hearing problem.

    b. Make certain to hold adequate pressure after the draw until bleeding stops.

    c. Speak extra loud in order to be certain that the patient can hear you.

    d. Tie the tourniquet extra tight to make the veins more prominent.

16. **Where is the tourniquet applied when drawing a hand vein?**

    a. A tourniquet is not required.

    b. Above the antecubital fossa.

    c. Just distal to the wrist bone.

    d. Proximal to the wrist bone.

17. **Specimen hemolysis can result from**

    a. filling tubes with a transfer device at an angle.

    b. leaving the tourniquet on until the last tube.

    c. mixing anticoagulant tubes several extra times.

    d. using a large-volume tube with a 23-gauge needle.

18. **Which of the following is the *least* effective way to immobilize a pediatric patient before a blood draw?**

    a. Allowing the child to sit with one arm bracing the other.

    b. Cradling the child close to the chest of the immobilizer.

    c. Grasping the child's wrist firmly in a palm-up position.

    d. Using two people: an immobilizer and a blood drawer.

19. **Criteria used to decide which needle gauge to use for venipuncture include**

    a. how deep the selected vein is.

    b. the size and condition of the vein.

    c. the type of test being collected.

    d. your personal preference.

20. **Which of the following is proper procedure when dealing with an elderly adult patient?**

    a. Address all questions to a relative or attendant if the patient is hard of hearing.

    b. Apply a pressure bandage in case the patient does not hold adequate pressure.

    c. Raise the pitch of your voice sharply to make certain you are heard properly.

    d. Refrain from drawing older adult patients if you have a cold, or else wear a mask.

Case Studies

 See the WORKBOOK for more case studies.

Case Study 8-1: Patient Identification

Jenny works with several other phlebotomists in a busy outpatient lab. This day has been particularly hectic, with many patients filling the waiting room. Jenny is working as fast as she can. Toward the end of the day, after Jenny has finished drawing blood from what seems like the millionth patient, she mentions to a coworker how extra busy it has been. The coworker says, "Yes it has, but it looks like there is only one patient left." Jenny grabs the paperwork and heads for the door of the waiting room. As her coworker has said, there is only one patient, an elderly woman, sitting there reading a book. The paperwork is for a patient named Jane Rogers. "You must be Jane," she says, glancing at the name on the paperwork. The patient looks up and smiles. "Have you been waiting long?" Jenny asks. The patient replies, "Not really," and Jenny escorts her to a drawing chair. The patient is a difficult draw, and Jenny makes two attempts to collect the specimen. The second one is successful. Jenny places the labels on the tubes, dates and initials them, bandages the patient, and sends her on her way. About 5 minutes later a somewhat younger woman appears at the reception window and says, "My name is Jane Rogers. I just stepped outside to make a phone call and was wondering if you called my name while I was gone." The receptionist notices that the patient's name is checked off the registration log. The receptionist turns around and asks if anyone had called a patient named Jane Rogers. "I already drew her," Jenny says as she walks over to the receptionist window. The woman at the window is not the one Jenny just drew; however, her information matches information on the requisition used to draw that patient.

QUESTIONS

1. What error did Jenny make in identifying the patient?

2. What assumptions did Jenny make that contributed to her drawing blood from the wrong patient?

3. Who might the other patient from whom Jenny mistakenly drew blood have been?

4. How can the error be corrected?

Case Study 8-2: Blood Draw Refusal

Two phlebotomists went to a pediatric ward to collect a blood specimen from a young boy they had drawn many times before. The child told them to go away and that he was not supposed to have any more blood tests. The boy's parents were not present, but in the past they had always given permission for blood draws over the child's objections. The phlebotomists ignored the child, and one of them collected the specimen while the other restrained him. It was later determined that the boy's parents had earlier filed a written request that the child was to have no more blood drawn.

QUESTIONS

1. What error did the phlebotomists make in drawing blood from the child?

2. What assumptions were made in deciding to draw blood from the child over his objections?

3. What might be the consequences of the phlebotomists' actions?

Bibliography and Suggested Readings

BD™ Blood Transfer Device product literature. BD Vacutainer Systems. Franklin Lakes, NJ:

Bishop ML, Fody EP, Schoeff LE. *Clinical Chemistry: Principles, Procedures, Correlations.* 7th ed. Philadelphia, PA: Lippincott Williams & Wilkins; 2013.

Clinical and Laboratory Standards Institute, GP33-A. *Accuracy in Patient and Sample Identification.* Wayne, PA: CLSI; 2010.

Clinical and Laboratory Standards Institute, GP41-A6. *Procedures for the Collection of Diagnostic Blood Specimens by Venipuncture.* 6th ed. Wayne, PA: CLSI; 2007.

College of American Pathologists (CAP) Publications Committee, Phlebotomy Subgroup. *So You're Going to Collect a Blood Specimen: An Introduction to Phlebotomy.* 14th ed. Northfield, IL: CAP; 2013.

Ernst DJ. *Applied Phlebotomy.* Baltimore, MD: Lippincott Williams & Wilkins; 2005.

Ernst DJ. *Blood Specimen Collection FAQs.* Corydon, IN: Center for Phlebotomy Education; 2008.

Food and Drug Administration (FDA). Allergic reactions to latex-containing medical devices. *FDA Med Alert.* 1991.

Graden M, Eriksson M, Holmqvist G, Holstein A, Schollin J. Pain reduction at venipuncture in newborns: Oral glucose compared with local anesthetic cream. *Pediatrics.* 2002;110:1053–1057.

Kronberger J, Woodson D. *Clinical Medical Assisting.* 4th ed. Philadelphia, PA: Lippincott Williams & Wilkins; 2012.

Lindh V, Wiklund U, Hakanssom S. Assessment of the effect of EMLA during venipuncture in newborn by analysis of heart rate variability. *Pain.* 2000;86:247–254.

Mitchell A, Waltman PA. Oral sucrose and pain relief for preterm infants. *Pain Manag Nurs.* 2003;4(2):62–69.

MEDIA MENU

Online Ancillaries (at http://thepoint.lww.com/McCall6e)

- Videos:
  - Blood Collection from a Hand Vein Using a Butterfly and ETS Holder
  - Collecting a Blood Specimen by Venipuncture Using the Evacuated Tube System
  - Collecting Blood from an Antecubital Vein Using a Needle and Syringe
  - Hand Washing/Hand Antisepsis
  - Introductory and Identification Processes Required Prior to Blood Specimen Collection
  - Poor and Good Workplace Ergonomics for Phlebotomy
  - Proper Tourniquet Application for Venipuncture
  - Specimen Labeling and Venipuncture Follow-up Procedures
  - Transferring Blood from a Syringe into ETS Tubes
- Interactive exercises and games, including Look and Label, Word Building, Body Building, Roboterms, Crossword Puzzles, Quiz Show, and Concentration
- Audio flash cards and flash card generator
- Audio glossary

Internet Resources

- Advance magazine for medical laboratory personnel: http://laboratorian.advanceweb.com/
- American Academy of Pediatrics: http://www.aap.org
- Center for Phlebotomy Education: http://www.phlebotomy.com
- National Institute for Safety and Health: http://www.cdc.gov/niosh

Other Resources

- McCall R, Tankersley C. *Student Workbook for Phlebotomy Essentials,* 6th ed. (available for separate purchase)
- McCall R, Tankersley C. *Phlebotomy Exam Review,* 6th ed. (available for separate purchase)

Chapter 9
Preanalytical Considerations

NAACLS Entry Level Competencies

4.4 List the general criteria for suitability of a specimen for analysis, and reasons for specimen rejection or recollection.

5.4 Describe substances that can interfere in clinical analysis of blood constituents and ways in which the phlebotomist can help to avoid these occurrences.

6.1 Identify potential sites for venipuncture and capillary (dermal) puncture.

6.4 List the effects of tourniquet, hand squeezing, and heating pads on specimens collected by venipuncture and capillary (dermal) puncture.

6.8 Explain the causes of phlebotomy complications.

6.9 Describe signs and symptoms of physical problems that may occur during blood collection.

7.5 Identify and report potential preanalytical errors that may occur during specimen collection, labeling, transporting, and processing.

Key Terms 📖 *Do Matching Exercise 9-1 in the WORKBOOK to gain familiarity with these terms.*

A-line
AV shunt/fistula/ graft
bariatric
basal state
bilirubin
CVAD
CVC

diurnal/ circadian
edema
exsanguination
hematoma
hemo- concentration
hemolysis
iatrogenic

icteric
implanted port
IV
jaundice
lipemic
lymphostasis
petechiae
PICC
preanalytical

reference ranges
reflux
saline lock
sclerosed
syncope
thrombosed
vasovagal
venous stasis

Objectives

Upon successful completion of this chapter, the reader should be able to:

1 Demonstrate basic knowledge of the preanalytical variables that influence laboratory test results, define associated terminology, and identify the tests most affected by each one.

2 Discuss problem areas associated with site selection including various vascular access sites and devices, and explain what to do when they are encountered.

3 Describe how to handle patient complications and conditions pertaining to blood collection, address procedural error risks, and specimen quality concerns, and analyze reasons for failure to draw blood.

Overview

The **preanalytical** (before analysis) or **preexamination** phase of the testing process begins for the laboratory when a test is ordered and ends when testing begins. Numerous factors associated with this phase of the testing process, if not properly addressed, can lead to errors that can compromise specimen quality, jeopardize the health and safety of the patient, and ultimately increase the cost of medical care. Since each blood collection situation is unique, a phlebotomist must have—in addition to the technical skills needed to perform a blood draw—the ability to recognize preanalytical factors and address them, if applicable, to avoid or reduce any negative impact. This chapter addresses physiological variables, problem venipuncture sites, various types of vascular access devices (VADs), patient complications and conditions, procedural errors, specimen quality issues, and how to troubleshoot failed venipuncture.

Reference Ranges/Intervals

Most tests are performed to confirm health or to screen for, diagnose, or monitor disease. To be properly evaluated, test results typically need to be compared with results expected of healthy individuals. Consequently, result values for most tests are established using specimens from normal, healthy individuals. Because results vary somewhat from person to person, the results used for comparison become a range of values with high and low limits, commonly called a **reference range** or **reference interval**. Test results within this range are said to be within normal limits, thus reference ranges are often called normal values. Most reference ranges are for healthy fasting individuals. Although less common, some tests have reference ranges that are age specific, or for certain illnesses or disorders such as diabetes.

Key Point One way a physician evaluates a patient's test results is by comparing them to reference ranges and, if available, previous results on the same patient. If a specimen has been compromised and the results are not valid, a physician could make a decision based upon incorrect information and thus jeopardize the patient's care.

Basal State

Basal state refers to the resting metabolic state of the body early in the morning after fasting for approximately 12 hours. A basal state specimen is ideal for establishing reference ranges on inpatients because the effects of diet, exercise, and other controllable factors on test results are minimized or eliminated. Basal state is influenced by a number of physiologic patient variables such as age, gender, and conditions of the body that cannot be eliminated.

Outpatient specimens are not basal state specimens and may have slightly different reference ranges (normal values).

Physiological Variables

Match physiological effects with lab tests in the Matching 9-2 activity in the WORKBOOK.

AGE

Values for some blood components vary considerably depending upon the age of the patient. For example, red blood cell (RBC) and white blood cell (WBC) values are normally higher in newborns than in adults. Some physiological functions such as kidney function decrease with age. For example, creatinine clearance, a measure of kidney function, is directly related to the age of the patient, which must be factored in when test results are being calculated. Hormone levels may also vary according to age (i.e., estrogen and growth hormone (GH), decrease with advanced age).

ALTITUDE

Test results for some blood analytes show significant variation at higher elevations compared with results at sea level. RBC counts are a prime example. RBCs carry oxygen. Decreased oxygen levels at higher altitudes cause the body to produce more RBCs to meet the body's oxygen requirements; the higher the altitude, the greater the increase. Thus RBC counts and related determinations such as hemoglobin (Hgb) and hematocrit (Hct) have higher reference ranges at higher elevations. Other analytes that increase at higher elevations include C-reactive protein and uric acid. Analytes that decrease in value at increased altitude include urinary creatinine (which in turn affects creatinine clearance tests) and plasma renin.

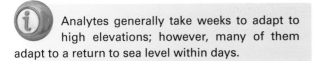 Analytes generally take weeks to adapt to high elevations; however, many of them adapt to a return to sea level within days.

DEHYDRATION

Dehydration (decrease in total body fluid), which occurs, for example, with persistent vomiting or diarrhea, causes **hemoconcentration**, a condition in which blood components that cannot easily leave the bloodstream become concentrated in the smaller plasma volume. Blood components affected include RBCs, enzymes, iron (Fe), calcium (Ca), sodium (Na), and coagulation factors. Consequently, results on specimens from dehydrated patients may not accurately reflect the patient's normal status. In addition, it is often difficult to obtain blood specimens from dehydrated patients.

DIET

Blood analyte composition can be altered by the ingestion of food and drink. As a result, blood specimens collected soon after a meal or snack are unsuitable for many laboratory tests. Diet effects on analytes are generally temporary and vary depending upon the amount and type of food or drink and the length of time between ingestion and specimen collection. Requiring a patient to fast or follow a special diet eliminates most dietary influences on testing. Patients are typically asked to fast approximately 8 to 12 hours, depending on the test. Fasting is normally done overnight after the last evening meal, with specimens collected the following morning before the patient has eaten.

⚠️ **CAUTION** Fasting beyond 12 hours can cause serious health problems, such as electrolyte imbalance and heart rhythm disturbances. Consequently fasting specimens, especially those requiring a 12-hour fast, should be collected promptly without unreasonable delay.

🔑 **Key Point** Patients are allowed to drink water during fasting unless they are NPO for another procedure (e.g., surgery). Refraining from drinking water while fasting can result in dehydration that can negatively affect test results and also make blood collection more difficult.

The following are examples of how some analytes can be significantly affected by the consumption of certain types of food or drink and the excess consumption of some fluids.

- Ammonia, urea, and uric acid levels may be elevated in patients on high-protein diets.
- Cortisol and ACTH levels have been shown to increase after drinking beverages containing caffeine.
- Glucose (blood sugar) levels increase dramatically with the ingestion of carbohydrates or sugar-laden substances but return to normal within 2 hours if the patient has normal glucose metabolism. Eating carbohydrates can also increase insulin levels.
- Hgb levels can decrease and electrolyte balance can be altered by drinking excessive amounts of water and other fluids.
- Lipid levels increase after eating foods such as butter or margarine, cheese, cream, and some enteral (tube feeding) preparations. (*Lipid* is a term meaning fat soluble that is used to describe certain fatty substances of animal or vegetable origin.) Abnormally increased blood lipid content is called **lipemia**. Lipids do not dissolve in water and thus high levels of lipids are visible in serum or plasma, causing it to appear milky (cloudy white) or turbid instead of transparent light yellow, and the specimen is described as being **lipemic** (Fig. 9-1).

🧠 **Memory Jogger** The word root *lip* means "fat." To associate lipemic with fat, think "fat lip" or visualize a big fat white cloud, because fats make the specimen appear cloudy white.

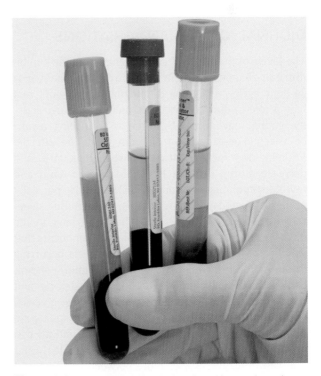

Figure 9-1 Left to right: Lipemic, icteric, and normal specimen.

Lipemia can be present for up to 12 hours, which is why accurate testing of triglycerides (a type of lipid) requires a 12-hour fast. In addition, some chemistry tests cannot be performed on lipemic specimens because the cloudiness interferes with the testing procedure.

Key Point Lipemia in a fasting specimen is rare. When a test requires a fasting specimen but the serum or plasma sample submitted is lipemic, it is a clue that the patient may not have been fasting.

- Some test methods that detect occult (hidden) blood in stool specimens also detect similar substances in meat and certain vegetables. Consequently, a special diet that eliminates these foods must be followed for several days before the specimen is collected.
- Triglycerides, certain liver enzymes, and other liver function analytes are increased by chronic consumption or recent ingestion of large amounts of alcohol, which can also cause hypoglycemia.

Malnutrition and starvation also affect the composition of blood analytes. Long-term starvation decreases cholesterol, triglycerides, and urea levels and increases creatinine, ketone, and uric acid levels.

DIURNAL/CIRCADIAN VARIATIONS

The levels of many blood components normally exhibit **diurnal** (happening daily) or **circadian** (having a 24-hour cycle) variations or fluctuations. Factors that play a role in diurnal variations include posture, activity, eating, daylight and darkness, and being awake or asleep. For example, melatonin levels are affected by light; they increase at night, when it is dark, and decrease during daylight hours. Maximum renin and thyroid-stimulating hormone (TSH) levels normally occur in the predawn hours of the morning during sleep, while peak cortisol levels normally occur later in the morning, around 8:00 A.M. Other blood components that exhibit diurnal variation with highest levels occurring in the morning include aldosterone, bilirubin, cortisol, hemoglobin, insulin, iron, potassium, testosterone, and RBCs. Blood levels of eosinophils, creatinine, glucose, growth hormone (GH), triglycerides, and phosphate are normally lowest in the morning. Diurnal variations can be large. For example, the levels of cortisol, TSH, and iron can differ by 50% or more between morning and late afternoon.

A change of several time zones can affect diurnal rhythm and the tests associated with it. Several days may be required to restore a normal rhythm.

Key Point Tests influenced by diurnal variation are often ordered as timed tests; it is important to collect them as close to the time indicated as possible.

DRUG THERAPY

Some drugs alter physiological functions, causing changes in the concentrations of certain blood analytes. The effect may be desired or an unwanted side effect or sensitivity. Consequently, it is not uncommon for physicians to monitor levels of specific blood analytes while a patient is receiving drug therapy. The following are just a few examples of drugs that can alter physiologic function and the analytes they affect:

- Chemotherapy drugs can cause a decrease in blood cells, especially WBCs and platelets.
- Many drugs are toxic to the liver, as evidenced by increased levels of liver enzymes such as aspartate aminotransaminase (AST)—also called serum glutamic-oxaloacetic transaminase (SGOT), alkaline phosphatase (ALP), and lactate dehydrogenase (LDH), and decreased production of clotting factors. Erythromycin and acetaminophen (e.g., Tylenol) can increase AST and bilirubin levels and give a false indication of abnormal liver function. Acetaminophen can also be a cause of abnormal liver function.
- Opiates such as morphine increase levels of liver and pancreatic enzymes.
- Oral contraceptives can affect the results of many tests. For example, they can elevate the erythrocyte sedimentation rate (ESR) and decrease levels of vitamin B_{12}.
- Steroids and diuretics can cause pancreatitis and an increase in amylase and lipase values.
- Thiazide diuretics (blood pressure medications) can elevate calcium and glucose levels and decrease sodium and potassium levels. Other thiazide-type medications that lower blood volume can increase blood levels of nitrogenous waste such as urea, a condition called azotemia.

Key Point Of special concern to phlebotomists are the anticoagulants warfarin and heparin, and over-the-counter drugs like aspirin that can cause prolonged bleeding after venipuncture.

Drugs can also interfere with the actual test procedure, causing false increases or decreases in test results. A drug may compete with the analyte for the same test sites in the reaction, causing a falsely low or false-negative result, or the drug may enhance the reaction, causing a falsely high or false-positive result.

> (i) An acronym for substances that interfere in the testing process is CRUD, which stands for "compounds reacting unfortunately as the desired."

Although it is ultimately up to the physician to prevent or recognize and eliminate drug interferences, this can be a complicated issue that requires cooperation between the physician, pharmacy, and laboratory to make certain that test results are not affected by medications. Phlebotomists can play a role in this effort by noting on the requisition when they observe medication being administered just prior to blood collection.

> **Key Point** According to CAP guidelines, drugs that interfere with blood tests should be stopped or avoided 4 to 24 hours prior to obtaining the blood sample for testing. Drugs that interfere with urine tests should be avoided for 48 to 72 hours prior to the urine sample collection.

EXERCISE

Exercise affects a number of blood components, raising levels of some and lowering levels of others. Effects vary, depending on the patient's physical condition and the duration and intensity of the activity. However, moderate to strenuous exercise appears to have the greatest effect. Levels typically return to normal soon after the activity is stopped. The following are examples of the effects of exercise on a number of blood components:

- Arterial pH and $PaCO_2$ levels are reduced by exercise.
- Glucose, creatinine, insulin, lactic acid, and total protein can be elevated by moderate muscular activity.
- Potassium (K^+) is released from the cells during exercise, increasing levels in the plasma. Levels generally return to normal after several minutes of rest.

> **CAUTION** The simple exercise of pumping the hand (i.e., repeatedly making and releasing a fist) during venipuncture is enough to erroneously increase potassium levels.

- Skeletal muscle enzyme levels are increased by exercise, with levels of creatine kinase (CK) and lactate dehydrogenase (LDH) remaining elevated for 24 hours or more.

> (i) Athletes generally have higher resting levels of skeletal muscle enzymes, and exercise produces less of an increase.

- Vigorous physical exercise shortly before blood collection can temporarily increase total cholesterol levels by 6% or more. Levels can remain elevated for up to an hour after the exercise has stopped. Vigorous or sustained exercise can also affect hemostasis. For example, an increased number of platelet clumps were seen in a study of runners evaluated immediately after running the Boston marathon.

FEVER

Fever affects the levels of a number of hormones. Fever-induced hypoglycemia increases insulin levels, followed by a rise in glucagon levels. Fever also increases cortisol and may disrupt its normal diurnal variation.

SEX

A patient's sex affects the concentration of a number of blood components. Most differences are apparent only after sexual maturity and are reflected in separate normal values for males and females. For example, RBC, Hgb, and Hct normal values are higher for males than for females.

INTRAMUSCULAR INJECTION

A recent intramuscular injection can increase levels of creatine kinase (CK) and the skeletal muscle fraction of LDH. Consequently, it is recommended that CK and LDH levels be drawn before intramuscular injection or at least 1 hour after injection. Muscular trauma from injuries or surgery can also increase CK levels.

JAUNDICE

Jaundice, also called **icterus**, is a condition characterized by increased **bilirubin** (a product of the breakdown of RBCs) in the blood, leading to deposits of yellow bile pigment in the skin, mucous membranes, and sclerae (whites of the eyes), giving the patient a yellow appearance (Fig. 9-2). The term **icteric** means relating to or marked by jaundice and is used to describe serum, plasma, or urine specimens that have an abnormal deep yellow to yellow-brown color due to high bilirubin levels (Fig. 9-1). The abnormal color can interfere with chemistry tests based on color reactions, including reagent-strip analyses on urine.

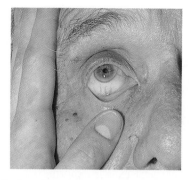

Figure 9-2 Jaundice. Note patient's yellow skin color in comparison with that of the examiner's hand.

> **Key Point** Although there are a number of different causes, jaundice in a patient may indicate liver inflammation caused by hepatitis B or C virus.

POSITION

Body position before and during blood collection can influence specimen composition. Going from supine (lying down on the back) to an upright sitting or standing position causes blood fluids to filter into the tissues, decreasing plasma volume in an adult up to 10%. Only protein-free fluids can pass through the capillaries; consequently the blood concentration of components that are protein in nature or bound to protein—such as aldosterone, bilirubin, blood cells, calcium, cholesterol, iron, protein, and renin—increases. In most cases the concentration of freely diffusible blood components is not affected by postural changes. Nevertheless, a significant increase in potassium (K^+) levels occurs within 30 minutes of standing; this has been attributed to the release of intracellular potassium from muscle. Other examples of the effects of posture changes include the following:

- A change in position from lying to standing can cause up to a 15% variation in total and high-density lipoprotein (HDL) cholesterol results, and 10% to 12% higher triglyceride results. Patients with congestive heart failure and hepatic disorders may exhibit even more pronounced positional effects.

> **Key Point** The National Cholesterol Education Program recommends that lipid profiles be collected in a consistent manner after the patient has been either lying down or sitting quietly for a minimum of 5 minutes.

- Plasma aldosterone and renin change more slowly but can double within an hour. Consequently patients are typically required to be recumbent (lying down) for at least 30 minutes prior to aldosterone specimen collection, and plasma renin activity levels require documentation of the patient's position during collection.

- The RBC count of a patient who has been standing for approximately 15 minutes will be higher than a basal state RBC count of that patient. The reverse happens when the patient lies down. In fact, the normal physiological response to a change in position from standing to lying down can cause a condition called **postural pseudoanemia** (posture related false anemia), a substantial decrease in hematocrit values due to an increase in plasma that could be mistaken for blood loss or acute anemia. Values return to normal when the patient has been sitting up for a while, as blood fluid moves back into the tissues. For proper interpretation of test results for analytes affected by positional changes, all test specimens for that analyte should be collected with the patient in the same position. Analytes most affected by positional changes typically have a recommended position for specimen collection, based upon the one used when their reference ranges were established.

> **Key Point** Calling outpatients into the drawing area and having them sit in the drawing chair while paperwork related to the draw is readied can help minimize effects of postural changes on some analytes.

PREGNANCY

Pregnancy causes physiologic changes in many body systems. Consequently results of a number of laboratory tests must be compared with reference ranges established for pregnant populations. For example, increases in body fluid that are normal during pregnancy, have a diluting effect on the RBCs, leading to lower RBC counts.

SMOKING

A number of blood components are affected by smoking. The extent of these effects depends upon the number of cigarettes smoked. Patients who smoke prior to specimen collection may have increased cholesterol, cortisol, glucose, growth hormone, and triglyceride levels as well as WBC counts. Chronic smoking often leads to decreased pulmonary function and increased RBC counts and hemoglobin levels. Smoking can also affect the body's immune response, typically lowering the concentrations of immunoglobulins IgA, IgG, and IgM but increasing levels of IgE.

> Skin-puncture specimens may be difficult to obtain from smokers because of impaired circulation in the fingertips.

STRESS

Emotional stress such as anxiety, fear, or trauma can cause transient (short-lived) elevations in WBCs. For example, studies of crying infants have demonstrated marked increases in WBC counts, which returned to normal within 1 hour after the crying stopped. Consequently CBC or WBC specimens on an infant are ideally obtained after the infant has been sleeping or resting quietly for at least 30 minutes. If they are collected while an infant is crying, this should be noted on the report.

> **(i)** Studies in psychoneuroimmunology (PNI)—a field that deals with the interactions between the brain, the endocrine system, and the immune system—have demonstrated that receptors on the cell membrane of WBCs can sense stress in a person and react by increasing cell numbers.

Stress is also known to decrease serum iron levels and increase adrenocorticotropic hormone (ACTH), catecholamine, and cortisol levels. Other hormones that can be affected include aldosterone and TSH, and GH in children.

TEMPERATURE AND HUMIDITY

Environmental factors such as temperature and humidity can affect test values by influencing the composition of body fluids. Acute heat exposure causes interstitial fluid to move into the blood vessels, increasing plasma volume and influencing its composition. Extensive sweating without fluid replacement, on the other hand, can cause hemoconcentration. Environmental factors associated with geographic location are generally accounted for when reference values are established.

> **(i)** Laboratory temperature and humidity are closely monitored to maintain specimen integrity and ensure equipment functions properly.

Problem Sites

> **After you finish this section, do Matching 9-3 in the WORKBOOK to see if you can match problem sites with possible drawbacks.**

BURNS, SCARS, AND TATTOOS

Avoid burned, scarred, and tattooed areas. Veins may be difficult to palpate or penetrate in burned and scarred areas. Healed burn sites and other areas with extensive scarring may have impaired circulation that could lead to erroneous test results. Newly burned areas are painful and susceptible to infection. Freshly tattooed areas may have an undetected infection or be more susceptible to infection. In addition, tattoos may mask problem areas and impair the ability to detect bruising, rashes, and other reactions to phlebotomy. Lastly, because of the value patients place in their tattoos, most do not want to have scarring or bruising anywhere near them.

> **(key)** **Key Point** If you have no choice but to draw in an area with a tattoo, try to insert the needle in a spot that does not contain dye.

DAMAGED VEINS

Some patients' veins feel hard and cord-like and lack resiliency because they are occluded or obstructed. These veins may be **sclerosed** (hardened) or **thrombosed** (clotted) from the effects of inflammation, disease, or chemotherapy drugs. Scarring caused by numerous venipunctures—as occurs in regular blood donors, persons with chronic illnesses, and illegal IV drug users—can also harden veins. Damaged veins are difficult to puncture, may yield erroneous (invalid) test results because of impaired blood flow, and should be avoided.

> **(key)** **Key Point** Use another site if possible, or draw below (distal to) damaged veins.

EDEMA

Edema is swelling caused by the abnormal accumulation of fluid in the tissues. It sometimes results when fluid from an IV infiltrates the surrounding tissues. Specimens collected from edematous areas may yield inaccurate test results owing to contamination with tissue fluid or altered blood composition caused by the swelling. In addition, veins are harder to locate, the stretched tissue is often fragile and more easily injured by tourniquet and antiseptic application, and healing may be prolonged in these areas. Another site should be chosen if possible.

> **(key)** **Key Point** Phlebotomists on early-morning rounds in hospitals or nursing homes are often the first to notice edema from infiltrated IVs and should alert the appropriate personnel.

HEMATOMA

A **hematoma** (Fig. 9-3) is a swelling or mass of blood (often clotted) that can be caused by blood leaking from

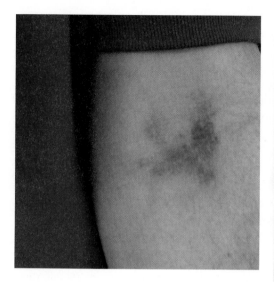

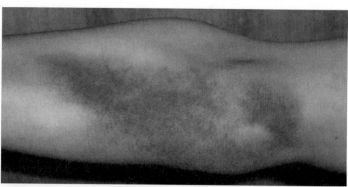

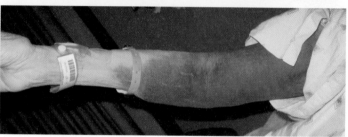

Figure 9-3 Examples of bruising resulting from hematomas that formed during or immediately following venipuncture. (Top right photo courtesy Monica Lewis. Bottom right photo courtesy Sue Kucera.)

a blood vessel during or following venipuncture. A large bruise eventually spreads over the surrounding area. Venipuncture through an existing hematoma is painful. If the draw is difficult, there is also the possibility that hemolyzed blood from the hematoma could be drawn into the tube or syringe, resulting in a specimen that is unsuitable for testing. Venipuncture in the immediate area surrounding a hematoma may also be painful. In addition, it is thought that obstruction of blood flow by the hematoma and the effects of the coagulation process could lead to inaccurate test results on the specimen.

CAUTION To ensure the collection of non-contaminated blood, never perform venipuncture through a hematoma. If there is no alternative site, perform the venipuncture distal to the hematoma to ensure the collection of free-flowing blood.

MASTECTOMY

Blood should never be drawn from an arm on the same side as a **mastectomy** (surgical breast removal) without first consulting the patient's physician. Lymph node removal, which is typically part of the procedure, may cause **lymphostasis** (obstruction or stoppage of normal lymph flow). Impaired lymph flow makes the arm susceptible to swelling, called lymphedema, and to infection. Lymphedema can cause range of motion limitations, pain, and weakness, or stiffness in the affected extremity. It has also been suggested that the effects of lymphostasis could change blood composition and lead to inaccurate test results.

Key Point When a mastectomy has been performed on both sides, the patient's physician should be consulted to determine a suitable site.

OBESITY

Obese (extremely overweight) patients often present a challenge to the phlebotomist. Veins of obese patients may be deep and difficult to find. Proper tourniquet selection and application is the first step to a successful venipuncture. Typical strap tourniquets, which are normally around 18 inches long, may be too short to fit around large arms without rolling and twisting, and being uncomfortably tight. **Bariatric** tourniquets (longer tourniquets designed for the obese) should be available. A bariatric or extra large size blood pressure cuff can also be used as long as it is inflated to just below the patient's diastolic pressure.

A euphemism is a word or expression substituted for one considered to be too blunt, hurtful, or embarrassing. Although bariatric means *pertaining to the treatment of obesity,* it is used as a euphemism to refer to individuals and items for individuals who are extremely overweight whether or not they are actually being treated for obesity.

Check the antecubital area first. Obese patients often have a double crease in the antecubital area with an easily palpable median cubital vein in the area (somewhat like a valley), between the two creases. If no vein is easily visible or palpable on tourniquet application, ask the patient what sites have been successful for past blood draws. Most patients who are "difficult draws" know what sites work best. If the patient has never had blood drawn before or does not remember, another site to try is the cephalic vein. To locate the cephalic vein, rotate the patient's arm medially, so that the hand is prone. In this position, the weight of excess tissue often pulls downward, making the cephalic vein easier to feel and penetrate with a needle.

PARALYSIS

Drawing blood from a paralyzed arm should be avoided if possible. Paralysis is the loss of muscle function. Paralysis can be temporary or permanent; localized in one area of the body, or widespread. Most paralysis is the result of a stroke or an injury to the spinal cord. Other causes include nerve damage and autoimmune disorders such as muscular dystrophy and amyotrophic lateral sclerosis (ALS).

> **Key Point** It should not be assumed that there is no feeling in a paralyzed arm. There is lack of feeling only if there is sensory damage.

An arm that has lost muscle function has also lost the muscle action that helps return blood to the heart. This can result in stagnation of blood flow and increase the chance of vein thrombosis. This chance is magnified because venipuncture disrupts the lining of the vein, which also increases the chance of thrombosis. If sensation is also lacking in that arm, there can be an inability to detect an adverse reaction such as nerve injury. If you have no choice but to draw from a paralyzed arm, follow strict venipuncture procedures (e.g., no probing or lateral needle redirection) and hold pressure over the site after the draw until you are certain that blood flow has ceased.

> When the lower part of the body and both legs are paralyzed it is called paraplegia. If both the arms and legs are paralyzed it is called quadriplegia.

Vascular Access Devices and Sites

Vascular access devices (VADs) are often used for patients who require frequent venous or arterial access. They are most commonly used for administration of medications, fluids, blood products and sometimes blood collection. As a general rule, venipuncture should not be performed on an extremity with a VAD. Follow facility policy. The following are the most common types of VADs that may be encountered by the phlebotomist.

> **Key Point** Only nurses and other specially trained personnel are allowed to draw blood specimens from vascular access devices (VADs). However, the phlebotomist typically assists by supplying the appropriate tubes, and if a syringe is used, transferring the blood to the tubes using a safety syringe transfer device.

INTRAVENOUS LINE

Intravenous means "of, pertaining to, or within a vein." An intravenous (IV) line, referred to simply as an **IV**, is a quick way to deliver fluids, medications, blood transfusion products, and other substances to patients. It consists of a catheter inserted in a peripheral vein. (Peripheral veins are veins that are located anywhere except the abdomen or chest). The catheter is typically connected to a line that is used to administer the fluid. The line is attached to a bag containing the substance being administered. An IV is often called an IV drip because it usually has a special drip chamber that prevents air from entering the tubing and allows the flow rate to be estimated and controlled.

It is preferred that blood specimens not be drawn from an arm with an IV (Fig. 9-4), as the specimens can be contaminated or diluted with the IV fluid, causing erroneous test results. This is especially true if specimens are drawn above the IV. When a patient has an IV in one arm, blood specimens should be collected from the other arm if possible. If a patient has IVs in both arms blood specimens can be collected below one of the IVs by following Procedure 9-1. If the other arm is also unavailable for some reason, some specimens can be collected by capillary puncture. If a specimen cannot be collected by capillary puncture it may have to be collected from an IV by a nurse or other specially trained person. Follow facility policy.

IV CATHETER LOCK

An IV catheter lock is a needleless connection device in the form of a stopcock (Fig. 9-5) or a cap that is connected to the hub of a catheter or cannula, by a short length of IV tubing. The cap or stopcock has a diaphragm (thin rubber-like cover) that provides access for administering medication or drawing blood. A lock is often placed in a vein in the lower arm above the back of the wrist and can be left in place for up to 48 hours. To keep it from clotting, the device is filled and also flushed with saline, and sometimes heparin. A device filled with saline is called a **saline lock**. One filled with heparin is called a heparin lock (heplock). Risks associated with using heparin, and the higher cost of heparin have resulted in the saline lock becoming the type most commonly used.

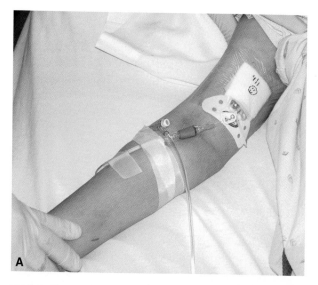

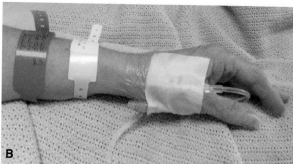

Figure 9-4 Arms with intravenous (IV) lines. **A:** IV in patient's upper arm. **B:** IV in patient's hand.

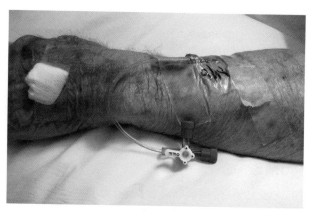

Figure 9-5 Saline lock with needleless entry stopcock.

Heparin readily adheres to surfaces; therefore it is difficult to remove all traces of it. Consequently a 5-mL discard tube should be drawn first when blood specimens are collected from a heparin lock or from a saline lock that has been flushed with heparin. Drawing coagulation specimens from them is also not recommended because traces of heparin or dilution with saline can negatively affect test results.

PREVIOUSLY ACTIVE IV SITES

Previously active IV sites present a potential source of error in testing. Blood specimens should not be collected from a known previous IV site within 24 to 48 hours of the time the IV was discontinued. Follow facility protocol.

Procedure 9-1: Performing Venipuncture Below an IV

PURPOSE: To obtain a blood specimen by venipuncture below an IV

EQUIPMENT: Applicable ETS or syringe system supplies and equipment

Step	Explanation/Rationale
1. Ask the patient's nurse to turn off the IV for at least 2 minutes prior to collection.	A phlebotomist is not qualified to make IV adjustments. Turning off the IV for 2 minutes allows IV fluids to dissipate from the area.
2. Apply the tourniquet distal to the IV.	Avoids disturbing the IV.
3. Select a venipuncture site distal to the IV and the tourniquet.	Venous blood flows up the arm toward the heart. Drawing below an IV affords the best chance of obtaining blood that is free of IV fluid contamination.
4. Perform the venipuncture in a different vein than the one with the IV if possible.	IV fluids can be present below an IV because of backflow and may still be there after the IV is shut off because of poor venous circulation.
5. Ask the nurse to restart the IV after the specimen has been collected.	IV flow rates must be precise, and starting or adjusting them is not part of a phlebotomist's scope of practice.
6. Document that the specimen was collected below an IV, indicate the type of fluid in the IV, and identify which arm was used.	This aids laboratory personnel and the patient's physician in the event that test results are questioned.

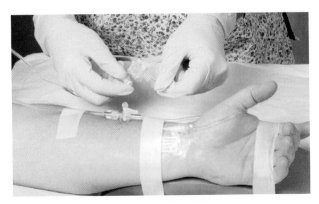

Figure 9-6 Nurse working with a patient's arterial line (A-line).

ARTERIAL LINE

📖 **Test your VAD knowledge with Matching Exercise 9-4 and Labeling Exercise 9-2 in the WORKBOOK.**

An **arterial line** (A-line or Art-line) is a catheter that is placed in an artery. It is most commonly located in the radial artery of the wrist (Fig. 9-6) and is typically used to provide accurate and continuous measurement of a patient's blood pressure. It may also be used to collect blood gas and other blood specimens and for the administration of drugs such as dopamine.

⚠️ **CAUTION** Never apply a tourniquet or perform venipuncture on an arm with an arterial line.

ARTERIOVENOUS SHUNT, FISTULA, OR GRAFT

An **arteriovenous (AV) shunt** (Fig. 9-7) is the permanent surgical connection of an artery and vein. Shunt means to move or force. An AV shunt bypasses the capillaries and forces arterial blood directly into a vein. A shunt created for dialysis use, commonly joins the radial artery and cephalic vein above the wrist on the underside of the arm. A dialysis shunt created by direct permanent fusion of the artery and vein is called a **fistula** (Fig. 9-7A) and is visible as a large bulging section of vein. A fistula has become the most common type of shunt used for dialysis. If the shunt was created using a piece of vein or tubing to form a loop from the artery to the vein that can be seen under the skin it is called a **graft** (Fig. 9-7B). When palpated a shunt has a distinctive buzzing sensation called a "thrill" that is the result of the pressure of the arterial blood flow meeting the passive flow of the vein. A temporary shunt with tubing on the surface of the skin can also be created.

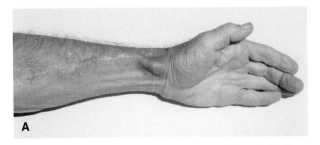

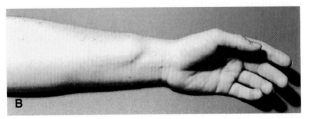

Figure 9-7 Arms with AV shunts; **A:** fistula **B:** graft.

⚠️ **CAUTION** A shunt is a dialysis patient's lifeline. Never apply a blood pressure cuff or tourniquet, or perform venipuncture, on an arm with any type of shunt.

BLOOD SAMPLING DEVICE

A needleless closed blood sampling device is sometimes connected to an arterial or central venous catheter (CVC) (see "Vascular-Access Devices") for the purpose of collecting blood specimens. These devices are said to reduce the chance of infection, prevent needlesticks, and minimize waste associated with line draws. One example is the VAMP® (Venous Arterial blood Management Protection system) from Edwards Lifesciences (Irvine, CA), shown in Figure 9-8.

CENTRAL VASCULAR ACCESS DEVICES

A **central vascular access device (CVAD)**, also called an **indwelling line**, consists of tubing inserted into

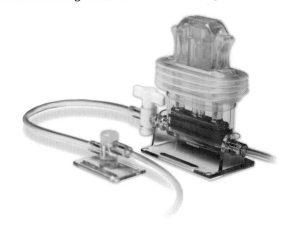

Figure 9-8 VAMP® blood sampling device. (Courtesy of Edwards Lifesciences, Irvine, CA.)

a main vein or artery. CVADs are used primarily for administering fluids and medications, monitoring pressures, and drawing blood. Having a CVAD is practical for patients who need IV access for an extended time and is especially beneficial for patients who do not have easily accessible veins.

> ⚠️ **CAUTION** Only specially trained personnel should access CVADs to draw blood. However, as with other VADs the phlebotomist may assist by transferring the specimen to the appropriate tubes using a blood transfer device.

Most CVADs are routinely flushed with heparin or saline to reduce the risk of thrombosis. To help ensure that the specimen is not contaminated with the flush solution, a small amount of blood must be drawn from the line and discarded before a blood specimen can be collected. The amount of blood discarded depends upon the dead-space volume of the line. Two times the dead-space volume is discarded for noncoagulation tests and six times (normally about 5 mL) is generally recommended

for coagulation tests, although it is preferred that specimens for coagulation tests not be drawn from CVADs. The three main types of CVADs are:

- **CVC** or **central venous line** (Fig. 9-9): a line inserted into a large vein such as the subclavian and advanced into the superior vena cava, proximal to the right atrium. The exit end is surgically tunneled under the skin to a site several inches away in the chest. One or more short lengths of capped tubing protrude from the exit site (Fig. 9-9A), which is normally covered with a transparent dressing. There are a number of different types of CVCs, including Broviac®, Groshong® (Fig. 9-9B), and Hickman® (Fig. 9-9C).

- **Implanted port** (Fig. 9-10): a small chamber attached to an indwelling line that is surgically implanted under the skin and most commonly located in the upper chest or arm (Fig. 9-10A). The device is located by palpating the skin and accessed by inserting a special needle through the skin into the self-sealing septum (wall) of the chamber (Fig. 9-10B). The site is not normally covered with a bandage when not in use.

- **Peripherally inserted central catheter (PICC)** (Fig. 9-11): a line inserted into the peripheral venous

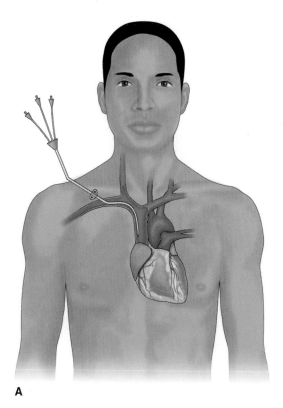

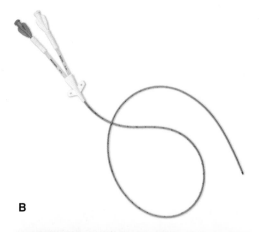

B

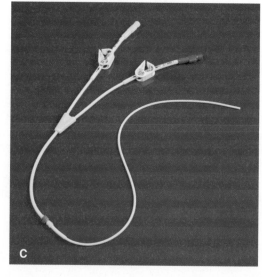

C

Figure 9-9 Central venous catheters (CVCs). **A:** CVC placement. (Reprinted with permission from Taylor CR, Lillis C, Lemone P. *Fundamentals of Nursing: The Art and Science of Nursing Care.* 6th ed. Philadelphia, PA: Lippincott Williams & Wilkins; 2008.) **B:** Groshong® CVC. **C:** Hickman® CVC. (Groshong® and Hickman® catheters courtesy BARD Access Systems, Inc., Salt Lake City, UT.)

A

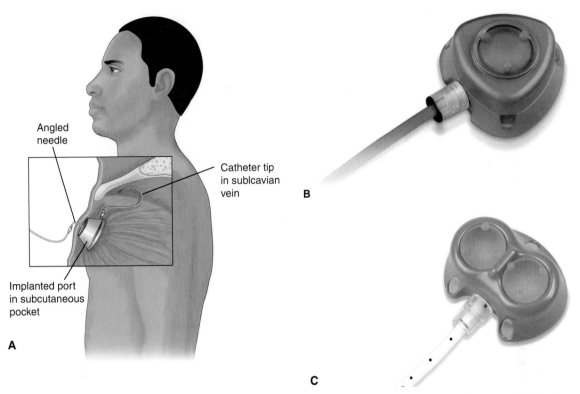

Angled
needle

Catheter tip
in sublcavian
vein

B

Implanted port
in subcutaneous
pocket

A

C

Figure 9-10 Implanted port. **A:** Port placement. (Reprinted with permission from Taylor CR, Lillis C, Lemone P. *Fundamentals of Nursing: The Art and Science of Nursing Care.* 6th ed. Philadelphia, PA: Lippincott Williams & Wilkins; 2008.) **B:** PowerPort® implanted port. (Courtesy Bard Access Systems, Inc., Salt Lake City, UT.) **C:** PowerPort® Duo implanted port. (Courtesy Bard Access Systems, Inc., Salt Lake City, UT.)

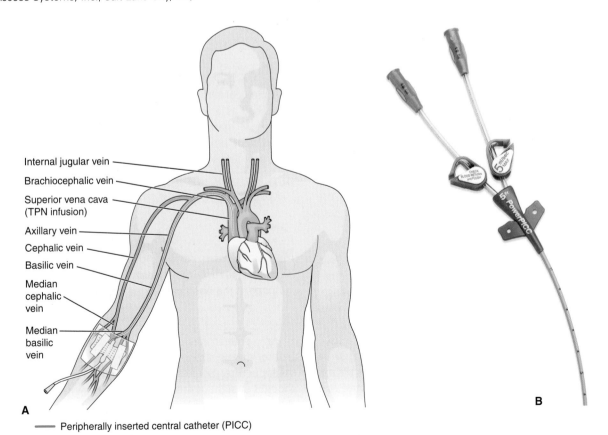

Internal jugular vein

Brachiocephalic vein

Superior vena cava
(TPN infusion)

Axillary vein

Cephalic vein

Basilic vein

Median
cephalic
vein

Median
basilic
vein

A

B

—— Peripherally inserted central catheter (PICC)

Figure 9-11 Peripherally inserted central catheter (PICC). **A:** PICC placement. (Reprinted with permission from Cohen BJ. *Medical Terminology.* 4th ed. Philadelphia, PA. Lippincott Williams & Wilkins; 2003.) **B:** PowerPICC® catheter. (Courtesy Bard Access Systems, Inc., Salt Lake City, UT.)

system (veins of the extremities) and threaded into the central venous system (main veins leading to the heart). It does not require surgical insertion and is typically placed in an antecubital vein just above or below the antecubital fossa (Fig. 9-11A). An example of a PICC is shown in Figure 9-11B.

> ⚠️ **CAUTION** Never apply a tourniquet or perform venipuncture above a PICC, as the line could be damaged by tourniquet pressure or needle puncture.

Patient Complications and Conditions

ALLERGIES TO EQUIPMENT AND SUPPLIES

Occasionally patients are encountered who are allergic to one or more of the supplies or equipment used in blood collection. Examples include the following.

Adhesive Allergy

Some patients are allergic to the glue used in adhesive bandages. One solution is to place a clean, folded gauze square over the site and wrap it with self-adherent bandaging material such as Coban™. Care must be taken not to wrap it too tightly, and the patient should be instructed to remove it in 15 minutes. If the patient is alert, mentally competent, and willing, another alternative is to instruct him or her to hold pressure for 5 minutes in lieu of applying a bandage.

Antiseptic Allergy

Occasionally, a patient is allergic to the antiseptic used in skin preparation prior to blood collection. (For example, many individuals are allergic to povidone–iodine.) Alternate antiseptics should be readily available for use in such cases.

Latex Allergy

Latex allergy involves a reaction to certain substances in natural rubber latex. Increasing numbers of individuals are allergic to latex. Some latex allergies are seemingly minor and involve irritation or rashes from physical contact with latex products. Other allergies are so severe that being in the same room where latex materials are used can set off a life-threatening reaction. There should be a warning sign on the door to the room of any patient known to have a severe latex allergy, and it is vital that no items made of latex be brought into the room whether collecting blood from the patient or a roommate. Fortunately, manufacturers have come up with latex-free alternatives to many items commonly used in health care such as gloves, bandages, and tourniquets. The result

is most healthcare facilities have abandoned the use of latex items where possible. However, there may be other medical items that still contain latex or latex parts and many nonmedical items such as balloons, rubber bands, and even the soles of some shoes that contain latex.

> 🔑 **Key Point** Patients with known allergies often wear special armbands or have allergy-specific warning signs posted in their hospital rooms.

EXCESSIVE BLEEDING

Normally, a patient will stop bleeding from the venipuncture site within a few minutes. Some patients, particularly those on aspirin or anticoagulant therapy, may take longer to stop bleeding. Pressure must be maintained over the site until the bleeding stops. If the bleeding continues after 5 minutes, the appropriate personnel should be notified.

> ⚠️ **CAUTION** Never apply a pressure bandage instead of maintaining pressure until bleeding has stopped, and do not dismiss an outpatient or leave an inpatient until bleeding has stopped or the appropriate personnel have taken charge of the situation.

FAINTING

The medical term for fainting is **syncope (sin'ko-pea)**, described as a loss of consciousness and postural tone (ability to maintain an upright posture) resulting from insufficient blood flow to the brain. It can last for as little as a few seconds or as long as half an hour.

thePoint* *View the How to Handle a Fainting Patient video at http://thePoint.lww.com/McCall6e.*

> 🧠 **Memory Jogger** To remember that syncope means fainting, look for the word *cope* in *syncope*. If the body can't cope, the patient faints.

Any patient has the potential to faint (Fig. 9-12) before, during, immediately following, or shortly after venipuncture. Some patients become faint at just the thought or sight of their blood being drawn, especially if they are ill or have been fasting for an extended period. Other contributing factors include anemia, dehydration, emotional problems, fatigue, hypoglycemia, hyperventilation, medications, nausea, needle phobia, and poor or compromised breathing.

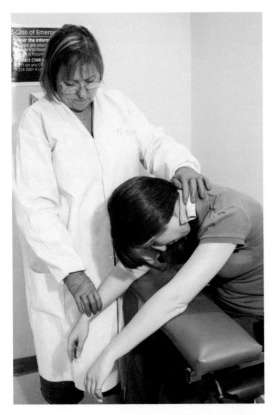

Figure 9-12 Phlebotomist caring for a patient who feels faint.

> 🔑 **Key Point** Sudden faintness or loss of consciousness caused by a nervous system response to abrupt pain, stress, or trauma is called **vasovagal** (relating to vagus nerve action on blood vessels) syncope.

Before beginning a venipuncture, phlebotomists should routinely ask patients if they have ever had a problem with a venipuncture. If the patient has felt faint or fainted on a prior venipuncture they will usually offer this information. A patient with a history of fainting should be asked to lie down for the procedure, no matter how long ago the fainting occurred.

> 🔑 **Key Point** A patient who appears to be extremely nervous, hyperventilates, or expresses fear or anxiety over the procedure should be considered at risk for fainting, nausea or vomiting.

A patient with a history of fainting should be asked to lie down for the procedure. Patients who feel faint just before or even after venipuncture should be asked to lie down until recovered. Inpatients, who typically are already lying down, rarely faint during blood draws. Outpatients are more likely to faint because they are usually sitting up during venipuncture.

Blood collection personnel should routinely ask patients how they are doing during a draw, watch for signs of fainting, and be prepared to protect them from falling. Signs to watch for include pallor (paleness), perspiration, and hyperventilation or an indication from the patient that he or she is experiencing vertigo (a sensation of spinning), dizziness, light-headedness, nausea, a darkening or constricting field of vision (tunnel vision), and sound fading into the background. Fainting can occur without any warning, so never turn your back on a patient. See Procedure 9-2 for steps to follow if a patient complains of feeling faint or exhibits symptoms of fainting during venipuncture.

> ⚠️ **CAUTION** Do not use ammonia inhalants to revive patients who have fainted as they can have unwanted side effects such as respiratory distress in asthmatic individuals.

When a patient who has fainted regains consciousness, he or she should remain in the area for at least 15 minutes. The patient should be instructed *not* to operate a vehicle for at least 30 minutes. It is important for the phlebotomist to document the incident (following institutional policy) in case of future litigation.

> 🔑 **Key Point** If a urine test is ordered along with blood tests on an outpatient, it is best to ask the patient to collect the urine specimen first. Otherwise, the patient could become faint after the venipuncture and pass out in the restroom with the door locked.

NAUSEA AND VOMITING

It is not unusual to have a patient experience nausea before, during, or after a blood draw. The patient may state that he or she is feeling nauseous or show signs similar to fainting, such as becoming pale or having beads of sweat appear on the forehead. A blood draw should not be attempted until the experience subsides. A blood draw that is in progress should be discontinued.

> 🔑 **Key Point** If the patient vomits during venipuncture, the procedure must be terminated immediately.

The patient should be reassured and made as comfortable as possible. A feeling of nausea often precedes vomiting, so it is a good idea to give the patient an emesis basin or wastebasket to hold as a precaution. Ask the patient to breathe slowly and deeply. Apply a

Procedure 9-2: Steps to Follow If a Patient Starts to Faint During Venipuncture

PURPOSE: To properly handle a patient who feels faint or shows symptoms of fainting during a blood draw

EQUIPMENT: Cold compress such as a washcloth dipped in cold water

Step	Explanation/Rationale
1. Release the tourniquet and remove and discard the needle as quickly and safely as possible.	Discontinuing the draw and safely discarding the needle protects the phlebotomist and patient from injury should the patient faint.
2. Apply pressure to the site while having the patient lower the head and breathe deeply.	Pressure must be applied to prevent bleeding or bruising. Lowering the head and breathing deeply helps get oxygenated blood to the brain.
3. Talk to the patient.	Diverts patient's attention, helps keep the patient alert, and aids in assessing the patient's responsiveness.
4. Physically support the patient.	Prevents injury in case of collapse.
5. Ask permission and explain what you are doing if it is necessary to loosen a tight collar or tie.	Avoids misinterpretation of actions that are standard protocol to hasten recovery.
6. Apply a cold compress or wet washcloth to the forehead and back of the neck	Is thought to hasten recovery.
7. Have someone stay with the patient until recovery is complete.	Prevents patient from getting up too soon and possibly causing self-injury.
8. Call first aid personnel if the patient does not respond.	Emergency medicine is not in the phlebotomist's scope of practice.
9. Document the incident according to facility protocol.	Legal issues could arise, and documentation is essential at that time.

cold, damp washcloth or other cold compress to the patient's forehead. If the patient vomits, provide tissues or a washcloth to wipe the face and water to rinse the mouth. If the patient is NPO for surgery, other procedures, or otherwise not allowed to have water, advise him or her to spit the water out after rinsing and not swallow any. Notify the patient's nurse, physician, or appropriate first aid personnel of the incident.

PAIN

A small amount of pain is normally associated with routine venipuncture and capillary puncture. Putting patients at ease before blood collection helps them relax and can make the procedure less painful. Warning the patient prior to needle insertion helps avoid a startle reflex. A stinging sensation can be avoided by allowing the alcohol to dry completely prior to needle insertion.

Key Point Excessive, deep, blind, or lateral redirection of the needle is considered probing. It can be very painful to the patient; risks injury to arteries, nerves, and other tissues; and should never be attempted.

Marked or extreme pain, numbness of the arm, a burning or electric shock sensation, or pain that radiates up or down the arm during a venipuncture attempt indicates nerve involvement and requires immediate removal of the needle. If pain persists after needle removal, the patient's physician or other appropriate personnel should be consulted and the incident documented. Application of an ice pack to the site after needle removal can help prevent or reduce inflammation associated with nerve involvement. Follow your healthcare facility's protocol.

CAUTION If you sense that the patient is in pain, or the patient complains of marked or extreme pain, or asks you to remove the needle for any reason, the venipuncture should be terminated immediately, even if there are no other signs of nerve injury.

PETECHIAE

Petechiae (Fig. 9-13) are tiny, nonraised red, purple, or brownish colored spots that appear on the patient's skin when a tourniquet is applied. The spots are minute drops of blood that escape the capillaries and come to

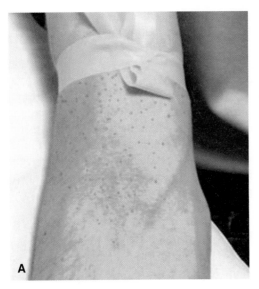

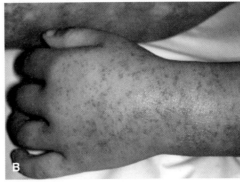

Figure 9-13 Petechiae. **A:** Adult arm. (Copyright Medical Training Solutions. Used with permission.) **B:** Hand of child with low platelet count. (Reprinted with permission from McConnell TH. *The Nature of Disease Pathology for the Health Professions.* Philadelphia, PA: Lippincott Williams & Wilkins; 2007.)

the surface of the skin below the tourniquet. Examples of causes include capillary wall defects, platelet abnormalities, certain medications such as aspirin, and some infectious and inflammatory diseases. They are not normally an indication that the phlebotomist has used incorrect procedure, unless the tourniquet has been incorrectly applied exceedingly tight. However, they are an indication that the venipuncture site may bleed excessively.

> ℹ️ Petechiae are generally less than 3 mm in diameter. Nonraised blood spots larger than 5 mm are called ecchymoses.

SEIZURES/CONVULSIONS

Seizures have been known to occur during venipuncture, although there is no evidence that they can be caused by venipuncture. In the rare event that a patient has a seizure or goes into convulsions during blood specimen collection, it is important to discontinue the draw immediately. Hold pressure over the site without restricting the patient's movement. Call for help to ease the patient to the floor and turn him or her to one side to keep the airway clear. Put something soft under the head. Loosen a tie, collar button, or anything else restrictive that could make breathing difficult. Try to protect the patient from self-injury without completely restricting movement of the extremities. Time the seizure and notify the appropriate first aid personnel.

> 🔑 **Key Point** Do not attempt to put anything into the patient's mouth to hold the tongue down. Contrary to popular belief, a person having a seizure cannot swallow the tongue.

Procedural Error Risks

HEMATOMA FORMATION AND BRUISING

Hematoma formation is the most common complication of venipuncture. It is caused by blood leaking into the tissues during or following venipuncture and is identified by rapid swelling at near or beneath the venipuncture site. (See Box 9-1 for situations that can trigger hematoma formation.)

Box 9-1

Situations That Can Trigger Hematoma Formation

- An artery is accidentally punctured
- Excessive or blind probing is used to locate the vein
- The vein is fragile or too small for the needle size
- The needle is only partly inserted into the vein
- The needle penetrates all the way through the vein
- The needle is removed while the tourniquet is still on
- Pressure is not adequately applied following venipuncture
- The arm is folded to hold the gauze in place after venipuncture

Match risks to procedural errors in the WORKBOOK activity Matching 9-5.

thePoint. *Watch a hematoma form in the Needle Positions, Bevel Partially into the Vein animation at http://thePoint.lww.com/McCall6e.*

⚠ CAUTION A rapidly forming hematoma may indicate that an artery has been accidentally hit. Discontinue the draw immediately and apply direct forceful pressure to the puncture site for a minimum of 5 minutes until active bleeding ceases.

A hematoma is painful to the patient, typically results in unsightly bruising (see Figure 9-3) and makes the site unacceptable for subsequent venipuncture. (See "Hematoma" under "Problem Sites".)

Continuing to draw blood while a hematoma is forming risks injury to the patient, as hematomas and large areas of pooled blood within the arm have been known to cause compression injuries to nerves and lead to lawsuits. The pooled blood can also migrate to lower areas of the arm (Fig. 9-3, bottom right photo) depending on the position of the arm. In addition, continuing the draw could potentially result in collection of a specimen contaminated with hematoma blood that has mixed with tissue fluids outside the vein. This is especially true if the draw is difficult and the needle is not correctly or completely within the vein.

If a hematoma forms during blood collection, the phlebotomist should discontinue the draw immediately and hold forceful pressure over the site for several minutes, and 3 to 5 minutes if accidental arterial puncture is suspected. A small amount of blood under the skin is relatively harmless and generally resolves on its own. If the hematoma is large and causes swelling and discomfort, the arm should be elevated, and the patient offered a cold compress or ice pack to relieve pain and reduce swelling. Follow facility protocol.

ⓘ Acetaminophen or ibuprofen can help to relieve discomfort from a hematoma. Ice applied in the first 24 hours helps manage the swelling and discomfort. After 24 hours, application of heat or warm, moist compresses can encourage the resorption of accumulated blood.

Bruising following venipuncture can be minimized by using adequate site compression after the draw and ensuring that bleeding has stopped not just on the surface of the skin, but at the vein site of needle entry as well.

IATROGENIC ANEMIA

Iatrogenic is an adjective used to describe an adverse condition brought on by the effects of treatment. Blood loss as a result of blood removed for testing is called iatrogenic blood loss. Removing blood on a regular basis or in large quantities can lead to iatrogenic anemia in some patients, especially infants.

 A primary reason for blood transfusion in neonatal ICU patients is to replace iatrogenic blood loss.

Blood loss to a point where life cannot be sustained is called **exsanguination**. Life may be threatened if more than 10% of a patient's blood volume is removed at one time or over a short period of time. Coordination with physicians to minimize the number of draws per patient, following quality assurance procedures to minimize redraws, collecting minimum required specimen volumes, especially from infants, and keeping a log of draws can help reduce iatrogenic blood loss.

There are a lot of new terms in this chapter. See how many you can unscramble in the WORKBOOK Knowledge Drill 9-2 Scrambled Words activity.

INADVERTENT ARTERIAL PUNCTURE

Inadvertent arterial puncture is rare when proper venipuncture procedures are followed. It is most often associated with deep or blind probing, especially in the area of the basilic vein, which is in close proximity to the brachial artery. If an inadvertent arterial puncture goes undetected, leakage and accumulation of blood in the area can result in compression injury to a nearby nerve. Such injuries are often permanent and can lead to lawsuits.

Signs of inadvertent arterial puncture include a rapidly forming hematoma and blood filling the tube very quickly. In the absence of these clues, arterial blood can be recognized by the fact that it spurts or pulses into the tube or by its bright red color if the patient's pulmonary function is normal. If arterial puncture is suspected, terminate the venipuncture immediately and apply direct forceful pressure to the site for 3 to 5 minutes and until bleeding stops.

Key Point If you think a specimen might be arterial blood, check with laboratory personnel to determine if a suspected arterial specimen is acceptable for testing, as opposed to redrawing more blood from the patient. If testing is permitted, identify the specimen as possible arterial blood, since some test values are different for arterial specimens.

INFECTION

Although a rare occurrence, infection at the site following venipuncture does happen. The risk of infection can be minimized by the use of proper aseptic technique, which includes the following:

- Do not open adhesive tape or bandages ahead of time or temporarily tape them to your lab coat cuffs or other contaminated objects.
- Do not preload (i.e., attach) needles onto tube holders to have a supply for many draws ready ahead of time. The sterility of the needle is breached once the seal is broken.
- Allow the alcohol to dry prior to needle insertion to achieve optimum bacteriostatic action.
- Before or during needle insertion, do not touch the site with your finger, glove, gauze, or any other non-sterile object after it has been cleaned.
- Try to minimize the time between removing the needle cap and performing the venipuncture.
- Remind the patient to keep the bandage on for at least 15 minutes after specimen collection.

NERVE INJURY

Though relatively rare, nerve injury is a serious phlebotomy complication that can result in permanent damage to motor or sensory nerve function of the arm or hand (Fig. 9-14) and the probability of a lawsuit. There

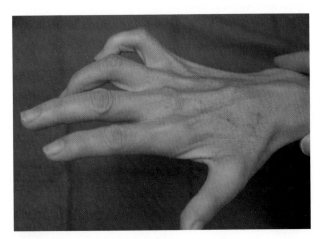

Figure 9-14 Abnormal hand position called "Claw hand" caused by ulnar nerve injury.

are two basic types of nerve injury as a consequence of venipuncture procedures. One involves the needle directly contacting the nerve in the form of a nick or puncture, the other results from a compression injury to the nerve rather than direct contact by the needle.

A nick or puncture to a nerve is usually the result of poor technique such as improper site or vein selection, inserting the needle too deeply or quickly, excessive or lateral redirection of the needle, or blind probing while attempting venipuncture. Another cause is startle reflex movement by the patient who has not been warned of imminent needle insertion. If initial needle insertion does not result in successful vein entry and slight forward or backward movement of the needle or use of a new tube does not result in blood flow, the needle should be removed and venipuncture attempted at an alternate site, preferably on the opposite arm. Knowledge of arm anatomy and CLSI venipuncture standards for site selection, vein selection, and venipuncture technique can minimize the risk of problems. Quick action in removing the needle if symptoms of nerve involvement do occur (see Caution) can minimize damage and help prevent permanent, painful disability. Application of an ice pack to the site after needle removal can help prevent or reduce inflammation associated with nerve involvement.

CAUTION Extreme pain, a burning or electric shock sensation, numbness of the arm, and pain that radiates up or down the arm are all signs of nerve involvement, and any one of them requires immediate termination of the venipuncture. Do not ask the patient if you should stop the draw. The patient may not understand the seriousness of the situation and allow you to continue.

Nerve compression injuries can occur from blood pooling and clotting beneath the vein as a result of accidental arterial puncture or blood leaking from the vein because the needle went all the way through it on initial needle entry. (See also Hematoma Formation and Bruising.) Nerve compression can also occur from a tourniquet that is too tight or left on too long. Although significant pain may be present at the time of venipuncture, a compression injury is harder for the phlebotomist to detect because swelling and numbness from nerve compression usually does not occur for 24 to 96 hours.

Key Point If significant pain or any other sign of nerve injury occurs, the incident should be documented, reported to the patient's healthcare provider, and the patient directed to seek the healthcare provider's advice should symptoms persist, according to facility protocol.

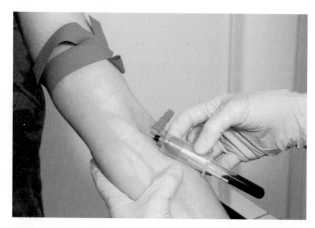

Figure 9-15 Correct filling of tube to avoid reflux.

REFLUX OF ADDITIVE

In rare instances, it is possible for blood to **reflux** (flow back) into the patient's vein from the collection tube during the venipuncture procedure. Reflux is thought to be caused by a normal variation in pressure in the patient's vein or the sudden drop in pressure on the vein when the tourniquet is released. Some patients have had adverse reactions to tube additives, particularly EDTA, that were attributed to reflux. Reflux can occur when the contents of the collection tube are in contact with the needle while the specimen is being drawn. To prevent reflux, the patient's arm must be kept in a downward position so that the collection tube remains below the venipuncture site and fills from the bottom up (Fig. 9-15). This prevents the tube holder end of the needle from being in contact with blood in the tube. Moving the tube in a manner that creates back-and-forth movement of blood in the tube should also be avoided until the tube is removed from the evacuated tube holder.

Key Point If the blood is flowing slowly into an anticoagulant tube and the phlebotomist feels the need to mix the tube to prevent clotting, it should be removed from the holder, mixed, and quickly replaced in the holder to continue the draw.

An outpatient can be asked to lean forward and extend the arm downward over the arm of the drawing chair to achieve proper positioning. Raising the head of the bed, extending the patient's arm over the side of the bed, or supporting the arm with a rolled towel or folded pillow can be used to help achieve proper positioning of a patient who is lying down.

thePoint *View the Reflux animation at* *http://thePoint.lww.com/McCall6e.*

Sometimes, when venipuncture is performed using a butterfly, blood initially flows into the tubing, but then some of it starts to disappear back into the vein before the tube is engaged. This is an example of reflux; however, since the tube is not engaged, there is no danger of additive reflux.

VEIN DAMAGE

Properly performed, an occasional venipuncture will not impair the patency of a patient's vein. Numerous venipunctures in the same area over an extended period of time, however, will eventually cause a buildup of scar tissue and increase the difficulty of performing subsequent venipunctures. Blind probing and improper technique when redirecting the needle can also damage veins and impair vein patency.

Specimen Quality Concerns

The quality of a blood specimen can be compromised by improper collection techniques. A poor-quality specimen will generally yield poor-quality results, which can affect the patient's care. Because it is not always apparent to the phlebotomist or testing personnel when the quality of a specimen has been compromised, it is very important for the phlebotomist to be aware of the following pitfalls of collection.

HEMOCONCENTRATION

Test your knowledge of hemoconcentration with Knowledge Drill 9-6 in the WORKBOOK.

Tourniquet application causes localized **venous stasis**, or stagnation of the normal venous blood flow. (A similar term for this is **venostasis**, the trapping of blood in an extremity by compression of veins.) In response, some of the plasma and filterable components of the blood pass through the capillary walls into the tissues. This results in hemoconcentration, a decrease in the fluid content of the blood with a subsequent increase in nonfilterable large molecule or protein-based blood components such as RBCs. Other abnormally increased analytes include albumin, ammonia, calcium, cholesterol, coagulation factors, enzymes, iron, potassium, and total protein. Changes that occur within 1 minute of tourniquet application are slight; however, prolonged tourniquet application can lead to marked changes.

Cholesterol levels can increase up to 5% after 2 minutes of tourniquet application and up to 15% after 5 minutes.

Heavy massaging of the site, probing for veins, long-term IV therapy, drawing blood from sclerosed or occluded veins, and vigorous hand pumping (making and releasing a fist) can also result in the collection of specimens affected by hemoconcentration.

> 🔑 **Key Point** Hand or fist pumping can increase blood potassium levels up to 20%. It is reported to be responsible for a third of all elevated potassium levels and may also increase lactate and phosphate levels.

Test results on hemoconcentrated specimens may not accurately reflect the patient's true status, so it is important to try to avoid them. A list of ways to prevent hemoconcentration during venipuncture is presented in Box 9-2.

thePoint *View the Hemolysis animation at http://thePoint.lww.com/McCall6e.*

HEMOLYSIS

Hemolysis results when RBCs are damaged or destroyed and the hemoglobin they contain escapes into the fluid portion of the specimen. The red color of the hemoglobin makes the serum or plasma appear pink (slight hemolysis), dark pink to light red (moderate hemolysis), to dark red (gross hemolysis), and the specimen is described as being "**hemolyzed**" (Fig. 9-16). Hemolyzed specimens can result from patient conditions such as hemolytic anemia, liver disease, or a transfusion reaction, but they are more commonly the result of procedural errors in specimen collection or handling that damages the RBCs. Hemolysis can erroneously elevate a number of analytes, especially

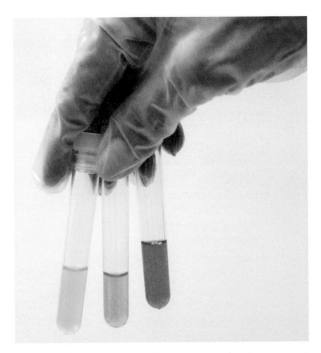

Figure 9-16 Left to right: Normal serum specimen, specimen with slight hemolysis, and grossly hemolyzed specimen.

potassium. (There is 23 times as much potassium in RBCs as in plasma.) Hemolysis also elevates ammonia, catecholamines, creatine kinase and other enzymes, iron, magnesium, and phosphate. RBC counts can be decreased by hemolysis. A specimen that is hemolyzed as a result of procedural error will most likely have to be redrawn. Box 9-3 lists procedural errors that can cause hemolysis.

> 🔑 **Key Point** A common procedural error by healthcare personnel that causes hemolysis is drawing blood through an IV valve. IV valves are designed to prevent backflow of IV solution by allowing fluid to move in only one direction. Consequently the force required to pull blood through a valve in the opposite direction can hemolyze the specimen.

PARTIALLY FILLED TUBES

ETS tubes should be filled until the normal amount of vacuum is exhausted. Failing to do so results in a partially filled tube (Fig. 9-17), referred to as a short draw. Inadvertent (unintentional) short draws are usually the result of difficult draw situations in which blood flow stops or vacuum is lost during needle manipulation. Short-draw serum tubes such as red tops and SSTs are generally acceptable for testing as long as the specimen is not hemolyzed and there is sufficient specimen to perform the test. Underfilled anticoagulant tubes and most other additive tubes, however, may not contain the blood-to-additive ratio for which the tube was designed.

Box 9-2

Ways to Help Prevent Hemoconcentration During Venipuncture

- Ask the patient to release the fist upon blood flow
- Choose an appropriate patent vein
- Do not allow the patient to pump the fist
- Do not excessively massage the area in locating a vein
- Do not probe or redirect the needle multiple times in search of a vein
- Release the tourniquet within 1 minute

Box 9-3

Procedural Errors That Can Cause Specimen Hemolysis

- Drawing blood through a hematoma
- Failure to wipe away the first drop of capillary blood, which can contain alcohol residue
- Forceful aspiration of blood during a syringe draw
- Forcing the blood from a syringe into an evacuated tube
- Frothing of blood caused by improper fit of the needle on a syringe
- Horizontal transport of tubes, which lets the blood slosh back and forth
- Mixing additive tubes vigorously, shaking them, or inverting them too quickly or forcefully
- Partially filling a normal-draw sodium fluoride tube
- Pulling back the plunger too quickly during a syringe draw
- Rough handling during transport
- Squeezing the site during capillary specimen collection
- Syringe transfer delay in which partially clotted blood is forced into a tube
- Using a large-volume tube with a small-diameter butterfly needle
- Using a needle with a diameter that is too small for venipuncture

Although in some cases underfilled additive tubes may be accepted for testing, the specimens can be compromised. For example:

- Excess EDTA in underfilled lavender-top tubes can shrink RBCs, causing erroneously low blood cell counts and hematocrits and negatively affecting the morphological examination of the RBCs on a blood smear. It can also alter the staining characteristics of the cells on a blood smear.

- Excess heparin in plasma from underfilled green-top tubes may interfere with the testing of some chemistry analytes.

- Excess sodium fluoride in underfilled gray-top tubes can result in hemolysis of the specimen.

- Underfilled coagulation tubes do not have the correct blood-to-additive ratio and will produce erroneous results.

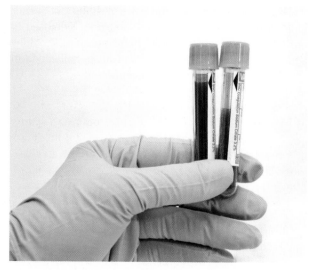

Figure 9-17 Light blue-top coagulation specimens. Tube on the left filled to the proper level. Tube on the right is underfilled.

 CAUTION Never pour two partially filled additive tubes together to fill one tube, as this will also affect the blood-to-additive ratio.

Phlebotomists sometimes underfill tubes on purpose when it is inadvisable to obtain larger quantities of blood, as when drawing from infants, children, or severely anemic individuals.

This is never advisable since partial vacuum tubes are available that are the same size as standard-fill tubes but designed to contain a smaller volume of blood. These tubes can be used in situations where it is difficult or inadvisable to draw larger amounts of blood. They are sometimes referred to as "short-draw" tubes, but when they are filled properly, the blood-to-additive ratio is correct even though they contain less blood. Some manufacturers' short-draw tubes have a line or arrow on the label to indicate the proper fill level (Fig. 9-18).

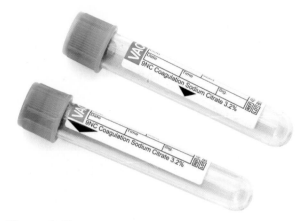

Figure 9-18 Normal-draw tube shown with "short-draw" tube designed for partial filling. Arrow on tube indicates proper fill level.

⚠ **CAUTION** Some phlebotomists underfill tubes to save time. This practice is never recommended.

SPECIMEN CONTAMINATION

Specimen contamination is typically inadvertent and generally the result of improper technique or carelessness, such as:

- Allowing alcohol, fingerprints, glove powder, baby powder, or urine from wet diapers to contaminate newborn screening forms or specimens, leading to specimen rejection.
- Filling tubes in the wrong order of draw. For example, drawing a potassium EDTA tube before a serum or plasma tube for chemistry tests can lead to EDTA contamination of the chemistry tube and cause false hyperkalemia (high potassium) and hypocalcemia (low calcium).
- Getting glove powder on blood films (slides) or in capillary specimens, resulting in misinterpretation of results. Calcium-containing powders can affect calcium results.
- Unwittingly dripping perspiration into capillary specimens during collection or any specimen during processing or testing. The salt in sweat, for example, can affect sodium and chloride levels.
- Using the correct antiseptic but not following proper procedure. For example, improperly cleaning blood-culture bottle tops or the collection site, touching the site after it has been prepped (cleansed), or inserting the needle before the antiseptic on the arm or bottle tops is dry. (Traces of the antiseptic in the culture medium can inhibit the growth of bacteria and cause false-negative results.) Performing capillary puncture before the alcohol is dry can cause hemolysis of the specimen and lead to inaccurate results or rejection of the specimen by the lab.
- Using the wrong antiseptic to clean the site prior to specimen collection. For example, using alcohol to clean the site can contaminate an ethanol (blood alcohol) specimen. Using povidone–iodine (e.g., Betadine) to clean a skin-puncture site can contaminate the specimen and cause erroneously high levels of uric acid, phosphate, and potassium.

WRONG OR EXPIRED COLLECTION TUBE

Drawing a specimen in the wrong tube can affect test results and jeopardize patient safety if the error is not caught before testing. The error may not be caught if the phlebotomist is also the one who processes the specimen, as it is impossible to visually tell serum from plasma, or one type of plasma from another, if the specimen has been removed from the cells and transferred to an aliquot tube. A phlebotomist who is not certain of the type of tube required for a particular test must consult the procedure manual before collecting the specimen.

Additives in expired tubes may not work properly. For example, expired anticoagulant may allow the formation of microclots. In addition expired tubes may have lost vacuum and result in short draws if used. Consequently, expiration dates of tubes must be checked routinely and expired tubes discarded.

Troubleshooting Failed Venipuncture

Failure to initially draw blood during a venipuncture attempt can be caused by a number of procedural errors. Being aware of these errors and knowing how to correct them may determine whether you obtain blood on the first try or have to repeat the procedure. If you fail to obtain blood after inserting the needle, stop all needle movement, remain calm so that you can clearly analyze and assess the situation, and correct the problem, which could be any one of the following situations.

🔑 **Key Point** Remember, to troubleshoot failed venipuncture the important steps are: STOP, ASSESS, & CORRECT.

📖 **Test your venipuncture troubleshooting abilities with the WORKBOOK Labeling Exercise 9-1.**

TUBE POSITION

Tube position is important. Check the tube to see that it is properly seated and the needle in the tube holder has penetrated the tube stopper. Reseat the tube to make certain that the needle sleeve is not pushing the tube off the needle.

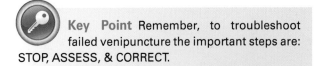 the**Point** *View the needle position animations at http://thePoint.lww.com/McCall6e.*

NEEDLE POSITION

Insertion of the venipuncture needle so that the bevel is correctly positioned within the vein is critical to the success of venipuncture. If the needle or bevel is incorrectly positioned, blood may not flow into the tube or syringe properly or at all. If blood flow is not established or the rate of flow is not normal, use visual cues to help determine if the needle is correctly positioned in the vein. Some problems are harder to discern than others. Eliminate any that you can and try the remedy for the others to see if one works. All needle adjustments must be made slowly and precisely to avoid injuring the patient. Correct needle position is shown in (Fig. 9-19A).

Needle Not Inserted Far Enough

If the needle is not inserted far enough, it may not penetrate the vein at all (Fig. 9-19B). This can happen if the vein is located more deeply than normal (e.g., if the patient is obese, or extremely overweight). In this case

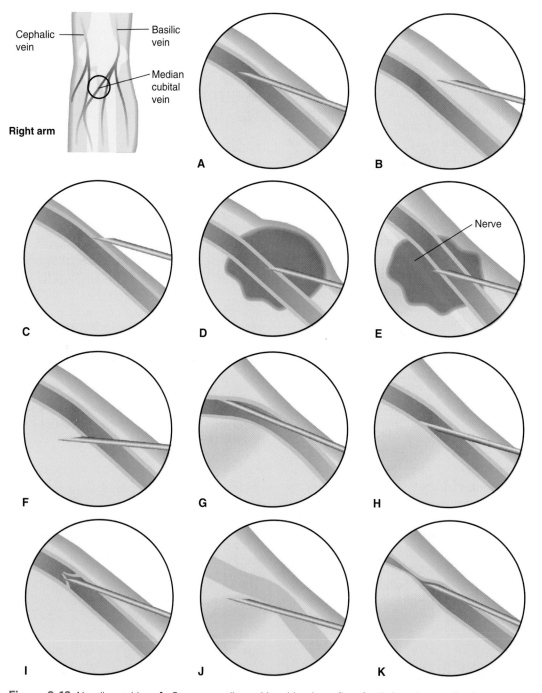

Figure 9-19 Needle position. **A:** Correct needle position; blood can flow freely into the needle. **B:** Needle not inserted far enough; needle does not enter vein. **C:** Needle bevel partially out of the skin; tube vacuum will be lost. **D:** Needle bevel partially into the vein; causes blood leakage into tissue. **E:** Needle bevel partially through the vein; causes blood leakage into tissue. **F:** Needle bevel completely through the vein; no blood flow obtained. **G:** Needle bevel against the upper vein wall prevents blood flow. **H:** Needle bevel against the lower vein wall prevents blood flow. **I:** Needle bevel penetrating a valve prevents blood flow. **J:** Needle beside the vein; caused when a vein rolls to the side, no blood flow obtained. **K:** Collapsed vein prevents blood flow despite correct needle position.

there will be no blood flow at all. To correct this problem, slowly advance the needle forward until blood flow is established.

> ⚠ **CAUTION** One must be very certain that needle depth is the issue before advancing the needle, as the deeper a needle goes, the greater the chance of injuring a nerve, artery, or other tissue.

Bevel Partially out of the Skin

If the needle bevel is not completely under the skin after it is inserted the tube will lose its vacuum when engaged and fail to fill with blood even if the bevel is mostly in the vein. This can happen with arm veins that are close to the surface of the skin as well as hand veins, especially if the angle of needle entry is too steep. Tube vacuum can also be lost if the bevel backs out of the skin slightly (Fig. 9-19C) during a draw; for example, if the holder is not held securely when the tube is removed from it. A short hissing sound is often heard as the vacuum is lost, and there may be a spurt of blood into the tube before blood flow stops. Discard the tube and advance the needle slowly until the bevel is under the skin before engaging a new tube. A hand vein may require you to thread the needle bevel within the lumen of the vein slightly. If the angle is too steep and the vein is small, the bevel may go through the vein before it is completely under the skin, in which case the venipuncture will have to be terminated and a new site chosen.

> ⓘ A patient who hears the hissing sound when the tube vacuum is lost during a draw may be alarmed and need reassurance that nothing harmful has happened.

Bevel Partially into the Vein

If the needle is not inserted deeply enough, the bevel may be beneath the skin but only partly through the upper vein wall (Fig. 9-19D), resulting in the blood filling the tube very slowly. Correct blood flow should be established by gently pushing the needle forward into the vein. If not corrected quickly, partial needle insertion can cause blood to leak into the tissue and form a hematoma. If this occurs, discontinue the draw immediately and hold pressure over the site.

> ⚠ **CAUTION** Continuing the draw while a hematoma is forming increases the risk of injury to the patient and the collection of blood from outside the vein; this blood would be contaminated with tissue fluids and is very likely to be hemolyzed.

Bevel Partially Through the Vein

If the needle is inserted too deeply, too quickly, or at an angle that is too steep, part of the bevel may go through the lower wall of the vein (Fig. 9-19E). If this is not corrected quickly, blood can leak into the tissue below the vein and result in hematoma formation, which may not be apparent until long after the draw is completed. If the needle appears to be inserted deeply and blood fills the tube slowly, this may be the case. Slowly pull the needle back until normal blood flow is established. If it appears that a hematoma has already formed, discontinue the draw immediately, and hold pressure over the site.

> ⚠ **CAUTION** Blood that pools beneath a vein can put pressure on underlying nerves, causing pain and the possibility of nerve damage.

Bevel Completely Through the Vein

If the needle has gone in too deep, the bevel may penetrate all the way through the vein (Fig. 9-19F). In this case, there may be a small spurt of blood into the tube as the bevel goes through the vein, or there may be no blood flow at all. This can happen on needle insertion, especially if the needle angle is too steep, or as a tube is pushed onto the needle if the tube holder is not held steady. To correct this problem, slowly withdraw the needle until blood flow is established. If the needle position is not corrected quickly, blood may leak out around the needle into the tissues and form a hematoma. Even after correction, blood may still leak out of the opening caused by the needle, especially if the tourniquet is left on throughout the draw. This too can result in a hematoma that is not apparent until long after the draw is completed. If a hematoma is visible, discontinue the draw.

Bevel Against a Vein Wall

Blood flow can be impaired if the needle bevel is up against the upper or lower wall of the vein. This can happen if the needle angle is wrong. For example, an angle that is too shallow can cause the needle bevel to contact the upper wall (Fig. 9-19G). This can also happen if the needle is inserted near a bend in the vein or at a point where the vein goes deeper into the skin. An angle that is too steep, or inserting the needle with the bevel down, can cause the needle to contact the lower wall (Fig. 9-19H). Most of these situations are hard to detect. Remove the tube from the needle in the holder to release vacuum pull on the vein and pull the needle back slightly. (Rotating the bevel slightly may also help.) Advance the tube back onto the needle. If blood flow is established, the problem most likely was an issue with the bevel and the vein wall.

⚠️ **CAUTION** Tube vacuum may hold the vein wall against the needle bevel. Do not rotate the bevel of the needle without first removing the tube and pulling the needle back slightly or the vein may be injured.

Bevel in a Valve

Since veins have valves it is possible that the needle bevel could hit a valve (Fig. 9-19I) during a blood draw. In fact, the needle bevel could be in the middle of the lumen where it should be and still come in contact with valve tissue. The needle bevel could be stuck in the valve, or the valve flaps could be drawn up against the needle bevel by tube vacuum. Some phlebotomists say contact with a valve is evidenced by a slight vibration or quiver of the needle caused by the valve attempting to open and close. This situation must be corrected quickly or the valve could be damaged and lead to collapse of the vein. If you are certain the needle is in the vein and no blood is flowing into the tube this could be the problem, regardless of whether or not you sense a needle vibration or quiver. This problem is corrected similar to when the bevel is up against a vein wall. Remove the tube from the needle in the holder to release vacuum pull on the valve tissue and pull the needle back slightly. Advance the tube back onto the needle. If blood flow is not established the needle may still be so close to the valve that the vacuum pull of the tube draws the valve back onto the needle. In this case, discontinue the draw and perform a second venipuncture on a new site, preferably the other arm.

Needle Beside the Vein

Vein walls are sometimes tough, and if a vein is not anchored well with the thumb, it may roll (move away) slightly and the needle may slip to the side of the vein instead of into it (Fig. 9-19J). Often the needle ends up beside the vein and slightly under it as well. (This is often the case with the basilic vein, which is not well anchored in the tissue to begin with.) If this happens, disengage the tube to preserve the vacuum, withdraw the needle slightly until just the bevel is under the skin, anchor the vein securely, redirect the needle into the vein, and reengage the tube. If redirection is unsuccessful, discontinue the draw and choose a new site. Do not search or probe for the vein or move the needle in a lateral (sideways) direction to find it.

ⓘ When phlebotomists "miss" veins, they often tell patients that they have "veins that roll." This leads patients to mistakenly believe that there is a problem with their veins, when more than likely the problem is the phlebotomist's technique.

COLLAPSED VEIN

A vein can collapse despite correct needle position. When a vein collapses, the walls draw together temporarily, shutting off blood flow (Fig. 9-19K). This can happen if the vacuum draw of a tube or the pressure created by pulling on a syringe plunger is too much for the vein. A vein can also collapse if the tourniquet is tied too tightly or too close to the venipuncture site. In this case, blood cannot be replaced as quickly as it is withdrawn, causing the vein to collapse. In addition, veins sometimes collapse when the tourniquet is removed during the draw. This is often the case in elderly patients, whose veins are fragile and collapse more easily.

ⓘ Stoppage of blood flow upon tourniquet removal does not necessarily mean that the vein has collapsed. It may be that the needle is no longer positioned properly and a slight adjustment is needed to reestablish blood flow.

A clue that a normally visible vein has collapsed is that it disappears as soon as the tube is engaged or when the tourniquet is removed. If the ends of the tourniquet are lying over the arm, grasp them with your free hand and twist them together to reintroduce pressure. That may be enough to reestablish blood flow. If the tourniquet cannot be retightened, use your finger to apply pressure to the vein several inches above the needle. (Do not apply pressure too close to the needle as this can be painful to the patient and dangerous to the phlebotomist if the patient should feel pain and jerk the arm so that the needle comes out.) Another tactic to try is to remove the tube from the needle and wait a few seconds for the blood flow to reestablish before reengaging it. Try using a smaller-volume tube or pull more slowly on the plunger if you are using a syringe. If the blood flow is not reestablished, discontinue the venipuncture and attempt a second venipuncture at another site.

Undetermined Needle Position

If you cannot determine the position of the needle and the above solutions do not help, you may have to use your finger to relocate the vein. Remove the tube from the holder needle and withdraw the needle until the bevel is just under the skin. Clean your gloved finger with alcohol and palpate the arm above the point of needle insertion to try to determine needle position and vein location. Be careful not to feel too close to the needle, as this can hurt. Once you have relocated the vein, pull the skin taut and redirect the needle into it. If you cannot relocate the vein (or if access to it would require lateral redirection of the needle), discontinue the draw and select a new site.

CAUTION *Do not* blindly probe the arm in an attempt to locate a vein. Probing is painful to the patient and can cause tears in the vein wall that result in hematoma formation, damage nerves, and other tissues, or lead to inadvertent puncture of an artery.

TUBE VACUUM

A tube can lose its vacuum during a venipuncture if the needle bevel is not completely under the skin. (See "Bevel Partially Out of the Skin," explained earlier, and Fig. 9-19C.) Tubes can also lose vacuum during shipping and handling, when they bump one another in trays, if they are dropped, or if they are pushed too far onto the needle prior to venipuncture. If you suspect that a tube has lost its vacuum, try using a new one. If you fail to establish blood flow during a draw and repositioning the needle does not help, try using a new tube before giving up on the draw, as it could be a vacuum problem.

Case Study 9-3 in the WORKBOOK concerns the issue of a dropped tube.

Key Point Tube vacuum problems at the start of a draw may be a sign that the tube is cracked or has been dropped. Cracked tubes present a safety hazard because they may leak or break with further handling. Never use a tube that has been dropped. Discard it instead.

To test your overall knowledge of this chapter check out Knowledge Drill 9-3 in the WORKBOOK.

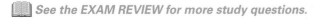

Study and Review Questions

📖 *See the EXAM REVIEW for more study questions.*

1. **Peak levels of this analyte typically occur around 08:00 hours.**
   a. Bilirubin
   b. Cortisol
   c. Eosinophil
   d. Glucose

2. **Which of these tests are most affected if the patient is not fasting?**
   a. CBC and protime
   b. Glucose and triglycerides
   c. RA and cardiac enzymes
   d. Blood culture and thyroid profile

3. **Veins that feel hard and cord-like when palpated may be:**
   a. collapsed.
   b. fistulas.
   c. thrombosed.
   d. venules.

4. **Tiny red spots that appear on a patient's arm when the tourniquet is applied are a sign that the**
   a. patient is allergic to nitrile.
   b. patient has anemia.
   c. site may bleed excessively.
   d. veins are sclerosed.

5. **When the arm of the patient is swollen with excess fluids, the condition is called**
   a. edema.
   b. hemolysis.
   c. icterus.
   d. syncope.

6. **A patient has several short lengths of IV-type tubing protruding from his chest. This is most likely a/an:**
   a. A-line.
   b. CVC.
   c. Port.
   d. PICC.

7. **Which of the following would be most likely to allow reflux to occur during venipuncture?**
   a. Filling the tube stopper end first
   b. Lateral redirection of the needle
   c. Tourniquet release on blood flow
   d. Using the wrong order of draw

8. **A patient complains of extreme pain when you insert the needle during a venipuncture attempt. The pain does not subside, but the patient does not feel any numbness or burning sensation. You know the needle is in the vein because the blood is flowing into the tube. You have only two tubes to fill, and the first one is almost full. What should you do?**

   a. Ask the patient if he or she wants you to continue the draw

   b. Discontinue the draw and attempt collection at another site

   c. Distract the patient with small talk and continue the draw

   d. Tell the patient to hang in there as you have only one tube left

9. **Which of the following situations can result in hemoconcentration?**

   a. Drawing a large tube with a small needle

   b. Leaving the tourniquet on over 1 minute

   c. Mixing the specimen too vigorously

   d. Partially filling a normal-draw tube

10. **You are in the process of collecting a specimen by venipuncture. You hear a hissing sound, there is a spurt of blood into the tube, and blood flow stops. What has most likely happened?**

    a. Reflux of tube contents

    b. The needle went too deep

    c. The vein has collapsed

    d. Tube vacuum escaped

11. **Most test result reference ranges are values for**

    a. healthy individuals.

    b. patients who are ill.

    c. people the same age.

    d. specific disorders.

12. **If a venipuncture fails to draw blood and the phlebotomist senses a slight vibration of the needle, this could be a sign that the needle**

    a. is up against a valve.

    b. penetrated a nerve.

    c. struck a hematoma.

    d. went through the vein.

13. **An arm that is paralyzed**

    a. has no muscle function.

    b. has sensory damage also.

    c. is a permanent condition.

    d. is the result of a stroke.

14. **A bariatric phlebotomy chair is designed for individuals who are**

    a. apt to faint.

    b. mentally ill.

    c. overweight.

    d. paralyzed.

15. **An AV fistula is most commonly used for**

    a. chemotherapy.

    b. dialysis access.

    c. drawing blood.

    d. fluid infusion.

Case Studies

 See the WORKBOOK for more case studies.

Case Study 9-1: Physiological Variables, Problem Sites, and Patient Complications

Charles is a phlebotomist who works in a physician's office laboratory. One morning shortly after the drawing station opens he is asked to collect blood specimens for a CBC and a glucose test from a very heavy set woman who appears quite ill. The patient tells Charles that she vomited all night and was unable to eat or drink anything. She also mentions that she has had a mastectomy on the left side and the last time she had blood collected she was stuck numerous times before the phlebotomist was able to collect the specimen.

QUESTIONS

1. What physiological variables may be associated with the collection of this specimen and how should they be dealt with?

2. What complications might Charles expect and how should he prepare for them?

3. How should Charles go about selecting the blood collection site?

4. What options does Charles have if he is unable to select a proper venipuncture site?

Case Study 9-2: Troubleshooting Failed Venipuncture

A phlebotomist named Sara is in the process of collecting a protime and CBC from a patient. The needle is in the patient's vein. As Sara pushes the first tube onto the needle in the tube holder, there is a spurt of blood into the tube and she hears a hissing sound. Then the blood stops flowing. She repositions the needle but is not able to establish blood flow.

QUESTIONS

1. Why did blood spurt into the tube and then stop?
2. What clues are there to determine what the problem is?
3. What can Sara do to correct the problem?

Bibliography and Suggested Readings

Baer DM, Ernst DJ, Willeford SI, Gambino R. Investigating elevated potassium values. MLO *Med Lab Obs.* 2006;38(11):24, 26, 30–31.

Bishop ML, Fody EP, Schoeff LE. *Clinical Chemistry: Principles, Procedures, Correlations.* 7th ed. Philadelphia, PA: Lippincott Williams & Wilkins; 2013.

Brigden ML, Heathcote JC. Problems in interpreting laboratory tests: What do unexpected results mean? *Postgrad Med.* 2000;107(7):145–146.

Burtis CA, Ashwood ER, Bruns DE. *Tietz Fundamentals of Clinical Chemistry and Molecular Diagnostics.* 7th ed. Philadelphia, PA: Elsevier/Saunders; 2015.

Cavalieri TA, Chopra A, Bryman PN. When outside the norm is normal: interpreting lab data in the aged. *Geriatrics.* 1992;47(5):66–70.

Clinical and Laboratory Standards Institute GP41-A7. *Procedures for the Collection of Diagnostic Blood Specimens by Venipuncture: Approved Standard.* 7th ed. Wayne, PA: CLSI; 2014.

Clinical and Laboratory Standards Institute GP42-A6. *Procedures and Devices for the Collection of Diagnostic Capillary Blood Specimens: Approved Standard.* 6th ed. Wayne, PA: CLSI; 2008.

College of American Pathologists (CAP). *So You're Going to Collect a Blood Specimen.* 14th ed. Northfield, IL: CAP; 2013.

Dale JC. Preanalytical variables in laboratory testing. *Lab Med.* 1998;29:540–545.

Dreskin SC. Urticaria and angioedema. In: Goldman L, Schafer AI, eds. *Goldman's Cecil Medicine.* Chapter 260. 24th ed. Philadelphia, PA: Saunders Elsevier; 2012.

Erickson VA, Pearson ML, Ganz PA, Adams J, Kahn KL. Arm edema in breast cancer patients. *J Natl Cancer Inst.* 2001;93(2):96–111.

Ernst DJ. *Applied Phlebotomy.* Baltimore, MD: Lippincott Williams & Wilkins; 2005.

Ernst DJ. *Blood Specimen Collection FAQs.* Ramsey, IN: Center for Phlebotomy Education; 2008.

Foran SE, Lewandrowski KB, Krantz A. Effects of exercise on laboratory test results. *Lab Med.* 2003;34:736–742.

Howanitz PJ. Errors in laboratory medicine: Practical lessons to improve patient safety. *Arch Pathol Lab Med.* 2005;129(10):1252–1261.

Lippi G, Salvagno GL, Montagnana M, Guidi GC. Short-term venous stasis influences routine coagulation testing. *Blood Coagul Fibrinolysis.* 2005;16(6):453–458.

Magee LS. Preanalytical variables in the chemistry laboratory. *Becton Dickinson Lab Notes.* 2005;15(1).

Mayo Foundation for Medical Education and Research. Postural and venous stasis–induced changes in total calcium. *Mayo Clin Proc.* 2005;80:1101.

McPherson RA, Pincus MR. *Henry's Clinical Diagnostics and Management by Laboratory Methods.* 22nd ed. Philadelphia, PA: Saunders; 2011.

Nursing 2008, upFront: Advice P.R.N.; Venipuncture, Armed with the facts. *Poststroke venipuncture sites.* 2008;38(6):10.

Rock RC. Interpreting laboratory tests: a basic approach. *Geriatrics.* 1984;39(1):49–50, 53–54.

Roda BF, Fritsma G, Doig K. *Hematology: Clinical Principles and Applications.* 3rd ed. Philadelphia, PA: Saunders; 2007.

Sharratt CL, Gilbert CJ, Cornes MC, Ford C, Gama R. EDTA sample contamination is common and often undetected, putting patients at unnecessary risk of harm. *Int J Clin Pract.* 2009;63(8):1259–1262.

Tryding N. *Drug Effects in Clinical Chemistry.* Washington, DC: AACC Press; 2007.

Tyndall L, Innamorato S. Managing preanalytical variability in hematology. *Becton Dickinson Lab Notes.* 2004;14(1).

Wians FH Jr. Clinical laboratory tests: which, why, and what do the results mean? *LabMed.* 2009;40:105–113.

Young DS. *Effects of preanalytical variables on clinical laboratory tests.* Washington, DC: AACC Press; 2007.

 MEDIA MENU

Online Ancillaries (at http://thepoint.lww.com/McCall6e)

- Animations:
  - Hemolysis
  - Needle positions:
    - Correct Needle Position
    - Needle Not Inserted Far Enough
    - Bevel Partially out of the Skin
    - Bevel Partially into the Vein
    - Bevel Partially Through the Vein
    - Bevel Completely Through the Vein
    - Bevel Against Upper Vein Wall
    - Bevel Against Lower Vein Wall
    - Bevel in a Valve
    - Needle Beside the Vein
    - Collapsed Vein
  - Reflux
- Videos:
  - How to Handle a Fainting Patient
- Interactive exercises and games, including Look and Label, Word Building, Body Building, Roboterms, Crossword Puzzles, Quiz Show, and Concentration
- Audio flash cards and flashcard generator
- Audio glossary

Internet Resources

- **BD Vacutainer (R) LabNotes-Preanalytical errors in the emergency department: http://www.bd.com/vacutainer/labnotes/Volume17Number1/**
- **Errors in Laboratory Medicine:** http://wwwn.cdc.gov/mlp/qiconference/Presentations/CDC%20Atlanta%20Plebani1.pdf
- **Preanalytical Variables:** http://www.thedoctorsdoctor.com/labtests/Preanalytical_variables.htm
- **Resource Center:** http://www.specimencare.com/
- **Troubleshooting Erroneous Potassium:** http://www.bd.com/vacutainer/pdfs/VS7048_troubleshooting_erroneous_potassiums_poster.pdf
- **Troubleshooting Hemolysis Issues in the Clinical Laboratory:** http://www.bd.com/vacutainer/labnotes/Volume16Number2/

Other Resources

- McCall R, Tankersley C. *Student Workbook for Phlebotomy Essentials.* 6th ed. (Available for separate purchase).
- McCall R, Tankersley C. *Phlebotomy Exam Review.* 6th ed. (Available for separate purchase.)

Chapter 10

Capillary Puncture Equipment and Procedures

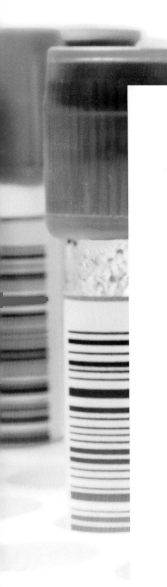

NAACLS Entry Level Competencies

3.6 Discuss the properties of arterial blood, venous blood, and capillary blood.

4.2 Describe the types of patient specimens that are analyzed in the clinical laboratory.

4.3 Define the phlebotomist's role in collecting and/or transporting these specimens to the laboratory.

4.4 List the general criteria for suitability of a specimen for analysis, and reasons for specimen rejection or recollection.

5.00 Demonstrate knowledge of collection equipment, various types of additives used, special precautions necessary, and substances that can interfere in clinical analysis of blood constituents.

5.5 List and select the types of equipment needed to collect blood by venipuncture and capillary (dermal) puncture.

5.6 Identify special precautions necessary during blood collections by venipuncture and capillary (dermal) puncture.

6.00 Follow standard operating procedures to collect specimens.

6.1 Identify potential sites for venipuncture and capillary (dermal) puncture.

6.3 Describe and demonstrate the steps in the preparation of a puncture site.

6.4 List the effects of tourniquet, hand squeezing, and heating pads on specimens collected by venipuncture and capillary (dermal) puncture.

6.6 Describe and perform correct procedure for capillary (dermal) collection methods.

6.7 Describe the limitations and precautions of alternate collection sites for venipuncture and capillary (dermal) puncture.

6.10 List the steps necessary to perform a venipuncture and a capillary (dermal) puncture in order.

6.12 Demonstrate a successful capillary (dermal) puncture following standard operating procedures.

Key Terms

 Do Matching Exercise 10-1 in the WORKBOOK to gain familiarity with these terms.

arterialized	calcaneus	differential	hypothyroidism
blood film/	CBGs	feather	interstitial
smear	cyanotic	galactosemia	fluid

intracellular fluid
lancet
microcollection
    containers

microhematocrit
    tubes
microtubes
neonatal screening

osteochondritis
osteomyelitis
PKU
plantar surface

posterior curvature
whorls

Objectives

Upon successful completion of this chapter, the reader should be able to:

1 Define and use capillary puncture terminology, identify capillary puncture equipment, and list the order of draw for capillary specimens and describe the theory behind it.

2 Describe capillary specimen composition, identify differences between capillary, arterial, and venous specimen composition and reference values, decide when capillary puncture is indicated, and demonstrate knowledge of site selection criteria.

3 Describe how to collect capillary specimens from adults, infants, and children, describe specimen collection procedures and explain the clinical significance of capillary blood gas, neonatal bilirubin, and newborn screening tests, and name tests that cannot be performed on capillary specimens and explain why.

4 Describe how to prepare both routine and thick blood smears, give reasons why they are sometimes made at the collection site, and identify tests performed on them.

Overview

Drops of blood for testing can be obtained by puncturing or making an incision in the capillary bed in the dermal layer of the skin with a lancet or other sharp device. Terms typically used to describe this technique include capillary, dermal, or skin puncture, regardless of the actual type of device or method used to penetrate the skin. The specimens obtained in this manner are respectively referred to as capillary, dermal, or skin puncture specimens. (To best reflect the nature and source of the specimen, and for simplification and consistency, the terms capillary specimen and capillary puncture are used in this chapter.) With the advent of laboratory instrumentation capable of testing small sample volumes, specimens for many laboratory tests can now be collected in this manner. This chapter covers capillary equipment, principles, collection sites, and procedures. Although steps may differ slightly, procedures in this chapter conform to CLSI Standards.

Key Point Capillary specimen collection is especially useful for pediatric patients in whom removal of larger quantities of blood by venipuncture can have serious consequences.

Capillary Puncture Equipment

In addition to blood collection supplies and equipment described in Chapter 7, the following special equipment may be required for skin puncture procedures.

LANCETS/INCISION DEVICES

A **lancet** is a sterile, disposable, sharp-pointed or bladed instrument that either punctures or makes an incision in the skin to obtain capillary blood specimens for testing. Lancets are available in a range of lengths and depths to accommodate various specimen collection requirements. Selection depends on the age of the patient, collection site, volume of specimen required, and the puncture depth needed to collect an adequate specimen without injuring bone. Lancets are specifically designed for either finger puncture (Fig. 10-1), or heel puncture (Fig. 10-2), and must have OSHA-required safety features.

Key Point An important OSHA-required lancet safety feature is a permanently retractable blade or needle point to reduce the risk of accidental sharps injury.

MICROCOLLECTION CONTAINERS/ MICROTUBES

Microcollection containers (Fig. 10-3), also called **microtubes**, are special small plastic tubes used to collect the tiny amounts of blood obtained from capillary punctures. They are often referred to as "**bullets**" because of their size and shape. Some come fitted with narrow plastic capillary tubes (Fig. 10-3B) to facilitate specimen collection. Most have color-coded bodies or caps/stoppers that correspond to color coding of ETS

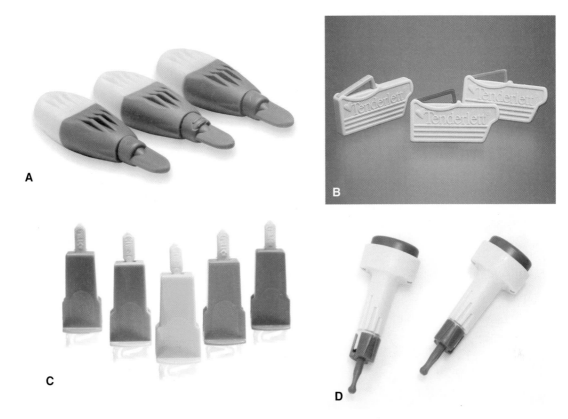

Figure 10-1 Several types of finger puncture lancets. **A:** BD Microtainer® contact activated lancets. (Courtesy Becton Dickinson, Franklin Lakes, NJ.) **B:** Tenderlett® toddler, junior, and adult lancets. (Courtesy ITC, Edison, NJ.) **C:** Capiject® safety lancets. (Courtesy Terumo Medical Corp., Somerset, NJ.) **D:** ACCU-CHEK® Safe-T-Pro Plus lancet with three depth settings. (Roche Diagnostics, Indianapolis, IN.)

blood collection tubes, and markings for minimum and maximum fill levels that are typically measured in microliters (μL), such as 250 μL and 500 μL, respectively (Fig. 10-3C). The BD Microtainer® MAP (Fig. 10-3E) has a penetrable septum for use with automated hematology systems. Some manufacturers print lot numbers and expiration dates on each tube.

> ⚠️ **CAUTION** Sometimes venous blood obtained by syringe during difficult draw situations is put into microtubes. When this is done, the specimen must be labeled as venous blood. Otherwise, it will be assumed to be a capillary specimen, which may have different reference ranges.

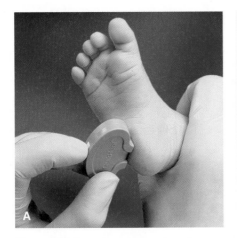

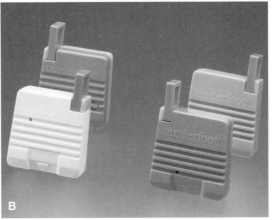

Figure 10-2 Several types of heel puncture lancets. **A:** BD QuikHeel™ infant lancet, also available in a preemie version. (Courtesy Becton Dickinson, Franklin Lakes, NJ.) **B:** Tenderfoot® toddler (*pink*), newborn (*pink/blue*), preemie (*white*), and micro-preemie (*blue*) heel incision devices. (Courtesy ITC, Edison, NJ.)

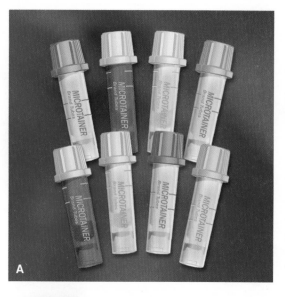

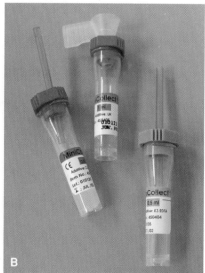

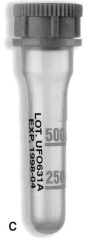

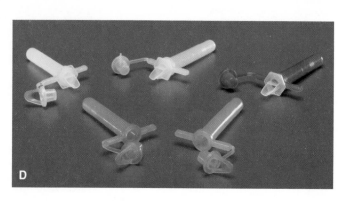

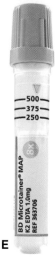

Figure 10-3 Examples of microcollection containers. **A:** Microtainer®. (Courtesy Becton Dickinson, Franklin Lakes, NJ.) **B:** MiniCollect® Capillary Blood Collection Tubes. (Courtesy of Greiner Bio-One International AG, Kremsmunster, Austria.) **C:** Capiject® EDTA Capillary Blood Collection Tube. (Terumo, Somerset, NJ.) **D:** Samplette™ capillary blood collection collectors. (Courtesy Tyco Healthcare, Kendall, Mansfield, MA.) **E:** BD Microtainer® MAP. (Courtesy Becton Dickinson, Franklin Lakes, NJ.)

MICROHEMATOCRIT TUBES AND SEALANTS

Microhematocrit tubes (Fig. 10-4) are disposable, narrow-bore plastic, or plastic-clad glass capillary tubes that fill by capillary action and typically hold 50 to 75 µL of blood. They are used primarily for manual hematocrit (Hct), also called packed cell volume (PCV), determinations. The tubes come coated with ammonium heparin, for collecting Hct tubes directly from a capillary puncture, or plain, to be used when an Hct tube is filled with blood from a lavender-top tube. Heparin tubes typically have a red or green band on one end; nonadditive tubes have a blue band. Smaller microhematocrit tubes designed for use with special microcentrifuges, such as those available from StatSpin, Inc. (Norwood, MA), require as little as 9 µL

of blood and are often used in infant and child anemia screening programs and pediatric clinics. Plastic, clay, or wax-type sealants that come in small trays are used to seal one end of microhematocrit tubes. Traditionally, the dry end of the tube was inserted into the clay to plug it. Because of safety concerns, it is now recommended that sealing methods be used that do not require manually pushing the tube into the sealant or products be used that measure Hct without centrifugation.

CAPILLARY BLOOD GAS EQUIPMENT

The following special equipment (Fig. 10-5) is used to collect **capillary blood gas (CBG)** specimens:

- *CBG collection tubes:* CBG collection tubes are long thin narrow-bore capillary tubes. They are normally

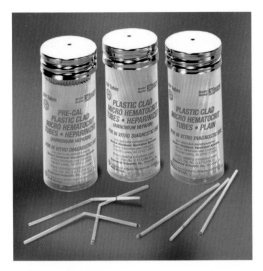

Figure 10-4 Plastic-Clad Microhematocrit tubes. (Courtesy Becton Dickinson, Franklin Lakes, NJ.)

plastic for safety and are available in a number of different sizes to accommodate volume requirements of various testing instruments. The most common CBG tubes are 100 mm in length with a capacity of 100 μL. The inside of the tube is coated with heparin, identified by a green band on the tube.

- *Stirrers:* Stirrers (e.g., small metal bars) are inserted into the tube after the blood is collected to aid in mixing the anticoagulant.
- *Magnet:* A magnet is used to mix the specimen after both ends of the tube have been sealed. The magnet typically has an opening in the center or side so that it can be slipped over the capillary tube and moved back and forth along the tube length, pulling the metal stirrer with it, and mixing the anticoagulant with the blood.

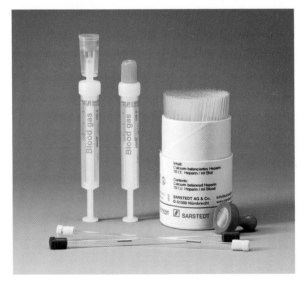

Figure 10-5 Capillary blood gas collection equipment displayed with arterial blood gas syringes. (Courtesy Sarstedt, Inc., Newton, NC.)

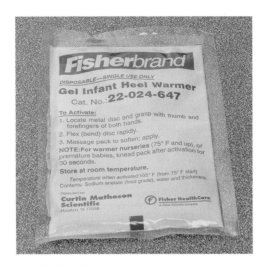

Figure 10-6 An infant heel warmer.

- *Plastic caps:* Plastic caps or closures are used to seal CBG tubes and maintain anaerobic conditions in the specimen. CBG tubes typically come with their own caps.

MICROSCOPE SLIDES

Glass microscope slides are occasionally used to make blood films for hematology determinations. (See Chapter 7, General Blood Collection Equipment and Supplies.)

WARMING DEVICES

Warming the site increases blood flow as much as seven times. This is especially important when performing heelsticks on newborns. Heel-warming devices (Fig. 10-6) are commercially available. To avoid burning the patient, the devices provide a uniform temperature that does not exceed 42°C. A towel or diaper dampened with warm tap water can also be used to wrap a hand or foot before skin puncture. However, care must be taken not to get the water so hot that it scalds the patient.

When you finish the chapter, have fun seeing how many types of equipment you can identify from among the crossword clues in the WORKBOOK.

Capillary Puncture Principles

COMPOSITION OF CAPILLARY SPECIMENS

Capillary specimens are a mixture of arterial, venous, and capillary blood, along with **interstitial fluid** (i.e., tissue fluid from spaces between the cells) and **intracellular**

fluid (fluid within the cells) from the surrounding area. Because arterial blood enters the capillaries under greater pressure than the venous pressure at the exits of the capillaries, capillary blood contains a higher proportion of arterial blood than venous blood. Consequently capillary blood resembles arterial blood in composition. This is especially true if the area has been warmed, because warming increases arterial flow into the area.

REFERENCE VALUES

Because the composition of capillary blood differs from that of venous blood, reference (normal) values may also differ. Most differences are minor, however clinically significant differences in some analytes have been reported. For example, the concentration of glucose and potassium are normally higher in capillary blood specimens, whereas bilirubin, calcium (Ca^{2+}), chloride, sodium, and total protein (TP) concentrations are lower.

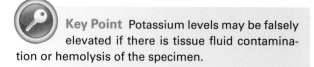 **Key Point** Potassium levels may be falsely elevated if there is tissue fluid contamination or hemolysis of the specimen.

INDICATIONS FOR CAPILLARY PUNCTURE

A properly collected capillary specimen can be a practical alternative to venipuncture when small amounts of blood are acceptable for testing.

Older Children and Adults

Capillary puncture can be an appropriate choice for older children and adults under the following circumstances:

- Available veins are fragile or must be saved for other procedures such as chemotherapy.
- Several unsuccessful venipunctures have been performed and the requested test can be collected by capillary puncture.
- The patient has thrombotic or clot-forming tendencies.
- The patient is apprehensive or has an intense fear of needles.
- There are no accessible veins (e.g., the patient has IVs in both arms or the only acceptable sites are in scarred or burned areas).
- To obtain blood for POCT procedures such as glucose monitoring.

Infants and Young Children

Capillary puncture is the preferred method of obtaining blood from infants and very young children for the following reasons.

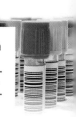

Table 10-1: Implications of a 10 mL Blood Draw in an Infant Population

Age	Weight (kg)	Total Blood Volume (%)
26-wk gestation	0.9	9.0
32-wk gestation	1.6	5.5
34-wk gestation	2.1	4.0
Term	3.4	2.5
3 mo	5.7	2.0
6 mo	7.6	1.6
12 mo	10.1	1.4
24 mo	12.6	1.0

Reprinted with permission from Bishop ML, Fody EP, Schoeff LE. *Clinical Chemistry, Principles, Techniques, and Correlations.* 7th ed. Philadelphia, PA: Lippincott Williams & Wilkins; 2013:722.

- Infants have a small blood volume; removing quantities of blood typical of venipuncture or arterial puncture can lead to anemia. According to studies, for every 10 mL of blood removed, as much as 4 mg of iron is also removed.
- Large quantities removed rapidly can cause cardiac arrest. Life may be threatened if more than 10% of a patient's blood volume is removed at once or over a very short period. Table 10-1 shows the percent of an infant's blood volume represented by a 10 mL blood draw in relation to age and weight.
- Obtaining blood from infants and children by venipuncture is difficult and may damage veins and surrounding tissues.
- Puncturing deep veins can result in hemorrhage, venous thrombosis, infection, and gangrene.
- An infant or child can be injured by the restraining method used while performing a venipuncture.
- Capillary blood is the preferred specimen for some tests, such as newborn screening tests.

 CAUTION Capillary puncture is generally *not* appropriate for patients who are dehydrated or have poor circulation to the extremities from other causes, such as shock, because specimens may be hard to obtain and may not be representative of blood elsewhere in the body.

TESTS THAT CANNOT BE COLLECTED BY CAPILLARY PUNCTURE

Although today's technology allows many tests to be performed on very small quantities of blood, and a wide selection of devices are available to make collection of skin puncture specimens relatively safe and easy, some tests cannot be performed on skin puncture specimens. These include most erythrocyte sedimentation rate methods, coagulation studies that require plasma specimens, blood cultures, and tests that require large volumes of serum or plasma.

> ⚠️ **CAUTION** Although light-blue–top micro-tubes are available from some manufacturers, they are not to be used for capillary specimens. They are intended to be used for venous blood collected by syringe in difficult draw situations.

ORDER OF DRAW

The order of draw for collecting multiple specimens by capillary puncture is not the same as for venipuncture. Puncturing the skin releases tissue thromboplastin, which activates the coagulation process in the blood drops. Specimens must be collected quickly to minimize the effects of platelet clumping and microclot formation and to ensure that an adequate amount of specimen is collected before the site stops bleeding. Hematology specimens are collected first because they are most affected by the clotting process. Serum specimens are collected last because they are supposed to clot. The CLSI order of draw (i.e., collection) for capillary specimens is as follows:

- Blood gas specimens
- EDTA specimens
- Other additive specimens
- Serum specimens

> 🔑 **Key Point** Specimens for newborn screening tests should be collected separately and from a separate puncture site.

NEW DIRECTIONS IN MICROSAMPLE TESTING

In today's healthcare environment, many factors, including the aging adult population, are pressuring the industry to be much more efficient and less costly. Consequently, companies that support medical services and laboratory testing are finding new cost efficient ways to do things quickly, accurately and easily. One such company is Theranos, a high-complexity CLIA-certified laboratory, presently located in Wellness Centers inside pharmacies in California and Arizona. Theranos addresses problems associated with collecting blood by venipuncture, especially from the typically small, fragile veins of geriatric and pediatric patients, by offering a test menu of over 100 tests that can be performed on a microsample collected by fingerstick. Many of the tests can be performed on a single drop of blood 1/1,000 the size of a typical blood draw. The results are stored in a secure database and sent to the physician in less than 3 days. The cost is considerably less, and major insurances as well as Medicare and Medicaid are accepted.

General Capillary Puncture Steps

Capillary specimens can be obtained from adults and children over the age of 1 year by puncturing a finger (fingerstick) and from infants less than a year old, and occasionally toddlers, by puncturing the heel (heelstick). Capillary punctures have the same general steps regardless of whether they are fingersticks or heelsticks. The first four steps are the same as Chapter 8 venipuncture steps 1 through 4.

STEP 1: REVIEW AND ACCESSION TEST REQUEST

STEP 2: APPROACH, IDENTIFY, AND PREPARE PATIENT

STEP 3: VERIFY DIET RESTRICTIONS AND LATEX SENSITIVITY

STEP 4: SANITIZE HANDS AND PUT ON GLOVES

STEP 5: POSITION PATIENT

Position is important to patient comfort and the success of specimen collection. For finger punctures, the patient's arm must be supported on a firm surface with the hand extended and palm up. Ask the patient which hand to use and select the nondominant hand if possible if the patient does not have a preference. A young child is typically held in the lap by a parent or guardian who restrains the child with one arm and holds the child's arm steady with the other. For heel punctures, an infant should be supine (lying face up) with the foot lower than the torso so the force of gravity can assist blood flow.

> 📖 **After reading Step 6 confirm that you know how to select a safe site by doing WORKBOOK Labeling Exercises 10-1 and 10-2.**

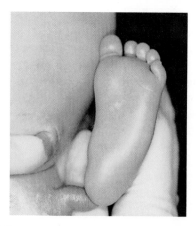

Figure 10-7 A type of cyanosis that commonly appears on the feet and hands of babies shortly after birth. (Reprinted with permission from Fletcher M. *Physical Diagnosis in Neonatology.* Philadelphia, PA: Lippincott-Raven Publishers; 1998.)

STEP 6: SELECT THE PUNCTURE SITE

General site selection criteria include one that is warm, pink or normal color, and free of scars, cuts, bruises, or rashes. It should not be **cyanotic** (bluish in color usually from a shortage of oxygen in the blood) (see Fig. 10-7), **edematous** (swollen), infected, or be a recent previous puncture site. Accumulated tissue fluid from swollen or previously punctured sites can contaminate the specimen and negatively affect test results. Puncturing such sites can also spread undetected infection. Specific locations for capillary puncture include fingers of adults and heels of infants.

Adults and Older Children

The CLSI-recommended site for capillary puncture on adults and children older than 1 year is the palmar

surface of the distal or end segment of the middle or ring finger of the nondominant hand. (Fingers on the nondominant hand are typically less calloused.) The puncture site should be in the central, fleshy portion of the finger, slightly to the side of center and perpendicular to the grooves in the **whorls** (spiral pattern) of the fingerprint (Fig. 10-8). Finger puncture precautions are summarized and explained in Table 10-2.

Key Point Some texts refer to the end segment of the finger as the distal phalanx. This is not to be confused with the use of the term phalanx (pl. phalanges) for finger bone.

CAUTION According to CLSI standards, capillary puncture *must not* be performed on the fingers or earlobes of newborns or other infants under 1 year of age.

Infants

The heel is the recommended site for collection of capillary puncture specimens on infants less than 1 year of age. However, it is important to perform the puncture in an area of the heel where there is little risk of puncturing the bone. Puncture of the bone can cause painful **osteomyelitis** (os'te-o-mi'el-i'tis), inflammation of the bone marrow and adjacent bone, or **osteochondritis** (os'te-o-kon-dri'tis), inflammation of the bone and cartilage, as a result of infection. Additional punctures must not be made through a current or previous puncture site as it can be painful. In addition if a previous site is inflamed

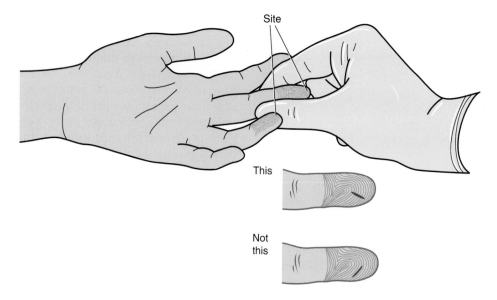

Figure 10-8 The recommended site and direction of finger puncture.

Table 10-2: Finger Puncture Precautions

Precaution	Rationale
Do not puncture fingers of infants and children under 1 year of age	The amount of tissue between skin surface and bone is so small that bone injury is very likely. Known complications include infection and gangrene
Do not puncture fingers on the same side as a mastectomy without permission from the patient's physician	The arm is susceptible to infection, and effects of lymphostasis can lead to erroneous results
Do not puncture parallel to the grooves or lines of the fingerprint	A puncture in line with a fingerprint groove makes collection difficult because it allows blood to run down the finger rather than form a rounded drop that is easier to collect
Do not puncture the fifth or little (pinky) finger	The tissue between skin surface and bone is thinnest in this finger, and bone injury is likely
Do not puncture the index finger	It is usually more calloused and harder to puncture, more sensitive so the puncture can be more painful, and it is typically used more, so a patient may notice the pain longer
Do not puncture the side or very tip of the finger	The distance between the skin surface and bone is half as much at the side and tip as it is in the central fleshy portion of the finger
Do not puncture the thumb	It has a pulse, indicating an artery in the puncture area, and the skin is generally thicker and more calloused, making it difficult to obtain a good specimen

or has an undetected infection, a repeat puncture can spread an infection.

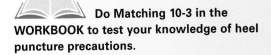

Do Matching 10-3 in the WORKBOOK to test your knowledge of heel puncture precautions.

Studies have shown that the **calcaneus** (kal-ka'ne-us) or heel bone of small or premature infants may be as little as 2 mm below the skin surface on the **plantar surface**, or bottom of the heel, and half that distance at the **posterior curvature** (back) of the heel. Punctures

deeper than this may cause bone damage. The vascular or capillary bed (Fig. 10-9) in the skin of a newborn is located at the dermal–subcutaneous junction between 0.35 and 1.6 mm beneath the skin surface, so punctures 2 mm deep or less will provide adequate blood flow without risking bone injury.

Key Point Deeper skin punctures are more painful because pain fibers increase in abundance below 2.4 mm deep. They are also totally unnecessary because the capillary bed in a full-term infant is richest in capillary loops above 1 mm deep.

According to CLSI, to avoid puncturing bone the only safe areas for heel puncture are on the plantar surface of the heel, medial to an imaginary line extending from the middle of the great toe to the heel or lateral to an imaginary line extending from between the fourth and fifth toes to the heel (Fig. 10-10). Punctures in other areas risk bone, nerve, tendon, and cartilage injury. Heel puncture precautions are summarized in Table 10-3.

Table 10-3: Heel Puncture Precautions

Precaution	Rationale
Do not puncture any deeper than 2 mm	Deeper punctures risk injuring the bone, even in the safest puncture areas
Do not puncture areas between the imaginary boundaries	The calcaneus may be as little as 2 mm deep in this area
Do not puncture bruised areas	It can be painful, and impaired circulation or byproducts of the healing process can negatively affect the specimen
Do not puncture in the arch and any other areas of the foot other than the heel	Arteries, nerves, tendons, and cartilage in these areas can be injured
Do not puncture sites that are swollen	Excess tissue fluid in the area could contaminate the specimen
Do not puncture the posterior curvature of the heel	The bone can be as little as 1 mm deep in this area
Do not puncture through previous puncture sites	This can be painful and can spread previously undetected infection

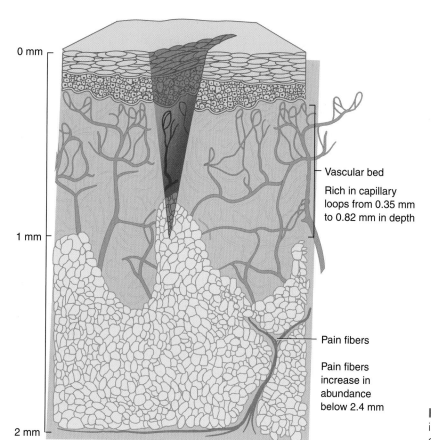

Vascular bed

Rich in capillary loops from 0.35 mm to 0.82 mm in depth

Pain fibers

Pain fibers increase in abundance below 2.4 mm

Figure 10-9 A cross-section of full-term infant's heel showing lancet penetration depth needed to access the capillary bed.

Memory Jogger One way to remember that the safe areas for heel puncture are the medial or lateral plantar surfaces of the heel is to think of the phrase "Make little people happy." Using the first letter of each word, "M" stands for medial, "L" stands for lateral, "P" stands for plantar, and "H" stands for heel.

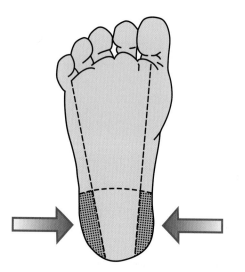

Figure 10-10 An infant heel. *Shaded areas indicated by arrows* represent recommended safe areas for heel puncture.

STEP 7: WARM THE SITE IF APPLICABLE

Warming increases blood flow up to sevenfold (seven times) and, except for PaO_2 levels, does not significantly alter results of routinely tested analytes. Increased blood flow makes specimens easier and faster to obtain and reduces the tendency to compress or squeeze the site, which can contaminate the specimen with tissue fluid and hemolyze red blood cells. Because the increase is caused by arterial flow into the area, a specimen obtained from a warmed site is described as being **arterialized**. Consequently, warming the site is essential when collecting capillary pH or blood gas specimens. Warming is typically recommended for heelstick procedures because infants normally have high red blood cell counts and other factors that result in relatively thick blood that flows slowly. Warming may also be required before fingersticks when patients have cold hands. Warming can be accomplished by wrapping the site for 3 to 5 minutes with a washcloth, towel, or diaper that has been moistened with comfortably warm water or using a commercial heel-warming device (Fig. 10-6).

⚠ **CAUTION** The temperature of the material used to warm the site must not exceed 42°C (108°F) because higher temperatures can burn the skin, especially the delicate skin of an infant.

STEP 8: CLEAN AND AIR-DRY SITE

The collection site must be cleaned with an antiseptic before puncture, so that skin flora (microorganisms on the skin) do not infiltrate the puncture wound and cause infection. The CLSI-recommended antiseptic for cleaning a capillary puncture site is 70% isopropanol.

> ⚠️ **CAUTION** *Do not* use povidone–iodine to clean skin puncture sites because it greatly interferes with a number of tests, most notably bilirubin, uric acid, phosphorus, and potassium.

> 🧠 **Memory Jogger** Help remember the tests affected by povidone–iodine by associating them with the word BURPP, where "B" stands for bilirubin, "UR" stands for uric acid, and the two "Ps" stand for phosphorous and potassium.

After cleaning, allow the site to air-dry to ensure maximum antiseptic action and minimize the chance of alcohol contamination of the specimen. Residual alcohol, in addition to causing a stinging sensation, causes rapid hemolysis of red blood cells. It has also been shown to interfere with glucose testing.

STEP 9: PREPARE EQUIPMENT

Select collection devices according to the tests that have been ordered and place them within easy reach, along with several layers of gauze or gauze-type pads. Select a new, sterile lancet according to the site selected, age of the patient, and amount of blood to be collected. Prepare equipment in view of the patient or guardian to provide assurance that it is new and being handled aseptically. Verify lancet sterility by checking to see that packaging is intact before opening. Open the package or protective cover in an aseptic manner and do not allow the lancet to rest or brush against any nonsterile surface. If the lancet has a protective shield or locking feature that prevents accidental activation, remove or release it per manufacturer's instructions. Gloves must be put on at this point if not put on in Step 4.

STEP 10: GRASP THE FINGER OR HEEL FIRMLY

To prepare for the puncture, use your nondominant hand to grasp the finger or heel firmly to prevent sudden movement by the patient. Hold the lancet between the thumb and index fingers of your dominant hand (or as described by the device manufacturer). Hold the patient's finger or heel as follows:

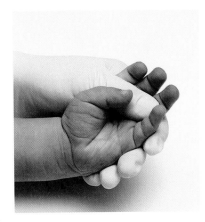

Figure 10-11 Holding a toddler's fingers prior to capillary puncture. (Courtesy ITC, Edison, NJ.)

- **Fingersticks:** Grasp the patient's middle or ring finger between your nondominant thumb and index finger. Hold it securely in case of sudden movement.

> 🔑 **Key Point** With very young children it is usually best to grasp three or four of the child's fingers (Fig. 10-11) between your fingers and thumb. If you grasp only one finger, the child may twist it trying to pull away. Although you are holding more fingers, it is still easy to puncture the middle finger because it is normally the longest and sticks out farthest.

- **Heelsticks:** Grasp the foot gently but firmly with your nondominant hand. Encircle the heel by wrapping your index finger around the arch and your thumb around the bottom. Wrap the other fingers around the top of the foot.

STEP 11: POSITION LANCET, PUNCTURE SITE, AND DISCARD LANCET

Place the lancet flat against the skin in an appropriate area described in Step 6. Use sufficient pressure to keep it in place without deeply compressing the skin. (Pressing too hard can result in a puncture that is deeper than intended). Warn the patient or parent/guardian if applicable, of the impending puncture. Activate the release mechanism to trigger the puncture. Remove the device from the skin following puncture and immediately discard it in a sharps container.

> 🔑 **Key Point** Most manufacturers of heel incision devices recommend puncturing the heel at a 90-degree angle to the length of the foot. This creates a "gap" puncture (i.e., a puncture that opens when pressure is applied).

STEP 12: LOWER FINGER OR HEEL AND APPLY GENTLE PRESSURE UNTIL A BLOOD DROP FORMS

Position the appendage downward and apply gentle pressure toward a heel puncture site or proximal to a finger puncture site to encourage blood flow. *Do not* squeeze. It may take a few moments for blood flow to start. Hold pressure until a large drop of blood forms at the site.

> ⚠️ **CAUTION** Double sticking (an immediate repeat puncture at the same site) is never acceptable. If blood does not flow or stops flowing at any time and cannot be restarted, a new puncture at a different site must be performed.

STEP 13: WIPE AWAY THE FIRST BLOOD DROP

Wipe away the first drop of blood with a clean, gauze pad. The first drop is typically contaminated with excess tissue fluid, and may contain alcohol residue that can hemolyze the specimen and also keep the blood from forming a well-rounded drop. In addition, there have been reports of isopropyl alcohol contamination causing errors in blood glucose testing.

> 🔑 **Key Point** Some POCT instruments may allow use of the first drop, so follow manufacturer's instructions.

STEP 14: FILL AND MIX TUBES/CONTAINERS IN ORDER OF DRAW

Continue to position the site downward to enhance blood flow and continue to apply gentle, intermittent pressure to assure the free flow of blood required for accurate test results. Allow a second drop to form.

> ⚠️ **CAUTION** *Do not* squeeze, use strong repetitive pressure, or "milk" the site, as hemolysis and tissue fluid contamination of the specimen can result.

Collect subsequent blood drops using microtubes or other devices appropriate for the ordered tests. To fill a collection tube or device, touch it to the drop of blood formed on the surface of the skin. Collect slides, platelet counts, and other hematology specimens first to avoid the effects of platelet aggregation (clumping) and clotting. Collect other anticoagulant microtubes next, and serum tubes last according to the CLSI order of draw for capillary specimens.

- If making a blood film, touch the appropriate area of the slide to the blood drop.
- The ability of a liquid to be automatically drawn into a narrow space or tube is called capillary action. A microhematocrit or narrow-bore capillary tube will fill automatically by capillary action if held in a vertical position above, or a horizontal position beside a blood drop and one end touched to the blood drop. While maintaining contact with the blood drop, the opposite end of the tube may need to be lowered slightly and brought back into position now and then as it fills. Do not remove the tube from the drop or continually hold or tip the tube below the site. This can result in air spaces in the specimen that cause inaccurate test results. When the tube is full, plug the opposite (dry end) with clay or other suitable sealant.
- To fill a microtube, hold it upright just below the blood drop. Touch the tip of the tube's collector device or "scoop" to the drop of blood and allow the blood to flow freely down the inside wall of the tube. The scoop should touch only the blood drop and not the surface of the skin. This allows blood to be collected before it runs down the surface of the finger or heel.

> ⚠️ **CAUTION** *Do not* use a scooping motion against the surface of the skin and attempt to collect blood as it flows down the finger. Scraping the scoop of the microtube against the skin activates platelets, causing them to clump, and can also hemolyze the specimen.

You may need to tap microtubes gently now and then to encourage the blood to settle to the bottom. When filled to the level required, immediately seal microtubes with the covers provided. Mix additive microtubes by gently inverting them 8 to 10 times or per manufacturer's instructions. If blood flow stops and you are unable to collect sufficient specimen, the procedure may be repeated at a new site with a new lancet.

> ⚠️ **CAUTION** Pay strict attention to fill levels of microtubes containing anticoagulants. Excess anticoagulant in underfilled microtubes can negatively affect test results. Overfilling can result in the presence of microclots in the specimen or even complete clotting of the specimen.

STEP 15: PLACE GAUZE, ELEVATE SITE, AND APPLY PRESSURE

After collecting specimens, apply pressure to the site with a clean gauze pad until bleeding stops. Keep the site elevated while applying pressure. An infant's foot should be elevated above the body while pressure is applied.

STEP 16: LABEL SPECIMENS AND OBSERVE SPECIAL HANDLING INSTRUCTIONS

Label specimens with the appropriate information (see Chapter 8). Include type and source of specimen according to facility policy. Label before leaving the patient's side or dismissing an outpatient. Label in view of the patient/parent/guardian, and affix labels directly to microcollection containers. Microhematocrit tubes can be placed in a nonadditive tube or an appropriately sized aliquot tube for transport and identifying information written on the label, or transport according to laboratory protocol. Follow any special handling required, such as cooling in crushed ice (e.g., ammonia), transportation at body temperature (e.g., cold agglutinin), or light protection (e.g., bilirubin).

STEP 17: CHECK THE SITE AND APPLY BANDAGE

The site must be examined to verify that bleeding has stopped. If bleeding persists beyond 5 minutes, notify the patient's physician, or appropriate healthcare provider. If bleeding has stopped and the patient is an older child or adult, apply a bandage and advise the patient to keep it in place for at least 15 minutes.

⚠️ **CAUTION** *Do not* apply bandages to infants and children under 2 years of age because they pose a choking hazard. In addition, bandage adhesive can stick to the paper-thin skin of newborns and tear it when the bandage is removed.

STEP 18: DISPOSE OF USED AND CONTAMINATED MATERIALS

Equipment packaging and bandage wrappers are normally discarded in the regular trash. Some facilities require contaminated items, such as blood-soaked gauze, to be discarded in biohazard containers. Follow facility protocol.

STEP 19: THANK PATIENT, REMOVE GLOVES, AND SANITIZE HANDS

Be sure to thank the patient, parent, or guardian. It is courteous and professional. Gloves must be removed in an aseptic manner and hands washed or decontaminated with hand sanitizer as an infection control precaution before leaving the site or proceeding to the next patient.

STEP 20: TRANSPORT SPECIMEN TO THE LAB PROMPTLY

Prompt delivery to the lab protects specimen integrity and is typically achieved by personal delivery, transportation via a pneumatic tube system, or a courier service.

Capillary Puncture Procedures

Most capillary punctures are fingersticks. Fingerstick procedure is illustrated in Procedure 10-1. Heel punctures are typically performed on infants under 1 year of age, although they are sometimes performed on toddlers using a lancet designed for use on toddlers. Heelstick procedure is illustrated in Procedure 10-2.

thePoint *Check out the Capillary Blood Specimen Collection video and the Introductory and Identification Processes Required Prior to Blood Specimen Collection video at http://thepoint.lww.com/McCall6e.*

Procedure 10-1: Fingerstick Procedure

PURPOSE: To obtain a blood specimen for patient diagnosis or monitoring from a finger puncture

EQUIPMENT: Nonlatex gloves, warming device (optional), antiseptic prep pad, safety finger puncture lancet, microtubes or other appropriate collection devices, gauze pads, sharps container, permanent ink pen, bandage

Step	Explanation/Rationale
1 to 4. See Chapter 8 Venipuncture steps 1 through 4.	See Chapter 8 Procedure 8-2: steps 1 through 4.
5. Position the patient.	CLSI standards require the patient to be seated or reclining in an appropriate chair, or lying down. The arm must be supported on a firm surface and the hand palm up.
	Note: A young child may have to be held on the lap and restrained by a parent or guardian.

Procedure 10-1: Fingerstick Procedure (Continued)

Step	Explanation/Rationale
6. Select the puncture site.	Selecting an appropriate site protects the patient from injury, allows collection of a quality specimen, and prevents spreading a previous infection.
7. Warm the site, if applicable.	Warming the site makes blood collection easier and faster, and reduces the tendency to squeeze the site. It is not normally part of a routine fingerstick unless the hand is cold, in which case, wrap it in a comfortably warm washcloth or towel for 3 to 5 minutes or use a commercial warming device.
8. Clean and air-dry the site.	Cleaning with 70% isopropyl alcohol removes or inhibits skin flora that could infiltrate the puncture and cause infection. Allowing the site to dry naturally permits maximum antiseptic action, prevents contamination caused by wiping, and avoids stinging on puncture and specimen hemolysis from residual alcohol.

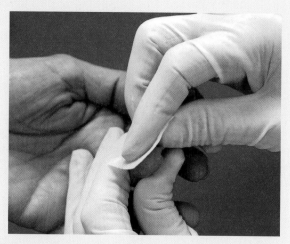

Step	Explanation/Rationale
9. Prepare equipment.	Selecting and preparing equipment in advance of use helps ensure that the correct equipment is ready and within reach for the procedure. Aseptically opening packaging aids in infection control.
10. Grasp finger firmly.	Grasping the finger firmly prevents sudden movement by the patient.
11. Position lancet, puncture site, and discard lancet.	Holding the lancet between the thumb and index fingers of your dominant hand (or as described by the device manufacturer) is required preparation for the puncture. Placing the lancet flat against the skin ensures good contact for the puncture. Discarding the lancet in a sharps container immediately after the puncture is a safety requirement that protects the patient, phlebotomist, and others from accidental injury or contamination from the lancet.

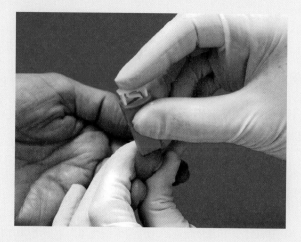

Procedure 10-1: Fingerstick Procedure (Continued)

Step	Explanation/Rationale
12. Lower finger and apply gentle pressure until a blood drop forms.	Lowering the appendage helps blood begin to flow freely. Gentle pressure encourages blood flow without compromising specimen integrity.

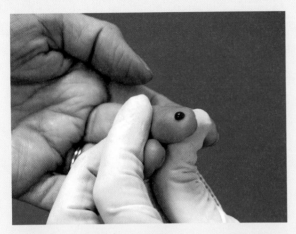

Step	Explanation/Rationale
13. Wipe away the first blood drop.	Prevents contamination of the specimen with excess tissue fluid and removes alcohol residue that could prevent formation of well-rounded drops and also hemolyze the specimen.

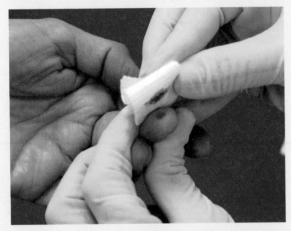

Step	Explanation/Rationale
14. Fill and mix the tubes/containers in order of draw.	Mixing tubes immediately after they are filled is necessary for proper additive function and to prevent clotting in anticoagulant tubes. Following the order of draw for capillary specimens minimizes negative effects of clotting on hematology specimens and other specimens collected in anticoagulant tubes.

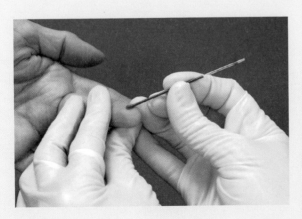

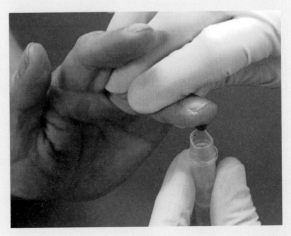

Procedure 10-1: Fingerstick Procedure (Continued)

Step	Explanation/Rationale
15. Place gauze, elevate site, and apply pressure.	Absorbs excess blood, and helps stop bleeding.
16. Label specimens and observe special handling instructions.	Prompt labeling (see Chapter 8) helps ensure correct specimen identification. Appropriate handling protects specimen integrity.
17. Check the site and apply bandage. **Note:** Do not apply a bandage to an infant or toddler.	Necessary to verify that bleeding has stopped. Bandaging keeps the site clean while the site heals. **Note:** If bleeding persists beyond 5 minutes, notify the patient's physician or designated healthcare provider.
18. Dispose of used and contaminated materials.	Equipment packaging, bandage wrappers, and other used materials must be discarded in the trash. Follow facility protocol for discarding contaminated items, such as blood-soaked gauze.
19. Thank patient, parent, or guardian, remove and discard gloves, and sanitize hands.	Thanking the patient, parent, or guardian is courteous and professional. Removing gloves aseptically and washing or decontaminating hands with sanitizer is an infection control precaution.
20. Transport specimen to the lab promptly.	Prompt delivery to the lab is necessary to protect specimen integrity.

Special Capillary Puncture Procedures

CAPILLARY BLOOD GASES

Capillary puncture blood is less desirable for blood gas analysis, primarily because of its only partial arterial composition and also because it is temporarily exposed to air during collection, which can alter test results. Consequently, specimens for **capillary blood gases (CBGs)** are rarely collected on adults. However, because arterial punctures can be hazardous to infants and young children, blood gas analysis on these patients is sometimes performed on capillary specimens.

CBG specimens are collected from the same sites as routine capillary puncture specimens. Warming the

Procedure 10-2: Heelstick Procedure

PURPOSE: To obtain a blood specimen for patient diagnosis or monitoring from a heel puncture

EQUIPMENT: Nonlatex gloves, warming device, antiseptic prep pad, safety heel puncture lancet, microcollection tubes or other appropriate collection devices, gauze pads, sharps container, permanent ink pen

Step	Explanation/Rationale
1 to 3. See Chapter 8 venipuncture steps 1 through 4.	See Chapter 8 Procedure 8-2: steps 1 through 4.
5. Position the patient.	The infant should be lying face up with the foot lower than the torso so gravity can assist blood flow.
6. Select the puncture site.	An acceptable heel puncture site is on the medial or lateral plantar surface of the heel, is warm, of normal color, and free of cuts, bruises, infection, rashes, swelling, or previous punctures.
7. Warm the site.	Warming makes blood collection easier and faster and reduces the tendency to squeeze the site. The heel should be warmed for 3 to 5 minutes by wrapping it in a comfortably warm wet washcloth, towel, or diaper, or use a commercial heel-warming device.

Procedure 10-2: Heelstick Procedure (Continued)

Step	Explanation/Rationale
8. Clean and air-dry the site. 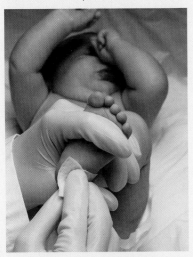	Cleaning with 70% isopropyl alcohol removes or inhibits skin flora that could infiltrate the puncture and cause infection. Allowing the site to dry naturally permits maximum antiseptic action, prevents contamination caused by wiping, and avoids stinging on puncture and specimen hemolysis from residual alcohol.
9. Prepare equipment. 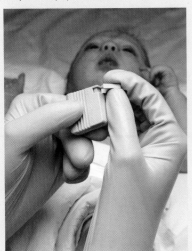	Selecting and preparing the equipment in advance of use helps ensure that the correct equipment is ready and within reach for the procedure, packaging is intact to ensure sterility, and appropriate devices are available and ready for use in collecting the ordered tests.
10. Grasp the heel firmly.	Helps prevent sudden unexpected movement by the patient.
11. Position lancet, puncture site, and discard lancet. 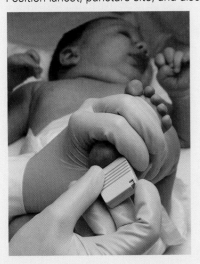	Holding the lancet between the thumb and index fingers of your dominant hand (or as described by the device manufacturer) is required preparation for the puncture. Placing the lancet flat against the skin ensures good contact for the puncture. Discarding the lancet in a sharps container immediately after the puncture is a safety requirement that protects the patient, phlebotomist, and others from accidental injury or contamination by the lancet.

Procedure 10-2: Heelstick Procedure (Continued)

Step	Explanation/Rationale
12. Lower heel and apply gentle pressure until a blood drop forms.	Helps blood begin to flow freely and encourages blood flow without compromising specimen integrity.

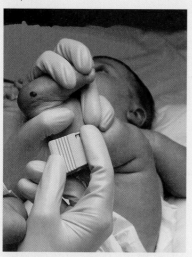

Step	Explanation/Rationale
13. Wipe away the first blood drop.	Prevents contamination of the specimen with excess tissue fluid and removes alcohol residue that could prevent formation of well-rounded drops and also hemolyze the specimen.

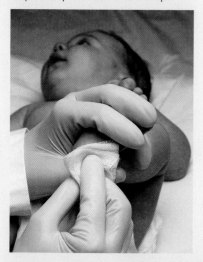

Step	Explanation/Rationale
14. Fill and mix tubes/containers in order of draw.	Necessary for proper additive function and to prevent clotting in anticoagulant tubes. Following the order of draw for capillary specimens minimizes negative effects of clotting on hematology specimens and other specimens collected in anticoagulants.

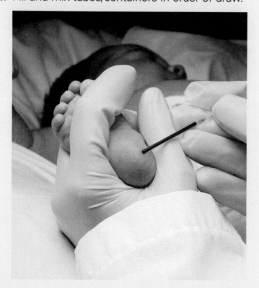

Procedure 10-2: Heelstick Procedure (Continued)

Step	Explanation/Rationale
15. Place gauze, elevate heel, and apply pressure. 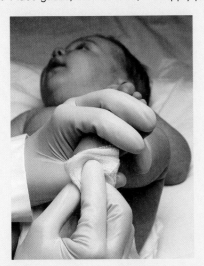	Absorbs excess blood and helps stop bleeding.
16. Label the specimen and observe special handling instructions.	Prompt labeling (see Chapter 8) helps ensure correct specimen identification. Appropriate handling protects specimen integrity.
17. Check the site.	Necessary to verify that bleeding has stopped. Applying a bandage to an infant is not recommended because it can become a choking hazard and can also tear the skin when removed. **Note:** If bleeding persists beyond 5 minutes, notify the patient's physician, or designated healthcare provider.
18. Dispose of used and contaminated materials.	Equipment packaging, bandage wrappers, and other used materials must be discarded in the trash. Follow facility protocol for discarding contaminated items, such as blood-soaked gauze.
19. Thank patient, parent, or guardian, remove gloves, and sanitize hands.	Thanking the patient, parent, or guardian is courteous and professional. Removing gloves aseptically and washing or decontaminating hands with sanitizer is an infection control precaution.
20. Transport specimen to the lab promptly.	Prompt delivery to the lab is necessary to protect specimen integrity.

site for 5 to 10 minutes before collection is necessary to increase blood flow and arterialize the specimen. Proper collection technique is essential to minimize exposure of the specimen to air. Collection of a capillary blood gas specimen by heel puncture is illustrated in Procedure 10-3.

📖📖 **Can you find "bilirubin" among the scrambled words in WORKBOOK Knowledge Drill 10-2?**

NEONATAL BILIRUBIN COLLECTION

Neonates (newborns) are commonly tested to detect and monitor increased bilirubin levels caused by overproduction or impaired excretion of bilirubin. Overproduction of bilirubin occurs from accelerated red blood cell hemolysis associated with hemolytic disease of the newborn (HDN). Impaired bilirubin excretion often results from temporary abnormal liver function commonly associated with premature infants. High levels of bilirubin result in jaundice (yellow skin color) (Fig. 10-12).

Procedure 10-3: Collection of a Capillary Blood Gas (CBG) Specimen by Heel Puncture

PURPOSE: To obtain a specimen for blood gas analysis by capillary puncture

EQUIPMENT: Nonlatex gloves, warming device, antiseptic prep pad, safety lancet, special capillary tube with caps, metal stirrer bar, magnet, sterile gauze pads, sharps container, permanent ink pen

Step	Explanation/Rationale
1 to 6. Same as fingerstick (adult) or heelstick (infant) procedures	See Fingerstick Procedure 10-1 or Heelstick Procedure 10-2, heelstick procedure steps 1 through 6.
7. Warm the site.	Warming the site is required to arterialize the specimen, makes blood collection easier and faster, and reduces the tendency to squeeze the site. Warming the site also makes blood collection easier and faster, and reduces the tendency to squeeze the site. The site can be warmed by wrapping it in a comfortably warm wet washcloth, towel, or diaper for 3 to 5 minutes or use a commercial heel-warming device.
8. Clean and air-dry the site.	Cleaning with 70% isopropyl alcohol removes or inhibits skin flora that could infiltrate the puncture and cause infection. Allowing the site to dry naturally permits maximum antiseptic action, prevents contamination caused by wiping, and avoids stinging on puncture and specimen hemolysis from residual alcohol.
9. Prepare equipment.	Selecting and preparing equipment in advance of use helps ensure that the correct equipment is ready and within reach for the procedure. The metal stirrer must be placed in the capillary tube before it is filled. Tube caps and magnet must be within easy reach. The puncture device must be opened aseptically.
10. Grasp the finger or heel firmly.	Grasping the finger or heel firmly prevents sudden movement by the patient.
11. Position lancet, puncture the site, and discard lancet.	Holding the lancet between the thumb and index fingers of your dominant hand (or as described by the device manufacturer) is required preparation for the puncture. Placing the lancet flat against the skin ensures good contact for the puncture. Discarding the lancet in a sharps container immediately after triggering the puncture is a safety requirement that protects the patient, phlebotomist, and others from accidental injury or contamination by the lancet.
12. Lower the site and apply gentle pressure until a blood drop forms.	Helps blood to begin to flow freely, without compromising specimen integrity.
13. Wipe away the first drop of blood.	Wiping the first drop prevents contamination of the specimen with excess tissue fluid and removes alcohol residue that could prevent formation of well-rounded drops and also hemolyze the specimen.
14. Quickly and carefully fill the capillary tube with blood.	The specimen must be collected quickly to minimize exposure of the blood drops to air, and carefully to prevent introduction of air spaces in the tube. A completely full tube with no air spaces is essential for accurate results.
15. Immediately cap both ends of the tube.	Sealing tubes as soon as possible prevents exposure to air and protects blood gas composition.

Procedure 10-3: Collection of a Capillary Blood Gas (CBG) Specimen by Heel Puncture (Continued)

Step	Explanation/Rationale
16. Mix the specimen with the magnet.	Running the magnet back and forth the full length of the tube several times, pulls the metal stirrer with it, mixes the blood with heparin, and prevents clotting.
17. Place gauze, elevate site, and apply pressure	Absorbs excess blood and helps stop bleeding.
18. Label the specimen	Immediate labeling with appropriate information ensures correct specimen identification.
19. Place the tube horizontally in ice slurry (or equivalent cooling device).	Cooling slows WBC metabolism and prevents changes in pH and blood gas values.
20. Check the puncture site. **Note:** Do not apply a bandage to an infant	Examining the site is necessary to verify that bleeding has stopped. If bleeding persists beyond 5 minutes, notify the patient's physician or designated healthcare provider.
21. Dispose of used and contaminated materials.	Follow facility protocol for discarding trash and contaminated items, such as blood-soaked gauze.
22. Thank patient, parent, or guardian, remove and discard gloves, and sanitize hands.	Thanking the parent or guardian is courteous and professional. Removing gloves aseptically and washing or decontaminating hands with sanitizer is an infection control precaution.
23. Transport specimen to the lab ASAP.	Prompt delivery to the lab is necessary to protect specimen integrity.

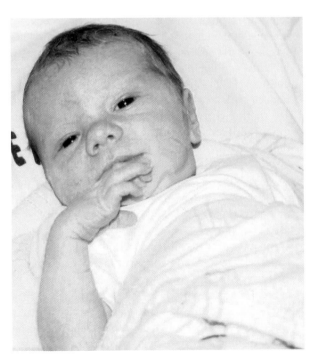

Figure 10-12 A newborn infant with jaundice. (Reprinted with permission from Carol Mattson Porth. *Pathophysiology Concepts of Altered Health States*. 7th ed. Philadelphia, PA: Lippincott Williams & Wilkins; 2005.)

Bilirubin can cross the blood–brain barrier in infants, accumulating to toxic levels that can cause permanent brain damage or even death. A transfusion may be needed if levels increase at a rate equal to or greater than 5 mg/dL/h or when levels exceed 18 mg/dL. Bilirubin breaks down in the presence of light. Consequently, jaundiced infants are often placed under special ultraviolet (UV) lights to lower bilirubin levels.

⚠️ **CAUTION** The UV light must be turned off when collecting a bilirubin specimen to prevent it from breaking down bilirubin in the specimen as it is collected.

Bilirubin specimens are normally collected by heel puncture. Proper collection procedure is crucial to the accuracy of results. Specimens must be collected quickly to minimize exposure to light and must be protected from light during transportation and handling. To reduce light exposure, specimens are typically collected in amber-colored microcollection containers (Fig. 10-13). Specimens must be collected carefully to avoid hemolysis, which could falsely decrease bilirubin results. Because determining the

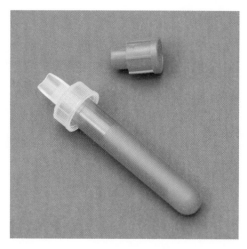

Figure 10-13 An amber-colored microcollection container used to protect a bilirubin specimen from effects of ultraviolet light.

rate of increase in bilirubin levels depends on accurate timing, specimens should be collected as close as possible to the time requested.

NEWBORN/NEONATAL SCREENING

There are serious health conditions that can be present at birth even though affected infants may not show symptoms of them at first. Fortunately, many of these conditions can be detected by **newborn/neonatal screening** (NBS), which is the state mandated testing of newborns to detect certain genetic (inherited), metabolic (chemical changes within living cells), hormonal, and functional disorders or conditions that can cause severe mental handicaps or other serious problems if not detected and treated early. Some states also screen for hearing loss, and for infectious agents, such as toxoplasma and HIV. All newborns in the United States get some type of newborn screening; however, the number and type of screening tests varies by state. Requirements for disorders to be included in NBS screening panels include benefits to early diagnosis, availability of accurate tests to confirm diagnosis, and better health as a result of early detection and treatment.

(i) For a fee, some labs will perform additional newborn screening tests that are not part of state-mandated testing.

The March of Dimes recommends that all newborns be screened for at least 31 health conditions for which there is effective treatment (Table 10-4). All states require newborn screening for at least 26 health conditions. So far, 42 states and the District of Columbia screen for 29 of the 31 conditions recommended by the March of Dimes. Some states screen for up to 50 or more health conditions.

(i) There are 25 other conditions that are often identified during NBS for which there is currently limited information or no treatment.

Screening for **phenylketonuria (PKU)**, **hypothyroidism**, and **galactosemia** is required by law in all 50 states and U.S. territories. Mandatory screening for cystic fibrosis (CF) is effective in all 50 states and the District of Columbia.

- *Phenylketonuria:* Phenylketonuria is a genetic disorder characterized by a defect in the enzyme that breaks down the amino acid phenylalanine, converting it into the amino acid tyrosine. Without intervention, phenylalanine, which is in almost all food, accumulates in the blood and is only slowly metabolized by an alternate pathway that results in increased phenylketones in the urine. PKU cannot be cured but normally can be treated with a diet low in phenylalanine. If left untreated or not treated early on, phenylalanine can rise to toxic levels and lead to brain damage and mental retardation. PKU testing typically requires the collection of two specimens, one shortly after an infant is born and another after the infant is 10 to 15 days old. The incidence of PKU in the United States is approximately 1 in 10,000 to 25,000 births.

- *Hypothyroidism:* Hypothyroidism is a disorder that is characterized by insufficient levels of thyroid hormones. If left untreated, the deficiency hinders growth and brain development. Some forms of neonatal hypothyroidism, although congenital (present at birth), are not inherited but temporarily acquired because the mother has the condition. Newborn screening tests detect both inherited and noninherited forms. In the United States and Canada, the newborn screening test for hypothyroidism measures total thyroxine (T_4). Positive results are confirmed by measuring thyroid-stimulating hormone (TSH) levels. The disorder is treated by supplying the missing thyroid hormone orally. The incidence of hypothyroidism is 1 in 4,000 births.

- *Galactosemia:* Galactosemia (GALT) is an inherited disorder characterized by lack of the enzyme needed to convert the milk sugar galactose into glucose needed by the body for energy. Within a week of birth, an infant with galactosemia will fail to thrive due to anorexia, diarrhea, and vomiting unless galactose and lactose (lactose breaks down to galactose and glucose) are removed from the diet. Untreated, the infant may starve to death. Untreated infants that survive typically fail to grow, are mentally handicapped, and have cataracts. Treatment involves removing all milk and dairy products from the infant's diet. Several less severe forms of galactosemia that may not need treatment can also be detected by newborn screening. The incidence of galactosemia is 1 in 60,000 to 80,000 births.

• *Cystic Fibrosis:* CF is a genetic disorder caused by one or more mutations in the gene that directs a protein responsible for regulating the transport of chloride across cell membranes. CF involves multiple organs, but primarily affects the lungs and pancreas. The mutation causes the body to produce thick, sticky mucus secretions that build up in the lungs and other organs. The mucus obstructs passageways in the lungs, leading to pulmonary infections. Mucus blockage of pancreatic enzymes needed for digestion can lead to malnutrition. Early diagnosis and treatment helps avoid respiratory distress and malnutrition, and has the potential to increase life expectancy. CF occurs in 1 of every 3,700 U.S. births. Prevalence at birth varies by race/ethnicity from 1 in 2,500 to 3,500 births among non-Hispanic whites, 1 in 4,000 to 10,000 among Hispanics, and 1 in 15,000 to 20,000 births among non-Hispanic blacks.

Most NBS tests are ideally performed when an infant is between 24 and 72 hours old. Because of early hospital release, some infants are tested before they are 24 hours old. Early testing for some tests (e.g., PKU) may not give accurate results, so some states require repeat testing approximately 2 weeks later. Specimens for NBS tests are collected by heel puncture and require a special state form. Newborn screening equipment is shown in Figure 10-14.

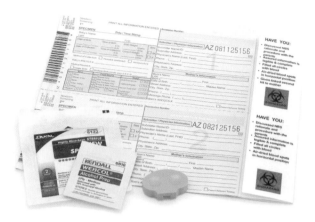

Figure 10-14 Newborn screening specimen collection equipment.

> ⚠ **CAUTION** If an infant requires a blood transfusion, newborn screening specimens should be collected before it is started, as dilution of the sample with donor blood invalidates test results.

ⓘ Online information on newborn screening can be found at the National Newborn Screening and Genetic Resource Center at http://genes-r-us.uthscsa.edu/

Blood Spot Collection

Newborn screening tests, except hearing tests, are typically performed on a few drops of blood obtained by heel puncture. The blood drops are collected by absorption onto circles printed on a special type of filter paper that is normally part of the NBS form (Fig. 10-15). The blood-filled circles are often referred to as blood spots. As many as 50 different disorders can be detected in the blood spots on one form. Table 10-4 on page 321 lists five groups of disorders that can be detected by newborn screening.

To fill the circles, heel puncture is performed, and the first blood drop is wiped away in the normal manner. The filter paper is brought close to the heel, and a large drop of free-flowing blood is applied to the center of the first circle on the printed side of the paper. The paper must not be allowed to touch the surface of the heel. This can result in smearing, blotting, and stoppage of blood flow and incomplete penetration of blood through the paper. The original position of the paper must be maintained and blood must continue flowing until it completely fills the circle on both sides of the paper. The same process is continued until all circles are filled. Unfilled or incompletely filled circles can result in inability to perform all required tests. Circles must be filled from one side of the paper only and by one large drop that spreads throughout the circle. Application of multiple drops or filling circles from both sides of the paper causes layering of blood and possible misinterpretation of results.

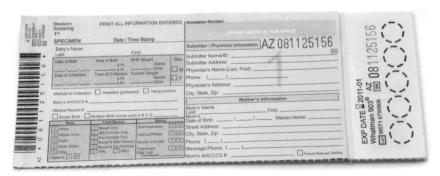

Figure 10-15 A newborn screening form with collection circles displayed.

⚠️ **CAUTION** Do not contaminate the filter paper circles by touching them with or without gloves or allowing any other object or substance to touch them before, during, or after specimen collection. Substances that have been identified as contaminants in newborn screening specimens include alcohol, formula, lotion, powder, and urine.

After collection, the specimen must be allowed to air-dry in an elevated, horizontal position away from heat or sunlight. Specimens should not be hung to dry or stacked together before, during, or after the drying process. Hanging may cause the blood to migrate and concentrate toward the low end of the filter paper and lead to erroneous test results on the sample. Stacking can result in cross-contamination between specimens, which also causes erroneous results. When dry, the requisition containing the sample is normally placed in a special envelope and sent to a state public health laboratory or other approved laboratory for testing. Results are sent to the infant's physician or other healthcare provider. The procedure for collecting blood spots for newborn screening is shown in Procedure 10-4.

ROUTINE BLOOD FILM/SMEAR PREPARATION

A **blood film/smear** (a drop of blood spread thin on a microscope slide) is required to perform a manual **differential** (Diff), a test in which the number, type, and characteristics of blood cells are determined by examining a stained blood smear under a microscope. A manual differential may be performed as part of a complete blood count or to confirm abnormal results of a machine-generated differential or platelet count. Two blood smears are normally prepared and submitted for testing. Although a common practice in the past, today blood smears are rarely made at the bedside. They are typically made in the hematology department from blood collected in an EDTA tube, either by hand or using an automated machine that makes a uniform smear from a single drop of blood.

🔑 **Key Point** Blood smears prepared from EDTA specimens should be made within 1 hour of collection to eliminate cell distortion caused by the anticoagulant.

Procedure 10-4: Newborn Screening Blood Spot Collection

PURPOSE: To obtain a newborn screening blood sample by heel puncture

EQUIPMENT: Gloves, warming device, antiseptic prep pad, safety lancet, newborn screening filter paper, sterile gauze pads, sharps container, permanent ink pen

Step	Explanation/Rationale
1 to 4. Follow Chapter 8 venipuncture steps 1 through 4.	See Chapter 8 Procedure 8-2: steps 1 through 4.
5. Position the patient.	See Heelstick Procedure 10-2: step 5.
6. Select the puncture site.	See Heelstick Procedure 10-2: step 6.
7. Warm the site, if applicable.	See Heelstick Procedure 10-2: step 7.
8. Clean and air-dry the site.	See Heelstick Procedure 10-2: step 8.
9. Prepare equipment.	See Heelstick Procedure 10-2: step 9.
10. Puncture site and discard lancet.	See Heelstick Procedure 10-2: step 10.
11. Wipe away the first blood drop.	See Heelstick Procedure 10-2: step 11.
12. Bring the filter paper close to the heel.	Ensures that drops fill the circles properly. The paper must not actually touch the heel; if it does, smearing, incomplete penetration of the paper, blotting, and stoppage of blood flow can result.
13. Generate a large, free-flowing drop of blood.	It takes a large, free-flowing blood drop to fill a circle. Small drops can result in incomplete filling and the tendency to layer successive drops in a circle to fill it.
14. Touch the blood drop to the center of the filter paper circle.	The drop must touch the center of the circle for blood to uniformly spread out to the perimeter.

Procedure 10-4: Newborn Screening Blood Spot Collection (Continued)

Step	Explanation/Rationale
15. Fill the circle with blood. 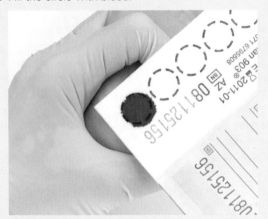	Blood drop position must be maintained until blood soaks through the circle, completely filling both sides of the paper. Caution: Do not fill spots from the reverse side to finish filling the circles because this causes layering and erroneous results.
16. Fill remaining blood spot circles. 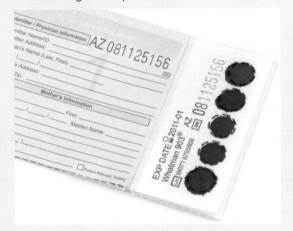	Fill all circles the same way. Unfilled or incompletely filled circles can result in inability to perform all required tests.
17. Place gauze, elevate site, and apply pressure.	Absorbs excess blood, and helps stop bleeding
18. Label specimen.	Immediate labeling with appropriate information helps ensures specimens are properly identified.
19. Check the site. **Note:** *Do not* apply a bandage to the infant.	Examining the site is necessary to verify that bleeding has stopped. *Do not* apply a bandage as it can become a choking hazard or tear the skin when removed. **Note:** If bleeding persists beyond 5 minutes, notify the patient's physician or designated healthcare provider.
20. Dispose of used materials	Follow facility protocol for discarding trash and contaminated items, such as blood-soaked gauze.
21. Allow the specimen to air-dry.	Air-drying in an elevated horizontal position away from heat or sunlight is required for newborn screening specimens. They must not be hung to dry or stacked with other specimens before, during, or after the drying process. Hanging or storage at a slant causes blood to migrate to the low end of the filter paper and leads to erroneous test results.
22. Dispatch specimen to testing facility.	When dry, the sample-containing requisition is normally placed in a special envelope and sent to the appropriate laboratory for testing.

A few special tests require evaluation of a blood smear made from a fresh drop of blood from a fingertip. An example is a leukocyte alkaline phosphatase (LAP) stain or score, which usually requires four fresh peripheral blood (blood from an extremity) smears. Skin puncture collection of peripheral smears is typically preferred. In addition, some hematologists prefer blood smears made from blood that has not been in contact with EDTA.

When collected with other skin puncture specimens, blood smears should be collected first to avoid effects of platelet clumping. Blood smear preparation from a capillary puncture is illustrated in Procedure 10-5.

To prepare a smear manually from an EDTA specimen, the tube of blood must first be mixed for a minimum of 2 minutes to ensure a uniform specimen. A plain capillary tube or pipet is then used to dispense a drop of blood from the specimen tube onto the slide. A device called DIFF-SAFE (Fig. 10-16A–C) (Alpha Scientific, Malvern, PA) allows a slide to be made from an EDTA tube without removing the tube stopper. The device is inserted through the rubber stopper of the specimen tube and then pressed against the slide to deliver a uniform drop of blood.

⚠️ **CAUTION** Blood smears are considered biohazardous or infectious until they are stained or fixed.

Making a good blood smear is a skill that takes practice to perfect. Improperly made blood smears may not contain a normal, even distribution of blood cells and can produce erroneous results. An acceptable smear covers about one-half to three-fourths of the surface of the slide and has no holes, lines, or jagged edges. It should show a smooth transition from thick to thin when held up to the light. The thinnest area of a properly made smear, often referred to as the **feather**, is one cell thick and is the most important area because that is where a differential is performed.

Smears that are uneven, too long (i.e., cover the entire length of the slide), too short, too thick, or too thin are not acceptable. The length and thickness of the smear can usually be controlled by adjusting the size of the drop or the angle of the spreader slide. Dirt, fingerprints, or powder on the slide, or fat globules and lipids in the specimen can result in holes in the smear.

Procedure 10-5: Preparing a Blood Smear from a Capillary Puncture

PURPOSE: To prepare two routine blood films (smears) for hematology or other studies using blood obtained by capillary puncture

EQUIPMENT: Gloves, alcohol prep pad, lancet/incision device, two plain or frosted glass slides free of cracks or chipped edges, gauze pads, bandage, and a pencil

Step	Explanation/Rationale
1. Perform capillary puncture.	Blood to make the slide can be obtained by normal finger or heel puncture, following applicable capillary puncture steps 1 through 11 until this point.
2. Wipe away first blood drop.	Wiping the first drop removes excess tissue fluid and alcohol residue that could distort cell morphology.
3. Touch a slide the next blood drop.	The drop should be 1 to 2 mm in diameter and centered on the slide adjacent to the frosted end or 1/2 to 1 inch from one end of a plain slide.

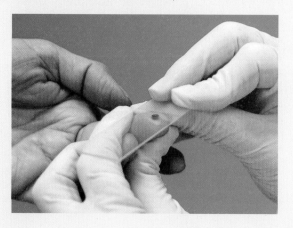

Procedure 10-5: Preparing a Blood Smear from a Capillary Puncture (Continued)

Step	Explanation/Rationale
4. Hold the blood drop slide between the thumb and forefinger of the nondominant hand. With the other hand, rest the second slide in front of the drop at an angle of approximately 30 degrees. 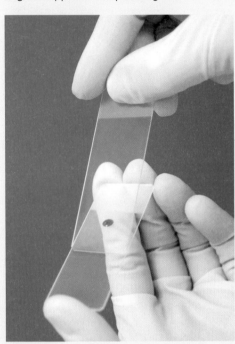	The second slide is called the pusher or spreader slide and is held at one end, between the thumb and index finger in either a vertical or horizontal position. If blood is of normal thickness, a 30-degree angle will create a smear that covers approximately three fourths of the remaining area of the slide.
5. Pull the spreader slide back to the edge of the blood drop. Stop it as soon as it touches the drop, and allow the blood to spread along its width. 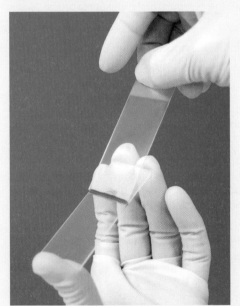	The blood must spread the width of the pusher slide or a bullet-shaped film will result.

Procedure 10-5: Preparing a Blood Smear from a Capillary Puncture (Continued)

Step	Explanation/Rationale
6. Push the spreader slide away from the drop in one smooth motion, carrying it the entire length and off the end of the blood drop slide.	Let the weight of the spreader slide carry the blood and create the film or smear. *Do not* push down on the spreader slide because this creates lines and ridges and an unacceptable blood film.

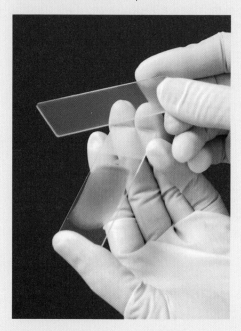

Step	Explanation/Rationale
7. Place the drop of blood for the second smear on the spreader slide. Use the slide with the first smear as the spreader slide for the second smear and make it in the same manner as the first one.	This way, two smears can be made using only two slides.
8. Place gauze over the wound and ask the patient to apply pressure.	A conscious, mentally alert patient can apply pressure; otherwise, the phlebotomist must apply pressure.
9. Label frosted blood slides by writing the patient information in pencil on the frosted area. If using a preprinted label, attach it over the writing or in the empty space at the blood drop end if it is a plain slide.	*Do not* use ink because it may dissolve during the staining process.
10. Allow the blood films to air-dry and place them in a secondary container for transport.	*Never* blow on a slide to dry it because red blood cell distortion may result. Be aware that unfixed slides are capable of transmitting disease and handle accordingly.
11. Thank patient, remove gloves, and sanitize hands.	Thanking the patients, parents, and guardians is courteous and professional. Remove gloves aseptically and wash hands or use a hand sanitizer as an infection control precaution.
12. Transport specimen to the lab.	Prompt delivery to the lab is necessary to protect specimen integrity.

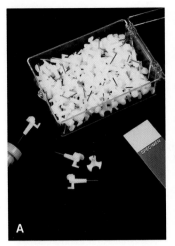
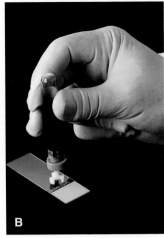
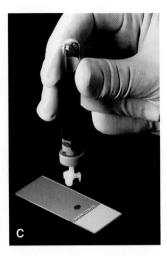

Figure 10-16 A: DIFF-SAFE blood drop delivery device. **B:** Applying a blood drop to a slide using a DIFF-SAFE device. **C:** Blood drop on slide. (Courtesy Alpha Scientific, Malvern, PA.)

A chipped pusher slide, a blood drop that has started to dry out, or uneven pressure as the smear is made can cause the smear to have ragged edges. Table 10-5 lists common problems associated with routine blood smear preparation.

THICK BLOOD SMEAR PREPARATION

Thick blood smears are most often requested to detect the presence of malaria, a disorder caused by four species of parasitic sporozoan (types of protozoa) organisms

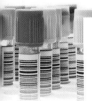

Table 10-4: Five Groups of Disorders That Can Be Detected by Newborn Screening

Disorder	Description	Consequence If Untreated	Example
Organic acid metabolism disorders	Inherited disorders that cause the inability to breakdown amino acids and other body substances, such as lipids, sugars, and steroids	Food is not metabolized correctly. Toxic acids build up in the body and can lead to coma and death within the first month of life.	IVA (isovaleric acidemia) GAI (glutaric acidemia) HMG (hydroxymethylglutaric aciduria) MCD (multiple carboxylase deficiency) MUT (methylmalonic acidemia from mutase deficiency) PROP (propionic acidemia)
Fatty acid oxidation disorders	Inherited defects in enzymes that are needed to convert fat into energy	The body is unable to change fat into energy when it runs out of glucose. This negatively affects the brain and other organs, and can lead to coma and death.	CUD (carnitine uptake defect) MCAD (medium-chain acyl-CoA dehydrogenase deficiency) VLCAD (very long-chain acyl-CoA dehydrogenase deficiency) TFP (trifunctional protein deficiency)
Amino acid metabolism disorders	A diverse group of disorders often involving lack of an enzyme needed to breakdown an amino acid, or the deficiency of enzyme needed to eliminate nitrogen from amino acid molecules	Amino acids (which help the body make protein) cannot be processed. Toxic levels of amino acids or ammonia can build up in the body, causing a variety of symptoms and even death. Symptom severity varies by disorder.	PKU (phenylketonuria) MSUD (maple syrup urine disease) HCY (homocystinuria) CIT (citrullinemia) ASA (argininosuccinic acidemia) TYR I (tyrosinemia type I)

(continued)

Table 10-4: Five Groups of Disorders That Can Be Detected by Newborn Screening (Continued)

Disorder	Description	Consequence If Untreated	Example
Hemoglobinopathies	Inherited disorders that affect red blood cells and result in anemia and other health problems	Anemias that vary in severity by disorder and by individual	Hb SS (sickle cell anemia) Hb S/Th (hemoglobin S/beta thalassemia) Hb S/C (hemoglobin S/C disease)
Other disorder	A miscellaneous group of inherited and noninherited disorders	Produces symptoms that vary from mild to life threatening, depending on the disorder.	BIOT (biotinidase deficiency) CH (congenital hypothyroidism) CCHD (critical congenital heart disease) GALT (classic galactosemia) HEAR (hearing loss) CF (cystic fibrosis) SCID (severe combined immunodeficiency)

called plasmodia. These organisms are transmitted to humans by the bite of infected female anopheles mosquitoes. Symptoms of malaria include serial bouts of fever and chills at regular intervals, related to the multiplication of certain forms of the organism within the red blood cells and the consequent rupture of those cells. The progressive destruction of red blood cells in certain types of malaria causes severe anemia.

Malaria is diagnosed by the presence of the organism in a peripheral blood smear. Diagnosis often requires the evaluation of both regular and thick blood smears. Presence of the organism is observed most frequently in a thick smear; however, identification of the species requires evaluation of a regular blood smear. Malaria smears may be ordered STAT or at timed intervals and are most commonly collected just before the onset of fever and chills.

To prepare a thick smear, a very large drop of blood is placed in the center of a glass slide and spread with the corner of another slide or cover slip until it is the size of a dime. The smear is allowed to dry for a minimum of 2 hours before staining with fresh diluted Giemsa stain, a water-based stain that lyses the red blood cells and makes the organism easier to see.

Table 10-5: Common Problems Associated with Routine Blood Smear Preparation

Problem	Probable Cause
Absence of feather	Spreader slide lifted before the smear was completed
Holes in the smear	Dirty slide Fat globules in the blood Blood contaminated with glove powder
Ridges or uneven thickness	Too much pressure applied to spreader slide
Smear is too thick	Blood drop too large Spreader slide angle too steep Patient has high red blood cell count
Smear is too short	Blood drop too small Spreader slide angle too steep Spreader slide pushed too quickly Patient has high red blood cell count
Smear is too long	Blood drop too large Spreader slide angle too shallow Spreader slide pushed too slowly Patient has a low hemoglobin
Smear is too thin	Blood drop too small Spreader slide angle too shallow Patient has a low hemoglobin
Streaks or tails in feathered edge	Blood drop started to dry out Edge of spreader slide dirty or chipped Spreader slide pushed through blood drop Uneven pressure applied to spreader slide

Study and Review Questions

📖 *See the EXAM REVIEW for more study questions.*

1. **Which of the following tests requires an arterialized specimen?**
   a. Bilirubin
   b. Blood gases
   c. Electrolytes
   d. Glucose

2. **Capillary puncture supplies include all of the following except**
   a. gauze pad.
   b. lancet.
   c. microcollection device.
   d. povidone–iodine pad.

3. **Capillary puncture blood contains**
   a. arterial blood.
   b. interstitial fluids.
   c. venous blood.
   d. all of the above.

4. **The concentration of this substance is higher in capillary blood than in venous blood:**
   a. Blood urea nitrogen
   b. Carotene
   c. Glucose
   d. Total protein

5. **Capillary puncture is typically performed on adults when**
   a. no accessible veins can be located.
   b. patients have thrombotic tendencies.
   c. veins are saved for chemotherapy.
   d. all of the above.

6. **If collected by capillary puncture, which of the following is collected first?**
   a. CBC
   b. Electrolytes
   c. Glucose
   d. Phosphorus

7. **Which of the following conditions disqualifies a site for capillary puncture?**
   a. Cyanotic
   b. Edematous
   c. Swollen
   d. All of the above

8. **Which of the following is the least hazardous area of an infant's foot for capillary puncture?**
   a. Central area of the heel
   b. Lateral plantar heel surface
   c. Medial area of the arch
   d. Posterior curvature of the heel

9. **According to CLSI, a heel puncture lancet should puncture no deeper than**
   a. 1.5 mm.
   b. 2.0 mm.
   c. 2.5 mm.
   d. 3.0 mm.

10. **Which of the following is a proper capillary puncture procedure?**
    a. Clean the site thoroughly with povidone–iodine.
    b. Milk the site to keep the blood flowing freely.
    c. Puncture parallel to fingerprint grooves.
    d. Wipe away the very first drop of blood.

11. **When making a routine blood smear, the "pusher slide" is normally used at an angle of how many degrees?**
    a. 15
    b. 30
    c. 45
    d. 60

12. **The blood specimen for this test is placed in circles on special filter paper:**
    a. Bilirubin
    b. CBGs
    c. PKU
    d. Malaria

13. **Which of the following fingers is the best choice for a capillary puncture?**
    a. Index
    b. Middle
    c. Pinky
    d. Thumb

14. **This test cannot be collected by capillary puncture and taken to the laboratory for processing and testing.**
    a. Bili
    b. Hgb
    c. Lead
    d. PTT

15. **Capillary action is a term used to describe how**
    a. arterial blood enters the capillaries.
    b. blood fills a microhematocrit tube.
    c. cells spread across a blood smear.
    d. warming can increase blood flow.

Case Studies

 See the WORKBOOK for more case studies.

Case Study 10-1: Capillary Puncture Procedure

A phlebotomist is sent to collect a CBC specimen on a 5-year-old pediatric patient. The patient has an IV in the left forearm. The right arm has no palpable veins so the phlebotomist decides to perform capillary puncture on the middle finger of the right hand. This is the phlebotomist's first job and, although he is quite good at routine venipuncture, he has not performed very many capillary punctures. The child is uncooperative and the mother tries to help steady the child's hand during the procedure. The phlebotomist is able to puncture the site, but the child pulls the hand away. Blood runs down the finger. The phlebotomist grabs the child's finger and tries to fill the collection device with the blood as it runs down the finger. The child continues to try to wriggle the finger free. The phlebotomist finally fills the container to the minimum level. When the specimen is tested, the platelet count is abnormally low. A slide is made and platelet clumping is observed. A new specimen is requested. Hemolysis is later observed in the specimen.

QUESTIONS

1. How might the circumstances of collection have contributed to the platelet clumping in the specimen?

2. What most likely caused the hemolysis?

3. What factors may have contributed to the specimen collection difficulties?

Case Study 10-2: Venous Blood and Microtubes

Casey is a phlebotomist in small rural hospital. Tonight he is working the night shift by himself. He has a major headache that won't quit, so he is not feeling his best. So far so good, though. It has been a quiet evening and all his draws have been patients with easy veins. Then he gets an order for STAT CBC, electrolytes and glucose on a patient in ICU. The patient has IVs in both arms and has tiny hand veins. Casey decides to perform a syringe draw on a hand vein. The vein blows and he has to discontinue the draw. There is a small amount of blood in the syringe so he decides to put half of it in a nonadditive microtube for the electrolytes and glucose, and the rest in an EDTA microtube. He is only able to fill each microtube part way. Just then he is paged for a STAT draw in the ER. He quickly finishes up with the patient, slaps labels on the microtubes, scribbles his initials on them, and heads to the lab to deliver them before proceeding to the ER.

QUESTIONS

1. Casey forgot to put something important on the labels of the microtubes. What was it and why is that a problem?

2. What effect could his forgetfulness have when the results of the electrolytes and glucose are reported? What is the reason for your answer?

3. One of the specimens is compromised even if the problem addressed by the first question had not happened. It might be compromised in another way also. Which specimen is it and describe why it is compromised for certain, and the second way that it also might be compromised.

Bibliography and Suggested Readings

Bishop ML, Fody EP, Schoeff LE. *Clinical Chemistry: Principles, Procedures, Correlations.* 7th ed. Philadelphia, PA: Lippincott Williams & Wilkins; 2013.

Clinical and Laboratory Standards Institute LA04-A5. *Blood Collection on Filter Paper for Newborn Screening Programs; Approved Standard.* 5th ed. Wayne, PA: CLSI/NCCLS; 2007.

Clinical and Laboratory Standards Institute, GP42-A6. *Procedures and Devices for the Collection of Capillary Blood Specimens; Approved Standard.* 6th ed. Wayne, PA: CLSI/NCCLS; 2007.

Clinical and Laboratory Standards Institute, GP43–A4. *Procedures for the Collection of Arterial Blood Specimens; Approved Standard.* 4th ed. Wayne, PA: CLSI/NCCLS; 2004.

Clinical and Laboratory Standards Institute, GP44-A4. *Procedures for the Handling and Processing of Blood Specimens; Approved Guideline.* 3rd ed. Wayne, PA: CLSI/NCCLS; 2010.

Fischbach F, Dunning MB. *A Manual of Laboratory & Diagnostic Tests.* 9th ed. Philadelphia, PA: Lippincott Williams & Wilkins; 2014.

Harmening D. *Clinical hematology and fundamentals of hemostasis.* 5th ed. Philadelphia, PA: FA Davis; 2008.

Hicks JM. Q & A: Blood volumes needed for common tests. *Lab Med.* 2001;32(4):187–189.

Turgeon ML. *Clinical Hematology.* 5th ed. Baltimore, MD: Lippincott Williams & Wilkins; 2012.

 MEDIA MENU

Online Ancillaries (at http://thepoint.lww.com/McCall6e)
- Videos:
  - Introductory and identification processes required prior to blood specimen collection
  - Capillary blood specimen collection
- Interactive exercises and games, including look and label, word building, body building, roboterms, crossword puzzles, quiz show, and concentration
- Audio flash cards and flash card generator
- Audio glossary

Internet Resources
- Advance magazine for medical laboratory personnel: http://laboratorian.advanceweb.com/
- American Academy of Pediatricians: http://www.aap.org
- Center for Phlebotomy Education: http://www.phlebotomy.com
- ITC Tenderfoot Heel Incision Device Video: http://www.itcmed.com
- National Newborn Screening and Genetic Resource Center: http://genes-r-us.uthsca.edu

Other Resources
- McCall R, Tankersley C. Student Workbook for Phlebotomy Essentials, 6th ed. (Available for separate purchase.)
- McCall R, Tankersley C. Phlebotomy Exam Review, 6th ed. (Available for separate purchase.)

Unit IV

Special Procedures

Chapter 11

Special Collections and Point-of-Care Testing

NAACLS Entry Level Competencies

4.5 Explain the importance of timed, fasting and stat specimens, as related to specimen integrity and patient care.

6.2 Differentiate between sterile and antiseptic techniques.

6.3 Describe the steps in the preparation of a puncture site.

7.3 Explain methods for transporting and processing specimens for routine and special testing.

7.6 Describe and follow the criteria for collection and processing of specimens that will be used as legal evidence, that is, paternity testing, chain of custody, blood alcohol levels, etc.

8.0 Demonstrate understanding of quality assurance and quality control in phlebotomy.

8.2 Identify policies and procedures used in the clinical laboratory to assure quality in the obtaining of blood specimens.

Key Terms

📖 *Do Matching Exercise 11-1 in the WORKBOOK to gain familiarity with these terms.*

AABB
ACT
aerobic
anaerobic
ARD
autologous
BAC
bacteremia
BNP
chain of custody
compatibility

CRP
EQC
ETOH
FAN
FUO
GTT
hCG
hyper/ hypoglycemia
hyper/ hypokalemia

hyper/ hyponatremia
hypoxemia
iCa^{2+}
INR
K^+
lactate
lookback
lysis
NIDA
peak level

POCT
PP
septicemia
TDM
TGC
TnI
TnT
trough level

Objectives

Upon successful completion of this chapter, the reader should be able to:

1 Demonstrate basic knowledge of special collection procedures, define the associated terminology, and understand importance for special labeling, equipment, collection, timing and handling of each procedure.

2 Describe patient identification and specimen labeling procedures required for blood bank tests and identify the types of specimens typically required.

3 Describe sterile technique in blood culture collection, explain why it is important, and list the reasons why a physician might order blood cultures.

4 Define point-of-care testing (POCT), explain the principle behind the POCT examples listed in this chapter, and identify any special equipment required.

Overview

This chapter describes special tests and point-of-care testing (POCT). Collecting specimens for these tests requires additional knowledge and may involve different preparation for collection and handling. POCT specimen types vary, and the small, portable, and often handheld testing devices that process the specimens bring laboratory testing to the location of the patient. Some of the most commonly encountered special blood test and POCT procedures are described in this chapter. Procedures in this chapter conform to CLSI standards.

Special Procedures

Most laboratory tests require blood specimens that are collected by routine venipuncture or capillary puncture procedures. Some tests, however, require specific and unique collection procedures or are performed on other body substances such as feces or urine. Collecting specimens for these tests may require special preparation, equipment, handling, or timing. Closely adhering to the specified instruction is necessary for quality results.

Blood Bank Specimens

Blood bank (BB) specimens yield information that determines which blood products can be transfused safely into a patient. Precise and consistent attention to protocol in collecting blood bank specimens is crucial to safe transfusions. It is important to always follow facility-specific procedures.

IDENTIFICATION AND LABELING REQUIREMENTS

Blood bank specimens require strict patient identification and specimen labeling procedures.

Key Point *The Joint Commission's top National Patient Safety Goal* (NPSG 01.01.01) is to improve the accuracy of patient identification by using at least two patient identifiers (neither to be the patient's room number) whenever administering medications or blood products; taking blood samples and other specimens for clinical testing, or providing any other treatments or procedures.

Specimens that have labeling errors of any kind or are unlabeled will not be accepted for testing. This pertains to specimens drawn in the emergency room or operating room as well. When someone outside of the laboratory personnel collects the specimen, the full name of that person or their assigned mnemonic, whether it is a physician or nurse, must be on the label. An error in specimen identification or labeling requires recollection of the specimen and causes a delay in patient treatment. An undetected error can result in administration of an incompatible blood product and the possibility of a fatal transfusion reaction. Typical labeling requirements for blood bank specimens are shown in Box 11-1.

SPECIAL IDENTIFICATION SYSTEMS

Blood bank ID bands are specifically designed to protect patients and healthcare facilities from potentially fatal errors made during identification and administration of blood products.

A variety of special blood bank identification products are available.

Some companies offer handwritten, self-carbon labels for the special BB bracelet (Fig. 11-1). Others provide preprinted patient labels with barcoded BBIDs that can be printed in the laboratory with the requisition or at the bedside. All bands contain a unique ID number on each patient's band to ensure that blood specimens are correctly identified with that one person only. The additional ID-numbered stickers from the bracelet or

Box 11-1

Typical Labeling Requirements for Blood Bank Specimens

- Patient's full name (including middle initial)
- Patient's hospital identification number (or other unique identifier)
- Patient's date of birth
- Date and time of collection
- Phlebotomist's ID number or full name
- Room number and bed number (optional)

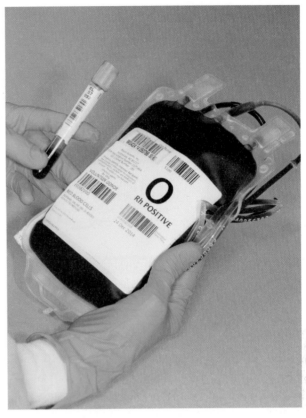

Figure 11-2 Prepared unit of blood with unique ID sticker that exactly matches that on the tube of blood collected for cross-match.

requisition are sent to the lab with the specimen to be used in the cross-match process. As soon as the testing begins the uniquely numbered sticker is attached to the unit of blood or other blood products used for transfusion as shown in Figure 11-2.

For more accuracy in the patient transfusion area, blood recipient patient ID *systems* have been created to reduce common transcription errors. These systems allow for the implementation of electronic ID and contain linear barcoded BBID numbers on all printed patient information, such as, requisitions, labels, and coded specimen stickers.

Key Point These special BBID systems allow for one-person verification for blood transfusions because they meet *The Joint Commission's National Patient Safety Goal* (NPSG 01.033.01) that states "Make certain that the correct patient gets the correct blood when they get a blood transfusion."

Figure 11-3 shows an example of a condensed Typenex FlexiBlood form, which accompanies the requisition when blood is being collected for patient cross-matching. This barcode system also has directions for proper overlabeling on specimen tubes, thereby making it possible for BB instrumentation to read the label correctly every time.

To gain familiarity with how to handle blood bank collections, try Labeling Exercise 11-2, in the WORKBOOK.

An example of an electronic blood bank ID system is the Siemens Patient Identification Check–Blood Administration workflow. Patient Identification Check provides positive identification safeguards for blood product administration, helping clinicians identify the right patient with the right blood product with barcode accuracy. The nurse initiates the blood product validation for a patient by gathering four key facts about the blood product in the presence of the patient.

- The healthcare provider's identity, scanned from the bar code on his or her identification card.

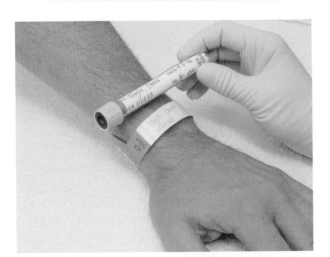

Figure 11-1 A phlebotomist compares a labeled blood bank tube with a blood bank ID bracelet.

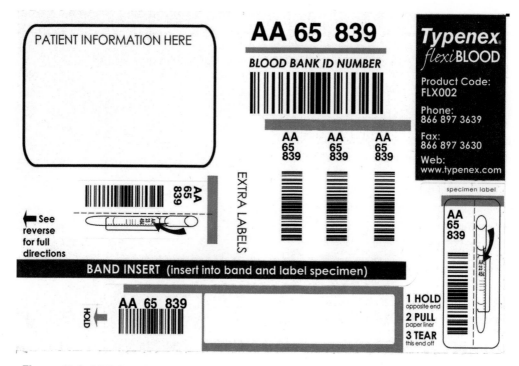

Figure 11-3 BBID form from the FlexiBlood System. (Courtesy Typenex Medical LLC, Chicago, IL.)

- The patient's identification scanned from the bar code on the patient's wristband as seen in Figure 11-4.
- The product's unique barcoded donor identifier on the blood unit.
- The blood product's bar code on the blood unit.

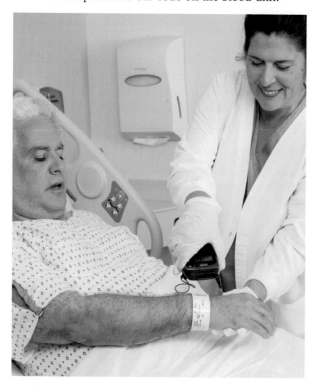

Figure 11-4 Using the Patient Identification Check to scan the patient ID band. (Courtesy Siemens Medical Solutions, Malvern, PA.)

Before the healthcare provider physically starts the transfusion, the Patient Identification Check may require a second nurse validation. Once all verification is complete, the unit is ready to be physically transfused by the clinician. Upon completion of the transfusion, the nurse updates the Patient Identification Check system, which in turn updates the blood bank system to reflect that the unit has been administered and logs the date and time of completion. This method helps to increase patient safety and provides accurate records for the blood administration workflow process.

SPECIMEN REQUIREMENTS

Blood bank tests require the collection of one or more lavender- or pink-top EDTA tubes. In some cases, a non-additive glass red-stoppered tube is used. Specimens collected for blood bank testing can be rejected if they:

- are not labeled exactly as described in the laboratory protocol.
- are grossly hemolyzed samples.
- contain IV fluid (note if drawn from opposite arm or below IV).
- have been collected longer than 72 hours before.

⚠️ **CAUTION** The BBID band needs to remain on the patient as long as it is still valid, usually 3 days. For example, the day the BB specimen is drawn is day "0" and is good until 23:59 of day "4."

TYPE, SCREEN, AND CROSS-MATCH

One of the most common tests performed by the blood bank is a blood type and screen. This test determines a patient's blood type (ABO) and Rh factor (positive or negative). When required, a cross-match is performed using the patient's type and screen results to help select a donor unit of blood. During a cross-match, the patient's plasma or serum and the donor's RBCs are mixed together to determine **compatibility** (suitability to be mixed). A transfusion of incompatible blood can be fatal because of **agglutination** (clumping) and **lysis** (rupturing) of the RBCs within the patient's circulatory system.

Blood Donor Collection

Blood donor collection involves screening and collecting blood to be used for transfusion purposes rather than for diagnostic testing. Blood is collected from volunteers in amounts referred to as units. Donor collection requires special training and exceptional venipuncture skills. Facilities that provide blood products for transfusion purposes are called Blood Donor Centers. Blood Centers follow guidelines set by the **American Association of Blood Banks (AABB)** for purposes of quality assurance and standardization. Regulation by the **U.S. Food and Drug Administration (FDA)** is required, since blood and blood products are considered pharmaceuticals.

Key Point All potential blood donors must be interviewed to determine their eligibility to donate blood as well as to obtain information for the records that must be kept on all blood donors.

DONOR ELIGIBILITY

According to the American Red Cross, persons wishing to donate blood must feel well and be in good general health. They must be at least 17 years old in most states and weigh at least 110 pounds. If allowed by state law, a 16-year old may donate and must have written permission from their parents. Adults over the age of 66 years may be allowed to donate at the discretion of the blood center physician. A brief physical examination as well as an extensive medical history is needed to determine the patient's health status. A check of the hemoglobin or hematocrit value is performed. Hemoglobin can be no less than 12.5 g/dL or 38% for the hematocrit. This information is collected each time a person donates, no matter how many times a person has donated before. All donor information is strictly confidential. In addition, the donor must give written permission for the blood bank to use his or her blood. The principles of donor unit collection are listed in Box 11-2.

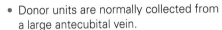

Box 11-2

Principles of Donor Unit Collection

- Donor units are normally collected from a large antecubital vein.
- The vein is selected in a manner similar to routine venipuncture and cleaned in a manner similar to blood culture collection (see Fig. 11-8).
- The collection unit is a sterile, closed system consisting of a bag to contain the blood connected by a length of tubing to a sterile 16- to 18-gauge needle.
- The bag fills by gravity and must be placed lower than the patient's arm.
- The collection bag contains an anticoagulant and preservative solution and is placed on a mixing unit while the blood is being drawn.
- The unit is normally filled by weight but typically contains around 450 mL of blood when full. Only one needle puncture can be used to fill a unit. If the unit only partially fills and the procedure must be repeated, an entire new unit must be used.

The anticoagulant and preservative CPD (citrate–phosphate–dextrose) or CPDA1 (CPD plus adenine) is typically used in collecting units of blood for transfusion purposes. The citrate prevents clotting by chelating calcium. A phosphate compound stabilizes the pH, and dextrose provides energy to the cells and helps keep them viable.

LOOKBACK PROGRAM

A unit of blood can be separated into several components: RBCs, plasma, granulocytes, platelets, and coagulation factors. All components of the unit must be traceable to the donor for federally required **lookback** program and this requires meticulous record keeping. Lookback can only occur when the blood service is made aware of the possibility of a transfusion-related infection. At that time, notification to all blood recipients is required and verification for all blood components previously collected and currently in inventory has been retrieved.

AUTOLOGOUS DONATION

Despite advances in blood bank procedures and identification processes, transfusions are risky; consequently,

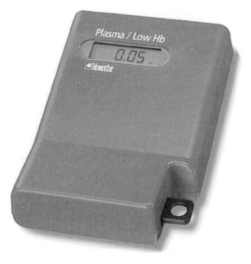

Figure 11-5 HemoCue® Plasma/Low Hb. (HemoCue, Inc., Mission Viejo, CA.)

many patients choose to take the safer route of autologous donations. **Autologous** donation is the process by which a person donates blood for his or her own use. This is done preoperatively for elective surgeries when it is anticipated that a transfusion will be needed. Using one's own blood eliminates many risks associated with transfusions, such as disease transmission and blood incompatibilities. Although blood is normally collected several weeks prior to the scheduled surgery, the minimum time between donation and surgery must be more than 72 hours. To be eligible to make an autologous donation, a person must have a written order from a physician and have a hemoglobin of at least 11 g/dL or a hematocrit equal to or greater than 33%.

CELL SALVAGING

Cell salvaging is a medical procedure designed to recover blood lost during surgery and reinfusing it back into the patient. It is a form of autologous blood transfusions. Prior to reinfusion, it is recommended that the salvaged blood be tested for residual free hemoglobin. A high free hemoglobin level indicates that too many red cells were destroyed during the salvage process and renal dysfunction could result if the blood were reinfused. Free hemoglobin can be detected using point-of-care instruments such as the HemoCue Plasma/Low Hemoglobin analyzer (Fig. 11-5).

Blood Cultures

It is known that bacteria can enter the body and cause disease. During the disease process, bacteria may also enter the circulatory system, causing **bacteremia** (bacteria in the blood) or **septicemia** (microorganisms or their toxins in the blood). Except when overwhelming infection is present, these organisms are generally cleared from the bloodstream by the body's immune system in minutes to hours. Sepsis (blood poisoning) can be life-threatening. Identifying the microorganisms in a patient's bloodstream has major diagnostic and prognostic importance. Blood cultures help determine the presence and extent of infection as well as indicating the type of organism responsible and the antibiotic to which it is most susceptible. They are also useful in assessing the effectiveness of antibiotic therapy once treatment is initiated.

INDICATIONS

Blood cultures should be ordered on the basis of whether the patient has a condition in which bloodstream invasion is possible and not only when a patient experiences a **fever of unknown origin (FUO)**. Some elderly patients and others with underlying conditions are often not capable of mounting good fever responses, even though they may be experiencing septicemia.

Key Point According to the American Society for Microbiology (ASM), laboratory diagnosis of bacteremia or fungemia (fungus or yeasts in the blood) depends on blood cultures, which are probably the most important cultures performed by the microbiology laboratory.

SPECIMEN REQUIREMENTS

Recommended Number and Timing

Recent literature of the **American Society for Microbiology (ASM)** states that two to four blood cultures are necessary to optimize the detection of bacteremia and fungemia.

One blood culture consists of blood from a single venipuncture inoculated into two separate bottles to accommodate the optimal blood-to-broth ratio.

Based on the patient's diagnosis and condition the following recommendations for time and number have been made.

- If it is an acute condition where rapid administration of antibiotics is important, two to three cultures, one right after another, from different sites immediately after the medical occurrence.
- For FUO, two to three cultures, one right after another from different sites. If these are negative after 24 to 48 hours, obtain two more cultures, as before from different sites.

- In suspected bacteremia or fungemia with persistent negative blood cultures, use alternative media to optimize the recovery of mycobacteria and fungi, that is, Myco/F Lytic media bottle.

Timing Considerations

- If the patient is in critical condition or an antibiotic must be given right away, the status of the patient will determine the timing of the blood cultures.
- When more than one set is ordered for collection at the same time, the second set should be obtained from a separately prepared site on the opposite arm if possible. In some cases, "second-site" blood cultures are more useful when drawn 30 to 60 minutes apart.
- If timing is not specified on the requisition, the phlebotomist should follow the laboratory protocol.

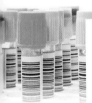

Key Point Blood cultures are typically ordered immediately before or during fever spikes when bacteria are most likely to be present. Timely collection is important, but volume is more important than timing in detecting the causative agent of septicemia.

Recommended Volume

The volume of blood drawn is the most important variable in detecting the causative agent. It has been shown that the identification of pathogens increases in direct proportion to the volume of blood cultured. ASM's recent recommendations for the amount of blood to be added to the culture media are based on weight as shown in Table 11-1.

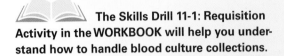

The Skills Drill 11-1: Requisition Activity in the WORKBOOK will help you understand how to handle blood culture collections.

SPECIMEN COLLECTION, TRANSPORTING, AND HANDLING

Blood culture specimens are most commonly collected in special bottles (Fig. 11-6) containing nutrient broth (referred to as medium) that encourages the growth of microorganisms. These specimens are typically collected in sets of two: one **aerobic** (with air) and one **anaerobic** (without air).

Key Point When a syringe is used to collect the blood, the anaerobic bottle is filled first. When a butterfly is used, it is preferable to fill the aerobic bottle first because air in the tubing will be drawn into it along with the blood.

Skin Antisepsis

The major difficulty in the interpretation of blood cultures is contamination by normal microbial flora on

Table 11-1: Recommended Volume of Blood to Be Cultured (by Patient Weight)

Recommended Volume of Blood to Be Cultured (by Patient Weight):

Weight	Vol in Pink-Capped Bottle	Vol in Blue-Capped Aerobic Bottles	Vol in Purple-Capped Anaerobic Bottles	Total for First Blood Culture Set (mL)	Total for Second Blood Culture Set (mL)	Total Vol Needed (mL)
	1–3 mL optimal; no less than 0.5 mL	8–10 mL optimal; no less than 3 mL	8–10 mL optimal; no less than 3 mL			
NICU patient	1 mL			1		1
<18 lb (<8 kg)	1 mL			1		1
18–29 lb (8–13 kg)	3 mL			3	3	6
30–88 lb (14–40 kg)		10 mL		10	10	20
>88 lb (>40 kg)		10 mL	10 mL	20	20	40

Courtesy of Judy Herrig, LabNM/Micro/SOP-Book1/Blood Culture Draw Procedure.

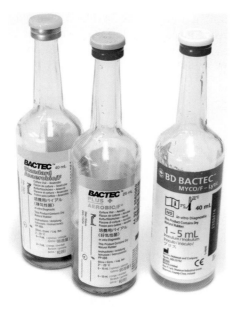

Figure 11-6 BACTEC blood culture bottles. Anaerobic/F, Aerobic/F, and Myco/F-lytic. (Becton Dickinson, Franklin Lakes, NJ.)

the skin. **Skin antisepsis**, the destruction of microorganisms on the skin, is a critical part of the blood culture collection procedure. Failure to carefully disinfect the venipuncture site can introduce skin-surface bacteria into the blood culture bottles and interfere with interpretation of results. The laboratory must report all microorganisms detected; it is then up to the patient's physician to determine whether the organism is clinically significant or merely a contaminant. If a contaminating organism is misinterpreted as pathogenic, it could result in inappropriate treatment. The best way to overcome this problem is by meticulous aseptic technique during preparation of the skin with the appropriate bactericidal agent.

Antiseptic or Sterile Technique

Blood culture collection varies slightly from one laboratory to another depending on the antiseptic used and the method selected. To minimize the risk of contamination by skin flora, collection sites require a 30- to 60-second friction scrub to get to the bacteria beneath the dead skin cells on the surface of the arm. Tincture of iodine, chlorhexidine gluconate, and a povidone/70% ethyl alcohol combination have all been shown to be effective.

Key Point It has been shown through recent research that cleansing the patient's skin with chlorhexidine or tincture of iodine is superior to using iodophors such as povidone–iodine in reducing contamination rate at BC collection sites.

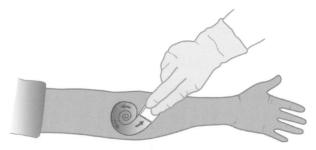

Figure 11-7 Pattern of concentric circles used in cleaning a blood culture site.

When using an ampule swab of chlorhexidine gluconate or tincture of iodine, the swab should be placed at the site of needle insertion and moved outward in concentric circles without going over any area more than once, as shown in Figure 11-7. The area covered should be at least 2.5 × 2.5 inches in diameter.

Because of the increasing incidence of iodine sensitivities, some healthcare facilities are using chlorhexidine gluconate/isopropyl alcohol antiseptic for blood cultures. They offer a one-step application and are effective with a 30-second scrub.

Key Point According to the CLSI, chlorhexidine gluconate is the recommended blood culture site disinfectant for infants 2 months and older and patients with iodine sensitivity.

Collection Procedure

The specimen collection procedure for blood culture is described in Procedure 11-1.

thePoint *View the video Collecting a Blood Culture Specimen at http://thePoint.lww.com/McCall6e.*

Key Point According to the latest OSHA revisions to the Blood-borne Pathogens Standard, employers will be cited and fined for failing to use engineering controls, such as plastic blood culture bottles that are considered much safer when sent through a pneumatic tube system or transported by courier.

PEDIATRIC BLOOD CULTURES CONSIDERATIONS

The collection of blood cultures from neonates and pediatric patients creates challenges not experienced with adult blood cultures. Besides the frequent difficulties in the collection of pediatric specimens, other challenges include the

Procedure 11-1: Blood Culture Specimen Collection

PURPOSE: Collect a blood culture specimen

EQUIPMENT: Gloves (sterile nitrile are suggested); suitable skin antiseptic; a set of blood culture bottles (aerobic and anaerobic); blood collection kit and blood culture tube holder or safety needle, syringe, and transfer device; isopropyl alcohol pads; bandage; permanent ink pen.

Although neither ASM nor CLSI standards require the use of sterile gloves for blood culture collection, using them can be beneficial during difficult draws if relocating the vein is necessary after the site has been cleaned.

Step	Explanation/Rationale
1. Follow normal identification protocol; explain collection procedure.	Patient must be properly identified and consent to the procedure.
2. Identify venipuncture site and release tourniquet.	Proper disinfection takes time; CLSI Standard GP41 states that the tourniquet should not be left on longer than 1 minute.

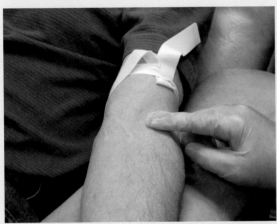

3. Aseptically select and assemble equipment.	Be very careful when removing the antiseptic sponge applicator from the packaging; keep the sponge sterile by touching only the handle. Aseptic technique in handling equipment aids in accurate diagnosis by reducing the risk of false-positive results due to contamination.

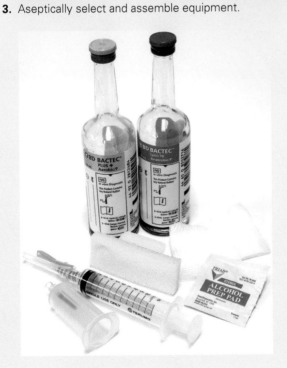

Procedure 11-1: Blood Culture Specimen Collection (Continued)

Step	Explanation/Rationale
4. Perform friction scrub.	Bacteria exist on the skin surface; they can be temporarily removed by vigorous scrubbing with an effective antiseptic solution for the amount of time designated by the procedure method. Maximum area of treatment by one applicator is approximately 2.5 × 2.5 inches. The applicator must be discarded after a single use.

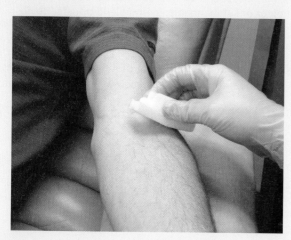

 CAUTION Do not scrub the skin of neonates too aggressively, as this may be abrasive and cause the skin to tear.

Step	Explanation/Rationale
5. Allow the site to dry.	Antisepsis does not occur instantly. The 30-second wait allows time for the antiseptic to be effective against skin-surface bacteria. Never blot, fan, or blow on the site.
6. Remove the flip-off cap and inspect the bottle for visible defects.	Inspect the bottle for contamination, excessive cloudiness, cracks, and bulging or indented septums. Make certain the bottle is in date and that the vacuum will draw at least 8 cc. Do *not* use if any defect is noted.

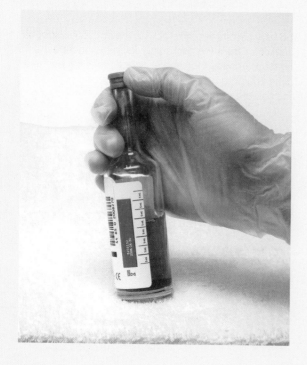

Procedure 11-1: Blood Culture Specimen Collection (Continued)

Step	Explanation/Rationale

7. Cleanse the culture bottle stoppers while the site is drying.

Top of the culture bottles must be free of contaminants when inoculated. They can be cleaned with 70% isopropyl alcohol after removing the flip-off cap. (Do not use iodine to disinfect the bottle tops). Allow to dry completely.

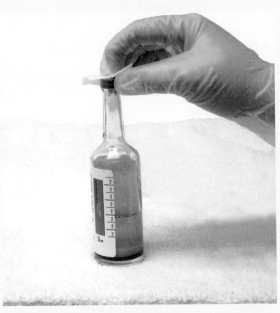

8. Mark the minimum and maximum fill on the culture bottles.

A blood culture bottle has a vacuum that usually exceeds 10 mL; consequently the user must carefully monitor how much blood is being added to the bottle. Most bottles have fill lines on the sides that can be marked. Marking the bottles ensures that enough but not too much blood enters the bottle. Typically, adult blood cultures require 20 mL per set, while pediatric blood cultures require 1 to 3 mL per set. (See Table 11-1) Consult manufacturer's instructions, as volume requirements may vary depending on the system used.

9. Reapply the tourniquet and perform the venipuncture without touching or repalpating the site.

The tourniquet must be reapplied to aid in venipuncture and care must be taken that the site is not recontaminated in the process. Ensuring antiseptic technique and sterility of the site is critical to accurate diagnosis. The site must not be repalpated. However, if the patient has "difficult" veins and a need to relocate the site is anticipated, sterile gloves are recommended, then repalpating should only be done above or below the site of needle entry.

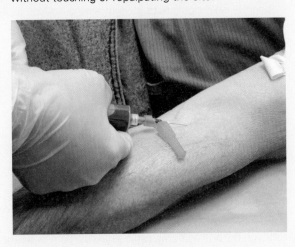

Procedure 11-1: Blood Culture Specimen Collection (Continued)

Step	Explanation/Rationale
10. Inoculate the medium as required. 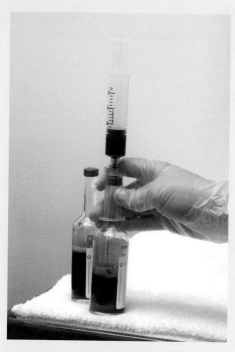	When using a butterfly, inoculation of the medium can occur directly into the bottle during specimen collection or after collection when a syringe is used. A bottle should never be inserted directly into an ETS holder used for normal specimen collection even though it may fit. There is a possibility that medium in the bottle could flow back into the patient's vein.
11. Invert the bottle several times.	The blood should be thoroughly mixed with the medium to prevent clotting and, if the bottle contains antibiotic adsorbing resin beads, to neutralize antibiotics in the patient's blood.
12. Clean the patient's skin if applicable.	If an iodine preparation was used to clean the arm, the iodine should be removed with alcohol or suitable cleanser. Iodine left on the skin can be irritating and even toxic to those with iodine sensitivity. Iodine contamination of a blood sample can also cause erroneous results for other tests.
13. Label the specimen containers with required identification information, including the site of blood collection.	Noting the collection site (e.g., right arm) or source, such as a catheter, is necessary in case there is a localized infection. Some facilities require that labeling information include the amount of blood added to each bottle. Document the date and time the culture was collected.
14. Dispose of used and contaminated materials.	Materials such as needle caps and wrappers are normally discarded in the regular trash. Some facilities require that contaminated items such as blood-soaked gauze be discarded in biohazard containers.
15. Thank the patient, remove gloves, and sanitize hands.	Thanking the patient is courteous and professional. Gloves must be removed in an aseptic manner and hands washed or decontaminated with hand sanitizer as an infection-control precaution.
16. Transport specimens to the lab as quickly as possible.	Prompt delivery to the lab protects specimen integrity, although BC bottles/tubes can be held at room temperature for a maximum of 4 hours after collections until processed. Refer to manufacturer's instruction for handling bottles that will be incubated in automated culture systems. Transportation is typically achieved by personal delivery, transportation via a pneumatic tube system, or by a courier service.

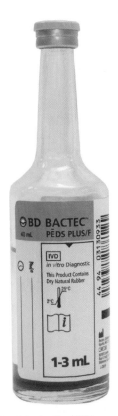

Figure 11-8 BACTEC Peds Plus™/F.

critical nature of pediatric pathogens such as *Streptococcus pneumoniae* and *Neisseria meningitidis,* and the common encounter with children having previously received broad-spectrum antibiotics. Because of these considerations, special blood culture bottles (Fig. 11-8) must be used for pediatric populations. These bottles are different from adult blood culture bottles in both the formulation of the broth and the volume. It is never advised to use pediatric blood culture bottles for adults. The small volume of blood and broth may result in false-negative results.

The same methods for skin antisepsis for adults apply to pediatric patients unless the antiseptic is tincture of iodine. It is recommended that in place of the iodine step, the site should be cleaned two additional times with separate preparation pads saturated with 70% iso-propyl alcohol or ethyl alcohol.

In general, for infants and younger children, the volume of blood collected for culturing should be from 1% to 4% of the patient's total blood volume. Pediatric blood culture bottles are designed to accommodate an inoculation of up to 4 mL of blood. See Box 11-1 for ASM's specific recommended volumes based on patient's weight.

CATHETER CONSIDERATIONS

Blood cultures should *not* be drawn through an indwelling intravenous (IV) or arterial catheter unless absolutely necessary. Draws from vascular lines are known to have a high contamination rate and may cause a

person to receive antibiotic therapy when not needed. When collecting blood cultures from a vascular access device (VAD), such as a catheter or IV, one set should be drawn percutaneously and one drawn through the catheter. This allows for the correct interpretation of a positive result since cultures drawn through any type of VAD may indicate bacterial growth in the device, and may not be representative of sepsis.

(i) Catheter-related bloodstream infections are common causes of healthcare-associated infections. Despite their frequent occurrence, catheter-related infections are difficult to diagnose.

MEDIA INOCULATION METHODS

Inoculation of media can occur in several different ways: directly into the bottle during specimen collection or after collection as when blood has been collected in a syringe. A third way is to use an intermediate collection tube to collect the sample for inoculation in the laboratory and not at the bedside.

Direct Inoculation

To collect the specimen directly into the blood culture medium, use a butterfly and specially designed holder (Fig. 11-9). Connect the special holder to the Luer

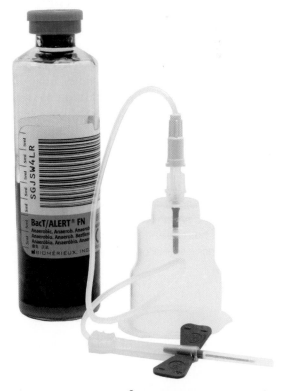

Figure 11-9 BacT/ALERT® anaerobic blood culture bottle and the specially designed holder to be used with a butterfly needle. (bioMerieux, Inc., Durham, NC.)

connector of the butterfly collection set. Fill the aerobic vial first, because the butterfly tubing has air in it. Avoid backflow by keeping the culture bottle or tube lower than the collection site and preventing the culture medium from contacting the stopper or needle during blood collection. Mix each container after removing it from the needle holder. After filling both containers and collecting blood for any other tests, remove the needle from the patient's arm, activate the safety device, and hold pressure over the site.

Key Point Blood culture specimens are always collected first in the order of draw to prevent contamination from other tubes.

Syringe Inoculation

When the syringe method is used, the blood must be transferred to the bottles after the draw is completed. Occupational Safety and Health Administration (OSHA) regulations require the use of a safety transfer device (see Fig. 7-25A) for this procedure. To transfer blood from the syringe to the culture bottles, activate the needle's safety device as soon as the needle is removed from the vein. Remove the needle and attach a safety transfer device to the syringe. Inoculate the aerobic bottle first and then the anaerobic. Push the culture bottle into the device until the needle inside it penetrates the bottle stopper. Allow the blood to be drawn from the syringe by the vacuum in the container being careful to only add the amount of blood recommended by the manufacturer. The plunger may have to be held back to keep from expelling too much blood into the bottle. Never push the plunger to expel the blood into the bottle. This can hemolyze the specimen and cause aerosol formation when the needle is removed.

CAUTION The practice of changing needles before transferring blood from a syringe into blood culture bottles is no longer recommended. Several studies have shown that changing needles has little effect on reducing contamination rates, and may actually increase risk of needlestick injury to the phlebotomist.

Intermediate Collection Tube

Blood is sometimes collected in an intermediate collection tube rather than blood culture bottles. A yellow-top sodium polyanethol sulfonate (SPS) tube (Fig. 11-10) is preferred for this purpose. In addition to being an anticoagulant, it reduces the action of a protein called complement which destroys bacteria. It can also slow down the

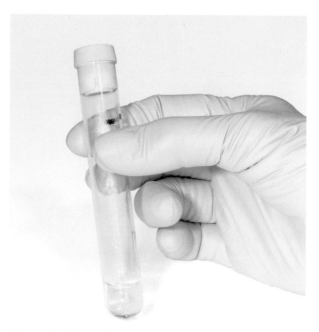

Figure 11-10 A yellow-top tube used for blood culture collection.

ingestion of bacteria by leukocytes and reduces the activity of certain antibiotics. Other anticoagulants—such as citrate, heparin, EDTA, and oxalate—may be toxic to bacteria and are not recommended. Use of an intermediate tube is discouraged, however, for the following reasons.

- SPS in the collection tube when added to the blood culture bottle increases the final concentration of SPS.
- Transfer of blood from the intermediate tube to the blood culture bottles presents another opportunity for contamination.
- Transfer of blood to the culture bottles presents an exposure risk to laboratory staff.

ANTIMICROBIAL NEUTRALIZATION PRODUCTS

It is not unusual for patients to be on **antimicrobial** (antibiotic) **therapy** at the time blood culture specimens are collected. Presence of the antimicrobial agent in the patient's blood can inhibit the growth of the microorganisms in the blood culture bottle. In such cases, the physician may order blood cultures to be collected in **fastidious antimicrobial neutralization (FAN)** (bioMerieux) or **antimicrobial removal device (ARD)** (Becton Dickinson) bottles (see Fig. 11-11). An ARD contains a resin that removes antimicrobials from the blood. FAN bottles contain activated charcoal, which helps to neutralize the antibiotic. The blood can then be processed by conventional technique with less possibility of antimicrobial therapy inhibiting the growth of microorganisms. ARDs and FANs should be delivered to the lab for processing as soon as possible.

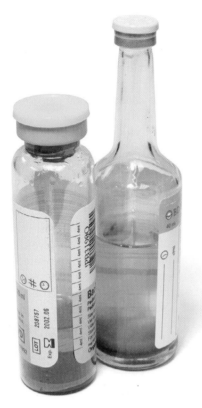

Figure 11-11 Left to right: FAN and ARD blood culture bottles.

> **Key Point** Blood cultures from patients who are already on antimicrobial therapy are typically ordered for a time when the antibiotic is anticipated to be at its lowest concentration in the blood.

Coagulation Specimens

The following are a number of important things to remember when collecting specimens for coagulation tests.

- Most coagulation tests are collected in light-blue-top sodium citrate tubes. Some special coagulation tests are collected in a light blue top called a CTAD (because it contains citrate, theophylline, adenosine, and dipyridamole). CTAD tubes are used to inhibit thrombocyte activation between collection of the specimen and testing.
- At one time it was customary to draw a "clear" or discard tube before drawing a light-blue-top tube if it was the first or only tube to be collected. A few milliliters of blood were drawn into a plain red-top tube to clear the needle of thromboplastin contamination picked up as it penetrated the skin. The clear tube was discarded if not needed for other tests. According to CLSI a clear tube is no longer necessary when collecting PT/INR,

PTT/aPTT, and some special coagulation tests. All other coagulation tests still require a clear tube.

> (i) Although CLSI says a discard tube is no longer necessary, a fairly large study in 2012 suggests that a discard tube *is* still necessary for coagulation testing. Follow facility protocol.

- If a light-blue-top is the first or only tube to be drawn using a winged blood collection set (butterfly), a discard tube must be collected first to prime the tubing. Otherwise, the air in the tubing will take the place of blood in the tube and result in an incomplete draw and an incorrect blood-to-additive ratio (see next bullet).
- Light-blue-top tubes for coagulation tests must be filled until the vacuum is exhausted to obtain a 9:1 ratio of blood to anticoagulant, which is critical to accurate test results. This ratio can be altered if the patient's hematocrit exceeds 55%, even if the tube is correctly filled. In such cases, laboratory personnel may request specimen collection in a special tube that has had the anticoagulant volume adjusted.

> ⚠ **CAUTION** All anticoagulant tubes must be gently inverted three or four times immediately after collection to avoid microclots, which can invalidate test results.

- Never pour two partially filled tubes together to create a full tube, as the anticoagulant-to-blood ratio will be greatly affected.
- Coagulation factors V and VIII are highly unstable. If these specimens cannot be tested within 4 hours, they must be centrifuged and the plasma frozen.
- Drawing a coagulation specimen from a VAD is not recommended. However, if there is no other choice, the specimen can be drawn by specially trained healthcare personnel following the procedure shown in Chapter 9 under Vascular Access Devices (VADs) and Sites. Coagulation specimens drawn from VADs require a discard volume of blood that is six times the deadspace volume of the tubing, or approximately 5 mL.

Two-Hour Postprandial Glucose

Postprandial (PP) means after a meal. Glucose levels in blood specimens obtained 2 hours after a meal are rarely elevated in normal persons but may be significantly increased in diabetic patients. Therefore

Box 11-3

Principles of 2-Hour PP Specimen Collection

- The patient fasts prior to the test. This means no eating, smoking, or drinking other than water for at least 10 to 12 hours before the test.
- A fasting glucose specimen may be collected before the start of the test.
- The patient is instructed to eat a high-carbohydrate breakfast (typically one containing the equivalent of 75 to 100 g of glucose) or given a measured dose of glucose beverage on the day of the test.
- After the meal, nothing else should be consumed before the test. Rest during the 2-hour waiting period; no exercise.
- A blood glucose specimen is collected 2 hours after the patient finishes eating.

a glucose test on a specimen collected 2 hours after a meal (**2-hour PP**) is an excellent screening test for diabetes and gestational diabetes. A 2-hour PP test is also used to monitor insulin therapy. Correct timing of specimen collection is very important. Glucose levels in specimens collected too early or late may be falsely elevated or decreased, respectively, leading to misinterpretation of results. If test results are abnormal, other tests that might be ordered are HbA1c or a glucose tolerance. The principles of the 2-hour PP procedure are shown in Box 11-3.

Glucose Tolerance Test

A **glucose tolerance test (GTT)** is used to diagnose problems of carbohydrate metabolism. The major carbohydrate in the blood is glucose, the body's source of energy. The GTT, also called the oral glucose tolerance test (OGTT), evaluates the body's ability to metabolize glucose by monitoring the patient's tolerance to high levels of glucose without adverse effects. The two major types of disorders involving glucose metabolism are those in which the blood glucose level is increased (**hyperglycemia**), as in diabetes mellitus, and those in which the blood glucose levels are decreased (**hypoglycemia**). Insulin, produced by the pancreas, is primarily responsible for regulating blood glucose levels. The GTT evaluates the insulin response to a measured dose of glucose by recording glucose levels on specimens collected at specific time intervals. Insulin levels are sometimes measured also. GTT length is typically 1 hour for gestational diabetes and 3 hours for other glucose metabolism evaluations. The test rarely exceeds 6 hours. Results are plotted on a graph, creating a so-called GTT curve (Fig. 11-12).

> **Experience setting up a GTT schedule and plotting a GTT curve in Knowledge Drill 11-4: Glucose Tolerance Test GTT in the WORKBOOK.**

There are a number of variations of the GTT procedure, involving different doses of glucose and timing of collections. The method used to collect the blood, however, should be consistent for all specimens. That is, if the first specimen is collected by venipuncture, all succeeding specimens should be venipuncture specimens. If skin

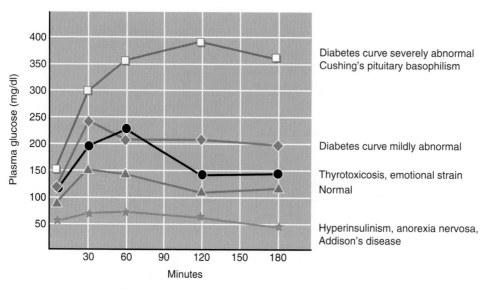

Figure 11-12 Glucose tolerance test (GTT) curves.

puncture is used to collect the first specimen, all succeeding specimens should also be skin puncture specimens.

GTT PREPARATION AND PROCEDURE

Preparation for a GTT is very important. Instruction should be followed exactly for accurate test results. While preparing for a GTT test, the patient must:

- eat balanced meals containing approximately 150 g of carbohydrate for 3 days before the test.
- fast for at least 8 hours but not more than 16 hours prior to the test.
- be allowed to drink water during the fast and during the test to avoid dehydration and because urine specimens may be collected as part of the procedure. No other foods or beverages are allowed.
- be discouraged from engaging in excessive exercise for 12 hours before the test.
- not smoke or chew gum, as these activities stimulate the digestive process and may cause erroneous test results.
- receive both verbal and written instructions to ensure compliance.

The GTT procedure is described in Procedure 11-2.

Procedure 11-2: GTT Procedure

PURPOSE: Perform a glucose tolerance test.

EQUIPMENT: Gloves, alcohol prep pads, ETS holder, tubes and needle, glucose beverage, urine containers (if applicable), bandage, permanent ink pen.

Step	Explanation/Rationale
1. Follow normal identification protocol, explain collection procedure, and advise patient that water *is* allowed but drinking other beverages, eating food, smoking, or chewing gum is *not* allowed throughout the test period.	Patient must be properly identified and must understand and consent to the procedure. Eating, drinking beverages other than water, smoking, and chewing gum all affect test results.
2. Draw fasting specimen and check for glucose.	If the fasting glucose result is abnormal, the patient's physician must be consulted before continuing the test. The test is not normally performed if the patient's blood glucose is over 200 mg/dL.
3. Ask the patient to collect a fasting urine specimen if urine testing has been requested.	The GTT can be requested with or without urine testing.
4. Give the patient the determined dose of glucose beverage.	A typical adult patient dose is 75 g. Children and small adults are given approximately 1 g of glucose per kilogram of weight. The dose for detecting gestational diabetes is normally between 50 and 75 g.
5. Remind the patient to finish the beverage within 5 minutes.	Results may be inaccurate if the patient takes longer to drink the beverage, as the glucose may start to be metabolized by the body, thus affecting test results.
6. Note the time that the patient finishes the beverage, start the timing for the test, and calculate the collection times for the rest of the specimens based on this time.	GTT specimens are typically collected 30 minutes, 1 hour, 2 hours, 3 hours, and so forth, after the patient finishes the glucose beverage.
7. Give a copy of the collection times to the patient.	Patients (especially outpatients) must be aware of the collection times so that they can be available for the draw.
8. Collect blood and urine specimens (if applicable) as close to the computed times as possible.	Timing of specimen collection is critical for computation of the GTT curve and correct interpretation of results.
9. Label all specimens with the exact time collected and the time interval of the test (1/2 hour, 1 hour, etc.) in addition to patient identification information.	Each specimen must be correctly identified for accurate computation of the GTT curve and interpretation of results. Actual time of collection must be recorded.
10. Deliver or send specimens to the lab as soon as possible.	Glucose specimens collected in gel barrier tubes must be separated from the cells or tested within 2 hours of collection for accurate results. Specimens collected in sodium fluoride are stable for 24 hours and are sometimes held and tested all together. Follow facility protocol.

> ⚠️ **CAUTION** If the patient vomits during a GTT procedure, his or her physician must be consulted to determine if the test should be continued.

In normal patients, blood glucose levels peak within 30 minutes to 1 hour following glucose ingestion. The peak in glucose levels triggers the release of insulin, which brings glucose levels back down to fasting levels within about 2 hours and no glucose spills over into the urine.

Diabetics have an inadequate or absent insulin response; consequently glucose levels peak at higher levels and are slower to return to fasting levels. If blood is not drawn on time, it is important for the phlebotomist to note the discrepancy so that the physician can take this into consideration.

Oral Glucose Challenge Test

Some pregnant women develop high blood glucose levels during pregnancy, a condition called gestational diabetes. The oral glucose challenge test (OGCT), also called a 1-hour glucose screening test or gestational glucose screening test, is a modified version of the OGTT that screens for gestational diabetes. To perform the test the patient is given a drink containing 50 g of glucose. A blood glucose specimen is collected 1 hour after the patient finishes the drink. If the glucose result on the specimen is greater than 140 mg/dL, it is suggested that the patient have a follow-up OGTT within 1 week.

Lactose Tolerance Test

A lactose tolerance test (Box 11-4) is used to determine if a patient lacks the enzyme (mucosal lactase) that is necessary to convert lactose, or milk sugar, into glucose and galactose. A person lacking the enzyme suffers from gastrointestinal distress and diarrhea following the ingestion of milk and other lactose-containing foods. Symptoms are relieved by eliminating milk from the diet.

A lactose tolerance test is typically performed in the same manner as a 2-hour GTT; however, an equal amount of lactose is substituted for the glucose. Blood samples are drawn at the same time as for a GTT. If the patient has mucosal lactase, the resulting glucose curve will be similar to a GTT curve, and the result is considered negative. If the patient is lactose intolerant (lacking the enzyme lactase), the glucose curve will be flat, rising no more than a few mg/dL from the fasting level. Some individuals normally have a flat GTT curve (resulting in a false-positive result); it is then suggested that they have a 2-hour GTT performed the day before

Box 11-4

Principles of Lactose Tolerance Testing

- It is suggested that a 2-hour GTT be performed the day before the lactose tolerance test.
- A 2-hour lactose tolerance test is performed in the same manner as the GTT; however, an equal amount of lactose is substituted for the glucose.
- Blood samples for glucose testing are drawn at the same time used in the previous GTT test.

Results

- If the patient has mucosal lactase, the resulting glucose curve will be similar to the GTT curve.
- If the patient lacks the enzyme (is lactose intolerant), glucose levels will rise only slightly from the fasting level, resulting in a "flat" curve.
- False-positive results have been demonstrated in patients with small bowel resections and disorders such as slow gastric emptying, Crohn disease, and cystic fibrosis.

the lactose tolerance test so that results can be evaluated adequately. False-positive results have also been demonstrated in patients with small bowel resections and with disorders such as slow gastric emptying, Crohn disease, and cystic fibrosis. The noninvasive, preferred test for lactose tolerance test is the hydrogen breath test. This test also requires the patient to drink high levels of lactose that if not properly digested will ferment in the colon and release larger than normal levels of hydrogen in the breath samples that are taken at regular intervals during the test (see Chapter 13).

Parentage/Paternity Testing

Parental testing is performed to determine the probability that two specific individuals have a genetic parent–child relationship. Parental testing can be used for determining either the alleged father or the alleged mother. However, most often it is used to determine paternity (i.e., whether a particular man is the father of a specific child). Generally, the paternity test results exclude the possibility of parentage rather than prove parentage. Testing may be requested by physicians, lawyers, child support enforcement bureaus, or individuals. Paternity testing requires a chain-of-custody protocol and specific identification procedures that may include fingerprinting. A photo identification document such as a passport is usually required. The mother, child, and alleged father are all tested. Blood samples are preferred for testing; however, buccal (cheek) swabs are increasingly being used.

Buccal samples are collected by rubbing a swab against the inside of the cheek to collect loose cells. DNA extracted from the cells is "mapped" to create a DNA profile. DNA profiles of the individuals involved are compared to determine the probability that the child's DNA was acquired from the person in question. If chain-of-custody procedures for the specimens are strictly followed the results can be used in a legal dispute.

Paternity testing can also be performed before the infant is born on specimens obtained by amniocentesis or by chorionic villus sampling, results of which are highly accurate. (Chorionic villi are projections of vascular tissue that have the same genetic makeup as the fertilized egg and become the fetal portion of the placenta.)

Therapeutic Drug Monitoring

Therapeutic drug dosage necessary to produce a desired effect varies widely among patients and may require oversight. **Therapeutic drug monitoring (TDM)**, the testing of drug levels in the bloodstream at specific intervals, is used

- to manage patients being treated with certain drugs in order to help establish a drug dosage.
- while adjusting the dosage when in combination with other drugs taken.
- in identifying noncompliant patients.
- in maintaining the dosage at a therapeutic (beneficial) level.
- to avoid drug toxicity.

Drugs that are monitored typically have a narrow therapeutic range, which means that the amount required to be effective is fairly close to the amount that can cause side effects or toxicity. Table 11-2 lists examples of categories of drugs that require monitoring.

When a patient takes a drug dose, the amount in the bloodstream rises initially. It eventually peaks and then falls, typically reaching its lowest or trough level just before the next dose is due. For a drug to be beneficial, the **peak (maximum) level** must not exceed toxic levels, and the **trough (minimum) level** must remain within the therapeutic range. Consequently, timing of specimen collection in regard to dosage administration is critical for safe and beneficial treatment and must be consistent. A team effort is essential and requires coordination with pharmacy, nursing, and the lab. The phlebotomist, a key player in this team effort, must understand the importance of peak and trough levels and collect the specimens in a timely manner.

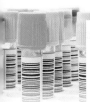

Table 11-2: Examples of Categories of Drugs That Typically Require Therapeutic Monitoring

Drug Category	Examples	Use
Antibiotics and antifungals	Aminoglycosides (e.g., gentamicin, tobramycin, amikacin), amphotericin, chloramphenicol, vancomycin	Treat infections caused by bacteria that are resistant to other antibiotics
Anticonvulsants	Carbamazepine (Tegretol), ethosuximide, phenobarbital, phenytoin, valproic acid	Epilepsy, seizure prevention, mood stabilization
Bronchodilators	Theophylline, caffeine	Asthma, chronic obstructive pulmonary disease (COPD), neonatal apnea
Cardiac drugs	Digitoxin, digoxin, procainamide, quinidine	Congestive heart failure (CHF), angina, arrhythmia
Chemotherapy drugs	Methotrexate. 5-fluorouracil	Psoriasis, rheumatoid arthritis (RA), non-Hodgkin lymphoma, osteosarcoma, systemic cancer
Immunosuppressants	Azathioprine, cyclosporine, sirolimus, tacrolimus	Autoimmune disorders, prevent organ transplant rejection
Protease inhibitors	Atazanavir, indinavir, lopinavir, nelfinavir, ritonavir, boceprevir, telaprevir	HIV/AIDS, hepatitis C
Psychiatric drugs	Antidepressants (e.g., imipramine, amitriptyline, nortriptyline, doxepin, desipramine), lithium, valproic acid	Bipolar disorder (manic depression), depression

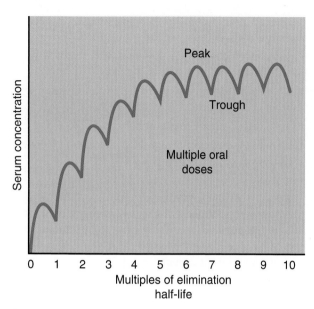

Figure 11-13 Dose–response curve after multiple oral doses of a drug were given each half-life.

- Peak levels screen for drug toxicity and specimens are collected when the highest serum concentration of the drug is anticipated. Peak times are influenced by many factors but typically occur approximately 30 minutes after IV administration, 60 minutes after intramuscular (IM) administration, and 1 to 2 hours after oral intake. Careful coordination of sample collection with dosing is critical.

- Trough levels are monitored to ensure that levels of the drug stay within the therapeutic range. Trough-level specimens are easiest to collect because they are collected when the lowest serum concentration of the drug is expected, usually immediately prior to administration of the next scheduled dose.

Collection timing is most critical for aminoglycoside drugs, such as amikacin, gentamicin, and tobramycin, which have short half-lives. A half-life is the time required for the body to metabolize half the amount of the drug. (Fig. 11-13 depicts a dose–response curve based on doses of drug given each half-life.) The timing is less critical for drugs that have longer half-lives, such as phenobarbital and digoxin.

The FDA has approved gel tubes from some manufacturers for all analytes, including TDM; however, other manufacturers' gel tubes may affect TDM results. Refer to the manufacturer's package inserts and test methodologies used in the laboratory for specific requirements.

Therapeutic Phlebotomy

Therapeutic phlebotomy involves the withdrawal of large volumes of blood usually measured by the unit (as in blood donation), or approximately 500 mL. It is performed by phlebotomists who have been specially trained in the procedure or in donor phlebotomy, as the procedure is similar to collecting blood from donors. It is used as a treatment for certain medical conditions such as polycythemia and hemochromatosis.

- *Polycythemia* is a disease involving the body's overproduction of RBCs, which is detrimental to the patient's health and the most common reason for performing therapeutic phlebotomy. The patient's RBC levels are monitored regularly, usually by the hematocrit test. Periodic removal of blood when the hematocrit exceeds a certain level is used to help keep the patient's RBC levels within the normal range.

- *Hemochromatosis* is a disease characterized by excess iron deposits in the tissues. It can be caused by a defect in iron metabolism or result from multiple blood transfusions or excess iron intake. Periodic removal of single units of blood from the patient gradually depletes iron stores, because the body then uses the iron to make new RBCs to replace those removed.

Toxicology Specimens

Toxicology is the scientific study of toxins (poisons). Clinical toxicology is concerned with the detection of toxins and treatment for the effects they produce. Forensic toxicology is concerned with the legal consequences of toxin exposure, both intentional and accidental. Toxicology tests examine blood, hair, urine, and other body substances for the presence of toxins, which often exist in very small amounts.

FORENSIC SPECIMENS

Increasingly law enforcement officials request the collection of a toxicology specimen for forensic or legal reasons. The tests most frequently requested are breath or blood for alcohol. Other requests include urine drug screens and blood specimens for drugs and DNA analysis. When forensic specimens are collected, a special protocol, referred to as the **chain of custody**, must be strictly followed. Chain of custody requires detailed documentation that tracks the specimen from the time it is collected until the results are reported. The specimen must be accounted for at all times. If documentation is incomplete, legal action may be compromised.

A chain-of-custody form is used to identify the specimen and the person or persons who obtained and processed it. Information on the form also includes the time, date, and place where the specimen was obtained, along with the signature of the person from whom the specimen was taken. Patient identification and specimen collection take place in the presence of a witness, frequently a law enforcement officer, in which case protocol and packaging are completed by the officer before the specimen is sent to a crime laboratory for analysis. Any person who is involved in drawing a blood alcohol specimen for legal reasons can be summoned to appear in court.

BLOOD ALCOHOL (ETHANOL) SPECIMENS

Normally a physician orders a blood alcohol (ethanol [ETOH]) test on a patient for medical reasons related to treatment or other clinical purposes. In such situations, there is no requirement for chain of custody, but the results of such analyses can ultimately become evidence in court. For that reason, the need for a standard protocol and well-documented handling becomes very important. Blood alcohol determinations for industrial purposes are becoming more common and may be required in connection with on-the-job injury, employee insurance programs, and employee drug screening. Occasionally a law enforcement agency may request a blood alcohol concentration (BAC) on an individual who has been involved in a traffic accident. Both industrial and legal samples require that chain-of-custody protocol be strictly followed. Refer to the specific state law for legal regulations and requirements.

Skin Preparation

The antiseptic used to clean the venipuncture site must not contain alcohol or other volatile organic substances that might compromise results. Therefore 70% isopropyl alcohol used for routine venipuncture site preparation or other alcohols such as methanol and ethyl alcohol cannot be used for a BAC collection. Tincture of iodine contains alcohol and likewise should not be used to clean the site. The most frequently used antiseptics for ETOH specimen collection is aqueous benzalkonium chloride (BZK), and some are still using aqueous povidone–iodine. If an alternative antiseptic is not available, regular soap and water can be used.

Specimen Requirements

A glass gray-top sodium fluoride tube, with or without an anticoagulant (depending upon the need for serum, plasma, or whole blood in the test procedure) is typically required for specimen collection. Because alcohol is volatile (easily vaporized or evaporated), the tube should be filled until the vacuum is exhausted and the stopper should not be removed. In today's environment, usage of synthetic stimulants, as well as some hallucinogenic drugs continues to increase. The phlebotomist may choose to draw other types of specimens at the same time for testing for these other drugs. The recommendation is light blue (citrate) for the synthetic stimulants and lavender for inhalants and DNA analysis.

Key Point Glass tubes are preferred for blood alcohol specimens because of the porous nature of plastic tubes.

DRUG SCREENING

Many healthcare organizations, sports associations, and major companies require workplace drug screening for pre-employment, prepromotion, postaccident or injury, random screening (without prior notice), reasonable suspicion, and for any other situation that they deem important. Tests may detect a specific drug or screen for up to 30 different drugs, depending upon the circumstance. Testing is typically performed on urine rather than blood because it is easy to obtain and a wide variety of drugs or their metabolites (products of metabolism) can be detected in urine for a longer period of time. See Table 11-3 for a list of illicit drugs commonly detectable by urine drug screening, along with the length of time after use that the drug is detectable in the body. An illicit drug is one that is prohibited by law to be used. The Triage TOX Drug Screen device (Biosite Incorporated, San Diego, CA) can rapidly and simultaneously test for up to 10 distinct classes of drugs of abuse. Illicit drugs detected include cocaine (crack), opiates (heroin), and amphetamines (ecstasy, speed, crystal), and tetrahydrocannabinol (pot). Table 11-4 lists some of the drugs commonly detected in blood and the length of time that they can be found following ingestion, insufflation, inhalation, or injection. The testing for drugs in the blood involves more sophisticated methods such as, gas chromatography-mass spectrometry (GCMS) and liquid chromatography-mass spectrometry (LCMS) that must be done at a forensic or clinical laboratory. It is important to note that detection times for drugs in blood and urine are dependent on many factors, including genetics, body size and composition, age, gender, history, and tolerance of the user. Also the user's disease state and accompanying drugs that may be in the user's system will definitely affect the detection times.

There are legal implications to drug screening, and a chain-of-custody protocol is required whether or not the test is being performed for legal reasons. One example of a chain-of-custody form is shown in Figure 11-14. Clinical laboratories also use this type of documentation for their facility's drug testing programs. The form is used to identify the specimen and the person or persons who obtained and processed it. Information on the form also includes the time, date, and place where the specimen was obtained, along with the signature of the person from whom the specimen was taken.

For a drug screening workplace program to be of value, the person who instructs and assists the donor

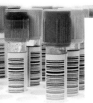

Table 11-3: Drugs Commonly Detectable at Urine Drug Screening

Drug or Drug Families	Common Names	Detectable (Time)	Comment
Alcohol		2–12 hr	
Amphetamines	Methamphetamine, speed, crystal, crank, ice	1–3 d 2–7 d	Single/light use Frequent/chronic use
Barbiturates	"Downers," Seconal, Fiorinal, Tuinal, phenobarbital	1–3 d	Varies considerably with drugs in this class
Benzodiazepines	Valium, Librium, Xanax, Dalmane, Serax	1–14 d	Varies considerably with drugs in this class
Cocaine (as metabolite)	Crack	1–3 d 3–14 d	Single/light use Frequent use/free base
Cannabinoids	Marijuana, grass, hash	1–7 d >30 d	Single/light use Habitual
Methadone	Dolophine	1–3 d	Single/light use
Opiates	Heroin, morphine, codeine, Dilaudid, hydrocodone	1–3 d >7 d	Single/light use Frequent/chronic use
Phencyclidine	PCP, angel dust	1–5 d >30 d	Single/light use Frequent/chronic use
Propoxyphene	Darvon, Darvocet	1–3 d >7 d	Single/light use Frequent/chronic use

Table 11-4: Drugs Commonly Detectable at Blood Drug Screening

Drug or Drug Families	Common Names	Detectable (Time)	Comment
Alcohol		2–12 hr	
Amphetamines	"Uppers", methamphetamine, speed, crystal, crank, ice, go, glass	1–3 d	
Barbiturates	"Downers," Seconal, Fiorinal, Tuinal, phenobarbital	24–52 hr	Varies significantly with drugs in this class
Benzodiazepines	Valium, Librium, Xanax, Dalmane, Serax	Up to 1 wk Metabolites up to 3 wk	Varies significantly with drugs in this class
Cocaine	Cocaine Benzoylecgonine (BE)	Less than 12 hr	
Cannabinoids	Marijuana, grass, hash D9-THC Hydroxy-THC Carboxy-THC	1–2 d Can be up to 7 d for metabolites	
Methadone	Dolophine	24–36 hr	
Opiates	Heroin Morphine Codeine Dilaudid, hydrocodone Oxycontin (extended release tab)	4–12 hr 6–12 hr 10–12 hr 12–24 hr 24–30 hr	
Inhalants	Aerosols Volatile Solvents Anesthetic Gases	30 min–6 hr 2–72 hr 5–60 min	Varies significantly with drugs in this class
Phencyclidine	PCP, angel dust	3–5 d	

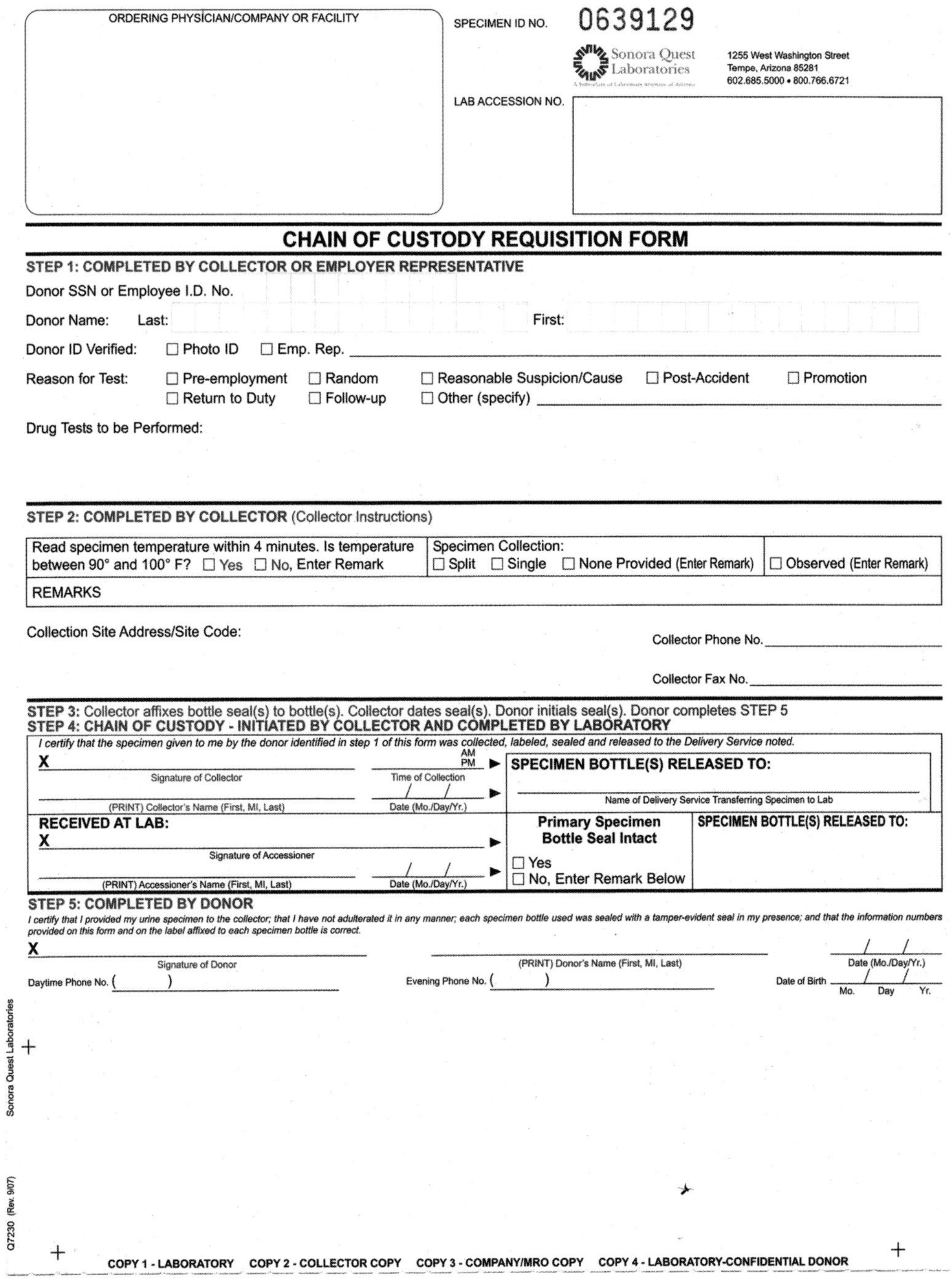

ORDERING PHYSICIAN/COMPANY OR FACILITY

SPECIMEN ID NO.   0639129

Sonora Quest Laboratories
A Subsidiary of Laboratory Sciences of Arizona

1255 West Washington Street
Tempe, Arizona 85281
602.685.5000 • 800.766.6721

LAB ACCESSION NO.

CHAIN OF CUSTODY REQUISITION FORM

STEP 1: COMPLETED BY COLLECTOR OR EMPLOYER REPRESENTATIVE

Donor SSN or Employee I.D. No.

Donor Name: Last: First:

Donor ID Verified: ☐ Photo ID   ☐ Emp. Rep. _____

Reason for Test: ☐ Pre-employment   ☐ Random   ☐ Reasonable Suspicion/Cause   ☐ Post-Accident   ☐ Promotion
                   ☐ Return to Duty   ☐ Follow-up   ☐ Other (specify) _____

Drug Tests to be Performed:

STEP 2: COMPLETED BY COLLECTOR (Collector Instructions)

Read specimen temperature within 4 minutes. Is temperature between 90° and 100° F? ☐ Yes ☐ No, Enter Remark	Specimen Collection: ☐ Split ☐ Single ☐ None Provided (Enter Remark)	☐ Observed (Enter Remark)
REMARKS		

Collection Site Address/Site Code:

Collector Phone No. _____

Collector Fax No. _____

STEP 3: Collector affixes bottle seal(s) to bottle(s). Collector dates seal(s). Donor initials seal(s). Donor completes STEP 5
STEP 4: CHAIN OF CUSTODY - INITIATED BY COLLECTOR AND COMPLETED BY LABORATORY

I certify that the specimen given to me by the donor identified in step 1 of this form was collected, labeled, sealed and released to the Delivery Service noted.

X _____
Signature of Collector

Time of Collection ___:___ AM/PM

SPECIMEN BOTTLE(S) RELEASED TO:

_____
(PRINT) Collector's Name (First, MI, Last)

Date (Mo./Day/Yr.)

Name of Delivery Service Transferring Specimen to Lab

RECEIVED AT LAB:

X _____
Signature of Accessioner

_____
(PRINT) Accessioner's Name (First, MI, Last)

Date (Mo./Day/Yr.)

Primary Specimen Bottle Seal Intact
☐ Yes
☐ No, Enter Remark Below

SPECIMEN BOTTLE(S) RELEASED TO:

STEP 5: COMPLETED BY DONOR

I certify that I provided my urine specimen to the collector; that I have not adulterated it in any manner; each specimen bottle used was sealed with a tamper-evident seal in my presence; and that the information numbers provided on this form and on the label affixed to each specimen bottle is correct.

X _____
Signature of Donor

_____
(PRINT) Donor's Name (First, MI, Last)

Date (Mo./Day/Yr.)

Daytime Phone No. ( )   Evening Phone No. ( )   Date of Birth   Mo. Day Yr.

Sonora Quest Laboratories

Q7230 (Rev. 9/07)

COPY 1 - LABORATORY   COPY 2 - COLLECTOR COPY   COPY 3 - COMPANY/MRO COPY   COPY 4 - LABORATORY-CONFIDENTIAL DONOR

Figure 11-14 Chain-of-custody requisition form for urine drug screen. (Courtesy Sonora Laboratory Sciences, Phoenix, AZ.)

in collecting the sample correctly must be articulate, detailed-oriented, and follow protocol meticulously with each and every donor. The collected specimen must be able to withstand all challenges to the validity of the results. The **Department of Transportation (DOT)** offers the online video, DOT's 10 Steps to Collection Site Security and Integrity, to help collectors and collection site managers appreciate their role in the integrity and security of the urine drug screening at their workplace. The 10 steps are listed in Box 11-5.

> The **National Institute on Drug Abuse (NIDA)** has a mission *to lead the nation in bringing the power of science to bear on drug abuse and addiction.* This undertaking will mean much research has to be done and then the sharing of the results of the research quickly and effectively so that drug abuse can be prevented, treated and policies can be formed on how to handle addiction and abuse.

Box 11-5

DOT's 10 Steps to Collection Site Security and Integrity

Drug Testing
Office of Drug and Alcohol Policy and Compliance
U.S. Department of Transportation
Updated: Tuesday, October 23, 2012

1. Pay careful attention to employees throughout the collection process.
2. Ensure that there is no unauthorized access into the collection areas and that undetected access (e.g., through a door not in view) is not possible.
3. Make sure that employees show proper picture ID.
4. Make sure employees empty pockets; remove outer garments (e.g., coveralls, jacket, coat, hat); leave briefcases, purses, and bags behind; and wash their hands.
5. Maintain personal control of the specimen and CCF at all times during the collection.
6. Secure any water sources or otherwise make them unavailable to employees (e.g., turn off water inlet, tape handles to prevent opening faucets, secure tank lids).
7. Ensure that the water in the toilet and tank (if applicable) has bluing (coloring) agent in it. Tape or otherwise secure shut any movable toilet tank top, or put bluing in the tank.
8. Ensure that no soap, disinfectants, cleaning agents, or possible adulterants are present.
9. Inspect the site to ensure that no foreign or unauthorized substances are present.
10. Secure areas and items (e.g., ledges, trash receptacles, paper towel holders, under-sink areas, ceiling tiles) that appear suitable for concealing contaminants.

www.dot.gov, accessed January 13, 2015.

Molecular Genetic Testing

Clinical molecular genetic testing provides for detection of genetic variations that offer the promise of revolutionizing personalized medicine and altering the way physicians diagnose and treat illness. At present, clinical molecular diagnostic technologies focus on

- identifying whether an individual has a certain genetic disease.
- determining whether an individual has an increased risk for a particular disease.
- classifying an individual's genetic makeup to determine whether a drug and dosage is suitable for that particular patient.
- examining the whole genome to discover genetic alterations that may cause disease.

Before specimen collection, essential information must be obtained. The patient's demographics are required and an informed consent form must be signed. Sterile whole-blood specimens for molecular genetic testing are generally collected in the lavender-top EDTA tubes or tubes specially designed for this type of diagnostic study, that is, white-top gel tubes from Greiner Bio-One. Other anticoagulant tubes used for genetic testing could contain ACD, sodium citrate or sodium heparin. When a test for RNA is ordered, the blood specimen must be sent for testing immediately or collected in a special stabilizing reagent. Blood specimens will be rejected if frozen, hemolyzed, or clotted. Ideal handling is to ship immediately at ambient temperature for overnight delivery. In hot weather a cool pack can be enclosed. Specimens for molecular genetic testing can be refrigerated up to 7 days before shipping. In this particular area of laboratory testing, major advances are being made daily. It is important for the HCW involved in collection and handling of this type of specimen stay current in facility protocol.

Trace Elements

Trace elements or metals include aluminum, arsenic, chromium, copper, iron, lead, mercury, and zinc. These elements are measured in such small amounts that traces of them in the glass, plastic, or stopper material of evacuated tubes may leach into the specimen, causing falsely elevated test values. For this reason, specimens for these tests must be collected in special trace-element–free tubes. These tubes are made of materials that have been specially manufactured to be as free of trace elements as possible. An insert with each carton of tubes gives a detailed analysis of residual amounts of metals contained in the tubes. These tubes are typically royal blue and contain EDTA, heparin, or no additive. The type of additive is indicated on the label (e.g., red for no additive, lavender for EDTA, and green for heparin). Tan-top tubes containing K_2ETDA are available for lead analysis.

In collecting trace elements, it is important to prevent introducing even the smallest amount of the contaminating substance into the tube, since the amounts being tested are in micro- or nanograms. Contaminants in the stoppers accumulate in the needle each time a different tube is pierced in a multiple tube collection. That accumulation can then carry over to the royal-blue–stoppered tube, changing the results. Consequently, when a trace-element test is ordered, it is best to draw it by itself if using a needle/tube assembly, or a syringe may be used. For best results, when using a syringe, change the transfer device before filling the royal-blue tube. Follow facility's collection guidelines.

Point-of-Care Testing

Bob Kaplanis, PBT, MT(ASCP), Systems Technical Director, POCT

Janet Vittori, BS, MT(ASCP), POC Specialist

Point-of-care testing (POCT)—also known as alternate site testing (AST) or ancillary, bedside, or near-patient testing—brings laboratory testing to the location of the patient. POCT has been made possible by advances in laboratory instrumentation that have led to the development of small, portable, and often handheld testing devices. Its benefits include convenience to the patient and a short turnaround time (TAT) for results that allow healthcare providers to address crucial patient needs, deliver prompt medical attention, and expedite patient recovery.

In addition to being able to operate the analyzer according to the manufacturer's instructions and possessing the phlebotomy skills required to collect the specimen, anyone who does POCT should be able to carry out the quality control (QC) and maintenance procedures necessary to ensure that results obtained are accurate. Everyone who performs POCT in a clinical setting must meet the requirements of the Clinical Laboratory Improvement Amendments (CLIA) for testing and the guidelines of the OSHA for specimen handling.

Quality and Safety in Point-of-Care Testing

It is important to have processes and systems in place to ensure that the testing that is being done at the bedside or at the patient's side is performed properly and that results correlate with the same test when performed in the main laboratory.

Monitoring the quality of the waived testing being done at bedside is a constant challenge for the laboratory, and each year more tests are classified as waived by the FDA. In addition, the POCT regulations that govern many institutions change periodically with the addition of new regulations and clarification of existing ones.

Waived tests do not require the same level of quality checks as tests classified as nonwaived or sometimes referred to as moderately complex tests. Not too long ago, all POCT required external QC to be performed daily if any patient testing was to be done that day. Today the College of American Pathologists (CAP) requires that external liquid control be performed only as specified by the manufacturer's instructions on many of the waived tests. In most cases that means performing liquid controls upon receipt of a new shipment of test kits and with each new testing personnel. If the kit is not stored properly or if patient results are questionable then controls must be performed before proceeding. The POCT regulations from CAP serve as a minimum guide that must be instituted. Some institutions choose to go beyond the minimum requirements because of past experiences and to be reassured that the testing is working properly.

Manufacturers have enhanced instruments to include **electronic QCs (EQCs)**, which can detect problems with the specimen (i.e., clotting, short samples, air bubbles) and electronic internal checks that can determine if the instrument is functioning properly. Although EQC has helped ease the regulatory requirements, it cannot check a very important part of the testing process, which is specimen collection and handling.

Some POC tests do not use instruments (often referred to as noninstrumented tests); for that reason the manufacturer or institution may require that daily external liquid QC be performed as a check on the technique used and the accuracy of the results. An example of such a test could be urine dipsticks that are read visually. At the bedside, this test does not use an instrument; instead, an individual compares the color pads on the dipstick (which has been dipped in urine) to a color chart on the strip vial. All control results must be recorded on some type of document, for example, a QC log and reviewed for consistency and acceptability. An example of a log listing high UA control results for urine specimens is shown in Figure 11-15. This log may be one or two pages: one page for recording low QC values and the other for the high QC.

In addition to the many quality assurance issues with the POC instruments in use in today's healthcare facilities, it has become evident that handheld POC analyzers carried between patients in a healthcare institution can be fomites for disease. One relevant publication from the Center for Disease Control (CDC) is entitled *Recommendations of CDC and the Healthcare Infection Control Practices Advisory Committee (HICPAC)*. The following quote from that document illustrates the important role medical equipment can play in the spread of infections.

"Although microbiologically contaminated surfaces can serve as reservoirs of potential pathogens, these surfaces generally are not directly associated with transmission of infections to either staff or patients. The transferral of microorganisms

POINT-OF-CARE TESTING
UA QC Log

Facility _General Hospital_   Instrument Serial #: _98157_

Month: _May_ Year: _2015_   Nursing Unit: _Pediatric Oncology_
High Control Lot # & Exp. Date _04489 4/2016_   Exp. Date at Room Temp: _June 1, 2016_
New High Control Lot # & Exp. Date_____   Exp. Date at Room Temp _____

Date	Sp. Gravity	pH	WBC	Nitrate	Protein	Glucose	Ketone	Urobil	Bilirubin	Blood	Signature
Write in QC Range to the right	1.005-1.030	7.0-8.5	1+ – 3+	Pos	1+ – 3+	Trace – 3+	1+ – 3+	2.0 – 8.0	1+ – 3+	Trace – 3+	
1	1.020	7.5	2+	Pos	2+	2+	2+	4.0	3+	3+	
2	1.015	7.5	2+	Pos	1+	3+	2+	4.0	2+	3+	
3	1.020	8.0	3+	Pos	1+	3+	2+	4.0	2+	3+	
4	1.020	7.5	2+	Pos	2+	3+	2+	4.0	2+	3+	
5	1.015	7.5	2+	Pos	2+	3+	2+	4.0	2+	3+	
6											
7											
8											
9											
10											
11											
12											
13											
14											
15											
16											
17											
18											
19											
20											
21											
22											
23											
24											
25											
26											
27											
28											
29											
30											
31											

Reagent Strip Lot and Expiration Date
New Reagent Strip Lot and Expiration Date
Two levels of control are run every day a patient sample is tested, if results do agree with patient results, if a strip vial is not stored properly, or if a new lot # of strips is used
Document corrective action for any out of range QC on reverse of this sheet
POCT Monthly Review Signature: Date: / /

Figure 11-15 Urinalysis QC log showing daily recorded results for the positive control.

from environmental surfaces to patients is largely via hand contact with the surface. Although hand hygiene is important to minimize the impact of this transfer, cleaning and disinfecting environmental surfaces routinely is fundamental in reducing their potential contribution to the incidence of healthcare-associated infections."

In an effort to reduce the possible transmission of microorganisms to patients, meter manufacturers have developed recommendations to disinfect their instruments. These vary by manufacturer; therefore, the specific recommendations for a particular device should be followed. Several manufacturers recommend cleaning the device with 10% bleach. It has been proven that a 1:10 bleach solution can effectively clean and disinfect POC instruments, but to be effective, such a solution must be mixed daily. A similar product available commercially is made up of individually wrapped EPA-registered bleach wipes designed to be used once and then thrown in the trash.

These wipes, shown in Figure 11-16, meet all OSHA and CDC regulations pertaining to devices that can be exposed to blood-borne pathogens. Because of their convenience, they have been found to encourage cleaning, thus reducing cross-contamination between patients

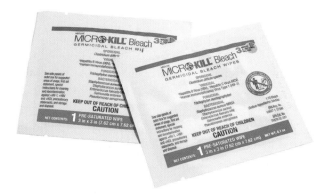

Figure 11-16 EPA registered bleach wipes for POCT instruments. (Medline Industries, Inc., Mundelein, IL.)

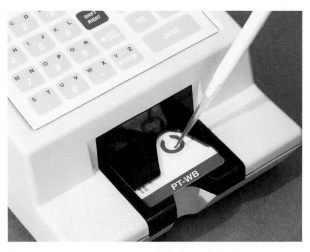

Figure 11-17 Whole-blood sample being added to the Cascade® POC barcoded assay card. (Courtesy Helena, Beaumont, TX.)

of various bacteria including *Clostridium difficile*, methicillin-resistant *Staphylococcus aureus* (MRSA), and vancomycin-resistant *Enterococcus* (VRE).

Coagulation Monitoring by POCT

Several different types of coagulation POCT analyzers can be used to measure and evaluate patient warfarin and heparin therapy. Some of the more common POCT coagulation tests monitored are as follows:

- Prothrombin time (PT) and international normalized ratio (INR)
- Activated partial thromboplastin time (aPTT or PTT)
- **Activated clotting time (ACT)**
- Platelet function

The numerous POCT instruments available to perform various coagulation tests include:

- Cascade POC—ACT, aPTT, PT/INR
- CoaguChek XS Plus—PT/INR
- GEM Premier 4000—ACT, aPTT, PT/INR
- i-STAT—ACT, PT/INR
- VerifyNow—Platelet function

ACT

The ACT test analyzes activity of the intrinsic coagulation factors and is used to monitor heparin therapy. Heparin is given intravenously to patients who have blood clots or whose blood is apt to clot too easily; it is also given as a precaution following certain surgeries. Effects on IV heparin administration are immediate but difficult to control. Too much heparin can cause the patient to bleed; therefore heparin therapy is closely monitored. Once a patient's condition is stabilized, the patient is placed on oral anticoagulant therapy (such as warfarin) and monitored by PT testing.

The ACT test has traditionally been a bedside test; however, timing and mixing were done manually and prone to error. With automated ACT analyzers, the mixing and timing are done automatically. An example of an analyzer used to perform this test is the Cascade POC (Helena, Beaumont, TX). To begin the testing process with the Cascade POC, the barcoded assay card is scanned by a reader on the instrument. This lets the instrument know which assay is requested and also the calibration details. The card is then placed into the instrument and, as shown in Figure 11-17, a whole-blood sample is added to the card for analysis. The data management system allows for the results to be sent directly to the laboratory information system (LIS) if desired.

PT/INR

The PT test is used to monitor warfarin (e.g., Coumadin) therapy. Many warfarin or anticoagulation clinics use POCT coagulation analyzers that perform **protime (PT)** and **international normalized ratio (INR)** tests on whole blood from a fingerstick to provide timely laboratory results. An example of a prothrombin time (PT/INR) meter that is frequently used is the **CoaguChek XS** (Roche Diagnostics, Indianapolis, IN) (Fig. 11-18).

The INR is derived from the mathematical formula below, which was developed to standardize the differences found between the various manufacturers' reagents.

$$INR = (PT_{patient}/PT_{normal})^{ISI}$$

$PT_{patient}$ = the patient's PT result expressed in seconds

PT_{normal} = the laboratory's geometric mean value for normal patients in seconds

ISI = international sensitivity index for the tissue factor in the manufacturer's reagent

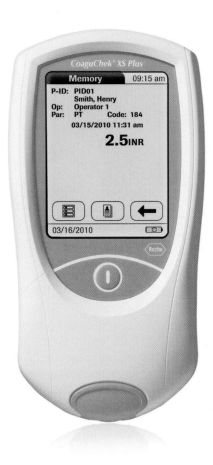

Figure 11-18 CoaguChek® XS Plus for PT/INR testing. (Courtesy Roche Diagnostics Corporation, Indianapolis, IN.)

Some POCT analyzers, such as CoaguChek, allow patients to perform protimes at home and transmit their results to the physician's office. The physician can then adjust medication over the phone and the patient does not have to make an office visit.

PTT

The aPTT/PTT test is used to screen for bleeding disorders prior to surgery, investigate bleeding or clotting disorders, detect clotting factor deficiencies, and monitor low-dose heparin therapy. Cascade POC is a point-of-care analyzer that has test functions for aPTT.

PLATELET FUNCTION

Platelet function testing allows the clinician to determine a patient's response to medication before open heart surgery or cardiac catheterization. This can help prevent excessive bleeding or blood clots. This testing can be done utilizing an automated analyzer with single-use, disposable assays called the VerifyNow® System (Accumetrics, San Diego, CA; Fig. 11-19). It uses whole-blood samples and gives measurements that correlate with laboratory testing.

Platelet function tests can measure the ability of an individual to respond to various antiplatelet medications. Patients respond differently to this type of medication; some are even very resistant. The VerifyNow System Aspirin Assay, which is CLIA waived, provides a measurement to determine whether or not a patient is responding to aspirin therapy.

Arterial Blood Gases and Electrolytes

Arterial blood gases (ABGs) and electrolytes are panels of tests that are often ordered in an emergency situation because of the critical balance in which these analytes must be maintained. ABG readings are used to determine the pH of blood which if outside the very narrow

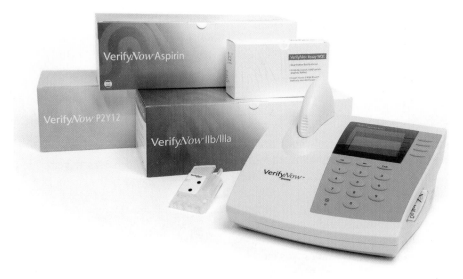

Figure 11-19 VerifyNow® automated analyzer for platelet function tests. (Courtesy Accumetrics, San Diego, CA.)

normal range threatens the patient's survival. Balance of the electrolytes is essential for normal function of cells and organs. POCT has proven to be invaluable in critical care challenges.

ARTERIAL BLOOD GASES

ABGs measured by POCT methods include **pH, partial pressure of carbon dioxide** (pCO_2), **oxygen saturation** (sO_2), and **partial pressure of oxygen** (pO_2).

- pH is an abbreviation for potential hydrogen, a scale representing the relative acidity or alkalinity of a solution. The arterial blood pH test is a measure of the body's acid–base balance and indicates his or her metabolic and respiratory status. The normal range for arterial blood pH is 7.35 to 7.45. Below-normal pH is referred to as acidosis and above-normal pH is referred to as alkalosis.

- The pCO_2 is a measure of the pressure exerted by dissolved CO_2 in the blood plasma and is proportional to the pCO_2 in the alveoli; therefore it is an indicator of how well air is being exchanged between the blood and the lungs. An abnormal increase in pCO_2 is associated with hypoventilation and a decrease with hyperventilation.

- The pO_2 is a measure of the pressure exerted by dissolved O_2 in the blood plasma and indicates the ability of the lungs to diffuse O_2 through the alveoli into the blood. It is used to evaluate the effectiveness of oxygen therapy.

- sO_2 is a measure of the percentage of hemoglobin binding sites occupied by oxygen in the bloodstream. It is used by physicians to determine a patient's oxygenation status. A normal, healthy individual will usually exhibit oxygen saturation around 98%. A person with an arterial sO_2 below 90% is said to have **hypoxemia** (a low oxygen level in the blood) and may be cyanotic.

ELECTROLYTES

The most common electrolytes measured by POCT are **sodium (Na^+), potassium (K^+), chloride (Cl^-), bicarbonate ion (HCO_3^-), and ionized calcium (iCa^{2+}).**

- Sodium is the most plentiful electrolyte in the blood. It plays a major role in maintaining osmotic pressure and acid–base balance and in transmitting nerve impulses. Reduced sodium levels are referred to as **hyponatremia**. Elevated levels are referred to as **hypernatremia**.

- Potassium is primarily concentrated within the cells, with very little found in the bones and blood. It is released into the blood when cells are damaged. Potassium plays a major role in nerve conduction, muscle function, acid–base balance, and osmotic

pressure. Decreased blood potassium is called **hypokalemia**. Increased blood potassium is called **hyperkalemia**.

- Chloride exists mainly in the extracellular spaces in the form of sodium chloride (NaCl) or hydrochloric acid. Chloride must be supplied along with potassium when hypokalemia is being corrected.

- Bicarbonate ion plays a role in transporting carbon dioxide (CO_2) to the lungs and in regulating blood pH. It is formed when carbonic acid is dissociated into H^+ and HCO_3^- ions. Decreased ventilation (hypoventilation) results in higher CO_2 levels and the production of more H^+ ions and can lead to acidosis. Hyperventilation decreases CO_2 levels and can lead to alkalosis.

- Ionized calcium (iCa^{2+}) accounts for approximately 45% of the calcium in the blood; the rest is bound to protein and other substances. Only ionized calcium can be used by the body for such critical functions as muscular contraction, cardiac function, transmission of nerve impulses, and blood clotting.

Multiple-Test-Panel Monitoring by POCT

Several small, portable, and in some cases handheld instruments are available that measure multiple test panels of commonly ordered stat tests such as BUN, glucose, lactate, hemoglobin, and potassium. The body normally maintains these analytes in specific proportions within a narrow range; any uncorrected imbalance can quickly turn life-threatening. POCT instruments in the ER or ICU play an important role at these times because of the immediate test result availability.

Examples of instruments that have a menu of several different tests are:

- GEM Premier
- i-STAT
- NOVA Stat Profile Analyzer
- ABL80 Flex

All the testing devices listed measure a multitude of analytes. Although they all have slightly different test menus, analytes that may be included are Na^+, K^+, Cl, and HCO_3^- as well as blood gas values for pH, pCO_2, pO_2, and sO_2, BUN, glucose, Hgb and Hct, ACT, lactate, and troponin.

The handheld i-STAT (Fig. 11-20A) (Abbott Diagnostics, Abbott Park, IL) is a versatile, portable system that measures a variety of tests. This system utilizes small test cartridges that contain sensitive biosensors on a silicon chip made to perform specific tests. After choosing the appropriate cartridge, two to three drops of either venous or arterial blood is applied and then the cartridge is inserted into the i-STAT. Some cartridges are for single tests, but

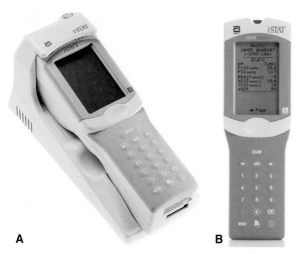

A

B

Figure 11-20 A: i-STAT® instrument with downloader. **B:** i-STAT® wireless that is not offered in all countries. (Courtesy Abbott Diagnostics, Abbott Park, IL.)

most can perform multiple tests on one cartridge. Many facilities are choosing to use the new wireless i-STAT (Fig. 11-20B) because it allows the meter to download test results into the patient's chart almost instantly from wherever it is located. The nonwireless must be taken to a download base which could be a good distance away making the process of documentation and the resulting

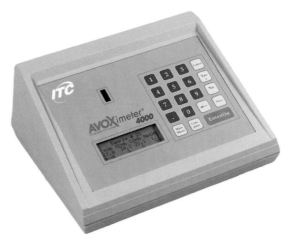

Figure 11-22 AVOXimeter® for blood gases. (Courtesy ITC, Edison, NJ.)

treatment take longer. Another POCT analyzer that measures blood gases and electrolytes is the GEM Premier 4000 (Instrumentation Laboratories, Lexington, MA) (Fig. 11-21). Test cartridges for this instrument also measure critical chemistry analytes, such as lactate, potassium, BUN, and creatinine, allowing for rapid "near-patient" screening for renal disease.

The AVOXimeter (ITC, Edison, NJ) (Fig. 11-22) provides physicians with quick results to aid in diagnosing carbon monoxide toxicity and methemoglobin status of patients. This instrument aids physicians in diagnosing

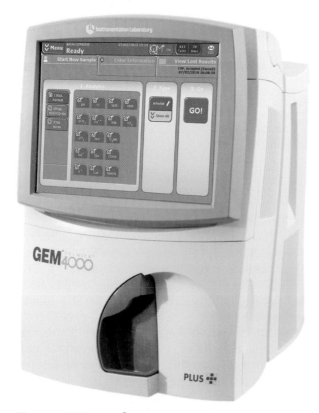

Figure 11-21 GEM® Premier™ 4000 now with Plus Technology used for rapid screening for renal disease. (Courtesy Instrumentation Laboratory, Lexington, MA.)

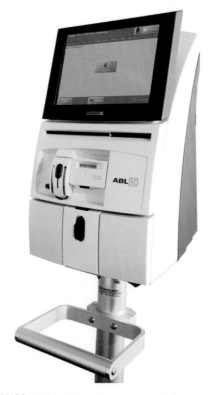

Figure 11-23 ABL80 Flex shown on a pole for portability in a hospital setting. (Courtesy of Radiometer America, Inc.)

and detecting intracardiac (within the heart) and great-vessel shunts. Because of its point-of-care availability, it can offer an evaluation of blood gases in approximately 10 seconds, enabling the physician to make critical decisions concerning care and treatment without delay.

The portable blood gas analyzer ABL80 Flex (Fig. 11-23) is used in primary clinics and full-service hospitals. The ABL80 series offers the ability to personalize diagnostic and test capabilities to suit the needs of a facility's acute care requirements.

Other Tests Performed by POCT

CARDIAC TROPONIN T AND I

Cardiac troponin T (TnT) and **troponin I (TnI)** are proteins specific to heart muscle. Blood levels of cardiac TnT begin to rise within 4 hours of the onset of myocardial damage and may stay elevated for up to 14 days. Cardiac TnI levels rise within 3 to 6 hours and return to normal in 5 to 10 days. Measurement of these proteins is a valuable tool in the diagnosis of acute myocardial infarction (AMI) or heart attack. TnT is also measured to monitor the effectiveness of thrombolytic therapy in cardiac patients. Cardiac troponin POCT analyzers include the following:

- The CARDIAC T Rapid Assay (Roche Corporation, Indianapolis, IN), a one-step, whole-blood test for cardiac TnT that uses disposable test kits to provide results in minutes.
- The Triage® Cardiac Panel (Alere, San Diego, CA), which provides results for three cardiac markers, TnI, CK-MB, and myoglobin.

LIPID TESTING

The Cholestech LDX® system (Alere, San Diego, CA) (Fig. 11-24) can perform cholesterol (TC), triglyceride, low-density lipoprotein (LDL), and high-density lipoprotein (HDL) tests. Non-HDL and TC/HDL ratio. Blood can be obtained by venipuncture or fingerstick and collected in a lithium heparin capillary tube for transfer into the testing cartridge. A quantitative result is obtained by the instrument's evaluation of the intensity of a colored bar.

B-TYPE NATRIURETIC PEPTIDE

B-type natriuretic peptide (**BNP**) is a cardiac hormone produced by the heart in response to ventricular volume expansion and pressure overload. It is the first objective measurement for congestive heart failure (CHF). BNP levels help physicians differentiate chronic obstructive pulmonary disease (COPD) and CHF. This facilitates early patient diagnosis and placement into the appropriate care plan. BNP blood concentrations increase with the increasing severity of CHF and have been shown to more accurately reflect final diagnosis than echocardiographic ejection fractions. BNP can be determined by the i-STAT® (Fig. 11-20) using a whole-blood or plasma specimen.

BILIRUBIN TESTING

The new Bilichek meter (Philips Healthcare) allows for a noninvasive, transcutaneous bilirubin measurement system for newborns. Using light from the meter on the baby's head or sternum, the meter can measure bilirubin levels across the depth of the skin and can be done wherever the newborn is, even in the mother's room. Instruments such as this take optical density readings that show a linear correlation with the serum total bilirubin concentration. The ability to measure total bilirubin levels in this manner means that the healthcare worker can assess the risk of hyperbilirubinemia quickly and easily with no pain to the infant.

C-REACTIVE PROTEIN

C-reactive protein (**CRP**) is a β-globulin found in the blood that responds to inflammation and can therefore be used as a sensitive though nonspecific marker of systemic inflammation disorders and associated diseases. The test can be performed on the Stratus® CS analyzer and is called hs-CRP (high-sensitivity CRP). It can be used as an aid in the detection and evaluation of infection, tissue injury, and inflammatory disorders. CRP also offers an independent marker for the identification of individuals at risk for the future cardiovascular disease. Owing to its high sensitivity, this test can detect low-grade inflammation and even CRP in asymptomatic individuals. Healthcare providers can use the Stratus® CS analyzer to measure this reactive protein within 14 minutes, using whole blood or plasma.

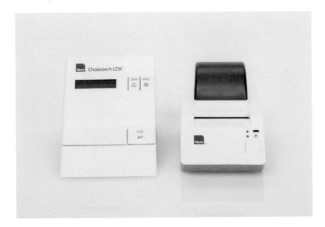

Figure 11-24 Cholestech LDX analyzer with printer. (Courtesy Alere, San Diego, CA.)

GLUCOSE

Glucose testing is one of the most common POCT procedures and is most often performed to monitor glucose levels of patients with diabetes mellitus. POCT glucose analyzers/meters are small, portable, and relatively inexpensive. Two different types of meters are made: one type for an individual's personal use and the other for use in healthcare settings. Hospital-approved glucose analyzers are equipped with data management systems and require various QC checks to monitor the performance of the meter and the operator. Glucose meters manufactured for home use do not have the same level of QC checks. It is common practice in hospitals not to use a patient's personal glucose meter for treatment decisions.

thePoint, *View the Finger Stick Glucose video at http://thepoint.lww.com/McCall6e.*

🔑 **Key Point** Regulatory guidelines and the CLSI recommend that a person receive institutional authorization to perform POCT glucose testing only after completing formal training in facility-established procedures, including maintenance and QC.

An example of some of the glucose meters that are available include:

- Accu-Chek Inform II System
- HemoCue Glucose 201 DM
- Precision Xceed Pro
- Nova BioMedical StatStrip

These analyzers require the use of special reagent test strips or microcuvettes that are unique to their meters. To prevent deterioration of the strips/microcuvettes, the containers they are stored in must be protected from excessive heat and moisture. Some strips/microcuvettttes are stored in vials, which should be tightly recapped after obtaining the necessary strip/microcuvette, while other strips are individually wrapped, like those used in Precision XceedPro. The Accu-Chek Inform II (Roche Diagnostics, Indianapolis, IN) (Fig. 11-25) has a code chip in the analyzer that must match the strip code number.

Glucose analyzers predominantly use whole-blood specimens obtained by routine skin puncture. Some will also accept heparinized venous specimens. To perform the test, a drop of blood is applied to the test strip/microcuvette. The analyzer determines the level of glucose in the blood, and the result appears on a display screen.

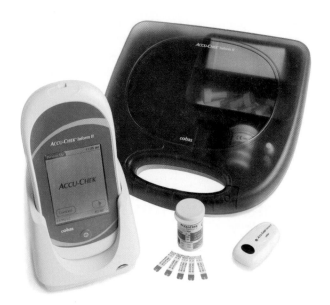

Figure 11-25 Accu-Chek® Inform II System kit. (Courtesy Roche Diagnostics, Indianapolis, IN.)

All of the analyzers approved for hospital use have the following in common.

- Sample types used may be venous, arterial, or capillary.
- They allow data for the glucose meter to be downloaded to a data management program.
- They require the use of a patient and/or authorized operator identification number.
- They require QC.

To download POCT test results from a remote location, an analyzer must either be linked to a downloader or have wireless connectivity like the StatStrip® Glucose meter (Fig. 11-26). Wireless connections to the facility's network is one of the more recent options used to transmit the patient's results to the EMR without any additional HCW intervention. The StatStrip has four

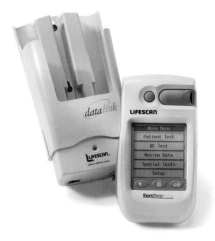

Figure 11-26 Nova BioMedical StatStrip® with wireless connectivity. (Courtesy Nova BioMedical, Waltham, MA.)

distinct areas on the test strip. Three are designed to reduce potential glucose measurement errors. One area measures hematocrit and corrects the glucose result for abnormal hematocrit levels. Two of the areas eliminate interferences from other substances, while the fourth area measures the glucose.

> **Key Point** QC should be repeated if the analyzer is dropped, the battery is replaced, or patient results or analyzer functioning are questioned.

The HemoCue Glucose 201 DM (HemoCue, Inc., Lake Forest, CA) Analyzer accepts arterial specimens as well as skin puncture and venous specimens. The test is performed using a microcuvette instead of a test strip. This unit is also a data management system that prompts the operator for identification, lot numbers, and other required QC information during analysis. The data are then transferred to the computer information system in the laboratory.

The Abbott Precision XceedPro (PXP) is designed to monitor patients at risk for diabetic ketoacidosis and can test both blood glucose and β-ketones on the same instrument. The system incorporates the latest technology to minimize the chance of error and to ensure patient safety in performing POCT. For example, the PXP is capable of scanning the patient's wrist band, the operator's badge, and the test strip's bar code (Fig. 11-27). The scan identifies the lot number and expiration date found on the strip and automatically calibrates the system. Each strip is individually wrapped so as to protect it from moisture and light until used. The patient name, date of birth, and gender is clearly displayed on the monitor to aid in patient identification.

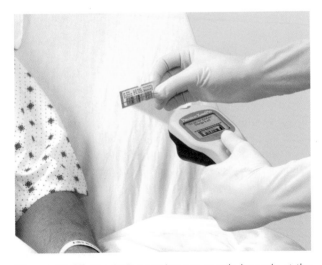

Figure 11-27 The PXP scanning a test strip barcode at the bedside. (Courtesy of Abbott Diabetes Care, Alameda, CA.)

Glycemic Index Control

Most institutions use a practice of intensive insulin therapy commonly referred to as **tight glycemic control (TGC)**. This may involve monitoring a patient's glucose level every half hour and the administration of insulin as required to keep glucose levels in a predetermined range and avoid hyperglycemia. TGC requires frequent and fast glucose results. Blood glucose monitors on a nursing unit are an integral part of this testing. It has been well documented that managing a patient's glucose level reduces infections, speeds healing, decreases length of stay, and lowers the costs of caring for a patient.

GLYCOSYLATED HEMOGLOBIN/HbA1c

HbA1c is the abbreviation used to describe the formation of a hemoglobin compound produced when glucose becomes chemically linked to the hemoglobin protein. The rate of formation of this hemoglobin compound is directly proportional to the plasma glucose amounts. Because glycosylation occurs at a constant rate during the 120-day life cycle of a red cell, glycosylated Hb levels reflect the average blood glucose level over the previous 2 to 3 months and thus can be used to evaluate the long-term effectiveness of diabetes therapy. In fact, it was recently accepted as a more accurate predictor than current techniques of a diabetic patient's likelihood of developing complications from the disease. Studies have shown that the clinical values obtained through regular measurement of HbA1c lead to changes in diabetes treatment and improvement of metabolic control as indicated by a lowering of the HbA1c values. The American Diabetes Association recommends measurement of HbA1c levels at least two times per year, and quarterly in patient who are not meeting their glycemic targets. One analyzer that measures glycosylated hemoglobin is the DCA Vantage® Analyzer (Siemens Healthcare Diagnostics, Inc., Tarrytown, NY) (Fig. 11-28). The instrument provides flexible data management and the convenience of an "on-board" printer. In addition, the clinician can see a patient's trend graph on the display screen for an immediate review of previous results; this also facilitates a discussion of compliance issues with the patient.

HEMATOCRIT

Hematocrit (Hct), also called packed cell volume (PCV), is a measure of the volume of RBCs in a patient's blood. It is calculated by centrifuging a specific volume of anticoagulated blood and determining the proportion of RBCs to plasma. Blood is collected in special microhematocrit capillary tubes. The tubes are sealed at one end with clay or a special stopper and placed in a special hematocrit centrifuge (Fig. 11-29). The StatSpin® CritSpin microhematocrit centrifuge provides complete

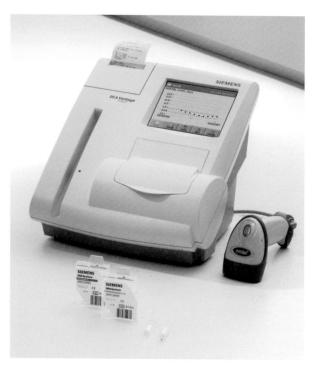

Figure 11-28 DCA Vantage® and two different A1c test cartridges. (Courtesy of Siemens Health Care Diagnostics, Deerfield, IL.)

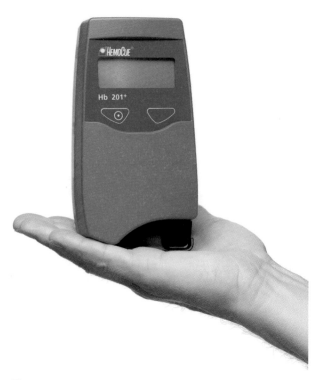

Figure 11-30 HB 201+ for measuring hemoglobin in arterial, venous, or capillary blood. (Courtesy of HemoCue, Inc., Mission Viejo, CA.)

cell packing in 2 minutes. The result is expressed as a percentage of cells to liquid.

Hematocrits are often performed in physician office labs (POLs), clinics, and blood donor stations to screen for anemia or as an aid in the diagnosis and monitoring of patients with polycythemia.

HEMOGLOBIN

The measurement of hemoglobin (Hb) levels is an important part of managing patients with anemia. A number of POCT analyzers measure hemoglobin. One example is the Hemocue HB 201+ Analyzer (Fig. 11-30) (HemoCue, Inc. Lake Forest, CA). It can determine hemoglobin levels in arterial, venous, or capillary blood specimens. A small amount of blood sample is placed in a special microcuvette and inserted into the machine for a reading. As part of the analyzer's electronic QC, the analyzer automatically verifies the performance of the optics every time it is turned on and every 2 hours while the analyzer is left on.

thePoint*⁂ **View the video Collecting Blood for Hemoglobin Determination at http://thepoint.lww. com/McCall6e.**

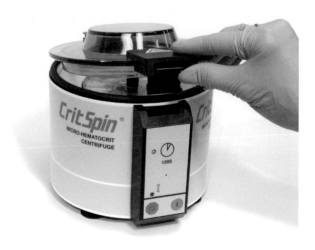

Figure 11-29 StatSpin® CritSpin microhematocrit centrifuge. (IRIS International, Inc., Chatsworth, CA.)

LACTATE

It has long been known that patients who are critically ill can exhibit metabolic acidosis. The accumulation of lactic acid (lactic acidosis) in blood has been identified as a cause of acid–base disorder (metabolic acidosis). Lactic acidosis is associated with major metabolic issues and is due to hyperlactatemia (increased lactate in the blood). Hyperlactatemia is usually present in patients with severe sepsis or septic shock.

The **lactate** level can be used as a marker of the severity of the condition and the patient's stress response. Patients who have an arterial lactate level of more than 5 mmol/L have a very poor prognosis; consequently it

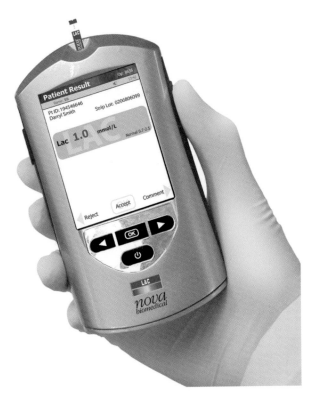

Figure 11-31 StatStrip Lactate analyzer. (Courtesy Nova Biomedical, Waltham, MA.)

is important to be able to obtain lactate results within minutes to effectively treat severe sepsis. If the test is to be performed in the laboratory, the sample must be transported on ice without delay and analyzed as soon as it arrives in the lab. Today the test can be performed at the bedside within a few seconds using the i-STAT or Nova Biomedical's StatStrip Lactate analyzer (Waltham, MA) (Fig. 11-31).

OCCULT BLOOD (GUAIAC)

Detection of occult (hidden) blood in stool (feces) is an important tool in diagnosing and determining the location of a number of diseases of the digestive tract, including gastric ulcer disease and colon cancer. Most tests that detect fecal blood make use of the peroxidase activity of the hemoglobin molecule to bring about a color change in the specimen being tested. For this reason, a patient's diet should be free of meat and vegetable sources of peroxidase, which may lead to false-positive results. Other sources of false-positive results may be certain drugs, vitamin C, alcohol, and aspirin.

Testing for occult blood in POCT settings typically involves the use of special kits containing cards on which small amounts of feces are placed. Hemoccult® II SENSA® (Beckman Coulter Inc., Brea, CA) offers easily used and safely transported cards for collection of the sample (Fig. 11-32). Hemoccult II SENSA has three numbered, connected cards so patients can collect serial

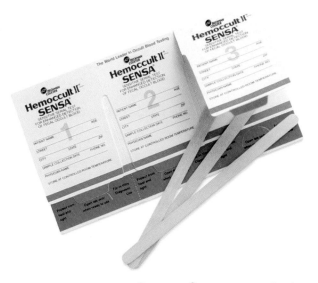

Figure 11-32 Hemoccult® II SENSA® occult blood collection cards. (Beckman Coulter, Fullerton, CA.)

specimens over 3 days, increasing the probability of detecting hidden blood from polyps and cancer. The specimen can be collected and tested on site or the cards can be sent home with the patient to collect the samples and mail back to the lab.

PREGNANCY TESTING

Most rapid pregnancy tests detect the presence of **human chorionic gonadotropin (hCG)**, a hormone produced by the placenta that appears in both urine and serum beginning approximately 10 days after conception. Most rapid pregnancy testing is performed on urine. Peak urine levels of hCG occur at approximately 10 weeks of gestation.

A number of manufacturers supply pregnancy testing kits. Two examples are the Beckman Coulter ICON® hCG (Beckman Coulter, Inc., Brea, CA) (Fig. 11-33) and

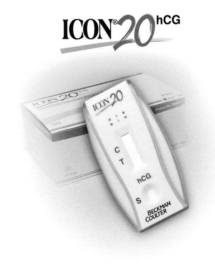

Figure 11-33 Icon® 20 hCG. (Beckman Coulter, Fullerton, CA.)

Quidel's (San Diego, CA) QuickVue+ hCG Combo test, both of which can use urine or serum to perform qualitative detection of hCG in urine or serum. Each manufacturer's kit has unique reagents, timing, and testing methods, and most test kits have a built-in control system. It is important to follow directions exactly. The steps in testing for hCG are outlined in Procedure 11-3.

After seeing all the POCT instruments in this portion of the book, try your hand at matching some of the instruments and devices with the tests they measure in Labeling Exercise 11-1 of the **WORKBOOK**.

Procedure 11-3: Pregnancy Testing

hCG Pregnancy Test Procedure

PURPOSE: To determine pregnancy status using a qualitative hCG urine test. The test checks to see if there is a hormone called human chorionic gonadotropin in the urine. HCG is a hormone normally present in serum and urine during pregnancy.

EQUIPMENT: Gloves, hCG test kit device, disposable dropper or other transfer device (usually supplied with test device), specimen collection cup, patient label, certified timer.

SPECIMEN REQUIREMENTS: No special patient preparation is necessary. Use a clean container to collect sample and keep at room temperature. First morning specimen is suggested because it generally contains the highest concentration of hCG, but any urine sample is suitable for testing.

NOTE: The pouch containing the hCG test kit must be at room temperature before it is opened.

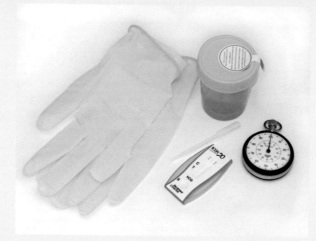

Step	Rationale
1. Identify the patient according to facility policy.	Correct ID is vital to patient safety and meaningful test results.
2. Label the specimen cup with the patient's label.	To avoid errors, the specimen cup should be labeled even if the specimen is the only one being tested at that time.
3. Obtain the patient's urine specimen.	If the patient will be collecting a urine specimen for the test, explain how to do so.
4. Remove the test device from the protective pouch and place it on a flat surface.	For correct results, the device should be absolutely flat so the urine will flow evenly onto the testing surface of the device.

NOTE: If the specimen appears to look watery, a specific gravity test should be performed.

Procedure 11-3: Pregnancy Testing (Continued)

Step	Rationale
5. Using the disposable dropper, add the required amount (three drops) of sample to the sample well (S) on the cassette.	Use the dropper supplied in the protective pouch for adding the sample. The size of the drops must be exactly as specified and consistent for results to be accurate.

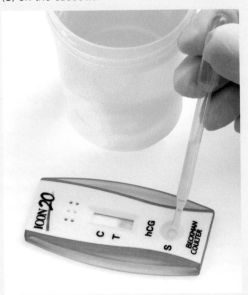

Step	Rationale
6. Set a timer for the time the hCG kit's manufacturer states a negative test must be read.	The reaction must be carefully timed with a certified timer. The test cassette should not be handled or moved until the test is ready to be read, and the results must be read at the specified time. Most manufacturers suggest reading their test after 3 minutes and to *not read* it after 10 minutes.
7. Read the cassette window's results when the timer goes off.	A positive result can be read as soon as lines at both the T and C areas of the test cassette window appear. A negative result is indicated by a line at the C area of the test cassette window only.

Negative Results

The test is negative if a colored line appears only in the control (C) position.

A negative result means, in most cases, that the person is not pregnant.

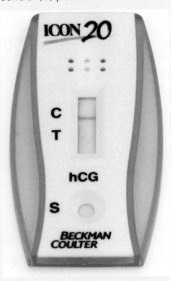

Once you have a negative test after 3 to 5 minutes, *throw out* the test. Any positive test appearing after that time is inaccurate and cannot be considered positive.

False negatives may occur when levels of hCG in the sample are below the sensitivity level of the test. If pregnancy is still suspected, the test can be repeated on a fresh sample collected 48 hours later. If results are questionable, a blood sample should be drawn and sent to the laboratory for testing. Most laboratories have hCG tests that are more sensitive than urine hCG tests.

False-negative results may occur when the sample is diluted due to a large amount of fluid consumption and a low specific gravity. A fresh morning sample will usually have the highest concentration of hCG.

If the results do not agree with other patient findings, a specimen should be sent to the laboratory for confirmation.

Procedure 11-3: Pregnancy Testing (Continued)

Step	Rationale

Positive Results

The test is positive if two colored lines appear, one at the test (T) position and one at the control (C) position. These lines may not be equally light or dark.

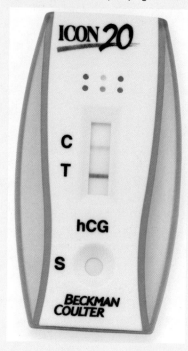

A positive result means, in most cases, that the person is pregnant.

- Some tests will produce a faint positive test result if read after the instructed time due to the formation of something called an "evaporation line."
- Expired tests can also lead to false-positive results. Always check the expiration date before testing.
- Certain rare medical conditions, such as ectopic pregnancy, and some drugs can give a false-positive pregnancy test.

Note: If a female receives shots of hCG for ovulation it is possible to have positive urine for 2 to 3 weeks after the shot and not be pregnant. After delivery or an abortion, hCG may remain detectable for a few days to several weeks.

Invalid Results

The test is considered invalid if there is no distinct visible line at the control (C) position, *even if a colored line appears in the test (T) position.*

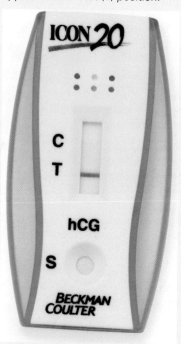

An invalid result means that the test should be repeated.

SKIN TESTS

Some laboratories offer skin testing services, especially for outpatients. Skin tests most often involve the intradermal (within the skin) injection of an allergenic substance (a substance that causes an immune response). Such tests are performed to determine whether an individual has come in contact with a specific allergen (antigen) and developed antibodies against it.

Skin Prick Test

This test is also called a puncture or scratch test and can check for allergic reactions to as many as 40 different substances at one time. This test is usually done to identify everyday allergens such as, pollen, dust mites, mold, foods, and pet dander. The pricks can be done on the forearm or back, and is usually performed in the physician's office.

Tuberculin Test

Many disease-producing microorganisms function as allergens, stimulating an antibody response in susceptible individuals. The tuberculin (TB) test is a skin test that determines whether an individual has developed an immune response to *Mycobacterium tuberculosis*, the microbe that causes tuberculosis. An immune response or reaction to the test can occur if someone currently has TB or has been exposed to it in the past. The procedure for administering a TB test is given in Procedure 11-4.

 Key Point ATB test is also called a PPD test after the purified protein derivative used in the test.

STREP TESTING

Numerous kits are available for the direct detection of group A streptococci on throat swab specimens; for example, the Acceava® Strep A test kit is shown in Figure 11-34. Performance of the test normally requires two steps. The first step involves extraction of the contents from the throat swab; the second step involves a rapid chromatographic immunoassay for the qualitative detection of Strep A antigen. Results are available in 5 minutes.

Procedure 11-4: TB Test Administration

PURPOSE: Administer a TB skin test.

EQUIPMENT: Gloves, alcohol pad, tuberculin syringe, 1/2-inch 27-gauge safety needle, TB antigen, permanent ink pen.

Step	Rationale
1. Identify the patient, explain the procedure, and sanitize hands.	Correct ID is vital to patient safety and meaningful test results. Proper hand hygiene plays a major role in infection control by protecting the phlebotomist, patient, and others from contamination. Gloves are sometimes put on at this point. Follow facility protocol.
2. Support the patient's arm on a firm surface and select a suitable site on the volar surface of the forearm, below the antecubital crease.	The arm must be supported to minimize movement during test administration. Areas with scars, bruises, burns, rashes, excessive hair, or superficial veins must be avoided as they can interfere with interpretation of the test.
3. Clean the site with an alcohol pad and allow it to air dry.	Cleaning with antiseptic and allowing it to air dry permits maximum antiseptic action.
4. Put on gloves at this point if you have not already done so.	Gloves are necessary for safety and infection control.
5. Clean the top of the antigen bottle and draw 0.1 mL of diluted antigen into the syringe.	The top of the bottle must be clean to prevent contamination of the antigen.
6. Stretch the skin taut with the thumb in a manner similar to venipuncture and slip the needle just under the skin at a very shallow angle (approximately 10 to 15 degrees).	The skin must be taut so the needle will slip into it easily. The fluid containing the antigen called tuberculin must be injected just beneath the skin for accurate interpretation of results.
7. Pull back on the syringe plunger slightly to make certain a vein has not been entered.	The antigen must not be injected into a vein.

Procedure 11-4: TB Test Administration (Continued)

Step	Rationale
8. Slowly expel the contents of the syringe to create a distinct, pale elevation commonly called a bleb or wheal.	Appearance of the bleb or wheal is a sign that the antigen has been injected properly.

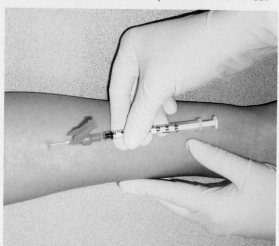

Step	Rationale
9. Without applying pressure or gauze to the site, withdraw the needle, activate the safety feature, and discard the needle. Features and prompt needle disposal minimize the chance of an accidental needlestick.	Applying pressure could force the antigen out of the site. Gauze might absorb the antigen. Both actions could invalidate test results. Activation of safety.
10. Ensure that the arm remains extended until the site has time to close. Do not apply a bandage.	A bandage can absorb the fluid or cause irritation, resulting in misinterpretation of test results.
11. Check the site for a reaction in 48 to 72 hours. This is called "reading" the reaction.	Maximum reaction is achieved in 48 to 72 hours. A reaction can be underestimated if read after this time.
12. Measure induration (hardness) and interpret the result. Do not measure erythema (redness).	A TB reaction is interpreted according to the amount of induration or firm raised area due to localized swelling.
Negative: induration absent or less than 5 mm in diameter.	The health status and age of the individual are important considerations when interpreting results.
Doubtful: induration between 5 and 9 mm in diameter.	Five millimeter of induration can be considered a positive test result in patients who are immunosuppressed due to chronic medical conditions.
Positive: induration 10 mm or greater in diameter.	

the Point. *View the video Rapid Detection of Strep at http://thepoint.lww.com/McCall6e.*

URINALYSIS

A routine urinalysis (UA) consists of a physical and chemical analysis of the specimen as well as microscopic analysis if indicated. A medical laboratory technician or technologist must perform a microscopic analysis.

Chemical composition is most commonly determined by use of an inert plastic reagent strip containing pads impregnated with reagents that test for the presence of bacteria, blood, bilirubin, glucose, leukocytes, protein, and urobilinogen; they measure pH and specific gravity as well. (Specific gravity can also be measured separately using an instrument called a refractometer.) A chemical reaction resulting in color changes to the strip takes place when the strip is dipped in urine. The results can be determined by comparing the strip visually against a code on the container, as shown in Figure 11-35, or by inserting the strip into a machine called a reflectance photometer, which reads the strip and prints out the results or offers connectivity by sending data directly to the LIS or EMR. Reflectance photometers include the Clinitek Advantus (Siemens Diagnostic, Deerfield, IL) and the CLIA-waived analyzers Clinitek Status Connect and Roche URISYS 1100 Urine Analyzers (Roche, Indianapolis, IN). The Clinitek Status Connect and Advantus both have lockouts that require the use of an authorized operator identification

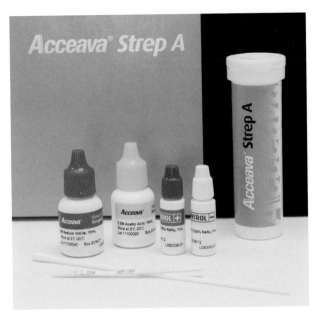

Figure 11-34 Acceava® Strep A test kit. (Alere Inc.,Waltham, MA.)

and can prevent patient testing until the QC has been accepted. These features are welcome additions to POCT urine instruments.

To ensure the integrity of the strips, they should remain tightly capped in their original containers when not in use so as to protect them from the deteriorating effects of light, moisture, and chemical contamination. The containers should also be protected from heat.

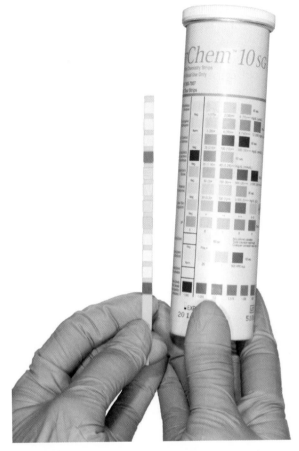

Figure 11-35 Technician comparing urine reagent strip with chart on reagent strip container.

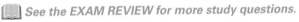

Study and Review Questions

📖 *See the EXAM REVIEW for more study questions.*

1. **When drawing a blood alcohol specimen, it is acceptable to clean the arm with**
   a. benzalkonium chloride.
   b. isopropyl alcohol.
   c. methanol prep.
   d. tincture of iodine.

2. **Which of the following is the most critical part of blood culture collection?**
   a. Adequately mixing the media vials
   b. Antisepsis of the collection site
   c. Selecting the collection site
   d. Timing of the second set of cultures

3. **TDM peak concentration may be defined as the**
   a. highest concentration of the drug during a dosing interval.
   b. lowest concentration of the drug during a dosing interval.

   c. concentration required for maximum drug effectiveness.
   d. none of the above.

4. **In performing a glucose tolerance test, the fasting specimen is drawn at 08:15 hours and the patient finishes the glucose beverage at 08:20 hours. When should the 1-hour specimen be collected?**
   a. 09:15 hours
   b. 09:20 hours
   c. 09:45 hours
   d. 09:50 hours

5. **What color is the stopper of a CTAD tube, for what type of test is it used and why?**
   a. Gray, blood alcohol, inhibits volatilization of alcohol.
   b. Lavender, molecular genetic testing, preserves DNA.
   c. Light blue; coagulation; to inhibit platelet activation.
   d. Orange; special chemistry, to decrease clotting time.

6. Removing a unit of blood from a patient and not replacing it is used as a treatment for
   a. arthritis.
   b. leukemia.
   c. polycythemia.
   d. tuberculosis.

7. Which of the following tests may require special chain-of-custody documentation when the specimen is collected?
   a. Blood culture
   b. Cross-match
   c. Drug screen
   d. TDM

8. What type of specimen is needed for a guaiac test?
   a. Blood
   b. Breath
   c. Feces
   d. Urine

9. Which of the following tests must have a 9:1 ratio of blood to anticoagulant in the collection tube?
   a. Two-hour PP
   b. Blood culture

   c. Electrolytes
   d. Protime

10. Which of the following tests are collected in a trace-element–free tube?
    a. ABGs
    b. Aluminum
    c. BUN
    d. Hemoglobin

11. Common chemistry tests performed by POCT instruments include
    a. Hgb and Hct.
    b. Na and K.
    c. PT and PTT.
    d. T_4 and TSH.

12. Which of the following is a test that measures packed cell volume?
    a. hCG
    b. Hct
    c. INR
    d. TnT

Case Studies

 See the WORKBOOK for more case studies.

Case Study 11-1: Performing a Glucose Tolerance Test

Nancy, a phlebotomist, helped Mr. Smith prepare for a glucose tolerance test over the telephone last week. Today Mr. Smith comes in to have his GTT performed. Nancy asks Mr. Smith if he ate regular, balanced meals for 3 days before today and did not eat, smoke, drink coffee or alcohol, or exercise strenuously for 12 hours before coming in. Mr. Smith answered that he had followed all the directions exactly. Nancy drew the fasting blood at 08:15. Mr. Smith was given the drink at 08:25.

QUESTIONS

1. How quickly must Mr. Smith completely finish the drink?

2. At what time would Nancy collect the 1-hour specimen?

3. If Mr. Smith's glucose was 300 at 30 minutes is this normal?

4. If Mr. Smith vomits after 45 minutes what should Nancy do?

Case Study 11-2: POCT in the ER

Due to the ever increasing demands on a crowded ED, point-of-care testing is used as much as possible for lab results and for quick TAT. The ED personnel receive formal training in POCT procedures, maintenance, and QC. This is done to ensure that the analyzers are properly handled and that the test results are correct. On this busy Friday morning, an elderly man arrives in the ED complaining of stomach cramps. The physician orders electrolytes to be performed. The blood is drawn by a nurse with a 3-cc syringe through the valve of an IV that was just inserted into the patient's left hand. The blood is then placed in the appropriate cartridge for running in the i-STAT. After a few minutes, the results are given to the physician and she immediately tells the nurse to redo the test because the other clinical findings do not support the potassium result of 6.7 mEq/L.

QUESTIONS

1. List four electrolytes that are normally ordered and may be performed on the i-STAT?

2. Can venous blood be used on a POC analyzer like the i-STAT?

3. What does a 6.7 mEq/L potassium result suggest to the physician if it is not supported by the other clinical findings?

4. Could the nurse affect the results by the way the specimen was collected?

Bibliography and Suggested Readings

American College of Obstetricians and Gynecologists. Gestational diabetes mellitus, Practice Bulletin NO. 137. *Obstet Gynecol.* 2013;122:406–416.

American Diabetes Association. Standards of medical care in diabetes – 2014. *Diabetes Care.* 2014;37(1 suppl):S14–S80.

Baron EJ, Weinstein MP, Dunne WM Jr, Yagupsky P, Welch DF, Wilson DM. In: Baron EJ, Coordinating ed. *Cumitech 1 C, Blood Cultures IV.* Washington, DC: ASM Press; 2005.

Bishop ML, Fody EP, Schoeff L. *Clinical Chemistry: Principles, Procedures, Correlations.* 7th ed. Philadelphia, PA: WoltersKluwer/Lippincott Williams & Wilkins; 2013.

Clinical and Laboratory Standards Institute, T/DM06-A. *Blood Alcohol Testing in the Clinical Laboratory: Approved Guideline.* Wayne, PA: CLSI/NCCLS; 1997;17(14) (reaffirmed September 2002).

Clinical and Laboratory Standards Institute POCT13-A2. *Glucose Monitoring in Settings without Laboratory support: Approved Guideline,* 2nd ed. Wayne, PA: CLSI; 2006.

Clinical and Laboratory Standards Institute, POCT04-A2. *Point-of-Care In Vitro Diagnostic (IVD) Testing: Approved Guideline.* 2nd ed. Wayne, PA: CLSI; 2006.

Clinical and Laboratory Standards Institute, H49-A. Point-of-Care Monitoring of Anticoagulation Therapy; Approved Guideline. Wayne, PA: CLSI; 2004.

Clinical and Laboratory Standards Institute M47-A. *Principles and Procedures for Blood Cultures; Approved Guideline.* 1st ed. Wayne, PA: CLSI; 2007.

Fischbach F, Dunning M. *A Manual of Laboratory & Diagnostic Tests.* 9th ed. Philadelphia, PA: Wolterskluwer/Lippincott Williams & Wilkins; 2014.

Garcia LS. *Clinical Microbiology Procedures Handbook.* Vol 1. 3rd ed. Washington, DC: ASM Press; 2010: p.3.4.1.1–3.4.1.4.

Harmening DM. *Clinical Hematology and Fundamentals of Hemostasis.* Philadelphia, PA: F. A. Davis; 2009.

Joint Commission. *Comprehensive Accreditation Manual for Pathology and Clinical Laboratory Sciences.* Oakbrook Terrace, IL: JCAHO; 2002–2003.

Morris LD, Pont A, Lewis SM. Use of a new HemoCue system for measuring haemoglobin at low concentrations. *Clin Lab Haematol.* 2001;23:91–96.

O'Grady NP, Alexander M, Dellinger EP, et al. Guidelines for the prevention of intravascular catheter-related infections. *MMWR Recomm Rep.* 2002;51(RR10):1–26.

Roback J, Grossman B, Harris T, Hillyer C. *Technical Manual.* 17th ed. (Technical Manual of the American Assoc of Blood Banks), AABB (American Association of Blood Banks); 2011.

Titchenal C, Hatfield K, Dunn M, Davis J. Does prior exercise affect oral glucose tolerance test results? *J Int Sport Nutr.* 2008; 5(1 suppl):P14.

U.S. Department of Transportation, Office of Drug and Alcohol Policy and Compliance, *DOT's 10 Steps to Collection Site Security and Integrity.* Updated: Tuesday, October 23, 2012, www.dot.gov, accessed January 13, 2015.

MEDIA MENU

Online Ancillaries (at http://thepoint.lww.com/McCall6e)

- Videos:
  - Collecting a Blood Culture Specimen
  - Collecting Blood for Hemoglobin Determination
  - Finger Stick Glucose
  - Rapid Detection of Strep
- Interactive exercises and games, including Look and Label, Word Building, Body Building, Roboterms, Crossword Puzzles, Quiz Show, and Concentration
- Audio flash cards and flash card generator
- Audio glossary

Internet Resources

- **Advance magazine for medical laboratory personnel:** http://laboratorian.advanceweb.com
- **Typenex Medical LLC:** www.typenex.com (video and guidelines)
- **Center for Phlebotomy Education:** www.phlebotomy.com
- **Genzyme Diagnostics:** www.osomtraining.com (procedureal training and printable certificate of completion)

Other Resources

- McCall R, Tankersley C. *Student Workbook for Phlebotomy Essentials.* 6th ed. (Available for separate purchase).
- McCall R, Tankersley C. *Phlebotomy Exam Review.* 6th ed. (Available for separate purchase).

Chapter 12

Computers and Specimen Handling and Processing

NAACLS Entry Level Competencies

4.4 List the general criteria for suitability of a specimen for analysis, and reasons for specimen rejection or recollection.

4.5 Explain the importance of timed, fasting and stat specimens, as related to specimen integrity and patient care.

7.3 Explain methods for transporting and processing specimens for routine and special testing.

7.4 Explain methods for processing and transporting specimens for testing at reference laboratories.

7.5 Identify and report potential preanalytical errors that may

occur during specimen collection, labeling, transporting, and processing.

7.6 Describe and follow the criteria for collection and processing of specimens that will be used as legal evidence, that is, paternity testing, chain of custody, blood alcohol levels, etc.

8.0 Demonstrate understanding of quality assurance and quality control in phlebotomy.

9.9 Demonstrate ability to use computer information systems necessary to accomplish job functions.

Key Terms

Do Matching Exercise 12-1 in the WORKBOOK to gain familiarity with these terms.

accession number	cursor	LIS	pre-centrifugation
aerosol	data	measurand	QNS
aliquot	DOT	menu	RAM
bar code	EMR	middleware	RFID
biobank	hardware	mnemonic	RNA
breach	HIS	network	ROM
central processing	IATA	output	software
centrifuge	icon	password	storage
cloud	ID code	post-centrifugation	terminal
	input	preanalytical	USB drive
	interface		

Objectives

Upon successful completion of this chapter, the reader should be able to:

1 Demonstrate basic knowledge of the elements of a computer system, define associated terminology and understand the flow of specimens through the laboratory information system.

2 Explain routine and special specimen handling procedures for laboratory

specimens, and identify preanalytical errors that may occur during collection, labeling, transporting, and processing.

3 Describe the steps involved in processing the different types of specimens, time constraints, and exceptions for delivery and list the criteria for specimen rejection.

4 Identify OSHA-required protective equipment worn when processing specimens.

Overview

Today many aspects of patient care are connected through computerized networking, even in the smallest clinic or physician's office. The phlebotomist is involved in certain aspects of the laboratory computer information system as it tracks patient specimens from the time they are collected until the results are reported. This chapter covers knowledge of computer components, general computer skills, and associated terminology. The chapter also addresses proper specimen handling and processing, including how to recognize sources of preanalytical error that may have occurred previous to receipt of the specimen by the laboratory. A thorough understanding of handling and processing helps the phlebotomist avoid preanalytical errors that can render the most skillfully obtained specimen useless and also helps ensure that results obtained on a specimen accurately reflect the status of the patient. Procedures in this chapter conform to CLSI standards.

Computers

Computerization in Health Care

Computers are an essential tool in health care. Various types of computer hardware and software are being used to manage **data** (information collected for analysis or computation), monitor patients, automate analyzers, and most recently, aid in diagnosis. In the laboratory, the phlebotomist should have the ability to use the laboratory information system (LIS) to accomplish all necessary assigned duties. Consequently, computer literacy is a required skill in all areas of health care. To be considered "computer literate," an individual must be able to do the following:

1. Know basic computer terminology (Table 12-1)

2. Understand the computer and the functions it performs

3. Perform basic operations using computers

4. Demonstrate willingness to adapt to the changes computers bring to our lives

Computers range in size from large supercomputers (found primarily in research settings) to desktop and laptop personal computers (PCs) to touchscreen tablets and **hand-held personal computers (HPCs)**. Hand-held devices are ideal for patient identification using bar code systems and paperless collection of data because they can go anywhere the patient may be.

COMPUTER NETWORKS

A computer **network** is a group of computers that are all linked for the purpose of sharing resources, which offers healthcare organizations a great advantage for coordinating data, communicating more efficiently, and sharing hardware and software. In a computer network, individual computer station, tablets, and even smartphones are called *nodes*. The network interconnection allows all the computers to have access through a special node called a server to each other's information or to a large database of information on a mainframe at a remote site. The computers can be connected by coaxial cables, fiber optics, standard telephone lines, the Ethernet, and wireless radiowave connections. When limited to a certain geographical area, these systems are also known as **local area networks (LANs)**.

Networking can take the form of simple interoffice connections or complex systems between several organizations in different cities or across continents. A good example of a large and complex system is the Internet, in which computers all over the world can access multiple sites and unlimited information.

Handhelds, laptops, mobile phones, tablets, datacards, and routers allow any user to connect to the Internet from wherever they are located if there is a wireless network supporting that device's technology. This connectivity and the immediate access it

Table 12-1: Common Computer Terminology

Term	Definition
Accession number	A unique number generated at the time the test request is entered into the computer
CPU	Central processing unit
Cursor	Flashing indicator on the monitor
Data	Information collected for analysis or computation
Hardware	Equipment used to process data
Icon	Image that represents a computer application (program or document)
ID code	A unique code used to identify a person for purposes of tracking
Input	Data entered into the computer
LIS	Laboratory information system
Logging on	Entering as a user on the system via a password
Middleware	Third party vendor software
Mnemonic	Memory-aiding code
Online	Computer is connected to the system and is operational
Output	Processed information generated by the computer
Password	Secret word or phrase used to enter the system
Peripherals	Additional devices, such as modem or printer, that work in conjunction with the computer
RAM	Random access memory; temporary storage of data in the memory of the CPU
ROM	Read-only memory; contains instruction for operation of the computer installed by the manufacturer
Software	Coded instructions required to control the hardware in the processing of data
Storage	A place for keeping data; outside the computer it is called secondary storage
Verify	To confirm or check for correctness of input

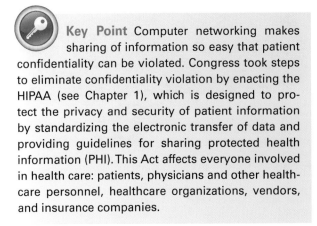

Key Point Computer networking makes sharing of information so easy that patient confidentiality can be violated. Congress took steps to eliminate confidentiality violation by enacting the HIPAA (see Chapter 1), which is designed to protect the privacy and security of patient information by standardizing the electronic transfer of data and providing guidelines for sharing protected health information (PHI). This Act affects everyone involved in health care: patients, physicians and other healthcare personnel, healthcare organizations, vendors, and insurance companies.

COMPUTER SECURITY

Today computer security violations are common place; consequently, large companies have learned to continually monitor for a data leak or **breach** (break in a security wall) in their database. So-called "cyber attacks" can occur from insiders with malicious intentions or through unintentional download of malware (software designed to damage or disable computer systems). There are reports that private information in healthcare facility patient records is quickly becoming a favorite target of hackers. Even the CMS database, which contains the PHI of millions of Medicare beneficiaries, has suffered from breaches and medical identity theft.

According to the MIT Technology Review, there are two reasons for the sharp increase in data breaches in healthcare facilities. Until recently, it was unknown how valuable the patient record information was for those who are uninsured and who would fraudulently use medical care that they could not otherwise afford, and, as happens with initial cyber attacks, the hospital networks were not adequately protected.

In order to help thwart security breaches, all healthcare information systems offer complete data encryption in addition to HIPAA and other regulatory requirements. Even so, it is important for every HCW to be aware of such attacks and use all measures possible to secure and protect this valued patient information.

COMPUTER COMPONENTS

When operating any type of computer, the user will employ the three basic components of any system. These components provide a means to input information, a way to process information, and a method to output information.

provides speeds up processing, increases productivity, and reduces costs. Most industries use this networking because of the advantages it offers in the competitive atmosphere of business. This is true of the healthcare industry and is one of the reasons ACOs and large managed care systems can grow and flourish.

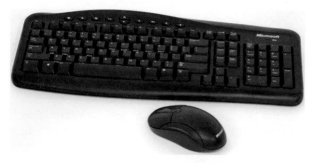

Figure 12-1 Wireless keyboard and mouse.

Input

There are several ways to **input** or enter data into a computer. The most common way is to use a keyboard, much like a typewriter keyboard with additional keys for computer functions (Fig. 12-1). Other methods of input include a light pen designed to read information on the computer screen; a "touchscreen" using a finger or pen for input; scanners programmed to read figures, letters, and bar codes; and a mouse (Fig. 12-1) or glide-pad (a touch-sensitive pad). There is also direct transfer or downloading from another device such as a CD/DVD or other external memory device.

Process

After information has been input, it is processed through a component called the **central processing unit (CPU)**. The CPU is made up of many electrical components and microchips. It is the thinking part of the computer that does comparisons and calculations and makes decisions. When you enter new data, the information will be stored in memory until the processor can execute the command. Memory may be of two types: **random-access memory (RAM)** and **read-only memory (ROM)**. RAM (main memory) serves as temporary storage for data that will be lost when the computer is shut off. If the information needs to be kept for a later date, the operator must transfer it to secondary storage in the form of a hard drive, **Universal Serial Bus (USB) drive** (Fig. 12-2), or compact disk (CD). ROM storage, installed by the manufacturer, instructs the computer to carry out operations requested by the user and is permanently stored inside the computer.

Output

Output describes the processed information or data generated by the computer to be received by the user or someone in another location. Just as there are several ways to input information, there are several means by which processed data can be received. One of the most common ways is through a printer. Data printed on paper is called "hard copy." Other output devices could be the computer screen or other nonpermanent media, such as smartphones or the Apple-iPad and

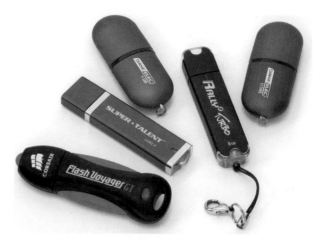

Figure 12-2 Assortment of USB drives.

tablet, which display the data as it is entered and during processing.

ELEMENTS OF THE COMPUTER

 Do the WORKBOOK Exercise Matching 12-3 to see if you recognize the different computer elements.

There are three elements that make up computer systems, hardware, software, and storage.

- **Hardware** is equipment used to process data; it includes the CPU and peripherals (any computer device that is external to the CPU) used for the input or output of information. Examples of hardware peripherals are keyboards, computer monitors or screens, bar code readers, scanners, PDAs, handhelds, facsimile machines, printers, modems, and routers that are used to transfer data to and from other computers. A computer screen and keyboard combination is called a "**terminal**." These are necessary peripherals for most computers and are found throughout the laboratory at workstations or directly connected to an analyzer, like the Sysmex Hematology system shown in Figure 12-3. Portable computers (laptops and handhelds) have the display and keypad built into the device.

- **Software** is the programming (coded instructions) designed to operate the computer hardware in the processing of data. Two basic types exist: systems software and applications software. Systems software is the built-in, preinstalled basics of the computer. It controls the normal operation of the computer and is the operating system that communicates between the hardware and the applications. Applications software refers to programs prepared by software companies or in-house programmers to perform specific tasks

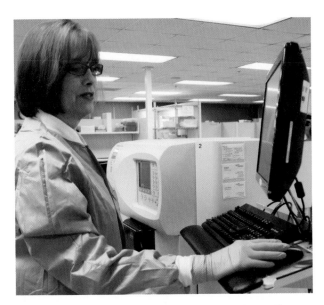

Figure 12-3 A computer terminal connected to a Sysmex Hematology Analyzer.

required by users. Software applications come in many different types: spreadsheets, communication systems, database systems, word processing, and graphics, for example. Packages that perform more than one application, such as word processing, spreadsheet, and database, are called integrated software. The advantage of integrating applications is that it allows the different functions to be easily merged in one document.

- A type of application software referred to as "**middleware**" is sometimes called "plumbing" because it connects two sides of an application and passes data between them. This type of software is becoming increasingly important for POCT analyzers and the laboratory. It is the middleware program that accepts data downloaded from POCT instruments and serves as an interface between the analyzers and the **hospital information system (HIS)**. Through this software the test results can be entered into a patient's electronic chart, and a charge can be submitted to the hospital financial software system that will capture the billing. Middleware in a healthcare setting can also be used as a conduit for data storage, report generation, operator competency tracking, instrument and interface monitoring, and even tracking of errors for quality control/improvement programs.
- **Storage** (preserving information) outside the CPU is necessary because RAM, as mentioned above, is limited temporary storage that will be lost when the computer is turned off. Storage outside the CPU primary storage is called secondary storage, which adds to the CPU's memory capacity by allowing information transfer from the secondary to primary when ready to be used. Examples of permanent secondary storage

devices for documents and programs are external back-up drives, Universal Serial Bus (USB) drives, CDs, DVDs, and storage in "the **cloud**." This relatively new term refers to saving data to an off-site storage system or hardware maintained by a third party. The benefit to cloud storage is that it gives the user unlimited disk space and the ability to connect from multiple devices in any location that has Internet capabilities.

LABORATORY INFORMATION SYSTEM

A **Laboratory Information System (LIS)**, sometimes referred to as a Laboratory Information Management System (LIMS), is a customized software package designed to manage a variety of workflow processes in the laboratory. This sophisticated software serves a variety of purposes, including operations and data management, security and quality control, interactive interface with instrumentation, information sharing with the HIS, **electronic medical records (EMRs)**, and interfaces with external information systems, such as national and regional reference laboratories. The advantages of using an LIS are faster turn-around time (TAT); reduced clerical and billing errors; flexible delivery options for reports, workload, and statistical reports; and increased efficiency with cost savings in all areas of the laboratory.

> (i) There are multiple vendors and types of laboratory information systems currently on the market. All provide the latest in technology to connect people, systems, and external sites, such as hospitals, other laboratories, physician's office and even the physician's home.

Extensive research goes into selecting the right computer system for specific laboratory needs. After selecting a vendor, it can take several months to a few years to bring a system online (make it operational). Usually one or two people are put in charge of the system's daily operation; they are called "system managers." These individuals are responsible for training other personnel in the laboratory and keeping them updated as changes are made to the software. They must readily develop troubleshooting skills as they solve day-to-day problems that develop after the system is installed.

Each type of LIS allows users to define their own parameters for terms and conditions that make the system unique to that facility. Several programs within the system allow phlebotomists and specimen processing personnel to do specific tasks, seemingly at the same time, such as (1) admit patients, (2) request test orders, (3) print labels, (4) evaluate and enter results, (5) inquire about results, and (6) generate reports. Each LIS user must have an ID code and password.

ID Codes

Laboratory computer users are given a unique identifier, which is typically a combination of numbers and letters, called an **ID code**. The security associated with an ID code determines what system functions can be accessed. An ID code is also logged with every transaction on the system, allowing the system manager to identify the person performing each transaction and for the purpose of accruing workload. ID codes are not always confidential because it is not always possible for phlebotomists to verify their own collections. A data entry clerk or central processor may verify all collections and must have access to the list of ID codes so that he or she can associate the proper phlebotomist with each draw.

Passwords

In addition to an ID code that identifies the person logging on, the user must also have a password. Just like online banking, the password uniquely identifies that person and allows him or her to become a system user. Passwords must be kept strictly confidential because they enable access to the LIS.

Icons and Mnemonic Codes

Some lab systems use **icons** or images to request the appropriate program or function necessary to enter data. Others may use a menu of **mnemonic** (memory-aiding) codes or an abbreviation for selecting a function.

A mnemonic code to identify the type and volume of tube required is always printed whenever a label is generated (Fig. 12-4). For example, if the phlebotomist knows that a CBC is ordered and the code on the label reads 5 mL LAV, he or she knows what tube type to choose and the amount of blood to draw. This demonstrates one of the benefits of computerized label generation; the label aids the phlebotomist in acquiring the proper specimen in a timely fashion. The generic steps used by the LIS for processing a typical specimen, from arrival in the lab through reporting of results, are shown in the flowchart in Figure 12-5.

Bar Codes

Most laboratory and POCT analyzers use bar code technology for specimen identification. A **bar code** is a parallel array of alternately spaced black bars and white spaces representing a code. The code may represent numbers or letters. Some of the uses of bar codes in health care include identification of patients (bar code ID bands), supply inventory, specimen identification, and pharmaceutical drug name, dose, and route. A bar code label, produced by the LIS on a bar code label printer as seen in Figure 12-6, is applied to collected specimens, making specimen processing in the laboratory more efficient. Hand-held

Figure 12-4 A computerized label generated when the requisition order is entered.

systems can be used to read patient ID bar code bands and generate the labels used for specimen collection at the patient's bedside. One system that performs this function is the Patient Identification Check from Siemens Healthcare, Malvern, PA (Fig. 12-7). While at the patient's bedside, the phlebotomist uses a wireless hand-held scanner, which identifies the patient, displays the collection tubes needed and the order of draw, scans the specimen container and automatically prints the correct label including the actual time of collection, and identifies the person who is performing the phlebotomy.

Radio Frequency ID

Another form of identification using computer technology is **radio frequency identification (RFID)**. RFID is a unique identifier that can be scanned to retrieve identifying information and track a product or person. This ID system is composed of a *reader* and a *tag* or *label* that serves the same purpose as a bar code or the magnetic strip on a credit card. In fact, the RFID tag looks very much like a bar code label, but is actually a silicon chip. One of the advantages of this wireless identification system is that it does not need to be in close proximity to the object being scanned because it communicates data by radio waves. It will work within a few feet and up to 100 feet away. The second advantage is that the RFID scanner can track more than one tag at a time and

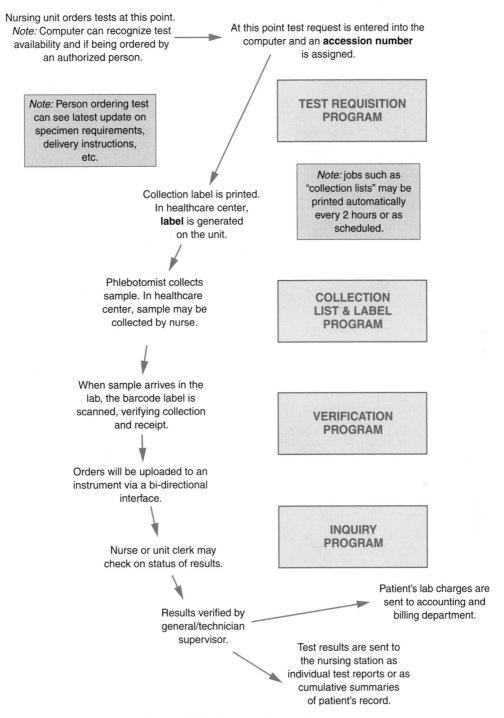

Nursing unit orders tests at this point. *Note:* Computer can recognize test availability and if being ordered by an authorized person.

At this point test request is entered into the computer and an **accession number** is assigned.

TEST REQUISITION PROGRAM

Note: Person ordering test can see latest update on specimen requirements, delivery instructions, etc.

Note: jobs such as "collection lists" may be printed automatically every 2 hours or as scheduled.

Collection label is printed. In healthcare center, **label** is generated on the unit.

Phlebotomist collects sample. In healthcare center, sample may be collected by nurse.

COLLECTION LIST & LABEL PROGRAM

When sample arrives in the lab, the barcode label is scanned, verifying collection and receipt.

VERIFICATION PROGRAM

Orders will be uploaded to an instrument via a bi-directional interface.

INQUIRY PROGRAM

Nurse or unit clerk may check on status of results.

Patient's lab charges are sent to accounting and billing department.

Results verified by general/technician supervisor.

Test results are sent to the nursing station as individual test reports or as cumulative summaries of patient's record.

Figure 12-5 Example of a work flow chart.

beyond the line of sight of the reader. In health care, it is used to identify and track specimens, equipment, records, and monitor patients.

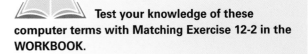

At present, barcodes are more accepted and less expensive, but with the standardization of the RFID industry and the cost of tags decreasing, the technology is becoming more commonplace in health care.

Test your knowledge of these computer terms with Matching Exercise 12-2 in the WORKBOOK.

GENERAL LABORATORY COMPUTER SKILLS

General skills that the phlebotomist must learn, regardless of what LIS is used, involve the following.

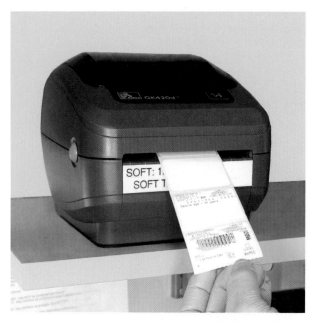

Figure 12-6 Bar code label printer in a laboratory.

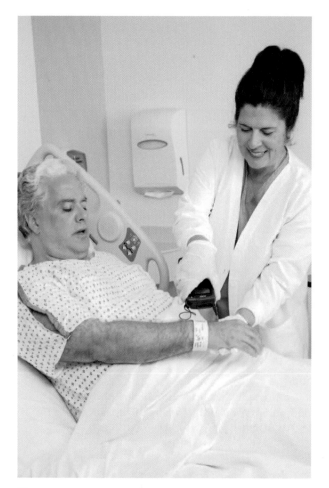

Figure 12-7 Siemens Patient Identification Check being used to scan a wristband. (Courtesy Siemens Healthcare, Malvern, PA.)

Logging on: A person who is allowed to access a computer system is given a username and **password**. The password uniquely identifies that person and allows him or her to become a system user. The process of entering a username and password to gain access to the system is called "logging on." When the log-on sequence is completed, a **menu** is displayed listing the options from which the user may choose. For security and authorization purposes, most systems are designed to allow users unique access to different menus or programs.

Cursor movement: After logging on, a flashing indicator on the screen, called the **cursor**, indicates the starting point for input. When entering patient information in an LIS, the cursor will automatically reset itself at the correct point for data input after the **Enter key** has been pressed.

Using icons: Access to documents and software programs can be initiated by using the mouse to click on a small representative image called an icon that opens a document or launches a software program.

Entering data: After necessary information has been input, the Enter key must be pressed for information to be processed. If an error in spelling or selection is made, it can easily be deleted by backspacing before pressing the Enter key. If the wrong information is entered, however, it is still possible to correct errors.

Correcting errors: This procedure is necessary to correct mistakes that are detected after the Enter key has been pressed. The procedure to delete errors is program-dependent and must be learned with each system. Some LIS programs use order verification, an additional step in the process, to allow a review of the information before it is accepted.

Verifying data: After all patient information has been entered, it will appear on the monitor screen as a complete order. At this point, the user can review the information again and can choose to modify, delete, or accept it. When all orders have been entered, the user can request an inquiry of the orders as another check.

Making order inquiries: Selecting an inquiry program allows the user to retrieve any or all of the test orders associated with a patient.

Canceling orders: If, after entering an order, a user finds that it is incorrect, he or she can request that the computer delete or cancel it.

COMPUTERIZED ANALYZERS

Computers are such accurate processors of information at incredible speeds that computerized laboratory analyzers are considered more efficient and cost-effective than relying on manual methods. Most laboratory analyzers have sophisticated computer systems designed to manage patient data and **interface** (connect for the purpose of interaction) with the LIS.

In the laboratory, multiple computers can connect to each other and share data. Two types of interfaces are used in the LIS. One is a unidirectional interface, which means data only go one way, from the analyzer to the LIS computer. The second interface is bidirectional, meaning data can upload (transfer from analyzer to LIS) or download (transfer from LIS to analyzer) between two systems.

(i) Major manufacturers of laboratory analyzers have the capability to connect their computer via the healthcare facility's Internet with an analyzer in their customer's laboratory to monitor the instrument's status and to troubleshoot. This Internet connection provides real-time intervention for those occasions when an analyzer malfunctions; therefore, greatly decreasing down time and the delay in test results.

INTERFACING AND INTEGRATING

Today's healthcare facility is quickly moving toward being totally **integrated** (connected) through networking of computers with the appropriate middleware. Some of the types of applications requiring interfaces are EMR, HIS, LIS, **Radiology Information System (RIS)**, Dietary, and Emergency Department.

An example of successful integration in the hospital setting is point-of-care testing. Because sophisticated testing is possible at the patient's side, the results need to be captured for appropriate treatment, accurate patient records, and documented in the EMR for access by the providers of care. While most point-of-care analyzers are interface capable, the decision to interface is based on the number of tests performed and the impact of the test to the patient. For example, a troponin result may need to be received by the physician immediately while the result of a creatinine is not that critical.

CONNECTIVITY INDUSTRY CONSORTIUM

To be used effectively, POC instruments must integrate with many different institutions' information systems. This requirement has led to formation of the Connectivity Industry Consortium (CIC), which was established to ensure that *any* point-of-care analyzer could talk to *any* LIS. A guideline for standardization was developed by POC analyzer manufacturers, LIS vendors, and healthcare providers that resulted in the *CLSI Point-of-Care Connectivity, Approved Standard-Second edition.*

COMPUTERIZATION AND CONNECTIVITY

Current trends in health care indicate that clinical laboratory operations will continue to decentralize, and that

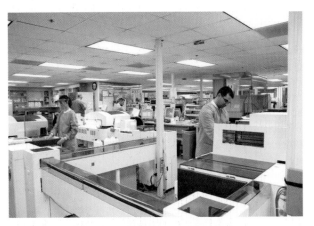

Figure 12-8 Roche Modular Pre-Analytics (MPA) system used in central processing.

POC testing will increase. The need for complete networking becomes even more apparent as remote laboratory testing facilities increase in numbers. Today large reference laboratories, totally separate from the healthcare facilities, can download results from automated instruments into patient charts and centralized databases. Computerization and instrumentation such as the Roche Modular Pre-Analytics (MPA) system (Fig. 12-8) make that possible. After the specimen has been collected and the recommended clot time has been met, a tube of blood can be placed in the MPA decapper/centrifuge module (Fig. 12-9) and through computer connections with the rest of the specimen processing modules and the specified analyzer in the laboratory, the test results arrive at a patient's EMR in the hospital or physician's office without any manual intervention required.

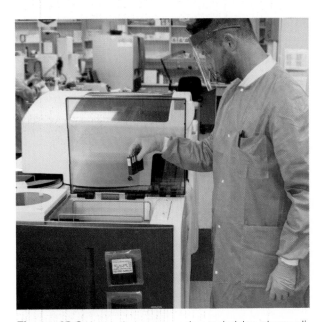

Figure 12-9 A specimen processing technician places aliquot tubes in the MPA.

Specimen Handling and Processing

As part of the computerization network that connects many aspects of patient care, the LIS tracks patient specimens from the time they are collected until the results are reported. This special technology increases efficiency and improves TAT, but cannot ensure quality results. The quality of results depends on correct procedures being followed in the three phases of the laboratory process: **preanalytical** (prior to analysis) or pre-examination phase, **analytical** (during analysis), and **postanalytical** (after analysis) or postexamination. Unfortunately, it is in the preanalytical phase, which begins when a patient is assessed and a test is ordered, where the majority of laboratory errors occur (see Box 12-1). Specimen handling and processing is a critical part of this phase. Correct handling and processing helps ensure that results obtained on a patient specimen accurately reflect the status of that patient. Improper handling or processing is a preanalytical error that can render the most skillfully obtained specimen useless or affect the analyte (substance undergoing analysis) or **measurand** (quantity being measured) in a way that causes erroneous (invalid) or misleading test results that can cause delayed or incorrect patient care. Proper specimen handling begins when a test is ordered and continues throughout the testing process until results are reported out. This section of the text, however, covers specimen handling from the time a blood specimen is drawn or a nonblood specimen is collected,

Box 12-1

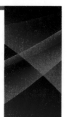

Possible Sources of Preanalytical Error

Before Collection

- Altitude
- Dehydrated patient
- Duplicate test orders
- Exercise
- Inadequate fast
- Incomplete requisition
- Medications
- Patient stress
- Pregnancy
- Smoking
- Strenuous exercise
- Treatments (e.g., intravenous medications, radioisotopes)
- Wrong test ordered

At Time of Collection

- Misidentified patient
- Antiseptic not dry
- Expired tube
- Failure to invert additive tubes properly
- Faulty technique
- Improper vein selection
- Inadequate volume of blood
- Inappropriate use of plasma separator tube (PST) or serum separator tube (SST)
- Incorrect collection tube
- Incorrect needle position
- Incorrect needle size
- Mislabeled tube

- Mixing tubes too vigorously
- Nonsterile site preparation
- Patient position
- Prolonged tourniquet application
- Underfilled tube
- Wrong collection time

During Specimen Transport

- Agitation-induced hemolysis
- Delay in transporting
- Exposure to light
- Failure to follow temperature requirements
- Transport method (e.g., hand vs. pneumatic tube)

During Specimen Processing

- Contamination (e.g., dust or glove powder)
- Delay in processing or testing
- Delay in fluid separation from cells
- Evaporation
- Failure to centrifuge specimen according to test requirements
- Failure to separate fluid from cells
- Incomplete centrifugation
- Mislabeled aliquot
- Multiple centrifugations
- Rimming of clots

During Specimen Storage

- Exposure to light
- Temperature change outside defined limits

throughout processing until testing begins, and during storage before and after testing. Storage after testing is part of the postanalytical phase but can become part of the preanalytical phase when repeat testing or additional tests are ordered on a specimen sometimes hours or even days later.

> Test your knowledge of preanalytical errors with WORKBOOK Labeling Exercise 12-3.

> **Key Point** It has been estimated that 50% to 70% of all laboratory errors occur prior to analysis.

Specimen Handling

It is not always easy to tell when a specimen has been handled improperly. Therefore, to ensure delivery of a quality specimen for analysis, it is imperative that all phlebotomists be adequately instructed in this area so that established policies and procedures are followed. In addition, to protect the phlebotomist and others from accidental exposure to potentially infectious substances, all specimens should be handled according to the standard precautions guidelines outlined in Chapter 3.

PATIENT IDENTIFICATION

The phlebotomist's role in specimen handling in the pre-analytical phase starts with the test order. The phlebotomist must prepare for test collection by having the right equipment for the test available, and to know of any special conditions required for its collection and handling. The most important part of collecting the specimen is patient identification (see Chapter 8). Obviously, if the patient has been misidentified, it doesn't matter how well the specimen is handled. Once the specimen is collected, patient identification must be reverified and a correct label placed on the tube or container for the entire process to lead to a valid result.

ROUTINE HANDLING

Mixing Tubes

Tubes with additives must be mixed gently by inversion (Fig. 12-10) as soon as they are drawn. All additives except sodium citrate require from 5 to 10 inversions depending on manufacturer instructions. Sodium citrate tubes require 3 to 4 inversions. (See the tube guides in

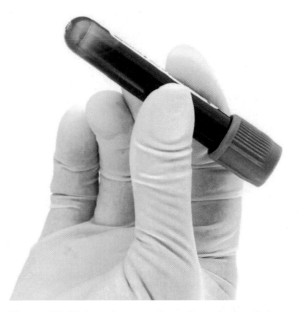

Figure 12-10 Inverting an anticoagulant tube to mix it.

Appendix F for tube inversion information from two major tube manufacturers.) Gentle inversion helps distribute the additive evenly for proper function, while minimizing the chance of hemolysis. Vigorous mixing can cause hemolysis and must be avoided.

> **Key Point** Tests that are seriously affected by hemolysis include potassium, plasma free hemoglobin, troponin I and T, AST, and LDH. Tests negatively affected by microclots include CBCs and related tests such as hemoglobin and hematocrit, platelet counts, and red and white blood cell counts.

Inadequate mixing of anticoagulant tubes, including plasma separator gel tubes, leads to microclot formation, which can cause erroneous test results, especially for hematology studies. Clotting may be incomplete in serum separator gel tubes that are not mixed properly because they also require 5 to 10 gentle inversions for the clot activator to function properly.

Labeling Specimens

Specimens must be labeled immediately after collection and before dismissing an outpatient or leaving the room of an inpatient. Reverification of patient information before the label is applied to the specimen is critical (see Chapter 8). Many laboratories now require the phlebotomist to show the labeled tube to the patient after collection and ask the patient to verify that the patient information on the label is correct. Some outpatient labs even have the patient initial or sign a document stating

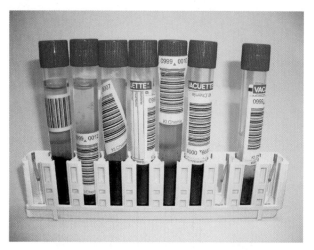

Figure 12-11 Correct and incorrect tube label application. Labels on the six tubes on the left have been incorrectly applied. The label on the tube to the far right was correctly applied. (Courtesy Greiner Bio-One International AG, Kremsmünster, Austria.)

that they were shown the labeled tube and that they verified that the information was correct. Placement of the label on the tube in the correct orientation (see Fig. 12-11) is also important, especially labels with barcodes that are scanned by analyzers.

TRANSPORTING SPECIMENS

It is important to handle and transport blood specimens carefully and deliver them as quickly as possible to the laboratory for processing. A delay in separating the blood cells from the plasma or serum can result in metabolic changes in the sample. Rough handling and agitation can hemolyze specimens, activate platelets, and affect coagulation tests as well as break collection tubes. According to CLSI, tubes should be transported vertically with the stopper up to reduce agitation that can cause red cell damage and lead to hemolysis in the specimen. The upright position also allows the blood to drain away from the tube stopper to minimize the chance of **aerosol** (a fine mist of specimen) release if the stopper is removed during processing or testing. In addition, the upright position aids clot formation in serum tubes and prevents the clot from sticking to the stopper. Blood in contact with tube stoppers in gel tubes may end up in the serum or plasma above the gel barrier after centrifugation. This can contaminate the specimen with blood cells that can affect test results, and fibrin strands that can cause blockages in instruments.

Key Point According to CLSI nonanticoagulant gel tubes should be placed in an upright position as soon as they have been mixed.

General Transportation Guidelines

Blood specimen tubes are typically placed in biohazard bags or containers for transportation to the laboratory. CLSI and OSHA guidelines require specimen transport bags to have a biohazard logo, a liquid-tight closure, and a slip pocket for paperwork (e.g., the requisition). Nonblood specimens should be transported in leak-proof containers with adequately secured lids. If the laboratory is on site, specimens are either hand delivered by the phlebotomist or other healthcare workers who have collected them, or sent to the laboratory by means of an automated internal transportation system such as a pneumatic tube, vertical track, or robot system (Fig. 12-12).

Automated Transportation Systems

All specimens transported through a pneumatic tube system (PST) or other type of automated transport system

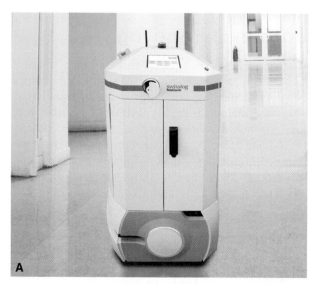

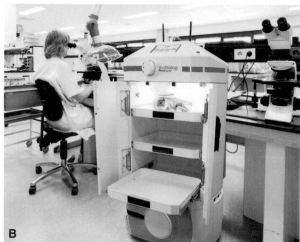

Figure 12-12 Robot specimen transportation system called the RoboCourier® Autonomous Mobile Robot. **A:** RoboCourier® in a lab after delivering a specimen. **B:** A RoboCourier® traveling down a hallway. (Courtesy Swisslog Healthcare Solutions North America, Denver, CO.)

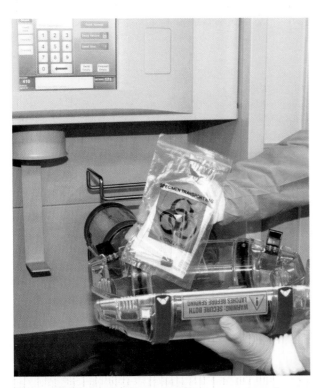

Figure 12-13 Specimen prepared for transport through pneumatic tube system.

Box 12-2

Tests That Are Not Affected by PTS Transport

- Albumin
- Alkaline phosphatase
- AST
- Chloride
- Creatinine
- Glucose
- Sodium
- Total bilirubin
- Total protein
- BUN
- Uric acid
- Thrombin time
- WBC concentration

within the facility should be considered biohazards and require strict protocol to prevent potential contamination issues. Specimens should be packaged correctly in leak-resistant containers, sealed in zipper-type plastic bags to contain spills (Fig. 12-13), and the carrier should be fitted with disposable clear plastic liners in case of leakage. Carriers must contain foam pads and special padded liners to provide containment and cushioning during transport.

Each facility's PST should be carefully evaluated for the effects of shock and vibration on the validity of laboratory test results. CLSI Guideline GP44-A4, states that in general, tests negatively affected by PTS transport are those influenced by red cell damage, and include potassium, plasma hemoglobin, acid phosphatase, and lactate dehydrogenase. Specimens that must be maintained at body temperature (e.g., cold agglutinin and cryoglobulin) are also not appropriate for PTS transport. Tests that are not affected by transport in tube delivery systems according to CLSI are shown in Box 12-2.

Key Point Unless specific documentation already exists, automated transport systems, pneumatic or otherwise, should be evaluated for any effects on laboratory testing. See CLSI document H21-A5 for specific recommendations regarding specimens for coagulation testing.

Off-Site Transportation

Many patient specimens are delivered to clinical laboratories from off-site locations such as physician offices, clinics, patient service centers, or private homes, or sent from these locations or healthcare facility laboratories to local or regional reference laboratories.

Local Courier or Mobile Phlebotomist

Specimens transported by a courier or mobile phlebotomist must be in a leak-proof–primary container (e.g., blood tube). This container is put in a zip closure plastic bag containing absorbent material such as paper towels, and placed in a plastic or metal cooler or transport box, which is the secondary container. Alternatively blood specimens can be placed upright in a rack that sits on top of absorbent material in the bottom of the transport box. The transport box must be closed to avoid spills and contamination in case it is jostled during transportation, properly labeled, and accompanied by forms containing specimen data and identification. The transport box should be placed on the floor of the vehicle, behind the driver's seat, where it has no direct exposure to the sun or air vents. If this is not possible it must be held in place on the back seat with a seat belt. Special care should be taken to protect specimens from the effects of extreme heat or cold.

Vehicles used to transport specimens on a routine basis must be used exclusively for this purpose. Specimens transported locally are exempt from most other **U.S.**

Department of Transportation (DOT) regulations unless they are known or suspected to be infectious.

Out-of-Area Transportation

Diagnostic specimens that are transported out of the area by public transportation are covered by **U.S. Department of Transportation (DOT),** and **International Air Transport Association (IATA)** regulations for transportation of infectious substances. DOT and IATA define two categories of infectious substances:

1. Biological Substance Category A; an infectious substance capable of causing permanent disability, or life-threatening or fatal disease in normally healthy humans (UN 2814) or animals (UN 2900).

2. Biological Substance Category B; an infectious substance that does not meet the criteria for Category A. Category B is assigned UN 3373, which includes laboratory specimens transported for diagnostic purposes.

Category B regulations require all diagnostic specimens transported by public carrier to have triple packaging. Packaging materials can be purchased that meet DOT requirements. Triple packaging requirements include the following:

- Specimens must be placed in watertight, positive-closure (e.g., screw-on cap) primary containers made of glass, metal, or plastic. Primary containers must be individually wrapped with sufficient absorbent material to accommodate their entire contents. Specimens must not exceed 500 mL (16.9 oz) if liquid, or 500 g (1.1 lb) if solid.

- The individually wrapped containers must be placed in a leak-proof–secondary container, such as a sealed plastic biohazard bag strong enough to withstand leakage.

- The primary and secondary containers must be placed in a sturdy third outer container made of wood, metal, rigid, plastic, or corrugated fiberboard with a minimum of one rigid side that is 4 inches wide. An itemized list of contents must be inserted between the secondary container and the outer container. Each complete package must be able to withstand a 4-foot (1.2 m) drop.

- Ice or dry ice must be placed outside the secondary container, within the outer container or as an overpack. There must be interior support to secure the secondary container if the ice or dry ice dissipates. The outer container must be leak proof if ice is used, and allow release of carbon dioxide if dry ice is used.

- Minimum required markings of the outer container include

  a. A UN 3373 label with the words "Biological Substance Category B."

  b. A Class 9 miscellaneous label if the package contains dry ice.

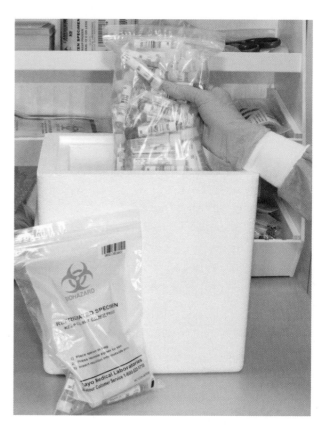

Figure 12-14 A specimen processing technician packing a specimen for send out.

  c. The name, address, and telephone number of the shipper and the receiver or consignee.

Diagnostic specimens can pose a danger if shipped improperly. Specimen processors (Fig. 12-14) and other personnel who package "infectious materials" to be transported by public carriers must show proof of training and be certified. Both IATA and DOT offer certification. DOT can inspect laboratories for compliance with shipping regulations, and severe penalties such as huge fines and even jail time can be imposed on anyone who knowingly or unknowingly violates them.

Time Limits

All specimens should be transported to the laboratory without delay. According to CLSI GP44-A4, *Procedures for the Handling and Processing of Blood Specimens,* serum or plasma should be physically separated from the cells as soon as possible unless there is conclusive evidence that a longer contact time will not contribute to error in test results. GP44-A4 also states that if an uncentrifuged blood specimen is sent to the laboratory from a blood drawing station, the separation of cells and plasma or serum must occur in a time limit to protect the stability of the analyte. If this cannot happen, the appropriate specimen processing must be done at the collection site and then delivered to the lab (see Specimen Processing covered later in this chapter).

Key Point CLSI guideline GP44-A4 sets 2 hours as the maximum time limit for separating serum and plasma from the cells for the following tests: catecholamines, homocysteine, lactic acid, and molecular tests targeting RNA. Studies cited by CLSI show that the 2-hour time limit also applies to glucose, ionized calcium, lactate dehydrogenase (LD or LDH), and potassium. Because tests for analytes with varying stabilities may be collected in a single specimen tube, many laboratories use 2 hours as the maximum time limit for separating all specimens as a general rule.

Prompt delivery and separation minimize the effects of metabolic processes, such as **glycolysis.** Unless chemically prevented by an additive, such as sodium fluoride (which can take as long as 4 hours for complete inhibition) glycolysis continues in a blood specimen, lowering glucose levels until the serum or plasma is physically separated from the cells. Cellular metabolism can also affect other analytes.

Find out how well you know other key points and cautions with WORKBOOK Knowledge Drill 12-1.

Key Point According to a 2013 article in the Journal of Environmental and Public Health, results of community outreach studies found that glycolysis by erythrocytes and leukocytes in blood specimens can falsely lower glucose values from 5% to 7% per hour.

Prompt delivery is easily achieved with an on-site lab, as in a hospital setting, but it is not always possible when specimens come to the lab from off-site locations, such as doctors' offices and nursing homes. Although specimens from these sites are typically picked up and transported to the testing site by a courier service on a regular basis, the time between collection and delivery can easily exceed 2 hours. Consequently, off-site locations should have a small processing area where blood specimens for tests that are performed on serum or plasma can be centrifuged (see Specimen Processing) and the serum or plasma separated and transferred to a leak-proof–secondary container for transport. Applicable temperature requirements for all specimens as well as any special handling requirements should be maintained until they are turned over to the courier service. The courier service then takes over the responsibility of seeing that all requirements for handling the specimens are met.

Time Limit Exceptions

"STAT" or "medical emergency" specimens take priority over all other specimens and should be transported, processed, and tested immediately. Examples of other exceptions to time limits include the following:

Ammonia Specimens

Blood ammonia levels increase rapidly at room temperature. Consequently, for accurate results, ammonia specimens must be immediately placed in ice slurry or a cooling tray after collection, transported stat, and separated from the cells within 15 minutes of collection.

Coagulation Specimens

The acceptable amount of time between coagulation specimen collection and testing depends on the test. In addition, sample stability is affected by a number of factors that can vary. Consequently, it is best if all specimens for plasma-based coagulation tests are processed as soon as possible after collection.

Ideally, PT and PTT (or aPTT) tests should be performed within 4 hours of specimen collection. However, according to CLSI, PT specimens can be held at room temperature either centrifuged with the plasma in contact with the cells, or uncentrifuged, for up to 24 hours after collection, provided the tubes have not been opened. PTT specimens from patients who are not on heparin can be held in the same manner, but only for up to 4 hours.

PT or PTT specimens that have been opened must be tested within 4 hours. If time limits for PT and PTT testing cannot be met the specimen's platelet-poor plasma (plasma carefully removed without disturbing the buffy coat) can be frozen at −20°C or below for up to 2 weeks or −70°C for longer storage.

PTT specimens for monitoring unfractionated heparin levels must be centrifuged within 1 hour of collection, and tested within 4 hours of specimen collection. If time constraints for samples from patients on unfractionated heparin cannot be met the specimen should be collected in a CTAD tube.

Glucose Specimens in Sodium Fluoride Tubes

Glucose specimens drawn in sodium fluoride tubes are stable for 24 hours at room temperature and up to 48 hours when refrigerated at 4°C to 8°C. However, inhibition of glycolysis may be inadequate in specimens from patients with abnormally high platelet, red blood cell, or white blood cell counts. In addition, complete inhibition of glycolysis by sodium fluoride can take as long as 4 hours during which time glucose levels can fall as much as 10 mg/dL even in samples with normal blood cell counts.

Pediatric Glucose Specimens

Glucose specimens from newborn and pediatric patients should be tested as soon as possible because it is difficult to inhibit glycolysis in newborn and pediatric specimens. Capillary specimens for glucose testing on pediatric patients should be collected in microcollection devices that contain a suitable antiglycolytic agent.

Hematology Specimens

- Blood smears made from EDTA specimens must be prepared within 1 hour of collection to preserve the integrity of the blood cells and prevent artifact formation due to prolonged contact with the anticoagulant.
- EDTA specimens for CBCs should be analyzed within 6 hours, but are generally stable for 24 hours at room temperature.
- EDTA specimens for erythrocyte sedimentation rate (ESR) determinations must be tested within 4 hours if left at room temperature or within 12 hours if refrigerated.
- EDTA specimens for reticulocyte counts are stable up to 6 hours at room temperature and up to 72 hours if refrigerated.

Molecular Test Specimens

Plasma preparation tubes (PPTs) for molecular testing, such as Hepatitis C qualitative or quantitative **ribonucleic acid (RNA)** must be transported, processed, and tested as soon as possible because RNA substances/materials are extremely unstable. If an RNA test must wait to be run in a batch, the plasma can be stored at 4°C, but only for 48 hours. If the plasma is not tested within that timeframe, it must be transferred from the PPT to an aliquot tube and frozen at −80°C.

Microbiology Specimens

Specimens collected for cultures, that is, blood, urine, throat, wounds, etc., should be transported to the laboratory as soon as possible. It is very important to properly transport and quickly attend to the microbiology specimens in order to preserve the microorganism present and identify it. After being accessioned, a sample is transferred to culture media or in the case of blood culture bottles, put immediately into an incubator. See Chapter 11 for more information on blood cultures.

Urine Specimens

The phlebotomist is often involved in transporting body fluids, such as urine, to the laboratory. Urines should be transported to the lab promptly. The time between collection and transport is of great importance because the quality of the test results is very dependent on the timeliness of the transport. If urine specimens are not tested promptly, urine components can change. For example,

cellular elements decompose, bilirubin breaks down to biliverdin, and bacteria multiply, leading to erroneous test results. Specimens that cannot be transported or analyzed promptly can be held at room temperature and protected from bright light for up to 2 hours. Specimens held longer should be refrigerated. Specimens that require both UA and C&S testing should be refrigerated if immediate processing is not possible. A urine specimen for cytology should be examined immediately after collection or a preservative such as ethanol added to avoid deterioration of the cells.

 Test your knowledge of special handling with WORKBOOK Labeling Activity 12-2.

SPECIAL HANDLING

When blood leaves the body it is exposed to the effects of temperature and light that can negatively affect analytes. Specimens for analytes that are significantly affected require special handling to protect them.

 Key Point It is important to know the following temperatures related to specimen handling:

- Body temperature: 36.4°C to 37.6°C (37°C average)
- Room temperature: 15°C to 30°C
- Refrigerated temperature: 2°C to 10°C
- Frozen temperature: −20°C or lower (some specimens require −70°C or lower)

Body Temperature Specimens

Some specimens will precipitate or agglutinate if allowed to cool below body temperature. These specimens need to be transported at or near the normal body temperature of 37°C. In addition, most of these specimens require collection in a tube that has been prewarmed to 37°C. Small, portable heat blocks that are kept in a 37°C incubator until needed are available for transporting body temperature specimens. The heat blocks hold this temperature for approximately 15 minutes after removal from the incubator. Temperature-sensitive specimens that can withstand slightly higher than 37°C can be wrapped in an activated heel warmer (Fig. 12-15). Follow facility protocol. Examples of specimens that need to be transported at body temperature are listed in Table 12-2.

Chilled Specimens

Blood cell metabolism continues in a blood specimen after collection. Chilling the specimen slows down blood

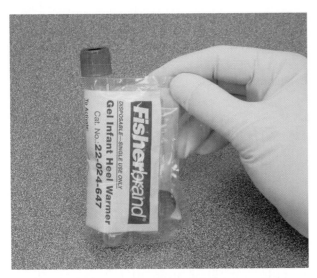

Figure 12-15 Temperature-sensitive specimen wrapped in an activated heel warmer.

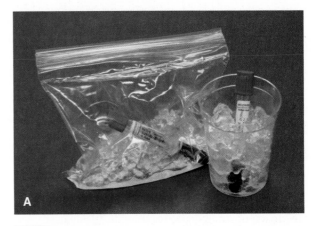

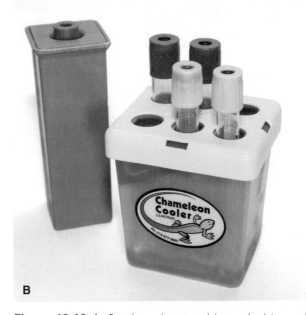

Figure 12-16 A: Specimen immersed in crushed ice and water slurry. **B:** Several specimens in a cooler rack.

cell metabolism and also protects **thermolabile** (i.e., altered or destroyed by heat) analytes. Blood specimens that require chilling should be completely immersed in a slurry of crushed ice and water (Fig. 12-16A) or put in a special cooling rack (Fig. 12-16B), and either tested immediately or refrigerated upon arrival in the laboratory. Large cubes or chunks of ice without water added do not allow adequate cooling of the entire specimen. Contact with a solid piece of ice can freeze parts of the specimen, resulting in hemolysis and possible analyte

breakdown. See Table 12-2 for examples of tests that require a chilled specimen.

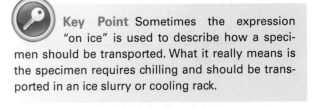 **Key Point** Sometimes the expression "on ice" is used to describe how a specimen should be transported. What it really means is the specimen requires chilling and should be transported in an ice slurry or cooling rack.

Specimens That Must Not Be Chilled

Some specimens are negatively affected by chilling during transportation. For example, most coagulation specimens must not be chilled before processing because it can activate clotting factors and disrupt platelet function. Potassium levels artificially increase if the specimen is chilled because cold inhibits glycolysis, which is what provides the energy to pump potassium into the

Table 12-2: Examples of Specimens That Require Special Handling[a]

Keep at 37°C	Chill in Ice Slurry or Cooling Rack	Protect from Light
Cold agglutinin	Adrenocorticotropic hormone (ACTH)	Bilirubin
Cryofibrinogen	Ammonia	
Cryoglobulins	Catecholamines	Beta-carotene
	Gastrin	Vitamin A
	Homocysteine (Red top): ice slurry OK	Vitamin B_2
	Homocysteine (Gel tube): cooler rack only	Vitamin B_6
	Lactic acid	Vitamin C
	Parathyroid hormone (PTH)	Urine porphyrins
	pH/blood gases (if indicated)	Urine porphobilinogen
	Pyruvate	
	RNA-based tests	

[a]Follow testing facility policy for the handling of all specimens.

cells. With glycolysis inhibited, potassium leaks from the cells into the serum or plasma, falsely elevating levels in the specimen.

> ⚠️ **CAUTION** If a potassium test is ordered with other analytes that require chilling, it should be collected in a separate tube.

Light-Sensitive Specimens

Some analytes are photosensitive (sensitive to light) and are broken down by light, resulting in falsely decreased values. The most common example is bilirubin, which can decrease by up to 50% after 1 hour of light exposure. An easy way to protect the blood in a collection tube from light is to wrap it in aluminum foil (Fig. 12-17). Amber tubes, biohazard bags, or light-blocking transport containers can also be used. Exposure to light can be especially damaging to infant bilirubin specimens collected by capillary puncture because the blood is directly exposed to light during collection, and light can easily penetrate the small amounts of blood collected as well. Consequently, light-blocking, amber-colored microcollection containers are available for collecting these specimens. Amber containers for urine specimen collection are also available. Light-blocking opaque secondary specimen transport containers are available for specimen aliquots as well. Table 12-2 lists examples of specimens that require protection from light.

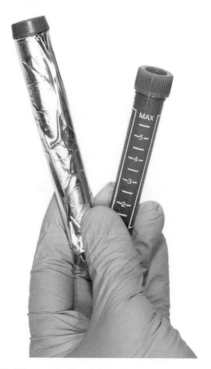

Figure 12-17 Specimen wrapped in aluminum foil to protect it from light and an amber aliquot or transport tube.

> 📖 **Now that you have finished this section, answer the study questions in Chapter 12 of the EXAM REVIEW to test your knowledge of specimen handling.**

Specimen Processing

Most off-site drawing stations have processing areas where specimens are centrifuged and separated from the cells to protect analyte stability before being sent to the testing site. Large laboratories may have a specific area, commonly called **central processing** or triage (screening and prioritizing area), where specimens are received and prepared for testing. Here the specimens are identified, logged/accessioned, sorted by department and type of processing required, and evaluated for suitability for testing.

> ⚠️ **CAUTION** OSHA regulations require those who process specimens to wear personal protective equipment (PPE), which includes gloves, fully closed fluid-resistant lab coats or aprons, and protective face gear, such as mask and goggles with side shields, or chin-length face shields.

SPECIMEN SUITABILITY

Suitable specimens are required for accurate laboratory results. Unsuitable specimens must be rejected for testing and new specimens obtained. The most frequently cited reason for rejection of chemistry specimens is hemolysis, followed by insufficient amount of specimen, or **QNS** (quantity not sufficient). The most frequent reason for rejection of hematology specimens is clotting. Clotting is also unacceptable for coagulation specimens. Coagulation specimens have a critical blood-to-additive ratio and also will be rejected if the tube is overfilled or underfilled.

Some suitability requirements depend on the individual tests ordered. Some rejection criteria, such as hemolysis, may not be identified until processing has begun or even completed. In the case of hematology specimens, hemolysis may not be noticed until after testing is complete and the specimen has separated while sitting in a specimen rack. In addition, microclots in hematology specimens might not be noticed unless the clot is drawn up by the instrument during testing, or abnormal platelet results are questioned.

Individual labs have specific policies concerning rejected specimens. If suitability questions arise the procedure manual should be consulted and facility policies followed. Examples of specimen rejection criteria are listed in Table 12-3. Generally, rejected specimens

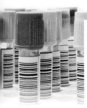

Table 12-3: Examples of Specimen Rejection Criteria

Rejection Criteria	Example
Body temperature (37°C) requirement not met	Cold agglutinin specimen delivered at room temperature
Chilling requirement not met	Ammonia specimen delivered at room temperature
Contaminated specimen	Urine C&S in an unsterile container
Delay in processing	Glucose specimen that was not separated from the cells until 4 hours after collection
Delay in testing	ESR specimen in an EDTA tube received 5 hours after it was collected
Exposure to light	Bilirubin specimen that was not protected from light
Hemolysis	Hemolyzed potassium specimen
Inadequate, inaccurate, or missing patient ID	Urine specimen that is not labeled
Microclots in the specimen	CBC that was not mixed properly
Outdated tube	Specimen collected in a tube that expired a month ago
QNS (quantity not sufficient)	Partially filled microtube submitted for multiple chemistry tests that require a minimum of 1 mL serum.
Specimen negatively affected by chilling	Potassium or protime specimen arrives on ice
Underfilled additive tube	Protime specimen in a partially filled light-blue–top tube lacks required blood-to-additive ratio
Wrong collection time	Therapeutic drug monitoring (TDM) specimen collected before the drug was given
Wrong tube	CBC collected in a red-top tube

are not discarded until the ordering physician or nursing unit has been notified.

 Test yourself on specimen rejection criteria with WORKBOOK Knowledge Drill 12-4.

Once suitability requirements are met, specimens that do not require additional central processing (e.g., centrifugation and separation) are promptly distributed to their testing areas where they may undergo more specific processing. Examples of specimens that can be distributed to their respective analysis areas without further processing or centrifugation include

- CBCs and other hematology specimens drawn in EDTA tubes
- Other whole-blood specimens for tests such as cyclosporine, hemoglobin A1c, and whole-blood lead analysis

 Specimens for cyclosporine, hemoglobin A1c, and whole-blood lead analysis should not be discarded if they are accidently centrifuged. The assay may still be possible after evaluation by a technologist.

- Cerebrospinal fluid (CSF), serous fluids, synovial fluid and bronchoalveolar lavage (BAL) specimens
- Microbiology specimens
- Urinalysis specimens

Specimens for tests performed on serum or plasma must be centrifuged before distribution. Specimens that arrive from off-site locations may have already been centrifuged; in which case they can proceed to the post-centrifugation stage after suitability requirements have been met.

PRECENTRIFUGATION

Anticoagulant tubes for plasma tests, including those that also contain gel (e.g., PSTs) can move on to the centrifugation phase without delay. Nonadditive, clot activator, and gel-containing tubes (e.g., SSTs) are used for serum tests and must clot in order for the serum to separate from the cells. If clotting is not complete when they are centrifuged, latent fibrin formation (Fig. 12-18) may form a clot in the serum after centrifugation. Residual fibrin can also be present as invisible fibrin strands or microfibers that can directly affect some tests (e.g., troponin) or cause problems with instrumentation. Consequently, serum tubes cannot be centrifuged until it is determined that clotting is complete.

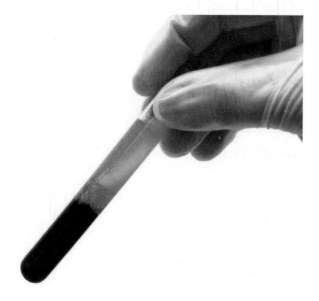

Figure 12-18 Fibrin clot and hemolysis in a centrifuged serum gel tube.

Tubes in the **precentrifugation** stage should be kept in an upright position with stoppers on. Removing the stopper from a specimen can cause loss of CO_2 and an increase of specimen pH, leading to inaccurate test results. For example, pH increases and ionized calcium and acid phosphatase levels decrease. In addition, leaving tube open exposes the specimen to evaporation and contamination. According to CLSI the practice of rimming the tube with an applicator stick to release the clot from the walls of the tube or the stopper before centrifuging the tube is a potential source of hemolysis and is not recommended.

> **Key Point** Stoppers must be left on tubes while awaiting and during centrifugation to prevent contamination, evaporation, **aerosol** (fine spray) formation, and pH changes.

CENTRIFUGATION

The ability of particles in a suspension (e.g., cells in a tube of blood) to settle to the bottom of a container over time due to the force of gravity is called sedimentation. A **centrifuge** (Fig. 12-19) is a machine that spins blood and other types of specimens at a high number of revolutions per minute (rpm). The part of the centrifuge that holds the tubes and spins is called the rotor. Carriers for holding the tubes are attached to the rotors. During operation the spinning rotor creates a force many times that of gravity. This accelerates the rate of sedimentation and results in the separation of particulate matter

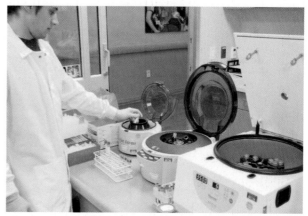

Figure 12-19 Clinical laboratory scientist loading a centrifuge in a STAT lab in the ER.

from the liquid in which it is suspended within minutes. Specimens for tests that require serum or plasma samples must be centrifuged to separate the cells from the liquid serum or plasma (Fig. 12-20).

The revolutions per minute describes how fast the rotor is spinning. The force applied to the substance being centrifuged is called gravities (g) or relative centrifugal force (RCF). This force is a function of the rotation speed of the centrifuge and the rotation radius, and

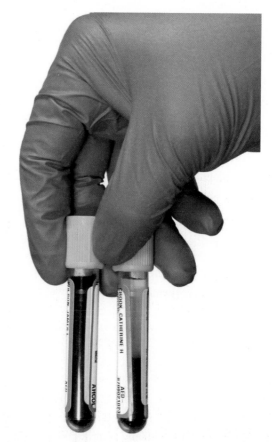

Figure 12-20 Sodium citrate tubes. **Right:** After being centrifuged. **Left:** Before being centrifuged.

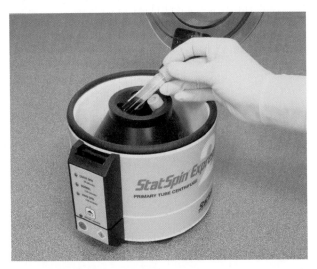

Figure 12-21 Prothrombin specimen after centrifugation in a StatSpin Express.

thus varies according to the size of the centrifuge. If the RCF (or g) required to spin the specimens is known, the radius of the centrifuge can be measured to determine the speed (rpm) setting that should be used. This can be calculated or determined from a graph called a nomogram. The speed and time of centrifugation are important specifications that each manufacturer and laboratory establishes. Generally, centrifuging blood specimens at a setting that creates a force of 1,000 g for 10 minutes will result in good separation of serum or plasma from the cells. Gel tubes may require a force of 1,000 to 1,300 g for 10 minutes. If a force of less than 1,000 g is used the gel may not function properly and the barrier it provides may be incomplete.

There are several designs for centrifuges, from small bench-top models to larger floor types. Some centrifuges such as the StatSpin Express (Fig. 12-21) have fixed angle rotors that are preferred for spinning coagulation tubes. Others have a swing-bucket design that is desired for gel tube separation because it produces a flat gel barrier.

> ⚠ **CAUTION** Because a centrifuge generates heat during operation, specimens requiring chilling should be processed in a temperature-controlled refrigerated centrifuge.

Centrifuging Plasma Specimens

Specimens for tests performed on plasma that are collected in tubes containing anticoagulants may be centrifuged without delay. For example, Figure 12-20 shows a prothrombin time (protime or PT) specimen collected in a light-blue–top sodium citrate tube that was immediately spun down using a StatSpin Express 2 centrifuge.

Although most chemistry tests traditionally have been performed on serum, STAT chemistry tests are sometimes collected in green-top heparin tubes to save time because plasma specimens can be centrifuged right away as opposed to serum specimens that must clot first. Some laboratories use heparinized plasma instead of serum for most chemistry tests, simply to reduce TAT. PSTs or other heparin-containing gel tubes are available to maintain specimen stability after centrifugation.

> ⚠ **CAUTION** There are different heparin formulations, and some of them cannot be used for certain tests. For example, lithium heparin cannot be used for lithium levels; ammonium heparin cannot be used for ammonia levels; and sodium heparin cannot be used for sodium levels.

Centrifuging Serum Specimens

Serum specimens should not be centrifuged until it is determined that clotting is complete. Complete clotting normally takes 30 to 60 minutes at room temperature (22°C to 25°C). Specimens from patients on anticoagulant medication, such as heparin or warfarin (i.e., Coumadin), specimens from patients with high white blood cell counts, and chilled specimens may take longer to clot. Serum separator tubes and other tubes containing clot activators usually clot within 30 minutes provided they are mixed adequately immediately after collection. Tubes containing thrombin such as the BD rapid serum tube (RST), normally clot in 5 minutes. Complete clotting can be determined by tilting or inverting the tube gently to see if a solid clot has formed. Some specimen processors set a timer to be sure they allow sufficient time for clotting to take place.

Centrifuge Operation

It is crucial that specimen tubes be "balanced" when loaded into a centrifuge. That means equal-size tubes with equal volumes of specimen must be placed opposite one another in the centrifuge (see Fig. 12-22). An unbalanced centrifuge may break the tubes, ruining specimens and causing the contents to form aerosols. A centrifuge that shakes, vibrates, or is noisier than usual when it is turned on may not be properly balanced and should be turned off immediately. Some centrifuges will automatically slow down or shut off if the load is not balanced.

The centrifuge lid must remain closed during operation and should not be opened until the rotor has come to a complete stop. A properly functioning modern centrifuge will not allow the user to open the lid prematurely.

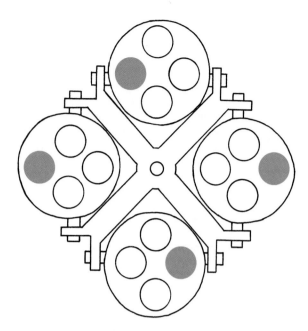

Figure 12-22 Illustration showing properly balanced centrifuge carriers assuming tubes contain equal volumes. Red circles equal counterbalanced positions for tubes.

Key Point A specimen should never be centrifuged more than once. Repeated centrifugation can cause hemolysis and analyte deterioration and alter test results. In addition, once the serum or plasma has been removed, the volume ratio of plasma or serum to cells changes.

Centrifuge Maintenance

To keep a centrifuge working properly, maintenance and calibrations must be done routinely. Daily cleaning maybe required for debris or spills that might occur during the processing of specimens. Otherwise, cleaning the interior of the centrifuge with soap and water followed by a bleach solution or approved surface disinfectant should be done on a routine basis. Regular maintenance should be scheduled according to manufacturer instructions to check the balance, braking mechanism, and the timer. On a routine basis, the gasket and cover latch should be inspected, and the brushes should be checked for wear and replaced as suggested by the manufacturer. The centrifuge service manual lists details on how to change brushes and the lubrication requirements. The speed of a centrifuge is easily checked using a strobe light or a tachometer, an instrument designed for measuring revolutions per minutes. Accreditation agencies require verification of periodic checks on the speed of the centrifuge.

thePoint *View the Balancing a Centrifuge video at http://thepoint.lww.com/McCall6e.*

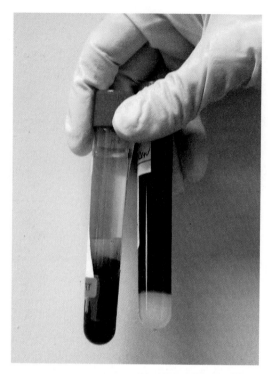

Figure 12-23 Serum gel tubes. **Right:** Before being centrifuged. **Left:** After being centrifuged.

POSTCENTRIFUGATION

In the **postcentrifugation** phase, the serum or plasma should be physically separated from the cells as soon as possible unless, according to CLSI, there is conclusive evidence that a longer contact time with the cells will not affect test results. Specimens in gel barrier tubes do not normally require manual separation because the separator gel lodges between the fluid and the cells during centrifugation, becoming a physical barrier that prevents glycolysis (see Fig. 12-23). Be sure to follow manufacturer recommendations. It also is important to visually inspect gel tubes for barrier integrity. This is especially important if the specimen is spun in a fixed angle centrifuge because the gel forms at a 45-degree angle. No red blood cells should be visible in the serum or plasma. If there is leakage around the gel, or the collection tube does not have a gel barrier, the serum or plasma should be removed from contact with the cells as soon as possible.

Key Point According to CLSI serum on gel barriers can be stored up to 48 hours at 4°C with the exception of specimens for analytes (e.g., estradiol, lidocaine, phenobarbital, phenytoin, quinidine, and tricyclic antidepressants), that can decrease as they are absorbed into the gel.

Stopper Removal

Some testing instruments sample, or aspirate, specimens directly through the tube stopper. Most of the time, however, the stopper has to be removed to obtain the serum or plasma needed for testing. Stoppers can be removed using commercially available stopper removal devices or by use of robotics. If robotic equipment is not used, the processor should be wearing a full-length face shield or the tube should be held behind a bench-top splash shield or in a safety cabinet when the stopper is removed.

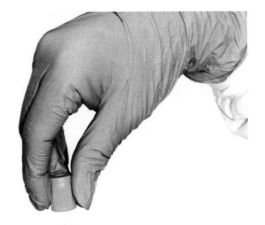

> **Key Point** Blood in contact with tube caps or stoppers can be a source of specimen contamination and can contribute to **aerosol** (a fine mist of specimen) formation during stopper removal.

Some tubes (e.g., Becton Dickinson Hemogard™ tubes and Greiner Bio-One Vacuette® tubes) have stoppers designed to contain spray and protect laboratory personnel from blood around the rim of the tube. With rubber stoppers (see the BD Vacutainer® Tube Guide in Appendix F) or other stoppers that lack such a safety feature, the stopper should be covered with a gauze or tissue to catch blood drops or aerosol that may be released as it is removed. Regardless of design, to prevent or minimize aerosols or blood spray, all tube stoppers should be pulled straight up and off (see Fig. 12-24) and not "popped" off using a thumb roll technique.

ALIQUOT PREPARATION

An **aliquot** is a portion of a specimen used for testing. Aliquots of specimens are sometimes created when multiple tests are ordered on a single specimen and the tests are performed on different instruments or in different areas of the testing department. Aliquots are prepared by transferring a portion of the specimen into one or more tubes labeled with the same ID information as the specimen tube.

thePoint* *Watch the Opening and Aliquoting a Specimen video at http://thepoint.lww.com/McCall6e.*

Before an aliquot can be prepared from a tube lacking a gel barrier, a plunger-type filter (plastic tube with a filter at the bottom) is typically used to separate the serum or plasma from the cells. When inserting the device into the specimen tube it is important to keep it from touching the clot or cells, which can be a source of hemolysis. This is accomplished by slightly withdrawing the device after it is inserted to create an air gap between the filter and the cell surface. The serum or plasma within the filtering device can then be transferred to the aliquot

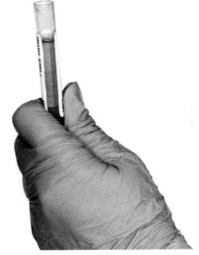

Figure 12-24 Example of a Vacuette closure tube. (Manufacturer of tube: Greiner Bio-One International AG, Kremsmunster, Austria.)

tube(s). Serum or plasma can be transferred directly from centrifuged gel tubes into aliquot tubes.

According to OSHA, "All procedures involving blood or potentially infectious materials shall be performed in such a manner as to minimize splashing, spraying, splattering, and generation of droplets of these substances." Consequently, disposable transfer pipettes should be used when transferring serum or plasma into aliquot tubes and all work should be done behind a bench-top splash shield (Fig. 12-25) or in a safety cabinet.

> ⚠️ **CAUTION** Pouring the serum or plasma into aliquot tubes is not recommended because it increases the possibility of aerosol formation or splashing.

Transfer of specimens into aliquot tubes has an inherent risk of error. Great care must be taken to match each specimen with the corresponding aliquot tube to avoid

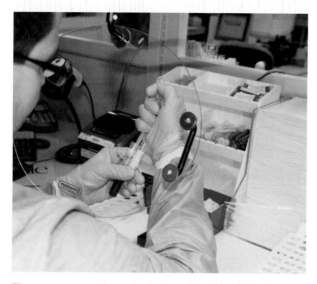

Figure 12-25 A sample being transferred from the collection tube to an aliquot tube.

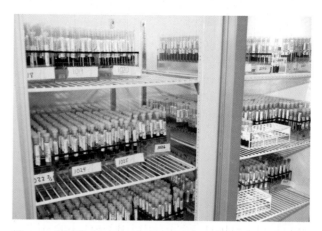

Figure 12-26 Storage of serum and plasma tubes for possible reuse.

misidentified samples. Different types of specimens (e.g., serum and plasma) for separate tests on the same patient can also present problems. Serum and plasma are virtually indistinguishable once they have been transferred into the aliquot tubes, so it is important to exactly match the specimen with both the aliquot tube of the requested test and the patient, and to indicate if the aliquot contains serum or plasma.

> ⚠ **CAUTION** Never put serum and plasma, or plasma from specimens with different anticoagulants, in the same aliquot tube.

Each aliquot tube should be covered or capped as soon as it is filled. According to CLSI, serum/plasma aliquots can remain at room temperature for no longer than 8 hours. If assays will not be completed within 8 hours, serum/plasma should be refrigerated (2°C to 8°C). If assays are not to be completed within 48 hours, or the separated serum/plasma will be stored beyond 48 hours, it should be frozen at or below −20°C. Some tests require the specimen to be refrigerated or frozen for analyte stability, especially if testing is to be delayed. Frozen samples should be thawed at room temperature and inverted 10 to 20 times after thawing before testing. It is important to consult the procedure manual for specific instructions.

> 🔑 **Key Point** Serum and plasma aliquots should not be frozen and thawed more than once. Refreezing can cause deterioration of the analytes to be measured. Freezers that are "frost-free" must not be used because they allow samples to partially thaw and then refreeze.

Specimen Storage

It is not unusual for certain specimens to be stored waiting for batch analysis or send out. It is standard procedure to refrigerate specimens after analysis (Fig. 12-26) in case other tests are ordered. Most chemistry tests can be performed on separated serum or plasma for up to 1 week. Studies have shown that significant stability of separated serum has been observed up to 14 days for some analytes. It is the responsibility of each laboratory to determine their own specimen stability criteria. To ensure the stability of the analyte while held, specific references should be consulted to determine the appropriate handling and storage conditions. Specimens must have a cover that is tightly secured and be stored in an upright position.

Serum and Plasma Aliquots

According to CLSI, serum and plasma that has been separated from the cells should not remain at room temperature for longer than 8 hours. If not tested before then, the aliquot should be refrigerated (2°C to 8°C).

Gel Tubes with Separator Devices

CLSI suggests that the manufacturer instructions be consulted when storing specimens in gel barrier tubes or with separator devices because there are limitations on how long serum or plasma can be in contact with the device or gel.

Body Fluids

CSF, bronchoalveolar lavage (BAL), serous, synovial, and other body fluids can be refrigerated after testing.

BioBanking

A **biobank** is a relatively new term used to describe a repository or bank where human biological samples such as, blood, saliva, plasma, skin cells, and organ tissues can be stored, preserved and cataloged for use in research for personalized medicine, for example. This type of storage facility offers scientists large amounts of genetic data in a single place allowing them the ability to test hundreds of thousands of samples instead of a few thousand. The quality of the results and research findings depend on how the specimen is processed and stored at the collection site. A sample can be processed for bio-banking if there is sufficient volume left after all clinical tests have been performed. Samples processed for bio-banking must have appropriate informed consent or the consent obligation must be waived by the Institutional Review Board/Independent Ethics Committee.

REPORTING RESULTS

Results are documented and reported in a number of ways. In fully automated laboratories with computerization, once the results are verified by testing personnel the LIS generates an electronic report that is shared with medical records and the HIS where it can be accessed by the ordering physician or other designated personnel. Results from national and reference laboratories can also be electronically transmitted to the HIS. In the absence of an automated reporting system, instrument printed reports can be distributed to the appropriate department or physician office. Stat and panic (i.e., critical) test results are reported directly to the physician or designated personnel as soon as possible, typically

Table 12-4: Examples of Tests That Commonly Appear on Panic Value Lists

Chemistry Tests	Coagulation Tests	Hematology Tests
Bilirubin	Protime/INR	Hemoglobin
Calcium	Partial thrombo-	Hematocrit
Carbon dioxide	plastin time/	Platelet count
Glucose	Activated partial	White blood cell
Magnesium	thromboplastin	count
Potassium	time	
Sodium		

by phone or pager. Panic values are significantly abnormal test results that considered a life-threatening situation that requires immediate attention by the physician. Examples of tests commonly found on panic value lists are shown in Table 12-4. Results in the panic range vary somewhat according to test methodology.

Key Point When phoning test results it is important to make certain the person receiving the results writes them down and then reads them back to you to confirm the accuracy of what was written. Verbal reports must be followed up with an electronic or hard copy of the report.

Study and Review Questions

 See the EXAM REVIEW for more study questions.

1. **Computer networking caused Congress to take steps to eliminate patient confidentiality violations by**
   a. eliminating cable connections
   b. enacting the HIPAA
   c. limiting the network size
   d. not using the Ethernet

2. **Logging on to most computer systems requires the use of a/an**
   a. accession number.
   b. bar code reader.
   c. modem.
   d. password.

3. **After arriving in the laboratory, all specimens are immediately**
   a. centrifuged to stop glycolysis.
   b. logged in or accessioned.
   c. refrigerated until processed.
   d. uploaded to testing instruments.

4. **Which of the following would be omitted from a lab-generated computer label?**
   a. Collector's initials
   b. Patient diagnosis
   c. Physician's name
   d. Time of collection

5. **Bar coding in this area of health care is unlikely at the present time.**
   a. CLIA documentation
   b. Drug administration
   c. Supply inventory
   d. Patient identification

6. **Which of the following specimens should be protected from light?**
   a. BUN
   b. CBC
   c. Bilirubin
   d. Glucose

7. **Which of the following is a type of machine used to separate the serum or plasma from blood cells in the sample?**
   a. Cholestech
   b. Glucometer
   c. Hemostat
   d. StatSpin

8. **After obtaining a specimen for a cold agglutinin test, the blood must be transported**
   a. as a "STAT" test.
   b. at body temperature.
   c. in a cooling rack.
   d. protected from light.

9. **Required PPE when processing specimens would exclude**
   a. chin-length face shields.
   b. disposable gloves.
   c. fluid-resistant lab coats.
   d. fluid-resistant shoe covers.

10. **Which of the following blood specimens should be transported in an ice slurry?**
    a. Beta-carotene
    b. Cold agglutinin
    c. Electrolytes
    d. Homocysteine

11. **A serum aliquot has a fibrin clot in it. The most likely cause is the specimen was**
    a. centrifuged before clotting was complete.
    b. from a patient with a high platelet count.
    c. hemolyzed from improper transportation.
    d. spun too long with the tube stopper off.

12. **Which of the following specimens would be acceptable for testing?**
    a. CBC collected in a lavender-top tube
    b. Potassium specimen that is hemolyzed
    c. Protime specimen in a partially filled tube
    d. Specimen lacking an identification label

13. **As a general rule serum or plasma should be removed from the cells within**
    a. 30 minutes.
    b. 60 minutes.
    c. 90 minutes.
    d. 120 minutes.

14. **Which of the following specimens can be centrifuged immediately?**
    a. Bilirubin collected in a red-top tube
    b. CBC collected in a lavender top
    c. Creatinine collected in an SST
    d. Electrolytes collected in a PST

15. **The difference between bar codes and radio frequency identification is**
    a. RFID is less expensive.
    b. RFID is not standardized.
    c. RFID can work up to 100 feet away.
    d. RFID cannot be used for specimen labeling.

16. **Most POC analyzers are interface capable, but the decision to do so is based on the**
    a. number of that analyzers available.
    b. impact the test result has to the patient.
    c. cost of the test being performed.
    d. type of POCT instrument being used.

17. **All blood specimens transported by a courier must be**
    a. centrifuged prior to transportation.
    b. placed in a refrigerated container.
    c. protected from direct sun exposure.
    d. transported horizontally for safety.

18. **Which federal agencies regulate the transporting of biological specimens off site?**
    a. CLIA and EPA
    b. DOT and IATA
    c. EPA and CLSI
    d. All of the above

19. **Which of the following test specimens can be analyzed without being centrifuged?**
    a. Bilirubin in an amber microtube
    b. Cholesterol in a gel barrier tube
    c. Hemoglobin A1c in an EDTA tube
    d. STAT potassium in a heparin tube

20. **A panic value is a/an**
    a. result that cannot be repeated.
    b. sign of instrument malfunction.
    c. significantly abnormal test result.
    d. test control that is out of range.

Case Studies

 See the WORKBOOK for more case studies.

Case Study 12-1: The Case of the Missing Results

Nurse Susan collected blood for blood urea nitrogen (BUN) and creatinine tests on patient Mr. Jones in bed 201 at 9:30 AM, and sent the specimen to the lab. At 10:30, Susan calls the lab and states she is not able to find Mr. Jones' results in the computer. The technologist, Frank, tells Susan he does not have a specimen with that name on it; however, he did run a BUN and creatinine on patient Betty Smith in bed 202 drawn at 9:30 AM by Susan. Susan says there could not have been an error because she labeled the specimen with the only label she found on the bar-coded label printer at the time.

QUESTIONS

1. What do you think has happened to Mr. Jones' specimen?

2. Why does the lab have results on Mrs. Smith?

3. What steps should Susan take to get the results on Mr. Jones?

4. What is to be done with the results on Mrs. Smith?

Case Study 12-2: A Cooled Specimen Gets a Chilly Reception

A new phlebotomist was working the early shift at a medical center and had already completed most of his assigned draws. He was then given a stat order for ammonia, electrolytes, and a CBC on a patient in ICU. Only one arm was available for the draw. The patient had lots of bruising and no palpable veins in the AC area so he decided to draw a hand vein. He couldn't remember if the ammonia required a green top or a purple top, so grabbed a green-top lithium heparin tube and two purple tops from his phlebotomy tray. The draw was successful, and although the blood flowed into the tubes slowly, he was able to fill all three tubes. He also remembered that the ammonia needed to be transported on ice so he went to the nurse's station and got a plastic bag of crushed ice and water. Since he wasn't sure which tube was needed for the ammonia, he put the green top and one of the purple tops in the ice slurry, just to be safe. He had only one more draw to do and the patient was on that same floor, so he quickly drew her, returned to the lab, and delivered the specimens to central processing. A short time later the central processing technician told him he needed to immediately redraw the stat electrolytes.

QUESTIONS

1. Were correct tubes drawn for the ordered tests?

2. Explain why you think the electrolyte specimen needed to be recollected.

3. How could this problem have been prevented?

Bibliography and Suggested Readings

Baer DM, Ernst DJ, Willeford SI, Gambino R. Investigating elevated potassium values. *MLO Med Lab Obs.* 2006;38(11):24, 26, 30–31.

Bishop ML, Fody EP, Schoef LE. *Clinical Chemistry: Principles, Procedures, Correlations.* 7th ed. Philadelphia, PA: Lippincott Williams & Wilkins; 2013.

Burtis CA, Ashwood ER, Bruns DE. *Tietz, Fundamentals of Clinical Chemistry and Molecular Diagnostics.* 7th ed. Philadelphia, PA: Elsevier/Saunders; 2015.

Clement N, Kendall B. Effects of light on vitamin B12 and folate. *Lab Med.* 2009;40:657–659.

Clinical and Laboratory Standards Institute. *GP33-A, Accuracy in Patient & Sample Identification.* 1st ed. Wayne, PA: CLSI; 2010.

Clinical and Laboratory Standards Institute. *GP34-A, Validation and Verification of Tubes for Venous and Capillary Specimens.* 1st ed. Wayne, PA: CLSI; 2010.

Clinical and Laboratory Standards Institute. *GP41-A6. Procedures for the Collection of Diagnostic Blood Specimens By Venipuncture.* 6th ed. Wayne, PA: CLSI; 2007.

Clinical and Laboratory Standards Institute. *GP42-A6. Procedures and Devices for the Collection of Diagnostic Capillary Blood Specimens by Venipuncture, Approved Standard.* 6th ed. Wayne, PA: CLSI; 2008.

Clinical and Laboratory Standards Institute. *GP44-A4. Procedures for the Handling and Processing of Blood Specimens, Approved Guideline.* Wayne, PA: CLSI; 2010.

Clinical and Laboratory Standards Institute. *POCT01-A2. Point of Care Connectivity, Approved Standard.* 2nd ed. Wayne, PA: CLSI; 2006.

Department of Transportation. Hazardous materials regulations; Title 49, Code of Federal Regulations, Parts 100–185; 2001.

Ernst D. *Applied Phlebotomy.* Philadelphia, PA: Lippincott Williams & Wilkins; 2005.

Fischbach F, Dunning M. *Laboratory Diagnostic Tests.* 9th ed Philadelphia, PA: Lippincott Williams & Wilkins; 2014.

Hammerling J. A review of medical errors in laboratory diagnostics and where we are today. *Lab Med.* 2012; 43(2):41–44.

HIPAA, Health Insurance Portability and Accountability Act. Federal Register; August 17, 2000.

Joint Commission. *Comprehensive Accreditation Manual for Laboratories and Point-of-Care Testing (CAMLAB).* Oakbrook Terrace, IL: Joint Commission Resources (JCR); 2010.

LabCorp test menu: www.labcorp.com/wps/portal/provider/testmenu; accessed November 16 2014.

McPherson RA, Pincus MR. *Henry's Clinical Diagnosis and Management of Laboratory Methods.* 22nd ed. Philadelphia, PA: W.B. Saunders; 2011.

Occupational Safety and Health Administration. Occupational exposure to bloodborne pathogens: Needlestick and other sharps injuries; final rule. 29 CFR 1910. *Fed Reg.* 2001;66(12):5318–5325.

O'Keane M, Cunningham S, Evaluation of three different specimen types (serum, plasma lithium heparin and serum gel separator) for analysis of certain analytes: Clinical significance of differences in results and efficiency in use. *Clinical Chem Lab Med.* 2006;44(5):662–668.

Plaut D. *The testing process lends itelf to designing a systematic approach to error detection and correction,* Advance for Administrators of the Laboratory.

Turchiano M, Nguygen C, Fierman A, Lifshitz M, Convit A. Impact of blood sample collection and processing methods on glucose levels in community outreach studies. *J Environ Public Health.* 2013;2013, Article ID 256151.

Wagar E. No Need to Panic – Critical Values in Your Laboratory. American Society for Clinical Pathology 2008 Annual Meeting, Session B112.

Winsten D. *RFID for Specimen Tracking.* Advance for Administers of the Laboratory, June 23, 2011.

 MEDIA MENU

Online Ancillaries (at http://thepoint.lww.com/McCall6e)

- Videos:
  - Balancing a Centrifuge
  - Opening and Aliquoting a Specimen
- Interactive exercises and games, including Look and Label, Word Building, Body Building, Roboterms, Crossword Puzzles, Quiz Show, and Concentration
- Audio flash cards and flash card generator
- Audio glossary

Internet Resources

- ClinLab Navigator
  http://www.clinlabnavigator.com/Links/detail/clinical-laboratory-science-internet-resources.html
- LabCorp (Laboratory Corporation of America): https://www.labcorp.com/wps/portal/provider/testmenu
- Quest Diagnostics test menu: http://www.questdiagnostics.com/hcp/qtim/testMenuSearch.do

Other Resources

- McCall R, Tankersley C. *Student Workbook for Phlebotomy Essentials.* 6th ed. (Available for separate purchase).
- McCall R, Tankersley C. *Phlebotomy Exam Review.* 6th ed. (Available for separate purchase).

Chapter 13

Nonblood Specimens and Tests

NAACLS Entry Level Competencies

4.00 Demonstrate understanding of the importance of specimen collection and specimen integrity in the delivery of patient care.

4.2 Describe the types of patient specimens that are analyzed in the clinical laboratory.

4.3 Define the phlebotomist's role in collecting and/or transporting these specimens to the laboratory.

4.4 List the general criteria for suitability of a specimen

for analysis, and reasons for specimen rejection or recollection.

4.5 Explain the importance of timed, fasting, and stat specimens, as related to specimen integrity and patient care.

7.2 Instruct patients in the proper collection and preservation for nonblood specimens.

7.3 Explain methods for transporting and processing specimens for routine and special testing.

Key Terms

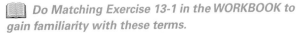 *Do Matching Exercise 13-1 in the WORKBOOK to gain familiarity with these terms.*

AFP	expectorate	O&P	suprapubic
amniotic fluid	FIT	occult blood	sweat chloride
buccal swab	FOBT	PCR	synovial fluid
C&S	gastric analysis	pericardial fluid	24-hour urine
C. difficile	*H. pylori*	peritoneal fluid	UA
catheterized	iontophoresis	pleural fluid	UTI
clean-catch	midstream	serous fluid	
CSF	NP	sputum	

Objectives

Upon successful completion of this chapter, the reader should be able to:

1 Demonstrate knowledge of nonblood specimens and tests, and define associated terminology.

2 Describe collection, labeling, and handling procedures for nonblood specimens.

Overview

Although blood is the specimen of choice for many laboratory tests, various other body substances are also analyzed. The phlebotomist may be involved in obtaining the specimens (e.g., throat swab collection), test administration (e.g., sweat chloride collection), instruction (e.g., urine collection), processing (accessioning and preparing the specimen for testing), or simply verifying, labeling, and transporting the specimens to the lab. As with other laboratory specimens standard precautions must be followed when handling nonblood specimens. This chapter addresses routine and special nonblood specimens and procedures, including the collection and handling of urine specimens and other nonblood body fluids and substances. A phlebotomist with a thorough understanding of all aspects of nonblood specimen collection helps ensure the quality of the specimens and the accuracy of test results.

Nonblood Specimen Labeling and Handling

Proper labeling helps avoid testing delays, which can compromise patient care. Nonblood specimens should be labeled immediately following collection, in the presence of the patient, using the same identifying information as blood specimens. In addition, since many body fluids are similar in appearance, labeling should include the type and/or source of the specimen. Because the lid is typically removed for testing, the label should be applied to the container, not the lid, to avoid misidentification. Follow facility protocol.

Key Point Phlebotomists are often asked to transport specimens to the lab that have been collected by other healthcare personnel. It is important for the phlebotomist to verify proper labeling before accepting a specimen for transport.

Nonblood specimens have various handling requirements. The phlebotomist must be familiar with these requirements to protect the integrity of the specimen and help ensure accurate test results. In addition, all body substances are potentially infectious, and standard precautions must be observed in handling them.

Nonblood Body-Fluid Specimens

Nonblood body fluids are liquid or semiliquid substances produced by the body and found in the intracellular and interstitial spaces and within various organs (e.g., the bladder) and body cavities (e.g., joints).

URINE

Urine, which has been studied since the very beginning of laboratory medicine, is the most frequently analyzed nonblood body fluid. It is readily available, easy to collect, and generally inexpensive to test; its analysis can provide information on many of the body's major metabolic functions. Analysis of urine can aid in monitoring wellness, the diagnosis and treatment of urinary tract infections, the detection and monitoring of metabolic disease, and determining the effectiveness or complications of therapy. Accurate results depend on collection method, container used, specimen transportation and handling, and timeliness of testing.

CAUTION If urine specimens are not tested promptly or preserved, urine components can change. For example, cellular elements decompose, bilirubin breaks down to biliverdin, and bacteria multiply, leading to erroneous test results.

Inpatient urine specimen collection is typically handled by nursing personnel. Outpatient urine specimen collection is often handled by phlebotomists. The phlebotomist must be able to properly explain urine collection procedures without embarrassing the patient, using language adapted to the patient's level of understanding.

Key Point Verbal urine specimen collection instructions for patients must be accompanied by written instructions, preferably with illustrations. In outpatient areas, written instructions are often posted on the wall in the restroom designated for patient urine collections.

The type of specimen preferred for many urine tests is the first urine voided (passed naturally from the bladder or urinated) in the morning, because it is the most concentrated. However, the type of urine specimen and method of collection vary depending on the type of test. The most common urine tests, types of specimens, and collection methods follow.

Common Urine Tests

Routine Urinalysis

A routine **urinalysis (UA)** is the most commonly requested urine test because it screens for urinary and systemic disorders. It may be ordered as part of a physical examination or at various times during hospitalization.

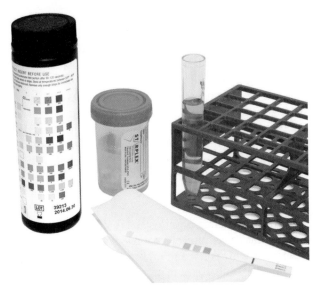

Figure 13-1 Urinalysis specimen collection kit (Container, transfer device, and preservative transport tube).

A routine UA typically includes physical, chemical, and microscopic analysis of the urine specimen. Urinalysis may be performed manually or using automated instruments like the Iris (see Chapter 1 Figure 1-11).

thePoint₃ *Watch the Routine Urinalysis video at http://thepoint.lww.com/McCall6e.*

- Physical analysis involves macroscopic observation and notation of color, clarity, and odor, as well as measurements of volume and specific gravity (SG) or osmolality. (SG and osmolality indicate urine concentration.) Physical analysis can also help explain or confirm chemical and microscopic results.
- Chemical analysis can detect bacteria, bilirubin, blood (red blood cells and hemoglobin), glucose, ketones, leukocytes, nitrite, protein, and urobilinogen, and measure pH and specific gravity. Analysis is commonly performed using a plastic reagent strip (often called a dipstick) (Fig. 13-1) that contains absorbent pads impregnated with test reagents. Each test has its own pad. The strip is dipped into a well-mixed urine specimen that is at room temperature. Excess urine is removed by lightly drawing the edge of the strip across the lip of the container as it is removed from the urine. The edge of the strip is then lightly blotted on absorbent tissue. The color reactions that take place on the pads are compared to a color chart, which is usually found on the label of the reagent strip container. Special timing, which is not the same for all tests, is involved in reading the results, which are reported in the manner indicated on the color chart. Results are typically reported using the terms *trace, 1+, 2+,* and so on to indicate the degree of a positive result, and *negative (neg)* or *(−)* when no reaction is noted. The strip is used once

and then discarded. Instruments are available that read the strips automatically.

- Microscopic analysis identifies urine components such as cells, crystals, casts, and microorganisms by examining a sample of urine sediment under a microscope. To obtain the sediment, a measured portion of urine is centrifuged in a special conical (tapered) plastic tube (see Fig. 13-1). After centrifugation, the supernatant, or top portion of the specimen, is discarded. A drop of the remaining sediment is placed either on a glass slide and covered with a small square of glass called a coverslip or placed in a special chamber. It is then examined under the microscope by a laboratory technologist or technician. There are also instruments that perform this function.

A random specimen is acceptable for routine urinalysis. However, to avoid contamination of the specimen by genital secretions, pubic hair, and bacteria surrounding the urinary opening, the ideal procedure for collecting a specimen for routine urinalysis is referred to as **midstream** collection. (See "Urine Collection Methods," for regular voided and midstream collection methods).

Routine UA specimens should be collected in clear, dry, chemically clean containers with tight-fitting lids. If a culture and sensitivity (C&S) is also ordered on the specimen, the container must be sterile. Urine specimens should be transported to the lab promptly. Specimens that cannot be transported or analyzed promptly can be held at room temperature and protected from light for up to 2 hours. Specimens held longer should be refrigerated or chemically preserved. Preservative tubes and urine transfer devices (Fig. 13-2) are available for specimens that cannot be processed within the 2-hour window (e.g., specimens sent to some off-site laboratories). Tubes must be filled to the indicated level for the proper

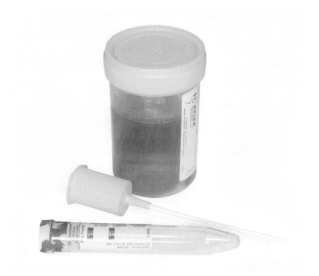

Figure 13-2 Urinalysis specimen, reagent strip for chemical testing, and urine in a conical tube ready to centrifuge for microscopic examination.

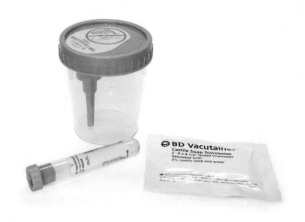

Figure 13-3 Sterile kit for urine culture and sensitivity (C&S) testing (Sterile Cup, preservative, urine tube, and castile soap towelettes).

urine-to-additive ratio. Specimens that require both UA and C&S testing should be refrigerated or chemical preservative added if immediate processing is not possible. (Urinalysis is also discussed under "Point-of-Care Testing" in Chapter 11.)

Urine Culture and Sensitivity

A urine **culture and sensitivity (C&S)** test may be requested on a patient with symptoms of **urinary tract infection (UTI)** such as a frequent urge to urinate, or pain or burning on urination. The culture involves placing a measured portion of urine on a special nutrient medium that encourages the growth of microorganisms, incubating it for 24 to 48 hours, checking it for growth, and identifying any microorganisms that grow. If a microorganism is identified, a sensitivity or antibiotic susceptibility test is performed to determine which antibiotics will be effective against the microorganism. Urine for C&S testing must be collected in a sterile container (Fig. 13-3), following midstream **clean-catch** (see "Urine Collection Methods") procedures to ensure that the specimen is free of contaminating matter from the external genital areas.

⚠️ **CAUTION** Urine specimens for C&S and other microbiology tests should be transported to the lab and processed immediately. If a delay in transportation or processing is unavoidable, the specimen should be refrigerated or preserved.

Urine Cytology Studies

Cytology studies on urine are performed to detect cancer, cytomegalovirus, and other viral and inflammatory diseases of the bladder and other structures of the urinary system. Cells from the lining of the urinary tract are readily shed into the urine, and a smear containing them can easily be prepared from urinary sediment or filtrate. The smear is typically stained by the Papanicolaou (PAP) method and examined under a microscope for the presence of abnormal cells. A fresh clean-catch specimen is required for the test. This should not be a first morning specimen as cells may have disintegrated in the bladder overnight. Ideally, the specimen should be examined as soon after collection as possible. If a delay is unavoidable, the specimen can be preserved by the addition of an equal volume of 50% alcohol. Follow facility protocol.

Urine Drug Screening

Urine drug screening is performed to detect illicit use of recreational drugs, use of anabolic steroids to enhance performance in sports, and unwarranted use of prescription drugs; it is also used to monitor therapeutic drug use in order to minimize withdrawal symptoms and to confirm a diagnosis of drug overdose. With the exception of alcohol, urine is preferred for drug screening, since many drugs can be detected in urine but not in blood.

Screening tests are typically performed in groups based on drug classifications or families (see Chapter 11, Table 11-2). A random sample in a chemically clean, covered container is required for the test. Specimens containing blood cells or having a high or low urine pH (highly alkaline or highly acid) or a specific gravity less than 1.003 or greater than 1.025 will yield erroneous results and will require recollection of the specimen. A strict chain of custody procedure may need to be followed. (For additional information, see "Forensic Specimens" in Chapter 11.)

Urine Alcohol Testing

Urine is not an ideal specimen for testing alcohol levels. Urine alcohol (ethanol or ETOH) levels can indicate if alcohol has been consumed within the past few hours if that is all that needs to be determined, but they do not necessarily correlate with blood alcohol levels. This makes them imprecise in evaluating an individual's degree of intoxication. Levels also vary depending on bladder function and mixing in the bladder with other liquids that may have been consumed. Ethanol is volatile and false negatives can result from uncapped specimens. False positives have resulted due to fermentation if the urine contains certain microorganisms such as *Candida albicans,* or if it has a high level of glucose. Measurement of ethyl glucuronide (EtG), a direct metabolite of alcohol, can demonstrate that alcohol was ingested long after it has been metabolized. However, according to the Substance Abuse and Mental Health Administration (SAMHSA) this test is too sensitive and can register positives in individual who have used alcohol-containing hand sanitizers, medications, hygiene products, cosmetics, foods, and other products that contain even small amounts of alcohol.

Urine Glucose and Ketone Testing

Urine reagent test strips are also used to screen for diabetes and monitor glucose and ketone levels in diabetics. The body breaks down carbohydrates to supply itself with glucose. Ketones are created when the body breaks down fat for energy because the diet is deficient in carbohydrates or when the body does not metabolize glucose properly. The testing of urine ketone levels can be used to diagnose diabetic ketoacidosis and help differentiate between diabetic and nondiabetic coma. Results are read by comparing color changes on the test strip to a color chart.

Urine Pregnancy Testing

Pregnancy can be confirmed by testing urine for the presence of human chorionic gonadotropin (HCG), a hormone produced by cells within the developing placenta, that appears in serum and urine approximately 8 to 10 days after conception, or fertilization. Although a random urine specimen can be used for testing, the first morning specimen is preferred because it is typically more concentrated and would therefore have the highest HCG concentration.

> (i) HCG may also appear in the urine of patients with melanoma, tumors of the ovaries or testes, and certain types of cancer, including breast, lung, and kidney.

Other Urine Tests

Numerous chemistry tests—including electrophoresis, tests for heavy metals (e.g., copper and lead), myoglobin clearance, creatinine clearance, and porphyrins—can be performed on urine specimens. Many of these tests require a pooled, timed specimen, such as a 24-hour collection.

Types of Urine Specimens

Random

Random urine specimens can be collected at any time. They are used primarily for routine urinalysis and screening tests. *Random* refers only to the timing of the specimen and not the method of collection.

First Morning/8-Hour Specimen

A first morning or 8-hour urine specimen (also called a first voided, overnight, or early morning specimen) is usually collected immediately upon awakening in the morning after approximately 8 hours of sleep. This type of specimen normally has a higher specific gravity, which means that it is more concentrated than a random specimen. For this reason, first morning specimens are often requested to confirm results of random specimens and specimens with low specific gravity.

Fasting

A fasting specimen is typically used for glucose monitoring. It differs from a first morning specimen in that it is the second specimen voided after a period of fasting. This helps assure that the specimen will not be affected by food consumed before fasting.

Timed

Some tests require individual urine specimens collected at specific times. Others require the collection and pooling of urine throughout a specific time period. Some of the most frequently encountered timed urine tests are as follows.

Two-Hour Postprandial Specimen. A 2-hour postprandial (PP) urine specimen is collected 2 hours after a meal and tested for glucose. It is primarily used to monitor the insulin therapy of patients with diabetes mellitus. The patient is instructed to void shortly before consuming a normal meal and to collect a specimen 2 hours later. Results are often compared with glucose results on fasting urine and fasting blood specimens.

Twenty-Four–Hour Specimen. A **24-hour urine** specimen is collected to allow quantitative analysis of a urine analyte. Collection of the specimen requires a large, clean, preferably wide-mouth container capable of holding several liters (Fig. 13-4). A special collection device that fits over the toilet and looks somewhat like an upside-down hat is sometimes provided to the patient to make collection of the specimen easier. Males may be given a plastic urinal. The specimen must be labeled at the time it is given to the patient.

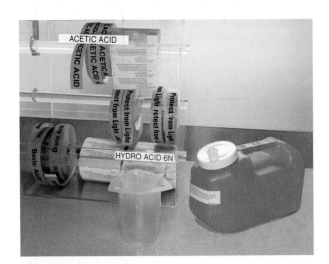

Figure 13-4 Twenty-four-hour urine specimen collection container with collection cup, and an assortment of labeling tapes and instruction stickers to be placed on collection containers.

The label should be affixed to the container, and not to the lid. In addition to standard patient identification, the label must also state it is a 24-hour specimen. Some 24-hour specimens require the addition of a preservative prior to collection. If so, the type of preservative should be clearly marked on the container, for example, using a special label that indicates the type of preservative added (see Fig. 13-4) and any precautions associated with it (e.g., some preservatives can burn the skin). A number of 24-hour specimens (e.g., creatinine clearance, quantitative porphyrins, and urine protein tests) must be kept refrigerated throughout the collection period. Some (e.g., quantitative porphyrins) also require protection from light. Others may have dietary restrictions. For example, when collecting a 24-hour urine specimen for 5-hydroxyindoleacetic acid (5-HIAA), a product of the breakdown of serotonin that is measured in the diagnosis of and monitoring of a particular type of tumor that produces serotonin, the patient must not eat certain foods that have a high serotonin content (including avocados, bananas, kiwi fruit, specific kinds of nuts, and tomato products) for a 72-hour period prior to and during collection. Certain drugs can also interfere with the 24-hour urine collections. Information on required procedure and proper handling for specific tests can be obtained by consulting the laboratory procedure manual.

Key Point If a preservative has been added to a urine collection container, patients must be instructed not to urinate directly into the container, to avoid being splashed with the preservative.

Collection and pooling of all urine voided during the designated 24-hour period is critical. The best time to begin a 24-hour collection is when the patient wakes in the morning, typically between 6 and 8 AM. The last specimen will be collected at the same time the following morning. The procedure begins and ends with an empty bladder. Consequently, the patient voids into the toilet and then begins the timing. The patient should be advised to set an alarm in order to awaken at the proper time the following morning. The patient then voids one last time and adds this specimen to the collection container. To prevent leaks, the patient should verify that the lid is securely tightened. The container should be transported to the laboratory as soon as possible, preferably in an insulated bag or disposable cooler to maintain specimen integrity during transportation, especially if the weather is warm or the specimen requires refrigeration. The procedure for 24-hour urine collection is shown in Procedure 13-1.

Test your knowledge of 24-hour urine collection with WORKBOOK Skills Drill 13-3.

Key Point A urine creatinine clearance test also requires collection of a blood creatinine specimen, which is ideally collected at the midpoint of urine collection (i.e., 12 hours into urine collection).

Double-Voided Specimen. A double-voided urine specimen is one that requires emptying the bladder and then waiting a specific amount of time (typically 30 minutes) before collecting the specimen. It is most commonly used to test urine for glucose and ketones. A fresh double-voided specimen is thought to more accurately reflect the blood concentration of the analyte tested, whereas a specimen that has been held in the bladder for an extended period may not.

Urine Collection Methods

Regular Voided Specimen

A regular voided urine collection requires no special patient preparation and is collected by having the patient void (urinate) into a clean urine container.

Midstream Specimen

A **midstream** urine collection is performed to obtain a specimen that is generally free of genital secretions, pubic hair, and bacteria that normally surround the urinary opening. To collect a midstream specimen, the patient voids the initial urine flow into the toilet. This initial flow helps flush contaminants from the urinary opening. The urine flow is interrupted momentarily and then restarted, at which time a sufficient amount of urine is collected into a specimen container. The last of the urine flow is voided into the toilet.

Check out WORKBOOK Knowledge Drill 13-4 to see if you know the rationale behind each step in the clean-catch procedure.

Midstream Clean-Catch Specimen

Midstream clean-catch urine is collected in a sterile container and yields a specimen that is suitable for microbial analysis or culture and sensitivity testing. Clean-catch procedures are necessary to ensure that the specimen is free of contaminating matter from the external genital areas. Special cleaning of the genital area is required before the specimen is collected. The cleaning methods vary somewhat depending upon whether the

Procedure 13-1: 24-Hour Urine Collection Procedure

PURPOSE: To provide instruction on how to properly collect a 24-hour urine specimen

EQUIPMENT: Requisition, specimen label, 24-hour urine container, preservative (if applicable), disposable ice chest (if required), copy of written instructions

Step	Explanation/Rationale
1. Void into toilet as usual upon awakening.	Removes all urine from the previous time period and ensures that the bladder is empty when timing starts.
2. Note the time and date on the specimen label, place it on the container, and begin timing.	Verifies the date, timing, and patient identification information of the specimen for the laboratory.
3. Collect all urine voided for the next 24 hours.	Ensures results are accurately based on the total amount of urine produced in 24 hours.
4. Refrigerate the specimen throughout the collection period if required. **Note:** Specimens can be kept cool in a refrigerator, or in a disposable ice chest placed in the bath tub, for example.	Preserves analyte integrity.
5. When a bowel movement is anticipated, collect the urine specimen before, not after it.	Prevents fecal contamination of the specimen.
6. Drink a normal amount of fluid unless instructed to do otherwise.	Prevents dehydration and facilitates specimen collection.
7. Void one last time at the end of the 24 hours and add it to the collection container.	Ensures the entire volume of urine produced in the 24 hours is collected. **Note:** The morning specimen is typically one of the largest by volume, the most concentrated and an important part of the 24-hour collection.
8. Seal the container, place it in a portable cooler unless instructed otherwise, and transport it to the laboratory ASAP.	Helps protect the integrity of the specimen.

patient is male or female. A phlebotomist must be able to explain the proper procedure to both male and female patients. The clean-catch urine collection procedure for females is described in Procedure 13-2. The procedure for males is described in Procedure 13-3.

Catheterized Specimen

A **catheterized** (cath) urine specimen is collected from a sterile catheter inserted through the urethra into the bladder. A catheterized specimen is collected when a patient is having trouble voiding or is already catheterized for other reasons. Catheterized specimens are sometimes collected on babies to obtain a specimen for C&S, on female patients to prevent vaginal contamination of the specimen, and on bedridden patients when serial specimen collections are needed.

Suprapubic Aspiration

Suprapubic collection of urine involves inserting a needle directly into the urinary bladder and aspirating

(withdrawing by suction) the urine directly from the bladder into a sterile syringe. The specimen is then transferred into a sterile urine container or tube. The procedure normally requires the use of local anesthesia and is performed by a physician. If the patient has a catheter, the specimen can be collected from the catheter by a nurse using a sterile needle and syringe. Suprapubic aspiration is used for samples for microbial analysis or cytology studies. It is sometimes used to obtain uncontaminated samples from infants and young children.

Pediatric Urine Collection

A plastic urine collection bag with hypoallergenic skin adhesive (Fig. 13-5) is used to collect a urine specimen from an infant or small child who is not yet potty trained. The patient's genital area is cleaned and dried before the bag is taped to the skin. The bag is placed around the vagina of a female and over the penis of a male. A diaper may be placed over the collection bag. The patient is checked every 15 minutes until an adequate specimen

Procedure 13-2: Clean-Catch Urine Collection Procedure for Women

PURPOSE: To instruct a female in how to properly collect a clean-catch urine specimen

EQUIPMENT: Requisition, specimen label, sterile urine container, special sterile antiseptic wipes, and copy of written instructions

Step	Rationale
1. Wash hands thoroughly.	Aids in infection control and helps avoid contamination of the site while cleaning.
2. Remove the lid of the container, being careful not to touch the inside of the cover or the container.	Helps ensure the lid and container will remain sterile for accurate interpretation of results.
3. Stand in a squatting position over the toilet.	Facilitates cleaning and downward flow of urine.
4. Separate the folds of skin around the urinary opening.	Allows proper cleaning of the area.
5. Cleanse the area on either side and around the opening with the special wipes, using a fresh wipe for each area and wiping from front to back. Discard used wipes in the trash.	Helps ensure thorough cleaning by using fresh wipes for each area in a way that carries bacteria away from the urethral opening.
6. While keeping the skin folds separated, void into the toilet for a few seconds.	Helps maintain site antisepsis while initial urination helps wash away antiseptic residue and any microbes remaining in the urinary opening.
7. Touching only the outside of the container and without letting it touch the genital area, bring the urine container into the urine stream until a sufficient amount of urine (30 to 100 mL) is collected.	Helps ensure sterility of the specimen and that a sufficient amount of urine to perform the test is collected.
8. Void any additional urine into the toilet.	Disposes of excess urine.
9. Cover the specimen with the lid provided, touching only the *outside* surfaces of the lid and container.	Helps maintain sterility of the specimen.
10. Clean any urine off the outside of the container with an antiseptic wipe.	Aids in infection control.
11. Wash hands.	Aids in infection control.
12. Hand specimen to phlebotomist or place it where instructed if already labeled.	Follow facility protocol.

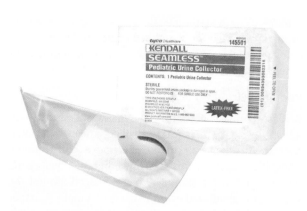

Figure 13-5 Urine collector for pediatric patients.

is obtained. The bag is then removed and sealed or the urine poured into a sterile container. The bag or container is labeled, and sent to the lab as soon as possible. A 24-hour specimen can be obtained by using a special collection bag with a tube attached that allows the bag to be emptied periodically.

AMNIOTIC FLUID

Amniotic fluid is the clear, almost colorless to pale-yellow fluid that fills the membrane (amnion or amniotic sac) that surrounds and cushions a fetus in the uterus. It is preferably collected after 15 weeks of gestation (pregnancy) and is obtained by a physician using a procedure called transabdominal amniocentesis. The procedure, which is typically performed with ultrasound guidance, involves inserting a needle through the mother's abdominal

Procedure 13-3: Clean-Catch Urine Collection Procedure for Men

PURPOSE: To instruct a male in how to properly collect a clean-catch urine specimen

EQUIPMENT: Requisition, specimen label, sterile urine container, special sterile antiseptic wipes, and copy of written instructions

Step	Rationale
1. Wash hands thoroughly.	Aids in infection control and helps avoid contamination of the site while cleaning.
2. Remove the lid of the container, being careful not to touch the inside of the cover or the container.	Helps ensure the lid and container remain sterile for accurate interpretation of results.
3. Wash the end of the penis with the special wipe (or soapy water), beginning at the urethral opening and working away from it in a circular motion (the foreskin of an uncircumcised male must first be retracted). Repeat the procedure with a clean wipe.	Carries bacteria away from the urethral opening, while repeating the process helps ensure thorough cleaning of the penis. Retracting the foreskin helps maintain antisepsis.
4. Keeping the foreskin retracted, if applicable, void into the toilet for a few seconds.	Helps maintain site antisepsis and helps wash antiseptic residue and any microbes remaining in the urinary opening into the toilet.
5. Touching only the *outside* of the container and without letting it touch the penis, bring the urine container into the urine stream until a sufficient amount of urine (30 to 100 mL) is collected.	Helps ensure sterility of the specimen and that a sufficient amount of urine needed to perform the test is collected.
6. Void the remaining urine into the toilet.	Disposes of excess urine.
7. Cover the specimen with the lid provided, touching only the *outside* surfaces of the lid and container.	Helps maintain sterility of the specimen.
8. Clean any urine spilled on the outside of the container with an antiseptic wipe.	Aids in infection control.
9. Wash hands.	Aids in infection control.
10. Hand specimen to phlebotomist or place where instructed if already labeled.	Follow facility protocol.

wall into the uterus and aspirating approximately 10 mL of fluid from the amniotic sac.

Amniotic fluid can be analyzed to detect genetic disorders such as Down syndrome, identify hemolytic disease resulting from blood incompatibility between the mother and fetus, and determine gestational age. However, the most common reasons for testing amniotic fluid are to detect problems in fetal development (particularly neural tube defects such as spina bifida) and assess fetal lung maturity.

Genetic disorders can be detected by chromosome studies done on fetal cells removed from the fluid, although the procedure has for the most part been replaced by studies on chorionic villi or placental tissue because it can be obtained earlier in the gestational period than amniotic fluid. Hemolytic disease can be detected by measuring bilirubin levels.

Although ultrasonography has become the accepted means of estimating gestational age, amniotic fluid creat-inine levels have also been used to estimate gestational age because these levels are related to fetal muscle mass.

Problems in fetal development can be detected by measuring **alpha-fetoprotein (AFP)**, an antigen normally present in the human fetus that is also found in amniotic fluid and maternal serum. Abnormal AFP levels may indicate problems in fetal development such as neural tube defects or the potential for Down syndrome. AFP testing is initially performed on maternal serum, and abnormal results are confirmed by amniotic fluid AFP testing. Because normal AFP levels are different in each week of gestation, it is important that the gestational age of the fetus be available or included on the specimen label.

 AFP is present in the blood of men and nonpregnant women in certain pathological conditions.

Fetal lung maturity can be assessed by measuring the amniotic fluid levels of substances called phospholipids, which act as surfactants to keep the alveoli of the lungs inflated. Results are reported as a lecithin-to-sphingomyelin (L/S) ratio. Lungs are most likely to be immature if the L/S ratio is less than 2. Amniotic fluid testing to assess fetal lung maturity may be ordered on or near the patient's due date and is often ordered stat when the fetus is in distress.

Amniotic fluid is normally sterile and must be collected in a sterile container. The specimen should be protected from light to prevent breakdown of bilirubin and delivered to the laboratory ASAP. Specimens for chromosome analysis must be kept at room temperature. Specimens for some chemistry tests must be kept on ice. Follow laboratory protocol.

CEREBROSPINAL FLUID

Cerebrospinal fluid (CSF) is the fluid that surrounds and helps cushion the brain and spinal cord. It is normally a clear, colorless liquid that has many of the same constituents as blood plasma. CSF specimens are obtained by a physician; most often through lumbar puncture (spinal tap).

Key Point A spinal tap is performed in the lower, lumbar region of the spine. The spinal cord ends near the first or second lumbar vertebrae. To avoid injury to the spinal cord, the needle used to withdraw the CSF is inserted between the third and fourth or the fourth and fifth lumbar vertebrae, well below where the spinal cord ends.

CSF analysis is used in the diagnosis and evaluation of bacterial or viral encephalitis, meningitis, fungal infections, and other disorders such as brain abscess, CNS cancer, and multiple sclerosis. Routine tests performed on spinal fluid include cell counts, chloride, glucose, and total protein. Other tests (e.g., cytology) are performed if indicated. CSF is generally collected in three or four special sterile screw top tubes (Fig. 13-6) specifically numbered in order of collection. Most tests require a minimum of 1-mL fresh fluid. Laboratory protocol dictates which tests are to be performed on each particular tube unless the physician indicates otherwise. Normally, the first tube is used for chemistry and immunology tests, the second for microbiology studies, the third for cell count and differential, because it is the least likely to be contaminated with blood cells introduced during the procedure. If a fourth tube is collected, it is typically used for cytology, other special tests, or as an extra tube. CSF should be kept at room temperature, delivered to the lab stat, and analyzed immediately.

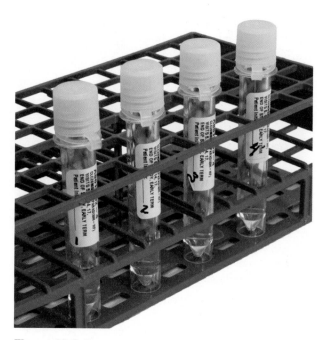

Figure 13-6 Four cerebrospinal fluid (CSF) tubes.

Proper handling and processing, and timely testing are crucial. CSF specimens are not easily recollected, and the procedure can be uncomfortable and costly. It also involves greater risk, and often produces a higher level of patient anxiety than the collection of most other types of laboratory specimens. If immediate testing is not possible chemistry and serology tubes are typically frozen, microbiology tubes can remain at room temperature, and hematology tubes are refrigerated. Follow facility protocol. Specimens that are over 24 hours old when delivered to the laboratory are normally considered unacceptable for testing and will most likely be rejected by the laboratory.

Want to have some fun? See if you can unscramble a word from this section in Knowledge Drill 13-2 in the WORKBOOK.

GASTRIC FLUID/GASTRIC ANALYSIS

Gastric fluid is stomach fluid. A **gastric analysis** examines stomach contents for abnormal substances and measures gastric acid concentration to evaluate stomach acid production. A basal gastric analysis involves aspirating a sample of gastric fluid by means of a tube passed through the mouth and throat (oropharynx) or nose and throat (nasopharynx) into the stomach after a period of fasting. This sample is tested to determine acidity prior to stimulation. After the basal sample has been collected, a gastric stimulant, most commonly histamine or pentagastrin, is administered intravenously and several more gastric samples are collected at timed intervals. All specimens are collected in sterile containers. The role of the phlebotomist in this procedure is to help label specimens and draw blood for serum gastrin (a hormone that stimulates gastric acid secretion) determinations.

NASOPHARYNGEAL SECRETIONS

The nasopharynx comprises the nasal cavity and pharynx. **Nasopharyngeal (NP)** secretions can be cultured to detect the presence of microorganisms that cause diseases such as diphtheria, influenza, meningitis, pertussis (whooping cough), and pneumonia. NP specimens are collected using a sterile Dacron or cotton-tipped flexible wire swab. The swab is inserted gently into the nose and passed into the nasopharynx. There it is gently rotated, then carefully removed, placed in a sterile tube containing transport medium, labeled, and delivered to the lab. (See Fig. 13-7 for an illustration of NP swab collection procedure.) NP aspirations can also be collected.

SALIVA

Saliva (fluid secreted by glands in the mouth) is increasingly being used to monitor hormone levels and detect alcohol and drug abuse because it can be collected quickly and easily in a noninvasive manner. In addition, detection of drugs in saliva indicates recent drug use (i.e., within the previous few days). Numerous kits are available for collecting and testing saliva specimens. Many are point-of-care tests. Saliva specimens for hormone tests, however, are typically refrigerated or frozen to ensure stability and sent to a laboratory for testing.

SEMEN

Semen (seminal fluid) is the sperm-containing thick yellowish-white fluid discharged during male ejaculation. It is analyzed to assess fertility or determine the effectiveness of sterilization following vasectomy. It is also sometimes examined for forensic (or legal) reasons (e.g., criminal sexual investigations). Semen specimens are collected in sterile or chemically clean containers and must be kept warm, protected from light, and delivered to the lab immediately.

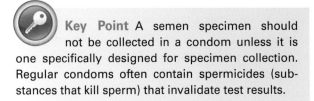 **Key Point** A semen specimen should not be collected in a condom unless it is one specifically designed for specimen collection. Regular condoms often contain spermicides (substances that kill sperm) that invalidate test results.

SEROUS FLUID

Serous fluid is the pale-yellow, watery, serum-like fluid found between the double-layered membranes enclosing the pleural, pericardial, and peritoneal cavities. It lubricates the membranes and allows them to slide past one another with minimal friction. The fluid is normally present in small amounts, but volumes increase when inflammation or infection is present or when serum protein levels decrease. An increase in fluid volume is called an effusion.

(i) Accumulation of excess serous fluid in the peritoneal cavity is called ascites (a-si' tez), and the fluid is referred to as ascitic fluid.

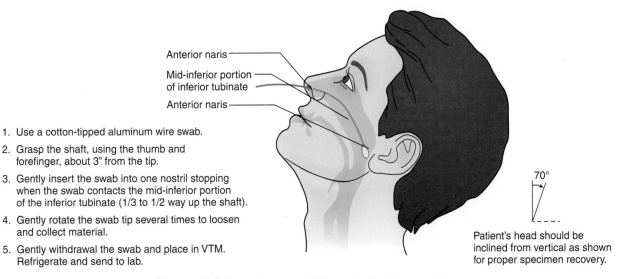

Anterior naris
Mid-inferior portion of inferior tubinate
Anterior naris

1. Use a cotton-tipped aluminum wire swab.
2. Grasp the shaft, using the thumb and forefinger, about 3" from the tip.
3. Gently insert the swab into one nostril stopping when the swab contacts the mid-inferior portion of the inferior tubinate (1/3 to 1/2 way up the shaft).
4. Gently rotate the swab tip several times to loosen and collect material.
5. Gently withdrawal the swab and place in VTM. Refrigerate and send to lab.

70°

Patient's head should be inclined from vertical as shown for proper specimen recovery.

Figure 13-7 Nasopharyngeal (NP) swab collection procedure.

Serous fluids can be aspirated for testing purposes or when increased amounts are interfering with the normal function of associated organs. A physician performs the procedure. Fluid withdrawn for testing is typically collected in EDTA tubes if cell counts or smears are ordered, in heparin or sodium fluoride tubes for chemistry tests, in nonanticoagulant tubes for biochemical tests, and in sterile heparinized tubes for cultures. The type of fluid should be indicated on the specimen label. Serous fluids are identified according to the body cavity of origin as follows:

• **Pleural fluid:** aspirated from the pleural space, or cavity, surrounding the lungs

• **Peritoneal fluid:** aspirated from the abdominal cavity

• **Pericardial fluid:** aspirated from the pericardial cavity surrounding the heart

> **Do you know what the word elements in pericardial mean? Practice your word-building skills with WORKBOOK Skills Drill 13-2.**

SPUTUM

Sputum is mucus or phlegm that is ejected from the trachea, bronchi, and lungs through deep coughing. Sputum specimens are sometimes collected in the diagnosis or monitoring of lower respiratory tract infections such as tuberculosis (TB), caused by *Mycobacterium tuberculosis*. Microorganisms in sputum can be detected and identified by C&S testing and by microscopic identification on a specially stained slide made from the sputum.

> **Key Point** The microbe that causes TB (*Mycobacterium tuberculosis*) is often referred to as an acid-fast bacillus (AFB) because it resists decolorizing by acid after it has been stained. Likewise, the sputum test for TB is often called an AFB culture, and the slide made from sputum is often called an AFB smear.

First morning specimens are preferred, as secretions tend to collect in the lungs overnight and a larger volume of specimen can be produced. It is also best to collect the specimen at least 1 hour after a meal to minimize the risk that the patient will gag or vomit. The patient must first remove dentures if applicable, then rinse his or her mouth and gargle with water to minimize contamination with mouth flora and saliva. The patient is instructed to take three or four slow, deep breaths, inhaling to full capacity and exhaling fully, then to cough forcefully on the last breath and **expectorate**

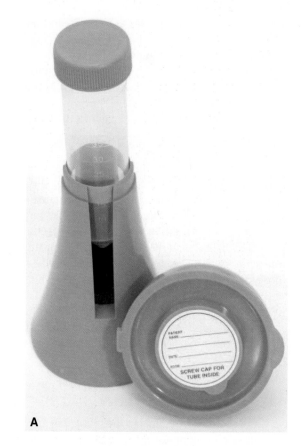

A

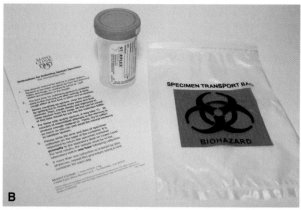

B

Figure 13-8 A: Specially designed sputum collection container. **B:** Sterile sputum collection kit (container, collection instructions, and biohazard bag for transport).

(cough up and expel sputum) into a special sterile container (Fig. 13-8). The process is repeated until a sufficient amount of sputum is obtained. A minimum of 3 to 5 mL is typically required for most tests.

> **Key Point** The patient must cough up material from deep in the respiratory tract and not simply spit into the container.

Specimens are transported at room temperature and require immediate processing upon arrival in the laboratory to maintain specimen quality.

SWEAT

Sweat is analyzed for chloride content in the diagnosis of **cystic fibrosis (CF)**, predominantly in children and adolescents under the age of 20. Cystic fibrosis is a disorder of the exocrine glands that affects many body systems but primarily the lungs, upper respiratory tract, liver, and pancreas. The sweat of patients with CF can be up to five times saltier than normal because their sweat contains two to five times the normal amount of chloride. The amount of chloride in sweat can be measured by the **sweat chloride** test. The test involves transporting pilocarpine (a sweat-stimulating drug) into the skin by means of electrical stimulation from electrodes placed on the skin, a process called **iontophoresis**. The forearm is the preferred site, but the leg or thigh may be used on infants or toddlers. Sweat is collected, weighed to determine its volume, and analyzed for chloride content. (The sweat chloride testing procedure is explained in Chapter 11 under "Point-of-Care Testing.")

> (i) Cystic fibrosis can also be diagnosed using DNA from cells collected from the inside of the cheek. (See Buccal/Oral Specimens.)

Sweat specimens can also be used to detect long-term illicit drug use when urine testing is not practical. The sweat is collected on patches placed on the skin for extended periods of time (up to 14 days) and then tested for drugs.

SYNOVIAL FLUID

Synovial fluid is a clear, straw (pale-yellow) colored, moderately viscous fluid that lubricates and decreases friction in movable joints. It normally occurs in small amounts but increases when inflammation is present. The procedure to collect synovial fluid is called arthrocentesis. The fluid may be removed for both therapeutic (removal can help relieve pain and pressure) and diagnostic purposes. Synovial fluid analysis may be performed to help diagnose the cause of joint inflammation and swelling, identify or differentiate inflammatory and noninflammatory arthritis, and evaluate and manage joint diseases such as septic arthritis, gout, and other inflammatory conditions. It is typically collected in three tubes: an EDTA or heparin tube for cell counts, identification of crystals, and smear preparation; a sterile tube for culture and sensitivity; and a nonadditive tube for macroscopic appearance, chemistry, and immunology tests and to observe clot formation.

Other Nonblood Specimens

BONE MARROW

Because it is the site of blood cell production, bone marrow is sometimes aspirated and examined to detect and identify blood diseases. A bone marrow biopsy may be performed at the same time. To obtain bone marrow, a physician inserts a special large-gauge needle into the bone marrow in the iliac crest (hip bone) or sternum (breastbone). Once the bone marrow is penetrated, a 10-mL or larger syringe is attached to the needle to aspirate 1 to 1.5 mL of specimen. A laboratory hematology technologist is typically present and makes special slides from part of the first marrow aspirated. Additional syringes may be attached to collect marrow for other tests such as chromosome studies or bacterial cultures. Part of the first sample may be placed in an EDTA tube for other laboratory studies. Remaining aspirate is sometimes allowed to clot and placed in formalin or another suitable preservative and sent to histology for processing and examination. In an alternate method, blood and particles from the EDTA tube are filtered through a special paper. The filtered particles are then folded in the paper and placed in formalin. If a bone marrow biopsy is collected at the same time, the cylindrical core of material obtained is touched lightly to the surface of several clean slides before being placed in a special preservative solution. The slides are air dried and later fixed with methanol and stained with Wright stain in the hematology department. The biopsy specimen and several slides are sent to the histology department for processing and evaluation. The remaining slides including biopsy touch slides are sent to the hematology department for staining and evaluation under the microscope.

BREATH SAMPLES

Breath samples are collected and analyzed in one type of lactose tolerance test, and to detect the presence of *Helicobacter pylori* (*H. pylori*). *H. pylori* is a type of bacteria that secretes substances that damage the lining of the stomach and causes chronic gastritis, which can lead to peptic ulcer disease.

> (i) Recent studies have shown that a number of chemical compounds unique to *Aspergillus fumigatus*, a type of fungus often responsible for pulmonary infections in certain patients (e.g., stem cell and organ transplant patients) can be detected in an infected patient's breath.

C-Urea Breath Test

A common test used to detect *H. pylori* is the **C-urea breath test (C-UBT)**. This test is based on the fact that

H. pylori produces urease, an enzyme that breaks down urea but is not normally present in the stomach. To perform the test, a baseline breath sample is collected, after which the patient drinks a special substance that contains synthetic urea. The synthetic urea contains a form of carbon called carbon-13. If *H. pylori* organisms are present, the urease they produce will breakdown the synthetic urea and in the process release carbon dioxide (CO_2) that contains carbon-13. The CO_2 will be absorbed into the bloodstream and exhaled in the patient's breath. The patient breathes into a special Mylar balloon or other collection device at specified intervals. The breath specimens are analyzed for carbon-13 content. If carbon-13 is found in amounts higher than those in the baseline sample, *H. pylori* is present in the stomach.

Hydrogen Breath Test

The hydrogen breath test measures the amount of hydrogen exhaled to help identify problems with the digestion of carbohydrates such as lactose (milk sugar) and fructose (fruit sugar) and is thought to be the most accurate lactose tolerance test. It can also be used to detect bacterial overgrowth in the small intestine.

Normally very little hydrogen gas is detectable in the breath. However, if the body does not properly digest lactose or certain other carbohydrates, intestinal bacteria in the colon will ferment them, producing larger than normal amounts of hydrogen. The hydrogen is absorbed into the bloodstream, transported to the lungs, and exhaled during normal breathing. The hydrogen breath test measures the amount of hydrogen exhaled and can detect the larger than normal amounts.

To prepare for the test, the patient must avoid certain foods for 24 hours before the test, not take antibiotics for at least 2 weeks before the test, and be fasting the day of the test. The patient is also required to refrain from vigorous exercise and smoking for 30 minutes prior to and during the test.

Breath samples are collected by having the patient exhale into a special bag or device. A baseline sample is collected first. Then the patient is given a drink that contains a measured amount of lactose or fructose (for lactose or fructose intolerance, respectively), or lactulose (to detect bacterial overgrowth). Additional breath samples are collected at regular intervals, typically, every 30 minutes for up to 3 hours, depending on the amount of hydrogen detected in the samples. For those given lactose or fructose, increased hydrogen levels in the breath samples respectively indicate faulty digestion and absorption of lactose or fructose. For those given lactulose, if bacterial overgrowth is present, increased hydrogen levels appear twice; the first time when the lactulose reaches bacteria in the small intestine and the second time when it reaches bacteria in the colon.

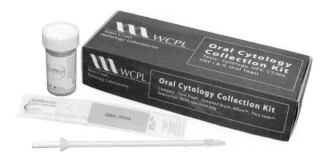

Figure 13-9 Buccal swab collection kit.

BUCCAL/ORAL SPECIMENS

Collection of a **buccal** (cheek) **swab** (Fig. 13-9) or oral specimen is a rapid, less invasive, and painless alternative to blood collection for obtaining cells for DNA analysis. (Plus, DNA is more easily extracted from buccal swabs than from blood samples.) Cells from the swab can be used for paternity testing and to identify viruses such as herpes simplex virus type 1 and type 2 (HSV-1 and HSV-2), oral human papillomavirus (HPV), and mumps virus. Because DNA analysis requires more DNA than is typically found in a buccal sample, a process called **polymerase chain reaction (PCR)** can be used to detect and amplify (i.e., make copies of) small segments of DNA. The process can target specific segments of DNA to aid in the particular analysis requested. The sample is typically collected by gently brushing or scraping the mucosa lining on the inside of the cheek and sometimes other areas of the mouth with a special swab or brush. Depending on the type of test, the swab may be placed in a transport container or envelope, or vigorously swirled in a preservative solution to release collected material, and then discarded. Follow manufacturer instructions.

> The polymerase chain reaction (PCR) process and other similar DNA identification methods can be used to identify DNA in many other types of specimens.

FECES (STOOL)

Examination of fecal specimens (feces or stool) can help identify disorders of the digestive tract, liver, and pancreas. Such disorders include GI bleeding, parasite, bacteria, fungus or virus infection, malabsorption syndrome, and cancer. A complete stool analysis typically includes evaluation of the amount, color, consistency, shape, and odor, and noting if mucus is present. In addition to evaluation of physical characteristics, stool analysis may also include chemical, microscopic, and microbiological tests.

- Chemical tests include pH, qualitative and quantitative **fecal fat**, urobilinogen, detection of proteolytic enzymes such as trypsin and chymotrypsin, and identifying the presence of **occult** (hidden) **blood**, which is blood that cannot be seen.

- Microscopic analysis can include looking for fecal fat (a qualitative fecal fat analysis) and muscle fibers, leukocyte detection, and **ova and parasite (O&P)** testing. O&P testing involves looking for parasites and their ova (eggs) or cysts. Examples of intestinal parasites include pinworms and *Giardia lamblia.*

- Microbiological analysis includes cultures to detect and identify infection with microorganisms such as **Clostridium difficile (C. difficile)**, *Salmonella*, *Shigella*, *Campylobacter*, enterohemorrhagic *Escherichia Coli* (EHEC).

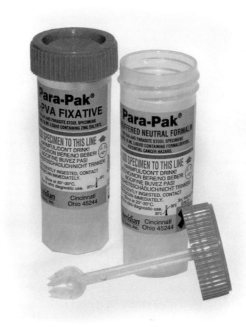

Clostridium difficile (*C. difficile*) is a bacterium that can inhabit the intestinal tract and multiply at the expense of normal bacteria in patients on antibiotic therapy. Although it is not commonly found in healthy adults, it is frequently found in hospitalized patients and is implicated as a causative agent of hospital-acquired diarrhea. Although cases are usually mild and subside when the antibiotic is discontinued, symptoms can persist and may become severe in some individuals.

Figure 13-11 Parasitology specimen collection containers with scoop.

Key Point Quantitative fecal fat analysis and urobilinogen are examples of tests that require 72-hour stool collection.

Stool Specimen Collection

Stool specimens are normally collected in clean, dry, wide-mouthed containers (Fig. 13-10) that must be sealed and sent to the laboratory immediately after collection. Special containers with preservative are available for ova and parasite collection (Fig. 13-11). Preserved specimens can usually be kept at room temperature. Large gallon containers, similar to paint cans, are used for 24-, 48-, and 72-hour stool collections. Multiple day stool collections must normally be refrigerated throughout the collection period.

Portions of a fecal specimen many need to be put in separate containers if several different tests are ordered, especially if the tests have different transport and handling conditions. Consult the facility procedure manual for test-specific collection and handling requirements.

A patient required to collect a stool specimen at home must be given the proper container, a biohazard transport bag, and written instructions. The instructions should include a warning against getting urine in the container since urine can kill microorganisms that might be present in the feces.

Although technically they are not fecal specimens, rectal swabs are sometimes collected for anal cytology tests, or to culture for microorganisms such as vancomycin-resistant enterococcus (VRE).

Fecal Occult Blood Tests

Fecal occult blood testing (FOBT) detects blood in feces and is used to screen for colorectal cancer and other lower digestive tract disorders that can result in bleeding such as such as diverticulosis, ulcerative colitis, and polyps. The traditional occult blood test is called a stool Guaiac test, named for a type of resin

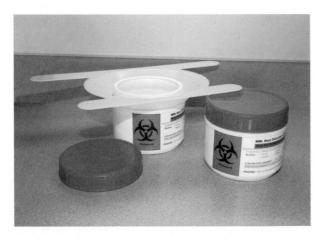

Figure 13-10 Stool specimen collection kit.

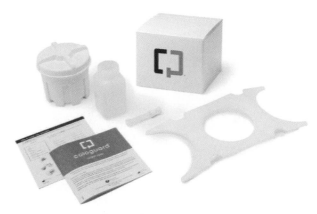

Figure 13-12 Cologuard® kit for colon cancer screening. (Courtesy Exact Sciences, Madison, WI.)

impregnated in the filter paper used for the test. It is also called a Guaiac smear test because the test is commonly performed on a smear of feces placed on the filter paper slide or test card. One example is the Hemoccult™ Fecal Occult Blood Slide (Beckman Coulter, Brea, CA). The test cards are often given to outpatients to collect the stool specimens at home. Patients are usually instructed to follow a meat-free diet for 3 days prior to the test. They then collect separate fecal specimens for 3 successive days. Cards can be mailed in or brought to the lab after collection. (See also Occult Blood in Chapter 11.)

A newer type of screening test for blood in stool is the **fecal immunochemical test (FIT)**, also called the immunochemical fecal occult blood test (iFOBT). These tests are based upon the immunochemical detection of the globin portion of human hemoglobin. Detection of globin in stool indicates bleeding in the colon or rectum because globin does not survive passage through the upper GI tract. The test has no diet restrictions, which is a big aid to patient compliance. The number of stool samples required depends upon the sensitivity of the test. One example of FIT is the InSure® FIT™, which requires only two samples, each from a separate bowel movement.

The newest fecal screening test for colon cancer, Cologuard® (Exact Sciences, Madison, WI) (Fig. 13-12) analyzes stool samples for altered DNA and blood biomarkers associated with colon cancer and precancerous polyps and lesions. Clinical trials found this test to be highly effective at detecting colon cancer in the early stages when it is most curable. This means the millions of individuals who have been avoiding colonoscopy as a means of detecting colon cancer, now have a noninvasive alternative to it. Patients collect stool samples at home as with FOBT and send the samples in sealed containers directly to Exact Sciences for testing.

HAIR

Hair samples can be used to detect alcohol and drugs of abuse such as amphetamines, opium, cocaine, or mari-

juana. Hair can also be used to identify poisoning by heavy metals such as lead and mercury, and for DNA analysis. Use of hair samples is advantageous because hair is easy to obtain, less invasive of privacy, and cannot easily be altered or tampered with provided chain of custody procedures are followed if required.

> **(i)** Hair analysis has been traditionally used to detect arsenic poisoning not only in forensic testing, but more commonly in agricultural workers as a result of inhaling fumes and dust from arsenic-containing insecticide sprays or dust.

An individual's hair keeps a record of alcohol or drug use for months. Because hair grows slowly, even hair close to the scalp can be weeks old. Consequently, hair shows evidence of chronic alcohol and drug use rather than very recent use. Depending on the length of hair sampled, it can show how long a person has been drinking alcohol, taking drugs, or been exposed to toxins. Reasons for DNA analysis of hair include paternity testing, and forensic analysis to help identify criminals. Forensic hair analysis can also include microscopic evaluation of hair structure.

The typical hair sample requirement is a lock of hair the width of a pencil and at least 3 inches in length. Hair samples are normally collected close to the scalp. For DNA analysis, the hair must include the root so samples must be plucked, not cut. Head hair is the preferred specimen, but beard, chest, mustache, or pubic hair can sometimes be used. Specimens are normally submitted at room temperature.

NAIL CLIPPINGS

Nail clippings can also be used for heavy metals testing. Clippings must be taken from all 10 nails (either fingernails or toenails). If both hair and nails are to be tested, they require separate containers and separate orders. Specimens are normally submitted at room temperature.

THROAT SWABS

Throat swab specimens are most often collected to aid in the diagnosis of streptococcal (strep) infections. A throat culture is typically collected using a special kit containing a sterile polyester-tipped swab in a covered transport tube containing transport medium (Fig. 13-13). Nursing staff usually collect throat culture specimens on inpatients. Phlebotomists commonly collect throat culture specimens on outpatients (see Fig. 13-14). The procedure for throat culture specimen collection is shown in Procedure 13-4. Throat swabs for rapid strep tests are collected in a similar manner.

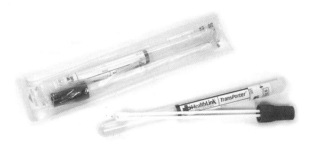

Figure 13-13 Throat swab and transport tube.

thePoint. *View the Throat Swab Collection and Rapid Detection of Strep procedure videos at http://thepoint.lww.com/McCall6e.*

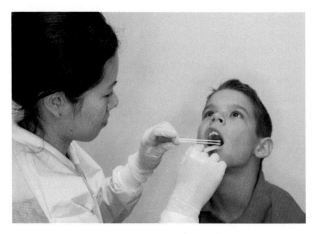

Figure 13-14 Phlebotomist collecting a throat swab specimen from a child.

Procedure 13-4: Throat Culture Specimen Collection

PURPOSE: To provide instruction in how to properly collect a throat culture specimen
EQUIPMENT: Requisition, specimen label, sterile container with swab and transport medium

Step	Rationale
1. Wash hands and put on gloves. The phlebotomist may wish to wear a mask and goggles. Follow facility protocol.	Aids in infection control. Protects the phlebotomist if the patient has a gag reflex or cough.
2. Open container and remove swab in an aseptic manner.	Helps maintain swab sterility for accurate interpretation of results.
3. Stand back or to the side of the patient.	Helps avoid contact with droplets if the patient coughs.
4. Instruct the patient to tilt back the head and open the mouth wide.	Allows adequate evaluation of the collection site and ease in specimen collection.
5. Direct light onto the back of the throat using a small flashlight or other light source.	Illuminates areas of inflammation, ulceration, exudation, or capsule formation.
6. Depress the tongue with a tongue depressor and ask the patient to say "ah."	Helps avoid touching other areas of the mouth and contaminating the sample during collection. Raises the uvula (soft tissue hanging from the back of the throat) out of the way.
7. Swab both tonsils, tonsillar crypts (crevasses), the back of the throat, and any areas of ulceration, exudation, or inflammation, being careful not to touch the swab to the lips, tongue, or uvula.	Follows standard protocol to enable sampling of problem areas. Avoids contaminating the swab with microbes from the oral cavity. Avoids a gag reflex that touching the uvula can cause.
8. Maintain tongue depressor position while removing the swab and then discard it.	Prevents the tongue from contaminating the swab.
9. Place the swab back in the transport tube, embed in media, and secure cover. (Follow instructions to crush ampule and release medium first if applicable.)	Keeps the microbes alive until they can be cultured in the laboratory.
10. Label specimen.	Prompt labeling is essential to ensure correct specimen identification.
11. Remove gloves and sanitize hands.	Proper glove removal and hand decontamination prevents the spread of infection.
12. Arrange transport or deliver to the laboratory as soon as possible.	Timely processing is necessary to prevent over growth of normal flora.

TISSUE SPECIMENS

Tissue specimens from biopsies may also be sent to the laboratory for processing. (A biopsy is the removal of a tissue sample for examination.) Most tissue specimens arrive at the laboratory in formalin or another suitable solution and need only be accessioned and sent to the proper department. However, with more biopsies being performed in outpatient situations, a phlebotomist in

specimen processing may encounter specimens that have not yet been put into the proper solution. It is important for the phlebotomist to check the procedure manual to determine the proper handling for any unfamiliar specimen. (For example, tissues for genetic analysis should *not* be put in formalin.) Improper handling can ruin a specimen obtained through a procedure that is, in all probability, expensive, uncomfortable for the patient, and not easily repeated.

Study and Review Questions

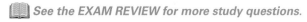 *See the EXAM REVIEW for more study questions.*

1. **Additional information typically required on a nonblood specimen label includes the**
   a. billing code.
   b. party to be charged.
   c. physician.
   d. specimen type.

2. **Which type of urine specimen is the best one for detecting UTI?**
   a. 24-hour
   b. First morning
   c. Clean-catch
   d. Random

3. **Which of the following statements describes proper 24-hour urine collection?**
   a. Collect the first morning specimen, start the timing, and collect all urine for the next 24 hours except the first specimen voided the following morning.
   b. Collect the first morning specimen, start the timing, and collect all urine for the next 24 hours including the first specimen voided the following morning.
   c. Discard the first morning specimen, start the timing, and collect all urine for the next 24 hours except the first specimen voided the following morning.
   d. Discard the first morning specimen, start the timing, and collect all urine for the next 24 hours including the first specimen voided the following morning.

4. **Which nonblood specimen is most frequently analyzed in the lab?**
   a. CSF
   b. Pleural fluid
   c. Synovial fluid
   d. Urine

5. **Which of the following fluids is associated with the lungs?**
   a. Gastric
   b. Peritoneal
   c. Pleural
   d. Synovial

6. **A procedure called iontophoresis is used in the collection of what specimen?**
   a. CSF
   b. Saliva
   c. Sweat
   d. Synovial fluid

7. **Saliva specimens can be used to detect**
   a. alcohol.
   b. drugs.
   c. hormones.
   d. all of the above.

8. **Which test typically requires a refrigerated stool specimen?**
   a. Fecal fat
   b. Guaiac
   c. Occult blood
   d. Ova and parasites

9. **A breath test can be used to detect organisms that cause**
   a. meningitis.
   b. peptic ulcers.
   c. tuberculosis.
   d. whooping cough.

10. **Which of the following is a type of serous fluid?**
    a. Amniotic fluid
    b. Pleural fluid
    c. Spinal fluid
    d. Synovial fluid

11. **A quick, noninvasive means of paternity testing is performed on cells from a**

    a. 24-hour urine.

    b. buccal swab.

    c. CSF specimen.

    d. feces sample.

12. **Which type of sample is commonly used to identify arsenic poisoning in agricultural workers?**

    a. Blood

    b. Feces

    c. Hair

    d. Saliva

13. **A positive FIT test indicates**

    a. bleeding in the colon or rectum.

    b. *C. diff* colonization of intestines.

    c. presence of intestinal parasites.

    d. sizeable fecal fat accumulation.

14. **A first morning specimen is unacceptable for urine cytology because**

    a. cells may have disintegrated in the bladder overnight.

    b. concentrated urine has many interfering substances.

    c. shedding of cells into the bladder at night is minimal.

    d. the pH level is usually too high for testing purposes.

15. **Alcohol testing of urine is problematic because**

    a. alcohol can evaporate from uncapped specimens.

    b. fermentation by bacteria can cause false positives.

    c. results may not correlate with blood alcohol levels.

    d. all of the above.

Case Studies

 See the WORKBOOK for more case studies.

Case Study 13-1: 24-Hour Urine Specimen Collection

A patient arrives at an outpatient lab with a 24-hour urine specimen. The specimen container is properly labeled and appears to hold a normal volume of urine. In speaking with the patient, however, the phlebotomist learns that the patient did not include the final morning specimen because he woke up several hours past the 24-hour collection deadline.

QUESTIONS

1. Should the phlebotomist accept the specimen? Why or why not?

2. Should the specimen have been accepted if the patient had included the specimen that was several hours late? Why or why not?

3. What can be done to ensure that future 24-hour collections are handled properly?

Case Study 13-2: DNA Specimen Collection

It is the last hour of work before a holiday at the All America Reference Laboratory and everyone is ready to leave, especially the phlebotomist in the receiving area

of Central Processing. A patient arrives at the lab and states he needs a DNA test. Unfortunately the person from the drawing area has left for the day. The central processing phlebotomist seems to remember that a DNA specimen requires whole blood, 7 mL green. Even though she hasn't collected blood in a few months, she prepares the patient and draws the necessary tube without problems. After the patient has been dismissed and gone from the lab, the phlebotomist reads the note attached to the request. It says the patient is a hemophiliac and cannot have blood drawn unless the physician is contacted. Immediately after that, the patient shows up at the door, bleeding down his arm and all over his clothes.

QUESTIONS

1. What did the phlebotomist do that was in error?

2. For a DNA order, can the specimen she collected be used? What specimen is preferred?

3. How should the phlebotomist handle the situation now that the patient has returned with an issue?

 You've finished the chapter. Time for some fun. Check out the crossword in the WORKBOOK.

Bibliography and Suggested Readings

Bishop M, Fody P, Schoeff L. *Clinical Chemistry.* 7th ed. Philadelphia, PA: Lippincott Williams & Wilkins; 2013.

Burtis C, Ashwood E, Bruns D. *Tietz Fundamentals of Clinical Chemistry, and Molecular diagnostics.* 7th ed. Philadelphia, PA: Saunders; 2015.

Clinical and Laboratory Standards Institute, GP-33A. *Accuracy in Patient and Sample Identification.* Approved Guideline. Wayne, PA: CLSI; 2010.

Clinical and Laboratory Standards Institute, C49-A. *Analysis of Body Fluids in Clinical Chemistry: Approved Guideline.* Wayne, PA: CLSI; 2007.

Clinical and Laboratory Standards Institute, H56-A. *Body Fluids Analysis for Cellular Composition: Approved Guideline Urinalysis.* vol. 26, no. 26. Wayne, PA: CLSI; 2006.

Clinical and Laboratory Standards Institute, C34-A3. *Sweat Testing: Sample Collection and Quantitative Chloride Analysis.* Approved Guideline, 3rd ed. Wayne, PA: CLSI; 2009.

Clinical and Laboratory Standards Institute, C52-A2. *Toxicology and Drug Testing in the Clinical Laboratory; Approved Guideline.* 2nd ed. Wayne, PA: CLSI; 2007.

Clinical and Laboratory Standards Institute, GP16-A3. *Urinalysis, Approved Guideline.* 3rd ed. Wayne, PA: CLSI; 2009.

Craven RF, Hirnle CJ, Jensen S. *Fundamentals of Nursing: Human Health and Function.* 7th ed. Phildelphia, PA: Lippincott Williams & Wilkins; 2013.

DuPont HL. Approach to the patient with suspected enteric infection. *Cecil Medicine.* 24th ed. Philadelphia, PA: Saunders Elsevier; 2011: chap 291.

Fischbach F, Dunning M. *A Manual of Laboratory & Diagnostic Tests.* 9th ed. Philadelphia, PA: Lippincott Williams & Wilkins; 2014.

Koneman E, Allen S, Janda W, et al. *Color Atlas and Textbook of Diagnostic Microbiology.* 6th ed. Philadelphia, PA: Lippincott Williams & Wilkins; 2005.

Mosby's Dictionary of Medicine, Nursing, & Health Professions. 9th ed. St. Louis, MO: Elsevier; 2012.

Poutanen S. Clostridium difficile–associated diarrhea in adults. *CMAJ.* 2004;171(1):51–58.

Skobe C. The Basics of specimen collection and handling of urine testing. *BD Labnotes.* 2004;14(2).

Stedman's Medical Dictionary for the Health Professions and Nursing. 7th ed. Philadelphia, PA: Lippincott Williams & Wilkins; 2011.

Turgeon M. *Linne & Ringsrud's Clinical Laboratory Science: The Basics and Routine Techniques.* 6th ed. St. Louis, MO: Mosby; 2011.

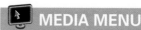

MEDIA MENU

Online Ancillaries (at http://thepoint.lww.com/McCall6e)
- Videos:
  - Rapid Detection of Strep
  - Routine Urinalysis
  - Throat Swab Collection
- Interactive exercises and games, including Look and Label, Word Building, Body Building, Roboterms, Crossword Puzzles, Quiz Show, and Concentration
- Audio flash cards and flash card generator
- Audio glossary

Internet Resources
- **Center for Phlebotomy Education:** http://www.phlebotomy.com/
- **Centers for Disease Control and Prevention (CDC): NP swab collection video.** http://www.cdc.gov/pertussis/clinical/diagnostic-testing/specimen-collection.html
- **Clinical Laboratory Science Internet Resources Website:** http://www.clinlabnavigator.com/Links/new-review/clinical-laboratory-science-internet-resources.html
- **LabCorp (Laboratory Corporation of America):** https://www.labcorp.com/wps/portal/provider/testmenu/
- **Mayo Medical Laboratories:** http://mayomedicallaboratories.com/it-mmlfiles/Urine_Preservatives10.pdf

Other Resources
- McCall R, Tankersley C. *Student Workbook for Phlebotomy Essentials.* 6th ed. (Available for separate purchase.)
- McCall R, Tankersley C. *Phlebotomy Exam Review.* 6th ed. (Available for separate purchase.)

Chapter 14

Arterial Puncture Procedures

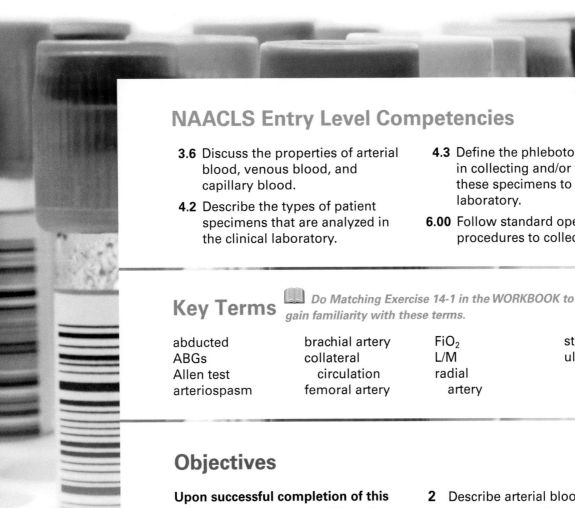

NAACLS Entry Level Competencies

3.6 Discuss the properties of arterial blood, venous blood, and capillary blood.

4.2 Describe the types of patient specimens that are analyzed in the clinical laboratory.

4.3 Define the phlebotomist's role in collecting and/or transporting these specimens to the laboratory.

6.00 Follow standard operating procedures to collect specimens.

Key Terms

Do Matching Exercise 14-1 in the WORKBOOK to gain familiarity with these terms.

abducted
ABGs
Allen test
arteriospasm

brachial artery
collateral
  circulation
femoral artery

FiO₂
L/M
radial
  artery

steady state
ulnar artery

Objectives

Upon successful completion of this chapter, the reader should be able to:

1 Demonstrate knowledge of practices, terminology, hazards, and complications related to arterial blood collection, and identify and analyze arterial puncture sites according to site-selection criteria and the advantages and disadvantages of each site.

2 Describe arterial blood gas (ABG) procedure including patient assessment and preparation, equipment and supplies, and commonly measured ABG parameters.

3 Perform the modified Allen test; explain how to interpret results and describe what to do based upon the results.

Overview

Arterial puncture is technically difficult and potentially more painful and hazardous than venipuncture. Consequently, arterial specimens are *not* normally used for routine blood tests, even though arterial blood composition is more consistent throughout the body than venous, which varies relative to the metabolic needs of the area it serves. The primary reason for arterial puncture is to obtain blood for **arterial blood gas (ABG)** tests. **ABGs** evaluate respiratory function. Arterial blood is the best specimen for evaluating respiratory function because of its normally high oxygen content and consistency of composition. Capillary blood, which is similar to arterial blood in composition provided that the puncture site is warmed prior to specimen collection, is sometimes used to test blood gases in infants (see Chapter 10).

Those who collect ABG specimens must have a thorough understanding of all aspects of collection in order to ensure accurate results and the safety of the patient. This chapter addresses advantages and disadvantages of using various arterial puncture sites, radial ABG procedures, ABG analytes, and arterial puncture hazards, complications, sampling errors, and specimen rejection criteria.

In addition to direct puncture of an artery, ABG specimens can be collected from an indwelling arterial line using a needleless blood sampling device such as the VAMP (see Chapter 9, Fig. 9-8) by personnel trained to do so.

ABGs

ABG evaluation is used in the diagnosis and management of respiratory disorders such as lung disease to provide information about a patient's oxygenation, ventilation (air entering and leaving the lungs), and acid–base balance, and in the management of electrolyte and acid–base balance in patients with diabetes and other metabolic disorders. ABG specimens are very sensitive to the effects of preanalytical errors; therefore accurate patient assessment and proper specimen collection and handling are necessary to ensure accurate results.

Key Point For accurate results, an ABG specimen must not be exposed to air. Consequently, the specimen must be collected in an anaerobic manner, which must be maintained throughout the collection, handling, and testing process.

Most ABG testing instruments directly measure hydrogen ion activity (pH), partial pressure of carbon dioxide ($PaCO_2$), and partial pressure of oxygen (PaO_2).

Other clinically useful analytes that may be measured include total hemoglobin (tHb), oxyhemoglobin saturation (O_2Hb), and saturation of abnormal hemoglobins such as carboxyhemoglobin (COHb) and methemoglobin (metHb). Values for plasma bicarbonate (HCO_3), base excess (or deficit), and oxygen (O_2) saturation can be determined by calculation.

Test yourself on these ranges with WORKBOOK Knowledge Drill 14-7.

See Table 14-1 for descriptions and normal ranges of commonly measured ABG analytes. Many instruments also measure other critical care analytes such as sodium, potassium, chloride, ionized calcium, and glucose on the same specimen.

Some references use the abbreviations PO_2 and PCO_2 instead of PaO_2 and $PaCO_2$. Although these abbreviations are interchangeable, the latter two are more specific, as they refer to the partial pressure of these gases in arterial blood.

Personnel Who Perform Arterial Puncture

Paramedical personnel (healthcare workers other than physicians) who may be required to perform arterial puncture include nurses, medical technologists and technicians, respiratory therapists, emergency medical technicians, and level II phlebotomists. Phlebotomists who collect arterial specimens must have extensive training involving theory, demonstration of technique, observation of the actual procedure, and performance of arterial puncture with supervision before performing arterial punctures on their own. Personnel who perform ABG testing are designated level I or level II depending on their formal education, training, and experience. Level II personnel supervise level I personnel and perform testing as well. For quality assurance purposes, individuals performing arterial puncture must undergo periodic evaluation. Those who do not meet acceptable standards must have remedial instruction and be reevaluated before being allowed to collect arterial specimens independently.

Site-Selection Criteria

Several different sites can be used for arterial puncture. The criteria for site selection include the following:

- Presence of **collateral circulation**, which means that the site is supplied with blood from more than one

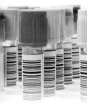

Table 14-1: Commonly Measured Arterial Blood Gas (ABG) Analytes

Analyte	Normal Range	Description
pH	7.35–7.45	A measure of the acidity or alkalinity of the blood; used to identify a condition such as acidosis or alkalosis.
PaO_2	80–100 mm Hg	Partial pressure of oxygen in arterial blood. A measure of how much oxygen is dissolved in the blood. Indicates if ventilation is adequate. Decreased oxygen levels in the blood increase the respiration rate and vice versa.
$PaCO_2$	35–45 mm Hg	Partial pressure of carbon dioxide in arterial blood. A measure of how much carbon dioxide is dissolved in the blood. Evaluates lung function. Increased CO_2 levels in the blood increase the respiratory rate and vice versa. *Respiratory* disturbances alter $PaCO_2$ levels.
HCO_3	22–26 mEq/L	Bicarbonate. A measure of the amount of bicarbonate in the blood. Evaluates the bicarbonate buffer system of the kidneys. *Metabolic* and *respiratory* disturbances alter HCO_3 levels.
O_2 saturation	97–100%	Oxygen saturation. The percent of oxygen bound to hemoglobin. Determines if hemoglobin is carrying the amount of oxygen it is capable of carrying.
Base excess (or deficit)	(–2)–(+2) mEq/L	A calculation of the nonrespiratory part of acid–base balance based on the $PaCO_2$, HCO_3, and hemoglobin.

artery, so that circulation can be maintained if one vessel is obstructed or damaged. Collateral circulation is the primary site-selection criterion. It can be evaluated using a portable ultrasound instrument (Fig. 14-1) or for the radial artery, by performing a simple test called the modified Allen test.

- Artery accessibility and size. The more accessible and larger an artery is, the easier it is to palpate and puncture.

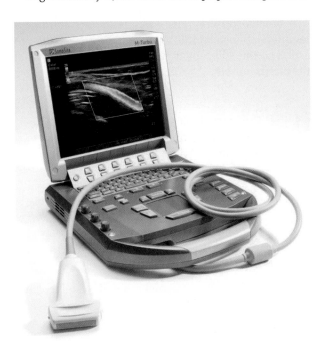

Figure 14-1 SonoSite M-Turbo® point-of-care ultrasound system displaying a brachial artery imaged with a high-frequency linear transducer. (Product photographs reprinted with permission from SonoSite; SonoSite M-Turbo® is a trademark owned by SonoSite, Inc.)

- Type of tissue surrounding the puncture site. The chosen artery should be in an area that poses little risk of injuring adjacent structures or tissue during puncture, helps fix or secure the artery to keep it from rolling, and allows adequate pressure to be applied to the artery after specimen collection.

- Absence of inflammation, irritation, edema, hematoma, lesion or a wound, an arterioventricular (AV) shunt in close proximity, or a recent arterial puncture at the site.

⚠️ **CAUTION** *Never* select a site in a limb with an AV shunt or fistula. It is a patient's lifeline for dialysis and should not be disturbed; also, venous and arterial blood mix together at the site.

Arterial Puncture Sites

THE RADIAL ARTERY

The first choice and most commonly used site for arterial puncture is the **radial artery**, located on the thumb side of the wrist (Fig. 14-2). Although smaller than arteries at other sites, it is easily accessible in most patients.

📖 See the arm labeling exercise in **WORKBOOK Labeling Exercise 14-1.**

ⓘ The radial pulse can be felt on the thumb side of the wrist approximately 1 in above the wrist crease.

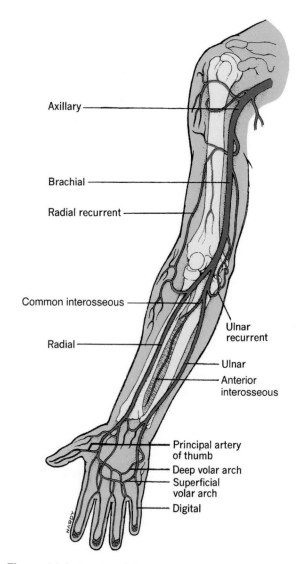

Figure 14-2 Arteries of the arm and hand.

Advantages

There are numerous advantages to using the radial artery to collect ABGs and other arterial specimens. For example:

- The biggest advantage of using the radial artery is the presence of good collateral circulation. Under normal circumstances, both the radial artery and the **ulnar artery** (Fig. 14-2) supply the hand with blood. If the radial artery were accidentally damaged as a result of an arterial puncture, the ulnar artery would still supply the hand with blood. Consequently the ulnar artery is normally off-limits for arterial specimen collection.

> 🔑 **Key Point** Adequate circulation via the ulnar artery must be verified before puncturing the radial artery. If ulnar blood flow is weak or absent, the radial artery should not be punctured.

- It is generally easy to palpate because it lies fairly close to the surface of the skin.
- There is less chance of hematoma formation following specimen collection because it can easily be compressed over the ligaments and bones of the wrist.
- There is a reduced risk of accidentally puncturing a vein or damaging a nerve because no major veins or nerves are immediately adjacent to the radial artery.

> ⓘ The radial artery is named after the radial bone in the lateral aspect (thumb side) of the lower arm, and the ulnar artery is named after the ulna, the large bone in the lower arm on the side opposite the thumb.

Disadvantages

Disadvantages of using the radial artery for collecting ABG and other arterial specimens include the following:

- Considerable skill is required to puncture it successfully because of its small size.
- It may be difficult or impossible to locate on patients with hypovolemia (decreased blood volume) or low cardiac output.

THE BRACHIAL ARTERY

The **brachial artery** (Fig. 14-2) is the second choice for arterial puncture. It is located in the medial anterior aspect of the antecubital fossa near the attachment of the biceps muscle.

> ⓘ The brachial pulse can be felt just above the bend of the elbow on the inside of the arm approximately in line with the ring finger.

Advantages

Advantages of using the brachial artery to collect ABGs and other arterial specimens include the following:

- It is large and can be relatively easy to locate and palpate.
- It is sometimes the preferred artery if a large volume of blood must be collected.
- It is often less painful than a radial artery puncture.

Disadvantages

Disadvantages of using the brachial artery to collect ABGs and other arterial specimens include the following:

- It has no direct collateral circulation and should be used with caution.
- It is deeper and can be harder to puncture than the radial artery.
- It may be difficult to palpate on obese patients.
- It lies close to the basilic vein, which could result in obtaining a venous sample by mistake.
- It also lies close to the median nerve, which, if accidentally hit by the needle, could cause the patient to experience extreme discomfort and possible nerve damage.
- Unlike the radial artery, there are no underlying ligaments or bone to support compression of the brachial artery, resulting in an increased risk of hematoma formation following the procedure. A hematoma in this area can cause compression injuries to the brachial artery and the median nerve.

Memory Jogger The median nerve lies medial to the brachial artery, which lies medial to the biceps tendon. The order from lateral to medial can be remembered by the mnemonic TAN, where T stands for tendon, A for artery, and N for nerve.

Key Point According to CLSI, the brachial artery in children, especially infants, is not commonly used because it is harder to palpate and lacks collateral circulation.

THE FEMORAL ARTERY

The **femoral artery** (Fig. 14-3) is the largest artery used for arterial puncture. It is located superficially in the groin, lateral to the pubic bone. Femoral puncture is performed primarily by physicians and specially trained emergency room personnel and is generally used only in emergency situations or when no other site is available.

 See the leg labeling exercise in the WORKBOOK.

Advantages

Advantages of using the femoral artery to collect ABGs and other arterial specimens include the following:

- It is large and easily palpated and punctured.
- It is sometimes the only site where arterial sampling is possible, especially on patients who are hypovolemic

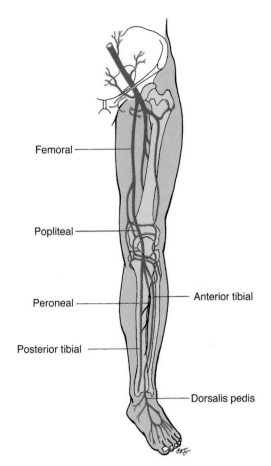

Figure 14-3 Arteries of the leg.

or have low cardiac output or during cardiac resuscitation.

Disadvantages

Disadvantages of using the femoral artery to collect ABGs and other arterial specimens include the following:

- It has poor collateral circulation.
- It lies close to the femoral vein, which may be inadvertently punctured and result in the collection of a venous specimen instead of an arterial one.
- There is increased risk of infection and difficulty in achieving aseptic technique because of its location and the presence of pubic hair.
- There is the possibility of dislodging plaque buildup from the inner artery walls of older patients.
- The femoral artery requires extended monitoring for hematoma formation or hemorrhage after puncture.

OTHER SITES

Other sites where arterial specimens may be obtained include the scalp, umbilical, and posterior tibial arteries in infants and the dorsalis pedis arteries in adults. The phlebotomist is not normally trained to perform arterial punctures at these locations or to obtain specimens from cannulas, catheters, or other indwelling devices at these or any other locations.

ABG Specimen Collection

TEST REQUISITION

As with any other test, a physician's order is needed before ABG specimens are collected. In addition to normal patient identification information, specific information concerning conditions at the time of collection—such as current body temperature, respiratory rate (respiration or breathing rate), ventilation status, and **fraction of inspired oxygen (FiO$_2$)**, which for room air is 0.21, or prescribed flow rate in **liters per minute (L/M)**—must be documented on the test requisition for meaningful interpretation of results. Required requisition information may vary according to regulatory requirements and institutional policy. Typical ABG requisition information is listed in Box 14-1.

EQUIPMENT AND SUPPLIES

Personal Protective Equipment

Personal protective equipment (PPE) needed by the blood drawer when collecting arterial specimens includes a fluid-resistant lab coat, gown, or apron; gloves; and face protection because of the possibility of blood spray during arterial puncture.

Specimen Collection Equipment and Supplies

ABG specimen collection equipment (Fig. 14-4) includes a safety needle, special heparinized syringe, and cap or other device to plug or cover the syringe after specimen collection so as to maintain anaerobic conditions.

Key Point Needles for radial ABG collection are typically 22 gauge or smaller, as larger-diameter needles may be too large to access the artery. Although smaller needles (e.g., 25 gauge) lessen pain and the likelihood of **arteriospasm** and hematoma, they can increase the chance of producing bubbles during the draw and specimen hemolysis.

ABG syringes typically contain special filters that vent residual air and seal upon contact with blood, or they may have air bubble removal caps that provide a safe way to remove bubbles from the specimen. ABG equipment is commonly available in sterile prepackaged kits that contain a heparinized syringe, capping device,

Box 14-1

Typical ABG Requisition Information

Required Information

- Patient's full name
- Medical record or identification number
- Age or date of birth
- Room number or other patient location
- Date and time of test collection
- Fraction of inspired oxygen (FiO$_2$) or flow rate in liters per minute (L/M)
- Body temperature
- Respiration rate
- Clinical indication for specimen collection (e.g., FiO$_2$ or mechanical ventilation change)
- Blood drawer's initials
- Requesting physician's name

Supplemental Information as Required by Institutional Policy or Regulatory Agencies

- Ventilation status (i.e., breathing spontaneously or mechanically supported)
- Method of ventilation (i.e., pressure support) or delivery (i.e., cannula or mask)
- Sampling site and type of procedure (i.e., arterial or capillary puncture or indwelling catheter)
- Patient activity and position
- Working diagnosis or ICD code

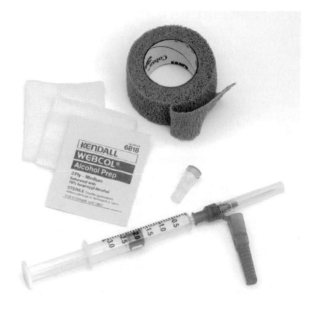

Figure 14-4 ABG equipment.

Box 14-2

ABG Collection Equipment and Supplies

- **Antiseptic** such as isopropanol or chlorhexidine sponges or pads for site cleaning.
- **Local anesthetic** to numb the site (optional); 1% lidocaine without epinephrine is recommended.
- **1- or 2-mL plastic syringe** with a 25- or 26-gauge ½–⅝-in long needle for administration of anesthetic solution (optional). Either the syringe or the needle should contain a safety device to prevent accidental needlesticks.
- **Sharp, short-bevel hypodermic needle** in 20–23 gauge or 25 gauge and ⅝–1½ in in length, depending on the collection site, the size of the artery, and the amount of blood needed. Typically, a 22-gauge 1-in needle is used for radial and brachial puncture and a 22-gauge 1½-in needle for femoral puncture. The needle should have a safety feature to prevent accidental needlesticks or be used with a safety syringe or other collection device with a safety feature.
- **Special glass or plastic 1- to 5-mL self-filling syringe** or other collection device (prefilled with the appropriate amount and type of lyophilized heparin salt) selected according to the type of tests ordered, the method of analysis, and the amount of blood required. The syringe or other collection device should contain a safety feature to prevent accidental needlesticks or be used with a safety needle.
- **Luer-tip normal or bubble removal cap** or other suitable device to cover the end of the syringe after needle removal to maintain anaerobic conditions within the specimen.
- (When applicable) **Coolant** capable of maintaining the specimen at a temperature between 1° and 5°C to slow the metabolism of white blood cells, which consume oxygen. (A container of crushed ice and water large enough to completely submerge the syringe barrel is typically used.)
- **2- by 2-in gauze squares** or pads to hold pressure over the site until bleeding has stopped.
- **Self-adhering gauze bandage** to wrap the site after collection.
- **Identification and labeling materials** such as waterproof labels and indelible ink pens or markers.
- **Puncture-resistant sharps container** to dispose off used needles and syringes.

and safety needle. ABG collection equipment and supplies are listed in Box 14-2.

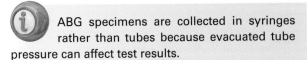

ABG specimens are collected in syringes rather than tubes because evacuated tube pressure can affect test results.

PATIENT PREPARATION

Identification and Explanation of Procedures

The blood drawer must properly identify the patient (see Chapter 8), explain the procedure, and obtain the patient's consent. The patient must be treated in a pleasant, professional, and reassuring manner to minimize apprehension or anxiety. Anxiety can lead to hyperventilation, breath-holding, or crying, which can compromise test results by lowering PaCO$_2$ and increasing pH.

Key Point The patient's anxiety can usually be minimized if the blood drawer is well organized and proceeds without delay.

Patient Preparation and Assessment

The patient must be relaxed and in a comfortable position. He or she should be lying in bed or seated comfortably in a chair for a minimum of 5 minutes or until breathing has stabilized. (Outpatients may take longer to stabilize.) Required collection conditions must be verified and documented on the requisition per institution policy. In addition, it should be determined whether or not the patient is on anticoagulant therapy. If an anesthetic is to be used, it should be confirmed that the patient is not allergic to it.

Steady State

Current body temperature, breathing pattern, and the concentration of oxygen inhaled affect the amount of oxygen and carbon dioxide in the blood. Consequently a patient should have been in a stable or **steady state** (i.e., no exercise, suctioning, or respirator changes) for at least 20 to 30 minutes before the blood gas specimen is obtained. This is especially important for patients with abnormal respiratory function, such as those with chronic lung disease. With the exception of certain emergency situations, ABG collection should not be performed until a steady state that meets required collection conditions has been achieved.

Modified Allen Test

It must be determined that the patient has collateral circulation before arterial puncture is performed. The modified **Allen test** is an easy way to assess collateral circulation before collecting a blood specimen from the radial artery. It is performed without the use of special equipment. If the test result is positive, arterial puncture can be performed on the radial artery. If the result is negative, arterial puncture should not be performed on that arm and the patient's nurse or physician should be notified of the problem. The procedure for the modified Allen test is described in Procedure 14-1.

 Do WORKBOOK Skills Drill 14-3 to reinforce your mastery of the steps of the Allen test procedure.

Procedure 14-1: Modified Allen Test

PURPOSE: To assess collateral circulation through the ulnar artery

EQUIPMENT: None

Step	Rationale/Explanation
1. Have the patient make a tight fist.	A tight fist partially blocks blood flow, causing temporary blanching until the hand is opened.
2. Use the middle and index fingers of both hands to apply pressure to the patient's wrist, compressing both the radial and ulnar arteries at the same time.	Pressure over both arteries is needed to obstruct blood flow, which is required to be able to assess blood return when pressure is released. Note: If the patient is unable to make a fist, the hand can be held above heart level for 30–60 seconds during steps 2 and 3.

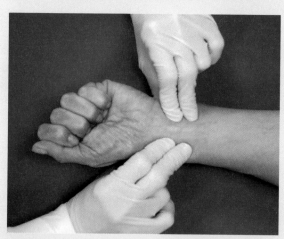

3. While maintaining pressure, have the patient open the hand slowly. It should appear blanched or drained of color.	Blanched appearance of the hand verifies temporary blockage of both arteries. Note: The patient must not hyperextend the fingers when opening the hand, as this can cause decreased blood flow and misinterpretation of results.

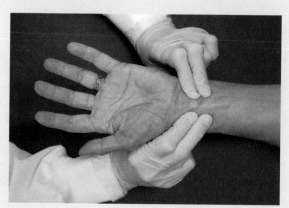

Procedure 14-1: Modified Allen Test (Continued)

Step	Rationale/Explanation
4. Lower the patient's hand and release pressure on the ulnar artery only.	The ulnar artery is released while the radial is still obstructed to determine if it will be able to provide blood flow should the radial artery be injured during ABG collection.
5. Assess Results:	
Positive Allen test result: The hand flushes pink or returns to normal color within 15 seconds.	A positive test result indicates return of blood to the hand via the ulnar artery and the presence of collateral circulation. If the Allen test result is positive, proceed with ABG collection.
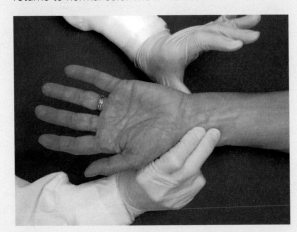	
Negative Allen test result: The hand *does not* flush pink or return to normal color within 15 seconds.	A negative test result indicates inability of the ulnar artery to adequately supply blood to the hand and therefore the absence of collateral circulation. If the Allen test result is negative, the radial artery should not be used and another site must be selected.
6. Record results on the requisition.	Verification that the Allen test was performed.

Administration of Local Anesthetic

The advent of improved thin-walled needles has made the routine administration of anesthetic (a drug that dulls pain by causing loss of sensation) prior to arterial puncture unnecessary. However, it may be a reassuring option for some patients, especially children, who are fearful of the procedure. A fearful patient may respond by breath-holding, crying, or hyperventilating, all of which may affect blood gas results. In addition to minimizing or preventing such patient reactions, local anesthesia may also prevent vasoconstriction. The recommended local anesthetic for ABG collection is 1% lidocaine without epinephrine; however, it may cause prolonged bleeding in patients on anticoagulant therapy. Consequently a physician's order is generally required before anesthetic is used. The procedure for preparing and administering local anesthetic is described in Procedure 14-2.

 Key Point Administration of lidocaine may dampen the strength of the palpable pulse.

 Check out Performing the Modified Allen test video at http://thepoint.lww.com/McCall6e.

 CAUTION Some individuals are allergic to lidocaine and its derivatives, so the absence of allergy must be determined before it is used.

RADIAL ABG PROCEDURE

Puncture of the radial artery can be performed only if it is determined that there is collateral circulation provided by the ulnar artery and the site meets other selection criteria previously described. The major points of radial ABG procedure are explained as follows:

Position the Arm

Position the patient's arm out to the side, away from the body (**abducted**) with the palm facing up and the wrist supported. (A rolled towel placed under the wrist

Procedure 14-2: Preparing and Administering Local Anesthetic

PURPOSE: Preparing and administering local anesthetic prior to arterial puncture

EQUIPMENT: Gloves, 25–26-gauge needle, 1-mL syringe[a], 1% epinephrine-free lidocaine[a], alcohol wipes, sharps container

[a]Either the needle or tube holder must have a safety feature to prevent needlesticks.

Step	Explanation/Rationale
1. Verify absence of allergy to anesthetic or its derivatives.	Allergy to lidocaine or its derivatives can cause a life-threatening reaction.
2. Sanitize hands and put on gloves.	Hand hygiene aids in infection control. Gloves provide a barrier to blood-borne pathogen exposure.
3. Attach the needle to the syringe.	A safety needle (or syringe with a safety device) must be used to reduce the chance of accidental needlestick.
4. Clean the stopper of the anesthetic bottle with an isopropyl alcohol wipe.	The stopper must be cleaned with an antiseptic to prevent contamination.
5. Insert the needle through the bottle stopper and withdraw anesthetic.	0.25–0.5 mL of lidocaine is adequate for most adult applications.
6. Carefully replace the needle cap and leave the syringe in a horizontal position.	Protects sterility of the needle and prevents contamination and leakage of the anesthetic.
7. Clean and air-dry the site.	Cleaning the site with antiseptic helps avoid contaminating the patient with skin-surface bacteria picked up during needle entry. Letting the site dry naturally permits maximal antiseptic action, prevents contamination caused by wiping, and avoids stinging on needle entry from residual alcohol.
8. Insert the needle of the anesthetic syringe into the intradermal layer of skin over the proposed arterial puncture site at an angle of approximately 10 degrees.	The anesthetic must be injected directly over the puncture site for optimal effect.
9. Pull back slightly on the plunger.	Verifies that a vein was not inadvertently penetrated. (If blood appears in the syringe, withdraw the needle, discard both needle and syringe, prepare a fresh needle and syringe, and repeat the procedure in a slightly different spot.)
10. Slowly expel the contents into the skin, forming a raised wheal.	Appearance of the wheal verifies proper application of the anesthetic.
11. Wait 1–2 minutes before proceeding with arterial puncture.	It takes 1–2 minutes for the anesthetic to take full effect. (The anesthetic wears off in 15–20 minutes.)
12. Note anesthetic application on the requisition.	Use of anesthetic must be documented on the requisition.

is typically used to provide support.) Ask the patient to extend the wrist at approximately a 30-degree angle to stretch and fix the tissue over the ligaments and bone of the wrist.

Locate the Artery

Use the index finger of your nondominant hand to locate the radial artery pulse proximal to the skin crease on the thumb side of the wrist. Palpate the artery to determine its size, direction, and depth. Take your time palpating the artery to verify optimal point of entry.

 CAUTION *Never* use the thumb to palpate, as it has a pulse that can be misleading.

Clean the Site

Prepare the site by cleaning with alcohol or another suitable antiseptic. Allow the site to air dry, being careful not to touch it with any unsterile object.

Prepare Equipment

Attach the safety needle to the syringe if not preassembled and set the syringe plunger to the proper fill level if applicable. Put on gloves if they were not put on in step 6 and clean the gloved nondominant finger so that it does not contaminate the site when relocating the pulse before needle entry.

Insert the Needle

Pick up and hold the syringe or collection device in your dominant hand as if you were holding a dart. Uncap and inspect the needle for defects. (Discard and replace it if flawed.) Relocate the artery by placing the index finger of the opposite hand directly over the pulse. Warn the patient of imminent puncture and ask him or her to relax the wrist as much as possible while maintaining its extended position. Direct the needle away from the hand, facing into the arterial blood flow, and insert it bevel-up into the skin at a 30- to 45-degree angle (femoral puncture requires a 90-degree angle) approximately 5 to 10 mm distal to the index finger that is locating the pulse.

Advance the Needle into the Artery

Slowly advance the needle, directing it toward the pulse beneath the index finger. When the artery is pierced, a "flash" of blood will appear in the needle hub. When the flash appears, stop advancing the needle. Do not pull back on the syringe plunger. The blood will pump, or pulse, into the syringe under its own power unless a needle smaller than 23 gauge is used, in which case a gentle pull on the plunger may be required. Hold the syringe very steady until the desired amount of blood is collected. If the artery is missed, slowly withdraw the needle until the bevel is just under the skin before redirecting the needle into the artery.

> ⚠ **CAUTION** *Do not* probe. Probing is painful and can cause hematoma or thrombus formation or damage the artery.

Withdraw the Needle and Apply Pressure

When the desired amount of blood has been obtained, withdraw the needle, immediately place a folded clean and dry gauze square over the site with one hand, and simultaneously activate the needle safety device with the other hand or place the needle in an approved needle removal safety device. Apply firm pressure to the puncture site for a minimum of 3 to 5 minutes. Longer application of pressure is required for patients on anticoagulant therapy.

> ⚠ **CAUTION** *Never* allow the patient to apply the pressure. A patient may not apply it firmly enough. In addition, *do not* replace use of manual pressure for the required length of time with the application of a pressure bandage.

Remove Air, Cap Syringe, and Mix Specimen

While applying pressure to the site with one hand, use your free hand to remove the safety needle and discard it in a sharps container. Handle the specimen carefully to avoid introducing air bubbles into it, as they can affect test results. If any air bubbles are present, immediately eject them from the specimen. If the equipment has an air bubble removal cap, follow manufacturer's instructions. Cap the syringe and gently but thoroughly mix the specimen by inversion or rotation to prevent clot formation. Label the specimen.

 Testing with a POCT instrument (e.g., i-STAT®) is performed according to manufacturer's instructions immediately after air bubble removal. Results are typically recorded by the instrument and transmitted to the lab automatically.

Check the Site

After applying pressure for 3 to 5 minutes, check the site. The skin below the site should be normal in color and warm to the touch, with no evidence of bleeding or swelling. If bleeding, swelling, or bruising is noted, reapply pressure for an additional 2 minutes. Repeat this process if necessary until you are certain that bleeding has stopped.

> ⚠ **CAUTION** *Never* leave the patient if the site is still bleeding. If bleeding does not stop within a reasonable time, notify the patient's nurse or physician.

If the site appears normal, wait 2 minutes and check it again. Then check the pulse distal to the site. If the pulse is absent or faint or the patient complains of numbness at the site, alert the patient's nurse or physician immediately, because a thrombus may be blocking blood flow. If the site appears normal and the pulse is normal, apply a pressure bandage and make a notation as to when the bandage may be removed.

Wrap-Up Procedures

Make certain the specimen has been properly labeled before leaving the patient's bedside. Dispose of used equipment properly. Remove gloves and face protection and wash or decontaminate hands with sanitizer. Thank the patient. If ABG testing has already been performed by POCT instrumentation, verify that the results have been recorded and transmitted to the lab and omit the last step (transportation and handling).

Complete Workbook Skills Drill 14-3 to see how well you know the steps of radial ABG collection.

Transportation and Handling

Transport the specimen according to laboratory protocol and deliver to the laboratory ASAP. According to CLSI, blood gas specimens collected in plastic ABG syringes can be transported at room temperature provided that the specimen will be analyzed within 30 minutes. If the patient has an elevated leukocyte or platelet count, the specimen should be analyzed within 5 minutes of collection. If a delay in analysis is expected beyond either of the above limits, the specimen should be collected in a glass syringe and cooled as soon as possible by placing it in ice slurry. Specimens for electrolyte testing in addition to ABG evaluation should not be cooled because cooling affects the diffusion of potassium (an electrolyte) in and out of the cells and makes potassium results unreliable. Such specimens should be transported and tested ASAP. The complete procedure for collection of radial ABGs is shown in Procedure 14-3.

Key Point WBCs and platelets in a blood specimen continue to consume oxygen. A high WBC or platelet count means that oxygen will be consumed at a higher rate than in a specimen with a normal WBC or platelet count. The rate of oxygen consumed depends upon handling temperature, length of time involved, and the amount of oxygen in the sample initially. Cooling slows down oxygen consumption by the cells.

Procedure 14-3: Radial ABG Procedure

PURPOSE: To obtain an ABG specimen from the radial artery by syringe

EQUIPMENT: Gloves, antiseptic prep pads, heparinized blood gas syringe, cap and appropriate needle, gauze pads, self-adhesive bandaging material, permanent ink pen, coolant if applicable, sharps container

Step	Explanation/Rationale
1. Review and accession test request.	The requisition must be reviewed for completeness of information (see Chapter 8: "Venipuncture Procedure," step 1) and required collection conditions, such as oxygen delivery system, and FiO_2 or L/M.
2. Approach, identify, and prepare patient.	Correct approach to the patient, identification, and preparation are essential. (See Chapter 8: "Venipuncture Procedure," step 2.) Preparing the patient by explaining the procedure in a calm and reassuring manner encourages cooperation and reduces apprehension. (Hyperventilation due to anxiety, breath-holding, or crying can alter test results.)
3. Check for sensitivities to latex and other substances.	Increasing numbers of individuals are allergic to latex, antiseptics, and other substances.
4. Assess steady state, verify collection requirements, and record required information.	Required collection conditions must be met and must not have changed for 20–30 minutes prior to collection. Test results can be meaningless or misinterpreted and patient care compromised if they have not been met. The patient's temperature, respiratory rate, and FiO_2 affect blood gas results and must be recorded along with other required information.
5. Sanitize hands and put on gloves.	Proper hand hygiene plays a major role in infection control, protecting the phlebotomist, patient, and others from contamination. Gloves provide a barrier to blood-borne pathogen exposure. Gloves may be put on at this point or later, depending on hospital protocol.

Procedure 14-3: Radial ABG Procedure (Continued)

Step	Explanation/Rationale
6. Assess collateral circulation. 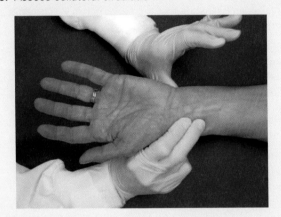	Collateral circulation must be verified by either the modified Allen test, an ultrasonic flow indicator, or both. Proceed if result is positive; choose another site if negative.
7. Position arm and ask patient to extend wrist.	The arm should be abducted, with the palm up and the wrist extended approximately 30 degrees to stretch and fix the soft tissues over the firm ligaments and bone. (Avoid hyperextension, as it can eliminate a palpable pulse.)
8. Locate the radial artery and clean the site.	The index finger is used to locate the radial pulse proximal to the skin crease on the thumb side of the wrist; palpate it to determine size, depth, and direction. An arterial puncture site is typically cleaned with alcohol or other suitable antiseptic and must not be touched again until the phlebotomist is ready to access the artery.
9. Administer local anesthetic (optional).	(See Procedure 14-2) Document anesthetic application on the requisition.
10. Prepare equipment and clean gloved nondominant finger.	Assemble ABG equipment and set the syringe plunger to the proper fill level if applicable. Gloves must be put on at this point if this has not already done, and the nondominant finger cleaned so that it does not contaminate the site when relocating the pulse before needle entry.
11. Pick up equipment and uncap and inspect needle.	The syringe is held in the dominant hand as if holding a dart. The needle must be inspected for defects and replaced if any are found.
12. Relocate radial artery and warn patient of imminent puncture.	The artery is relocated by placing the nondominant index finger directly over the pulse. The patient is warned to prevent a startle reflex and asked to relax the wrist to ensure smooth needle entry.
13. Insert the needle at a 30- to 45-degree angle, slowly direct it toward the pulse, and stop when a flash of blood appears. 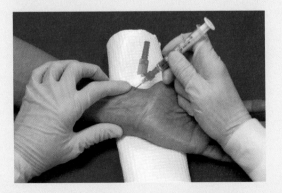	A needle inserted at a 30–45-degree angle, 5–10 mm distal to the finger that is over the pulse; it should contact the artery directly under that finger. When the artery is entered, a flash of blood normally appears in the needle hub or syringe. Note: If a needle smaller than 23 gauge is used, it may be necessary to pull gently on the syringe plunger to obtain blood flow.

Procedure 14-3: Radial ABG Procedure (Continued)

Step	Explanation/Rationale
14. Allow the syringe to fill to proper level.	Blood will normally fill the syringe under its own power, which is an indication that the specimen is indeed arterial blood (see exception in step 13).
15. Place gauze, remove needle, activate safety feature, and apply pressure.	A clean folded gauze square is placed over the site so firm manual pressure can be applied by the phlebotomist immediately upon needle removal and for 3–5 minutes thereafter. The needle safety device must be activated as soon as possible to prevent an accidental needlestick.
16. Remove and discard syringe needle.	For safety reasons, the specimen must not be transported with the needle attached to the syringe. The needle must be removed and discarded in the sharps container with one hand while site pressure is applied with the other.
17. Expel air bubbles, cap syringe, mix and label specimen. 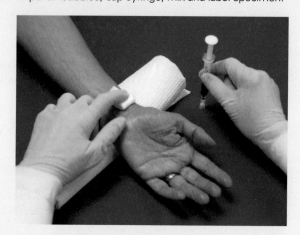	Air bubbles in the specimen can affect test results and must be expelled per manufacturer's instructions. While still holding pressure, the specimen must be capped to maintain anaerobic conditions, mixed thoroughly by inversion or rotating to prevent clotting, labeled with the required information, and if applicable, placed in coolant to protect analytes from the effects of cellular metabolism.
18. Check patient's arm and apply bandage.	The site is checked for swelling or bruising after pressure has been applied for 3–5 minutes. If the site is warm and appears normal, pressure is applied for 2 more minutes, after which the pulse is checked distal to the site to confirm normal blood flow. If pulse and site are normal, a pressure bandage is applied and the time at which it should be removed is noted. Note: If the pulse is weak or absent, the patient's nurse or physician must be notified immediately.
19. Dispose of used and contaminated materials, remove gloves, and sanitize hands.	Used and contaminated items must be disposed of per facility protocol. Gloves must be removed and hands sanitized as an infection control precaution.
20. Thank patient and transport specimen to the lab ASAP.	Thanking the patient is courteous and professional behavior. Prompt delivery of the specimen to the lab protects specimen integrity.

ABG COLLECTION FROM OTHER SITES

Collection of ABGs from brachial, femoral, and other sites is similar to the procedure for radial ABGs. Because phlebotomists are not normally trained to collect specimens from these sites, specific procedures are not given in this text. Phlebotomists may, however, be asked to provide the equipment and assist in labeling and transporting specimens collected from these sites by others (e.g., an emergency room physician).

Hazards and Complications of Arterial Puncture

There are hazards and complications associated with arterial puncture, as with any invasive procedure. Most can be avoided with proper technique, while some cannot be avoided. Complications or other adverse events observed by the blood drawer should be documented and reported to the patient's nurse or physician according to facility protocol. Examples of hazards and complications include the following:

Quiz yourself on these important points by doing WORKBOOK Knowledge Drill 14-4.

ARTERIOSPASM

Pain or irritation caused by needle penetration of the artery muscle and even patient anxiety can cause a reflex (involuntary) contraction of the artery referred to as an **arteriospasm**. The condition is transitory but may make it difficult to obtain a specimen. To help minimize the chance of arteriospasm, reassure the patient by fully explaining the procedure and its purpose and answering questions to help relieve patient anxiety.

ARTERY DAMAGE

Repeated punctures at the same site can damage the vessel, resulting in swelling, which can lead to partial or complete blockage of the vessel. In rare cases, repeated punctures have led to aneurysm of the artery.

DISCOMFORT

Some discomfort is generally associated with arterial puncture, even with the use of a local anesthetic. Usually this is minor and temporary. Extreme pain during arterial puncture may indicate nerve involvement, in which case the procedure should be terminated.

INFECTION

Localized infection can result from improper site preparation, contamination of the site prior to specimen collection, or choosing a site where inflammation or infection is present. Careful site selection, proper antiseptic preparation of the site, and avoiding activities that can contaminate the site prior to specimen collection minimize the chance of infection.

HEMATOMA

Blood is under considerable pressure in arteries and initially more likely to leak from an arterial puncture site than a venipuncture site. Fortunately, arterial puncture sites tend to close more rapidly because of the elastic nature of the arterial wall. The probability of hematoma formation is greater in older patients, because arterial elasticity normally decreases with age, and in patients receiving anticoagulant therapy. Multiple punctures to a single site also increase the chance of hematoma formation and should be avoided. Proper site selection, precise needle insertion, and adequate pressure applied by the phlebotomist following needle withdrawal are essential to minimize the risk of hematoma formation.

Key Point Needle size also plays a role in hematoma formation. The greater the needle diameter, the larger the puncture opening, the greater the chance of leakage, and the greater the need for precise needle insertion.

NUMBNESS

Numbness of the hand or wrist can be a sign of impaired circulation or nerve irritation or damage due to an error in technique, such as improper redirection of the needle when the artery is missed. Numbness must be addressed immediately by alerting the patient's nurse or physician.

THROMBUS FORMATION

Injury to the intima or inner wall of the artery can lead to thrombus or clot formation. A thrombus may grow until it blocks the entire lumen of the artery, obstructing blood flow and impairing circulation. A thrombus can also be the source of an embolus, which may cause a thrombus, clot, or embolism to appear in another area of the body. If thrombus formation is suspected, the patient's nurse or physician must be alerted immediately.

VASOVAGAL RESPONSE

A vasovagal response—faintness or loss of consciousness related to hypotension caused by a nervous system response (increased vagus nerve activity)—or abrupt pain or trauma can occur during arterial puncture. If a patient feels faint or faints during arterial puncture, remove the needle immediately, activate the safety device, hold pressure over the site, and follow the syncope procedures discussed in Chapter 9.

> **Have some fun and see if you can find vasovagal among the scrambled words in WORKBOOK Knowledge Drill 14-2.**

Sampling Errors

A number of factors can affect the integrity of a blood gas sample and lead to erroneous results. These factors include the following:

AIR BUBBLES

Air bubbles must be immediately and completely expelled from the sample or oxygen from the air bubbles can diffuse into the sample, CO_2 can escape from the sample, and test results can be compromised.

> **Key Point** Secure attachment of the needle to the syringe can help minimize the chance of air bubble production.

DELAY IN ANALYSIS

Blood cells continue to metabolize or consume oxygen and nutrients and to produce acids and carbon dioxide in the specimen at room temperature. If the specimen remains at room temperature for more than 30 minutes, the pH, blood gas, and glucose values will not accurately reflect the patient's status. Processing the specimen as soon as possible after it is obtained helps ensure the most accurate results. Optimal time of analysis is within 10 minutes of collection.

IMPROPER MIXING

Inadequate or delayed mixing of the sample can lead to clotting, making the sample unacceptable for testing. Undetected microclots can lead to erroneous results and ABG instrument malfunction.

IMPROPER SYRINGE

Use only syringes especially designed for ABG procedures. The use of regular plastic syringes will lead to erroneous values. Use of commercially available ABG kits can eliminate this source of error.

OBTAINING VENOUS BLOOD BY MISTAKE

Markedly inaccurate ABG values will result if a venous sample is obtained by mistake. Normal arterial blood is bright red in color. Venous blood is a darker bluish-red color. However, it is sometimes difficult to distinguish between arterial and venous blood in poorly ventilated patients because their arterial blood may appear as dark as venous blood. The best way to be certain that a specimen is arterial is if the blood pulses into the syringe. In some instances, such as low cardiac output, a specimen may have to be aspirated. In these cases it is hard to be certain that the specimen is truly arterial.

USE OF IMPROPER ANTICOAGULANT

Heparin is the accepted anticoagulant for blood gas specimens. Oxalates, EDTA, and citrates may alter results, especially pH. Use of commercially available ABG kits, which come with heparinized syringes, eliminates this problem.

USE OF TOO MUCH OR TOO LITTLE HEPARIN

Too much heparin in the syringe can result in acidosis of the specimen and cause erroneous results. Too little

Box 14-3

Typical Criteria for Rejection of ABG Specimen

- Air bubbles in the specimen
- Clotted specimen
- Hemolysis of the specimen (if electrolytes are ordered)
- Improper or absent ID or other labeling requirements
- Improper transportation temperature
- Inadequate volume of specimen for the test (QNS)
- Prolonged delay in delivery to the lab
- Wrong type of syringe used

heparin can result in clotting of the specimen. Use of commercially available kits containing preheparinized syringes can eliminate this source of error.

Criteria for ABG Specimen Rejection

ABG specimens that have been improperly collected, handled, or transported can produce erroneous results that can negatively affect patient care. Consequently specimens with obvious problems will be rejected by laboratory personnel. Examples of typical criteria used to reject ABG specimens for analysis are shown in Box 14-3.

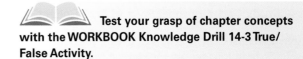 **Test your grasp of chapter concepts with the WORKBOOK Knowledge Drill 14-3 True/ False Activity.**

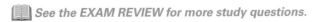

Study and Review Questions

See the EXAM REVIEW for more study questions.

1. **The primary reason for performing arterial puncture is to**
   a. determine hemoglobin levels.
   b. evaluate blood gases.
   c. measure potassium levels.
   d. obtain calcium values.

2. **The first-choice location for performing arterial puncture is the**
   a. brachial artery.
   b. ulnar artery.
   c. femoral artery.
   d. radial artery.

3. **ABG supplies include**
   a. 18-gauge needles.
   b. heparinized syringes.
   c. tourniquets.
   d. all of the above.

4. **Commonly measured ABG parameters include**
   a. pH.
   b. $PaCO_2$.
   c. O_2 saturation.
   d. All of the above.

5. **A phlebotomist has a request to collect an ABG specimen while the patient is breathing room air. When the phlebotomist arrives to collect the specimen, the patient is still on a ventilator. What should the phlebotomist do?**
   a. Call the phlebotomy supervisor and ask how to proceed.
   b. Consult with the patient's nurse to determine what to do.
   c. Draw the ABG and note the oxygen setting on the request.
   d. Take the patient off the ventilator and draw the specimen.

6. **The purpose of the modified Allen test is to determine**
   a. blood pressure in the ulnar artery.
   b. if collateral circulation is present.
   c. if the patient is absorbing oxygen.
   d. the clotting time of both arteries.

7. **Which of the following is an acceptable angle of needle insertion for radial ABGs?**
   a. 10 degrees
   b. 20 degrees
   c. 45 degrees
   d. 90 degrees

8. **Which of the following complications are associated with arterial puncture?**
   a. Arteriospasm
   b. Hematoma
   c. Infection
   d. All of the above

9. **Which of the following can cause erroneous ABG values?**
   a. The presence of air bubbles in the specimen
   b. Delay in analysis exceeding 30 minutes
   c. Inadequate mixing results in microclots
   d. All of the above

10. **Which of the following would cause you to suspect that a thrombus had formed in the artery while you were collecting an ABG?**
    a. A hematoma quickly forms at the site.
    b. The patient complains of extreme pain.
    c. The pulse distal to the site is very weak.
    d. All of the above.

Case Study

 See the WORKBOOK for more case studies.

Case Study 14-1: Complications of ABG Collection

A phlebotomist has a requisition to collect an ABG specimen from a patient in the cardiac care unit (CCU). The phlebotomist identifies the patient and records the required requisition information. The patient has an IV in the left arm in the area of the wrist, so the phlebotomist chooses the right arm. The patient is having difficulty breathing and appears quite restless and agitated. The phlebotomist performs the modified Allen test. The result is positive. The phlebotomist attempts puncture of the radial artery. The patient moves his arm as the needle is inserted and it misses the artery. The phlebotomist redirects the needle several times and finally hits the artery. The blood pulses into the syringe but is dark reddish-blue in color. The phlebotomist completes the draw, removes the needle, holds pressure over the site, and at the same time activates the needle safety device, removes the needle, and caps the syringe, being careful not to introduce air bubbles into it. After holding pressure for 5 minutes, the phlebotomist checks the pulse distal to the site. The pulse is barely discernible.

QUESTIONS

1. What should the phlebotomist do next?
2. What might be affecting the pulse?
3. How might the patient have contributed to the problem?
4. How might the phlebotomist's technique have contributed to the problem?
5. Can the phlebotomist be certain that the specimen is arterial?

Bibliography and Suggested Readings

Bishop M, Fody E, Schoeff L. *Clinical Chemistry, Principles, Procedures, Correlations.* 7th ed. Philadelphia, PA: Lippincott Williams & Wilkins; 2013.

Broaddus VC, Mason RJ, Martin T, King T. *Murray and Nadel's Textbook of Respiratory Medicine.* 5th ed. Philadelphia, PA: Saunders; 2010.

Burtis C, Ashwood E, Bruns D. *Tietz Fundamentals of Clinical Chemistry, and Molecular Diagnostics.* 7th ed. Philadelphia, PA: Saunders; 2015.

Clinical and Laboratory Standards Institute (CLSI), GP43-A4. *Procedures for the Collection of Arterial Blood Specimens: Approved Standard.* 4th ed. Wayne, PA: CLSI/NCCLS; 2004.

Kacmarek RM, Stoller JK, Huer AH. *Egan's Fundamentals of Respiratory Care.* 10th ed. St. Louis, MO: Elsevier/Mosby; 2012.

MEDIA MENU

Appendix A

Laboratory Tests

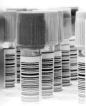

Table A-1: Alphabetical Listing of Laboratory Tests

Test	Abbreviation	Sample Considerations	Dept.	Clinical Correlation
Acid-fast bacillus culture (blood)	AFB	Green-top tube, isolator tube, or gel-barrier tube. Special cleaning for site and tube stopper.	M	Isolate and identify mycobacteria
Acid phosphatase	Acid p'tase	Gel-barrier tube. Centrifuge, separate, and freeze serum immediately. Transport frozen.	C	Cancer of the prostate
Alanine aminotransferase	ALT (SGPT)	Gel-barrier tube. Centrifuge for complete separation as soon as possible and refrigerate.	C	Evaluate hepatic disease
Alcohol	ETOH	Gray (preferred) or gel-barrier tube. Use nonalcohol germicidal solution to cleanse skin. Chain-of-custody required if for legal purposes.	C	Intoxication
Aldosterone		Plain red top; gel-barrier tube unacceptable. Centrifuge, separate, and refrigerate serum. Draw "up-right" sample at least ½ hr after patient sits up.	C	Overproduction of this hormone
Alkaline phosphatase	Alk phos or ALP	Gel-barrier tube. Centrifuge for complete separation as soon as possible. Fasting 8–12 hr is required.	C	Liver function
Alpha-fetoprotein	AFP	Gel-barrier tube. Avoid hemolysis; can be performed on amniotic fluid.	C	Fetal abnormalities, adult hepatic carcinomas
Aluminum	Al	Royal-blue tube; no additive. Avoid all sources of external contamination.	C	Trace metal contamination, dialysis complication
Ammonia	NH3	Lavender-top tube placed immediately on ice slurry. Centrifuge within 15 min without removing stopper; separate plasma and freeze in plastic vial.	C	Evaluates liver function. High levels in the blood lead to a problem known as hepatic encephalopathy.
Amylase		Gel-barrier tube. Centrifuge, and refrigerate serum. Avoid hemolysis and lipemia.	C	Acute pancreatitis
Antibody screen	Coombs test, indirect	Collect whole blood (lavender); special ID procedure.	I	Identifies any atypical antibodies present
Antinuclear antibodies (screen or titer)	ANA	Gel-barrier tube, refrigerated serum. Avoid hemolysis and lipemia.	S	Systemic lupus erythematosus and other autoimmune connective tissue diseases

(continued)

Table A-1: Alphabetical Listing of Laboratory Tests (Continued)

Test	Abbreviation	Sample Considerations	Dept.	Clinical Correlation
Anti-Rh antibody preparation		Special ID procedure.	I	Administered to Rh-negative mothers to prevent Rh immunization
Antistreptolysin O test	ASO	Refrigerate or freeze serum if not performed immediately.	S	Streptococcal infection
Antithrombin III activity	AT-III	Light-blue top, invert 3 to 4 times. Centrifuge, separate, and freeze plasma immediately in plastic vials. Transport frozen.	CO	Clotting factor deficiency
Apolipoprotein B	ApoB	Gel barrier. Centrifuge and refrigerate serum as soon as possible.	C	Primary component of LDL, coronary artery disease
Aspartate aminotransferase	AST, GOT, SGOT	Gel-barrier tube. Centrifuge for complete separation and refrigerate.	C	Acute and chronic liver disease
B_{12} and folate		Gel-barrier tube. Centrifuge, separate, and refrigerate. Protect from light.	C	Macrocytic anemia
Basic metabolic panel	BMP	Gel-barrier tube or red top. Refrigerate unopened spun-barrier tube. Separate within 45 min of venipuncture. Fasting 8–12 hr is required.	C	A designated number of tests covering certain body systems
Bilirubin, total and direct	Bili	Gel-barrier tube. Spin and separate within 45 min. Wrap in foil to protect from light. Refrigerate.	C	Increased with types of jaundice (i.e., obstructive, hepatic, or hemolytic; hepatitis or cirrhosis)
Blood culture	BC	Whole blood inoculated into two blood culture bottles: one anaerobic and one aerobic from two different sites or yellow tube. Do not refrigerate.	M	Isolate and identify potentially pathogenic organisms causing bacteremia or septicemia
Blood group and Rh type	ABO and Rh	Dedicated lavender top or pink top. Special ID procedure.	I	Detection of ABO and Rh antigens on the red blood cells
Calcitonin		Plain red. Allow to clot for 1–4 hr in an ice bath. Centrifuge, separate, and freeze immediately in plastic vial.	C	Evaluate suspected medullary carcinoma of the thyroid and is characterized by hypersecretion of calcitonin
Carbon monoxide (carboxyhemoglobin)	CO level	Fill lavender tube completely. Refrigerate immediately. Submit original, full, unopened tube.	C	Carboxyhemoglobin intoxication
Carcinogenic antigen	Ca 125	Serum gel tube. Refrigerate; freeze if testing is delayed.	C	Tumor marker primarily for ovarian carcinoma
Calcium, ionized	iCa++	Gel-barrier tube. Centrifuge with cap on; do not pour over; refrigerate. Place a piece of tape over the top of tube, write "do not open."	C	Bone cancer, nephritis, multiple myeloma
Carcinoembryonic antigen	CEA	Gel-barrier tube. Refrigerated serum.	C	Monitoring of patients with diagnosed malignancies; malignant or benign liver disease; indicator of tumors

Table A-1: Alphabetical Listing of Laboratory Tests (Continued)

Test	Abbreviation	Sample Considerations	Dept.	Clinical Correlation
Carotene, beta		Gel-barrier tube. Transport in amber plastic tube with amber stopper, if available. Wrap in aluminum foil to protect from light. Freeze.	C	Carotenemia
Chlamydia antibodies		Gel-barrier tube. Refrigerate serum collected using aseptic technique. Centrifuge and separate serum from clot within 4 hr of collection.	M	For trachoma, psittacosis, LGV, and pneumonia
Cholesterol and HDL ratio	Chol HDL	Gel-barrier tube. Separate as soon as possible; refrigerate serum.	C	Evaluates risk of coronary heart disease (CHD)
Chromium	Cr level	Royal blue—no additive; metal free, separate and refrigerate immediately.	C	Associated with diabetes and aspartame toxicity
Cold agglutinins		Gel-barrier tube. Must be kept warm; incubate at 37°C and allow it to clot at 37°C before separation. Store and ship at room temperature.	S	To diagnose viral and atypical pneumonia caused by *Mycoplasma pneumoniae*
Complete blood count	CBC	Lavender top. Invert gently 6 to 8 times immediately after drawing; includes WBC, RBC, Hgb, Hct, indices, platelets, and diff.	H	Blood diseases
Copper	Cu level	Royal blue—no additive; metal free. Separate and transfer to a plastic transport tube immediately.	C	Wilson disease or nephritic syndrome
Cord blood		Refrigerate serum.	I	Group and type baby's blood to detect the presence of incompatibilities, or mother for possible Rh immune globulin
Cortisol, timed		Gel-barrier tube. Refrigerated serum. Clearly note time drawn.	C	Cushing syndrome
Creatine kinase	CK	Gel-barrier tube. Refrigerated serum.	C	Muscular dystrophy and trauma to skeletal muscle
Creatine kinase MB	CK-MB	Gel-barrier tube. Refrigerated serum.	C	Organ differentiation and to rule out myocardial infarction
Creatinine	Creat	Gel-barrier tube or red top. Separate as soon as possible; refrigerate serum.	C	Kidney function
C-reactive protein high sensitivity	Hs-CRP	Gel-barrier tube. Refrigerated serum.	C	Chronic inflammation
Cryoglobulin		Gel-barrier tube. Draw and process at room temperature. Separate from cells immediately.	C	Associated with immunological diseases (i.e., multiple myeloma or rheumatoid arthritis)
Cyclosporin		Whole blood or serum from SST. Refrigerated. NOTE: Use same type of specimen each time analyte is measured.	C	Immunosuppressive drug for organ transplants
Culture		Collect the appropriate fluid or tissue using culture swab transport media. Indicate on the requisition location of culture.	M	Identification of infective agent and appropriate antibiotic treatment

(continued)

Table A-1: Alphabetical Listing of Laboratory Tests (Continued)

Test	Abbreviation	Sample Considerations	Dept.	Clinical Correlation
Cytomegalovirus antibody	CMV	Gel-barrier tube. Separate as soon as possible; refrigerate serum.	I	Screens donors and blood products for transplant programs
D-dimer	D-D1	1-mL frozen citrated plasma from a completely filled light-blue tube. Separate and freeze plasma immediately in plastic vials. Transport frozen.	CO	DIC and thrombotic episodes such as pulmonary emboli
Differential	Diff	Blood smear stained with Wright stain.	H	Classifying types of leukocytes, describing erythrocytes, and estimation of platelets
Direct antiglobulin test	DAT, Coombs test, direct	Dedicated lavender top. Special ID procedure.	I	Detects antibodies attached to the patient's red blood cells
Disseminated intravascular coagulation panel	DIC panel	Light-blue top completely filled. Centrifuge, separate, and freeze plasma immediately in plastic vials. Transport frozen.	CO	Distortion of the normal coagulation and fibrinolytic mechanisms
Drug monitoring	See individual drugs listed below	Sample consideration for all drugs listed below are the same. Use plain red; do not use gel-barrier tube. Centrifuge and separate within 1 hr and transfer to plastic transfer tube.		
Amikacin			C	Broad-spectrum antibiotic
Carbamazepine	*(Tegretol)*		C	Mood-stabilizing drug in bipolar affective disorder
Digoxin	*(Lanoxin)*		C	Heart stimulant
Dilantin	*(Phenytoin)*		C	Treatment of epilepsy
Gentamicin			C	Broad-spectrum antibiotic
Lithium			C	Manic-depression medication
Phenobarbital	*(Barbiturates)*		C	Anticonvulsant for seizures
Salicylates	*(Aspirin)*		C	Evaluation of therapy
Theophylline	*(Aminophylline)*		C	Asthma medication
Tobramycin			C	Broad-spectrum antibiotic
Valproic acid	*(Depakote)*		C	Seizures and symptomatic epilepsy
Vancomycin	*(Vancocin)*		C	Broad-spectrum antibiotic
Electrolytes	Na, K, Cl, CO_2, lytes	Gel-barrier tube. Centrifuge within 30 min after drawing. Do not remove stopper. Avoid hemolysis and lipemia.	C	Fluid balance, cardiotoxicity, heart failure, edema
Eosinophil	Eos	Lavender top. Invert gently 6 to 8 times immediately after drawing.	H	Allergy studies
Epstein–Barr virus panel	EBV	Gel-barrier tube. Store serum at 2 to 8 degrees.	S	Mononucleosis
Erythrocyte sedimentation rate	ESR	Lavender top. Invert gently 6 to 8 times immediately after drawing.	H	

Table A-1: Alphabetical Listing of Laboratory Tests (Continued)

Test	Abbreviation	Sample Considerations	Dept.	Clinical Correlation
Factor assays		Light-blue top. Invert 3 to 4 times; centrifuge, separate, and freeze plasma immediately in plastic vials. 1-mL aliquot for each factor.	C	To detect coagulation factor deficiency
Febrile agglutinin panel		Gel-barrier tube, random serum specimen. Avoid gross hemolysis and lipemia.	S	Screens for *Salmonella, Tularemia, Rickettsia,* and *Brucella* organism antibodies
Ferritin		Gel-barrier tube. Refrigerated serum.	C	Hemochromatosis, iron deficiency
Fibrinogen		Completely filled light-blue top. Invert 3 to 4 times; centrifuge 15 min, separate, and freeze immediately. Place in plastic vial and transport frozen.	CO	To investigate suspected bleeding disorders
Fibrin split products/ fibrin degradation product	FSP/FDP	One light-blue top, completely filled and inverted six times. Immediately centrifuge for 15 min, separate and freeze. Transport frozen.	CO	DIC and thrombotic episodes, valuable early diagnostic sign of increased rate of fibrin deposition
Fluorescent treponemal antibody absorption	FTA-ABS	Gel-barrier tube. Refrigerated serum.	S	Syphilis
Gamma-glutamyl transpeptidase	GGT	Gel-barrier tube. Spin and separate as soon as possible; refrigerate serum.	C	Assists in the diagnosis of liver problems; specific for hepatobiliary problems
Gastrin		Gel-barrier tube. Separate serum from cells within 1 hr after collection; freeze serum. Overnight fasting is required.	C	Stomach disorders
Glucose, fasting	FBS	Gel-barrier tube. Separate from cells within 1 hr or use gray-top tube.	C	Diabetes, hypoglycemia
Glycosylated hemoglobin	Hgb A1c	Lavender tube.	C	Monitoring diabetes mellitus
Glucose-6-phosphate dehydrogenase	G-6-PD	Lavender tube. Do not freeze.	C	Drug-induced anemias
Gonorrhea screen	GC	Taken from the urethra of male or endocervical canal from female.	M	Sexually transmitted disease
Hematocrit	Hct	Lavender top. Invert gently 6 to 8 times immediately after drawing.	H	Anemia
Hemoglobin	Hgb	Lavender top. Invert gently 6 to 8 times immediately after drawing.	H	Anemia
Hemoglobin A1c See glycosylated hemoglobin				
Hemoglobin electrophoresis		Refrigerated lavender top. Invert gently 6 to 8 times immediately after drawing.	C	Hemoglobinopathies and thalassemia
Hepatitis B surface antibody	HBsAb	Gel-barrier tube. Refrigerated serum.	S	Determination of previous infection and immunity by hepatitis B

(continued)

Table A-1: Alphabetical Listing of Laboratory Tests (Continued)

Test	Abbreviation	Sample Considerations	Dept.	Clinical Correlation
Hepatitis B surface antigen	HBsAg	Gel-barrier tube. Refrigerated serum.	S	Diagnosis of acute or some chronic stages of infection and carrier status of hepatitis B
Homocysteine	Hcy	Gel-barrier tube. Specimens must be centrifuged and separated within 2 hr of draw.	C	Elevated levels indicate increased risk of atherosclerosis
Human immunodeficiency virus antigen	HIV-1	Gel-barrier tube. Refrigerated serum—do not ship in glass tubes. Protect patient's confidentiality by using a code number in place of patient's name.	S	Screen for donated blood and plasma as an aid in the diagnosis of HIV-1 infection
Human leukocyte antigen-B 27	HLA-B27	Yellow-top (ACD) tubes; unopened tube required. Do not freeze or refrigerate; ethnic origin must be included.	I	Tested for disease association, matching prior to organ transplantation, platelet transfusion, and paternity and forensic evaluation
Human chorionic gonadotropin	HCG	Gel-barrier tube. Refrigerated serum.	C	Pregnancy, testicular cancer
Immunoglobulins	IgA IgG IgM	Gel-barrier tube. Refrigerated serum.	C	Measurement of proteins capable of becoming antibodies, chronic liver disease, myeloma
Indices	MCV, MCH, MCHC	Lavender top. Invert gently 6 to 8 times immediately after drawing.	H	Indicates mean cell hemoglobin (MCH), hemoglobin concentration (MCHC), and volume (MCV)
Iron and total iron-binding capacity	TIBC and Fe	Gel-barrier tube. Refrigerated serum. Separate from cells within 1 hr of collection. Fasting morning specimen is preferred.	C	Assist in differential diagnosis of anemia
Lactic acid (blood lactate)		Draw whole blood from a stasis-free vein into a gray-top tube. Centrifuge and separate plasma within 15 min of collection.	C	Measurement of anaerobic glycolysis due to strenuous exercise; increased lactic acid can occur in liver disease
Lactic dehydrogenase	LD	Gel-barrier tube. Avoid hemolysis—do not freeze or refrigerate.	C	Cardiac injury and other muscle damage
Lead	Pb	Royal blue EDTA or tan-top lead-free tube. Use of other evacuated tubes or transfer tubes may produce falsely elevated results due to contamination.	C	Lead toxicity, which can lead to neurologic dysfunction and possible permanent brain damage
Lipase		Gel-barrier tube. Refrigerated serum.	C	Used to distinguish between abdominal pain and that owing to acute pancreatitis
Lipoproteins		Gel-barrier tube. Refrigerated serum.	C	
High-density lipoprotein	HDL	Must be fasting a minimum of 12 hr.		Evaluates lipid disorders and coronary artery disease risk
Low-density lipoprotein	LDL	Must be fasting a minimum of 12 hr.		Evaluates lipid disorders and coronary artery disease risk

Table A-1: Alphabetical Listing of Laboratory Tests (Continued)

Test	Abbreviation	Sample Considerations	Dept.	Clinical Correlation
Magnesium	Mg	Gel-barrier tube. Separate from cells within 45 min. Maintain specimen at room temperature.	C	Mineral metabolism, kidney function
Mononucleosis screen	Mono-test	Gel-barrier tube. Refrigerated serum.	S	Infectious mononucleosis
N-Terminal proBrain natriuretic peptide	NT-proBNP	Gel-barrier tube. Separate from cells within 45 min, refrigerate.	C	Cardiovascular assessment
Partial thromboplastin time (activated PTT)	PTT/aPTT	Completely filled blue top. Invert 3 to 4 times immediately after drawing. Do not centrifuge or freeze if the sample will not be tested within 24 hr.	CO	Clotting factor deficiency, monitoring heparin therapy
Phosphorus	P, PO4	Gel-barrier tube. Separate from cells within 45 min. Maintain specimen at room temperature.	C	Thyroid function, bone disorders, and kidney disease
Plasminogen		Blue top. Centrifuge, separate, and freeze plasma immediately in plastic vials. Transport frozen.	CO	Fibrin clot formation prevention
Platelet aggregation	Plt. agg	4–5-mL sodium citrate tubes. Invert 3 to 4 times. Do not centrifuge. Do not refrigerate. Notify the lab before collection. Specimen must be received within 1 hr of collection.	H	Hemostasis and thrombus formation
Platelet count	Plt. ct	Lavender top, invert gently 6 to 8 times immediately after drawing.	H	Bleeding disorders
Prostate-specific antigen, total and free	PSA	Gel-barrier tube. Separate and freeze serum immediately in a plastic vial. Transport frozen.	C	Screen for the presence of prostate cancer, to monitor the progression of the disease and monitor the response to treatment for prostate cancer
Prothrombin time	PT	Completely filled blue top. Invert 3 to 4 times immediately after drawing. Do not centrifuge or freeze if the sample needs to be transported.	CO	Clotting factor deficiency, monitoring warfarin therapy
QuantiFERON® TB gold	QFT-GIT	Must be collected in special QFT, received by the lab within 12 hr and incubated by lab within 16 hr of collection.		Screens for latent tuberculosis infection
Red cell count	RBC	Lavender top. Invert gently 6 to 8 times immediately after drawing.	H	Anemia
Reticulocyte count	Retic	Lavender top. Invert gently 6 to 8 times immediately after drawing.	H	Anemia
Rheumatoid factor	RF	Gel-barrier tube. Refrigerated serum. Overnight fasting is preferred.	S	Arthritic conditions
Rapid plasma reagin	RPR	Gel-barrier tube. Refrigerated serum. Hemolysis and lipemia may alter test results.	S	Syphilis
Sedimentation rate, Westergren	ESR	Lavender top. Invert gently 6 to 8 times immediately after drawing.	H	Abnormal protein linkage
Serum protein electrophoresis	SPEP or PEP	Gel-barrier tube. Refrigerated serum.	C	Abnormal protein detection

(continued)

Table A-1: Alphabetical Listing of Laboratory Tests (Continued)

Test	Abbreviation	Sample Considerations	Dept.	Clinical Correlation
Sputum screen		True sputum, not saliva—early morning sample.	M	Tuberculosis
Streptococcus screen	Strep	Submit culturette.	M	Strep throat
Sweat chloride or electrolytes (iontophoresis)		Fluid collected is sweat.	C	Cystic fibrosis
Thyroid profile (comprehensive)	FTI, T_3, T_4, TSH	Gel-barrier tube or red-stoppered tube that must be separated to plastic transfer tube.	C	Hyper- or hypothyroid conditions
Triglycerides		Gel-barrier tube. Refrigerated serum. Strict fasting 12–14 hr is required (water only).	C	Used to evaluate risk of coronary heart disease
Blood group and Rh		Dedicated lavender top or pink. Special ID procedure—hand label with special band.	I	Group and type and detect atypical antibodies for prenatal screen or crossmatch
Urea nitrogen	BUN	Serum gel tube. Centrifuge for complete separation, and refrigerate.	C	Kidney function
Uric acid		Serum gel tube or red-stoppered tube that must be separated within 45 min; maintain specimen at room temperature.	C	Gout
White cell count	WBC	Lavender top. Invert gently 6 to 8 times immediately after drawing.	H	Infection (viral or bacterial)
Zinc	Zn	Royal blue. No additive or EDTA. If serum should be separated within 45 min and transferred to plastic transport tube.	C	Liver dysfunction

Codes for related departments to listed tests are as follows: I, immunohematology/blood bank; C, chemistry; CO, coagulation; H, hematology; M, microbiology; S, immunology/serology.

Appendix B
Laboratory Mathematics

The Metric System

The system of measurement used in the healthcare industry is the metric system, which derives its name from its fundamental unit of distance, the meter (M or m). In this system, the meter is the basic unit of linear measure, the gram (G or g) is the basic unit of weight, and the liter (L or l) is the basic unit of volume. The metric system is a decimal system (a system based on the number 10), in which units larger or smaller than the basic units are arrived at by multiplying or dividing by 10 or powers of 10.

In the metric system, prefixes added to the basic units indicate larger or smaller units. Prefixes are the same whether or not the units are meters, grams, or liters. Table B-1 shows prefixes commonly used in the medical laboratory. Basic metric units (meters, grams, liters) can be converted to larger units by moving the decimal point to the left according to the appropriate multiple. The multiple is the value of the exponent, which is a number indicating how many times the number is multiplied by itself. For example, a kilogram is 1,000, or $10 \times 10 \times 10$, or 10^3 g. The multiple, determined by the exponent, is 3.

EXAMPLE: Convert 100 grams to kilograms

From Table B-1 we determine that 1 kg is equal to 1,000, or 10^3 g. The multiple is 3. Therefore, to convert 100 grams to kilograms, move the decimal point three places to the left:

$$100 \text{ g} = 100.0 = 0.1 \text{ kg}$$

To convert basic metric units to smaller units, move the decimal point to the right according to the appropriate multiple.

EXAMPLE: Convert 100 g to mg

From Table B-1, we see that 1 mg is equal to 10^{-3} g. The multiple is minus 3. We therefore move the decimal point three spaces to the right:

$$100 \text{ g} = 100.00 = 100,000.00 \text{ mg}$$

Metric units other than basic units can be converted to larger units by moving the decimal point to the left according to the appropriate multiple, determined by subtracting the value of the exponent of the desired unit from the value of the exponent of the existing unit.

EXAMPLE: Convert 200 mg to kg

From Table B-1, we determine that 1 mg is 10^{-3} and 1 kg is 10^3. The desired unit is kilograms; therefore, we subtract −3 from 3 to determine the multiple:

$$3 - (-3) = 3 + 3 = 6$$

We are going from a smaller unit to a larger unit, so the decimal point moves to the left six spaces.

$$200 \text{ mg} = 000200.00 = 0.0002 \text{ kg}$$

Metric units other than basic units can be converted to smaller units by moving the decimal point to the right according to the appropriate multiple, determined by subtracting the value of the exponent of the desired unit from the value of the exponent of the existing unit.

EXAMPLE: Convert 25 cm to μm

From Table B-1, we determine that 1 cm is 10^{-2} and 1 μm is 10^{-6}. The desired unit is micrometers; therefore, we subtract −6 from −2 to determine the multiple:

$$-2 - (-6) = -2 + 6 = 4$$

We are going from a larger unit to a smaller unit, so the decimal point moves to the right four spaces.

$$25 \text{ cm} = 25.00 = 250,000.00 \text{ μm}$$

It is often necessary to convert the units of our English system to metric units. Table B-2 lists English units and their metric equivalents that are commonly encountered in the healthcare setting.

To convert from English units to metric units, multiply by the factor listed. Metric units can be converted back to English units by dividing by the same factor or multiplying by the factor in the metric conversion chart.

EXAMPLE: Convert 200 lb to kg

1 lb is equal to 0.454 kg

Therefore, multiply 200×0.454 to arrive at 90.8 kg

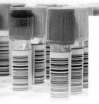

Table B-1: Commonly Used Measurement Prefixes

Multiple	Meter (m)	Gram (g)	Liter (l)	Prefix
Kilo- (k)	1,000 (10^3)	km	kg	kL
Deo- (d)	1/10 (10^{-1})	dm	dg	dL
Centi- (c)	1/100 (10^{-2})	cm	cg	cL
Milli- (m)	1/1,000 (10^{-3})	mm	mg	mL
Micro- (µ)	1/1,000,000 (10^{-6})	µm	µg	µL

Table B-3 shows the common equivalents for converting metric units to English units. To convert metric units to English units, multiply by the factor listed. To convert English units back to metric, divide by the same factor or multiply by the factor in the English unit conversion chart.

EXAMPLE: Convert 15 mL to tsp

1.0 mL is equal to ⅕ tsp

Therefore, multiply 15 × ⅕ to arrive at ¹⁵⁄₅

or 3 tsp (or 15 × 0.2 = 3.0 tsp)

Military Time

Most hospitals use military (or European) time, which is based on a clock with 24 numbers instead of 12 (Fig. B-1). Twenty-four-hour time eliminates the need for designating A.M. or P.M. Each time is expressed by four digits. The first two digits represent hours and the second two represent minutes. 1200 hours is noon and 2400 hours is midnight. One A.M. is 0100, 2 A.M. is 0200, and so on.

Noon is 1200; 1 P.M. is 1300

To convert regular (12-hour) time to 24-hour time, add 12 hours to the time from 1 P.M. on.

EXAMPLE: 1:00 P.M. becomes 1:00 + 12 hours
= 1300 hours

5:30 P.M. becomes 5:30 + 12 hours = 1730 hours

To convert 24-hour time to 12-hour time, subtract 12 hours after 1 P.M.

EXAMPLE: 1300 hours becomes 1300 − 12 hours
= 1:00 P.M.

Temperature Measurement

Two different temperature scales (Fig. B-2) are used in the healthcare setting. The Fahrenheit (F) scale is used to measure body temperature, whereas the Celsius (C) scale, also known as the centigrade scale, is used to measure temperatures in the laboratory.

- Fahrenheit: The freezing point of water is 32°F and the boiling point is 212°F. Normal body temperature expressed in Fahrenheit is 98.6°F.
- Celsius/centigrade: The freezing point of water is 0°C and the boiling point is 100°C. Normal body temperature expressed in the Celsius scale is 37°C.

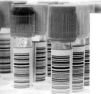

Table B-2: English–Metric Equivalents

	English		Metric
Distance	Yard (yd)	=	0.9 meters (m)
	Inch (in)	=	2.54 centimeters (cm)
Weight	Pound (lb)	=	0.454 kilograms (kg) or 454 grams (g)
	Ounce (oz)	=	28 grams (g)
Volume	Quart (qt)	=	0.95 liters (L)
	Fluid ounce (fl oz)	=	30 milliliters (mL)
	Tablespoon (tbsp)	=	15 milliliters (mL)
	Teaspoon (tsp)	=	5 milliliters (mL)

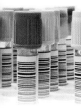

Table B-3: Metric–English Equivalents

	Metric		**English**
Distance	Meter (m)	=	3.3 feet/39.37 inches
	Centimeter (cm)	=	0.4 inches
	Millimeter (mm)	=	0.04 inches
Weight	Gram (g)	=	0.0022 pounds
	Kilogram (kg)	=	2.2 pounds
Volume	Liter (L)	=	1.06 quarts
	Milliliter (mL)	=	0.03 fluid ounces
	Milliliter (mL)	=	0.20 or 1/5 tsp

Note: A milliliter (mL) is approximately equal to a cubic centimeter (cc), and the two terms are often used interchangeably.

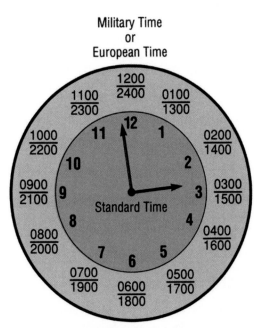

Figure B-1 Clock showing 24-hour (military) time.

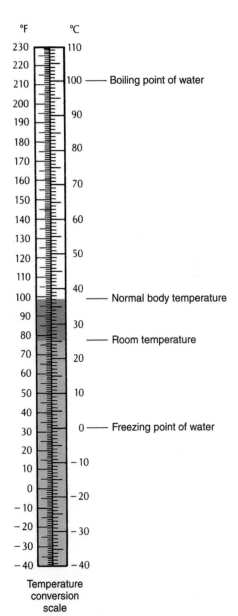

Figure B-2 Thermometer showing both Fahrenheit and Celsius degrees. (Courtesy of R. L. Memmler, B. J. Cohen, and D. L. Wood.)

The following formulas can be used to convert from one temperature scale to the other:

$$\text{Celsius temperature} = \frac{5}{9}\ (°F - 32)$$

$$\text{Fahrenheit temperature} = \frac{9}{5}\ (°C + 32)$$

Roman Numerals

In the Roman numeral system, letters represent numbers. Roman numerals may be encountered in procedure outlines, in physicians' orders or prescriptions, and in the identification of values or substances such as coagulation factors.

The basic Roman numeral system consists of the following seven capital (or lowercase) letters:

I	(i)	=	1	C	(c)	=	100
V	(v)	=	5	D	(d)	=	500
X	(x)	=	10	M	(m)	=	1,000
L	(l)	=	50				

GUIDELINES FOR INTERPRETING ROMAN NUMERALS

1. When numerals of the same value follow in sequence, the values should be added. There should never be more than three of the same numeral in a sequence.

   EXAMPLE: III = 1 + 1 + 1 = 3

   XX = 10 + 10 = 20

2. When a lower-value numeral precedes a numeral with a higher value, the lower value should be subtracted from the higher value. Numerals V, L, and D are never subtracted. No more than one lower-value number should precede a higher-value number.

   EXAMPLE: IV = 5 − 1 = 4

   IX = 10 − 1 = 9

3. When a numeral is followed by one or more numerals of lower value, the values should be added.

   EXAMPLE: XI = 10 + 1 = 11

   VII = 5 + 1 + 1 = 7

4. When a lower-value numeral comes between two higher-value numerals, it is subtracted from the numeral following it.

   EXAMPLE: XIX = 10 + 10 − 1 = 19

   XXIV = 10 + 10 + 5 − 1 = 24

5. Roman numerals are written from left to right in order of decreasing value (except for numerals that are to be subtracted from subsequent numerals).

   EXAMPLE: XXVII = 10 + 10 + 5 + 1 + 1 = 27

   MCMXCII = 1,000 + (1,000 − 100)

   + (100 − 10) + 1 + 1 = 1992

6. A line over a Roman numeral means multiply the numeral by 1,000.

   EXAMPLE: $\bar{\text{V}}$ = V × 1,000 = 5,000

Percentage

Percent means "per 100" and is represented by the symbol %. Two values are involved when a number is expressed as a percentage. They are the number itself and 100.

   EXAMPLE: 10% means 10 per 100 or 10 parts in a total of 100 parts. To change a fraction to a percentage, multiply by 100 and add a percent sign to the result.

   EXAMPLE: Change ¾ to a percentage

$$\frac{3}{4} \times \frac{100}{1} = \frac{300}{4} = 4\overline{)300}^{\,75} = 75\%$$

Dilutions

The concentration of laboratory reagents is often expressed as a percentage. For example, a solution of 70% isopropyl alcohol is used in skin cleansing before blood collection.

A 10% dilution of bleach (5.25% sodium hypochlorite) is used to disinfect countertops and other surfaces. A 10% dilution of bleach means that there are 10 parts of bleach in a solution containing a total of 100 parts. This dilution can also be expressed as a ratio, showing the relationship between the part of the solution and the total solution. A 10% solution is also a 1:10 (1 to 10) solution or one part bleach in a total of 10 parts solution. A dilution of 10 parts in a total of 100 parts is the same as 1 part in a total of 100 parts, or a 1:10 dilution. A 10% dilution of bleach can be prepared by adding 10 mL of bleach to 90 mL of water, resulting in a total of 100 mL of bleach solution. The same percentage dilution would result from adding 1 mL of bleach to 9 mL of water, 20 mL of bleach to 180 mL of water, and so on.

Blood Volume

Blood volume in adults is generally stated as 5.0 quarts or 4.75 liters (L). Because people come in different sizes, common sense tells us that they should not all have 5 quarts of blood. Actual blood volume is based on weight. Blood volume can be calculated for any size person from infant to adult as long as the person's weight is known. If the volume is calculated for adults and infants, it is important to realize that the value is not exact because the calculation is based on averages.

 Key Point CLSI lists the following blood volumes for infants and children:

Premature infants	115 mL/kg
Newborns	80–100 mL/kg
Infants and children	75–100 mL/kg

ADULT BLOOD VOLUME CALCULATION

Average adult blood volume is 70 mL per kg of weight.

EXAMPLE: Calculate the blood volume of a man who weighs 250 lb.

1. Change the weight in pounds to kilograms.
   Because 1 lb = 0.454 kg, you must multiply 250 lb by 0.454 to arrive at 113.5 kg.

2. Next, multiply the number of kilograms by 70 because there are 70 mL of blood for each kg of weight.

$$113.5 \text{ kg} \times 70 \text{ mL/kg} = 7,945 \text{ mL}$$

3. Because blood volume is reported in liters rather than milliliters, divide the total number of mL by 1,000 (1 liter = 1,000 mL).

$$\text{Blood volume} = 7,945 \text{ mL/1,000 mL} = 7.945 \text{ L}$$
$$\text{or } 7.9 \text{ L (rounded)}$$

CALCULATION OF INFANT BLOOD VOLUME

Estimating Blood Volume

When asked to collect a blood specimen from an infant, the phlebotomist must be able to make a quick mental estimate of the patient's blood volume in order to avoid causing harm. This can be accomplished by dividing the patient's weight in pounds by 2 to convert them to kilograms and multiplying the kilograms by 100 to get estimated blood volume. This estimate will always be higher than the true value. (The ability to convert pounds to kilograms is also needed in deciding how much of a glucose beverage to give a child during a GTT).

It is very important to be able to calculate the blood volume of an infant, especially if that infant is in an intensive care unit, where blood samples may be taken several times a day. A very small infant can become anemic if not monitored closely. Removal of more than 10% of an infant's blood volume in a short period of time can lead to serious consequences, such as iatrogenic anemia or cardiac arrest.

An average infant's blood volume is 100 mL per kg.

EXAMPLE: Calculate the blood volume of a baby that weighs 5.5 lb.

1. Change the weight from pounds to kilograms, using the same formula as for adults.

$$5.5 \text{ lb} \times 0.454 = 2.5 \text{ kg}$$

2. Multiply 2.5 kg by 100 for total blood volume in milliliters.

$$2.5 \text{ kg} \times 100 = 250 \text{ mL}$$

3. Change blood volume in mL/kg to liters.

$$250 \text{ mL/1,000 mL} = 0.25 \text{ L}$$

Appendix C

Conversational Phrases in English and Spanish

Although English is our official language, a variety of other languages are spoken in the United States, and prominent among them is Spanish. The following English-to-Spanish table has been prepared to help healthcare workers develop a better rapport with patients who speak only Spanish by using the translated remarks or sentences when conversing with them. Before approaching the patient, you should say these basic phrases aloud several times to someone who can correct the pronunciation if necessary. This is important, because if said incorrectly, the meanings of the phrases could be changed enough to insult or bewilder the patient.

The first column of the table is the phrase or word in English. The second column lists the phrase or word in Spanish, and the third column offers a phonetic pronunciation. The syllable in each word to be accented is printed in italic type. Even if you are not proficient in English-to-Spanish, your Spanish-speaking patients will appreciate your efforts to converse in their language if only to say "por favor" and "gracias." If you find that you have difficulty pronouncing the words, you can write them down or point to the Spanish phrase in the textbook.

English Phrase/Word	Spanish Phrase/Word	Phonetic Pronunciation
Hello.	¡Hola	(ō-lah)
Good morning.	Buenos días.	(bwā-nos dē-ahs)
Good afternoon.	Buenas tardes.	(bwā-nahs tahr-dās)
Good evening.	Buenas noches.	(bwā-nahs no-chās)
My name is	Me llamo	(mā yah-mō)
I am from the laboratory.	Soy del laboratorio.	(soy dāl lah-bō-rah-tō-rē-ō)
I am here to take a blood sample.	Estoy aquí para tomarle una prueba de sangre.	(ās-toy ah-kē pahr-ah tō-mahr-lā un-ah prū-bah dā sahn-grā⁻)
May I see your wristband?	¿Me permite ver su identificación?	(mā pār-mē-tā vār sū ē-dān-tē-fē-cah-sē-ōn?)
Do you understand me?	¿Me entiende?	¿Me ayn-tee-ayn-day?
What is your name?	¿Como se llama?	(cō-mō sā yah-mah?)
How old are you?	¿Cuántos años tienes?	¿Kwan-tohs ahn-yos tee-aynjays?
Speak slower.	Habla más despacio.	Ah-blah mahs days-pah-see-oh
It is necessary.	Es necesario.	Ays neh-say-sah-ree-oh.
Your doctor ordered this.	Su doctor ordeno.	(sū dōc-tor or dā-nō esto ās-to⁻)
Mr. or Sir	Señor	(sā-nyor)
Mrs. or Madame	Señora	(sā-nyō-rah)
Ms. or Miss	Señorita	(sā-nyō-rē-tah)
Okay.	Muy bien.	(mū-ē- byān)
Sit here.	Siéntese aquí.	(syān-tā-sā ah-kē)
You are the person I need.	Usted es la persona que necesito.	(ūs-tēd ās lah pār-sōn-ah)

(continued)

English Phrase/Word	Spanish Phrase/Word	Phonetic Pronunciation
Have you eaten?	¿Ha comido?	(ah cō-*mē*-dō)
I need . . .	Yo necesito	(kā na-sā-*sē*-tō)
I am going to . . .	Voy a . .	(voy ah)
I am going to put a tourniquet on your arm.	Le voy a poner un torniquete en el brazo.	(lā voy ah pō-*nār* ūn tor-n ē -*kā*-tā ān el *brah*-sō)
Please	Por favor	(por fah-*vor*)
Close your hand.	Cierra la mano.	(syā-rah lah *mah*-nō)
Make a fist.	Haga un puño.	(*hah*-ga ūn pun yo)
Open your hand.	Abra la mano.	(*ah*-brah lah *mah*-nō)
Straighten your arm.	Enderezca el brazo. OR Estire su brazo.	(en-dār-*āz*-kah el *brah*-sō) (ās-*te*—rā sū *brah*-sō)
Relax.	Relájese.	(rā-lah *hā*-sā)
It will hurt a little.	Le dolerá un poco.	(lā dō-lā-*rah* ūn pō-kō)
How do you feel?	¿Cómo se siente?	(¿Kob-moh say see-*ayn*-tay?)
It is important to . . .	Es importánte que . . .	(Ays eem-por-*tahn*-tay kay . . .)
You need to ask your doctor.	Necesita preguntarle a su doctor.	(nā-sā-*sē*-tah prā-gūn-*tahr*-lā ah sū dōc-*tor*)
Thank you.	¡Gracias!	(*grah*-syahs)
Have a good day.	Que le vaya bien.	(kā lā *vī*-yah byān)
Someone will be back in a few minutes.	Alguien regresará en un momento.	(ahl-*gwē*-ān rā-grā-sah-*rah* ān ūn mō-*mān*-tō)
I will get the nurse.	Buscaré a la enfermera.	(būs-cah-*rā* ah lah ām-fār-*mā*-rah)

Additional Phrases/Words	Spanish Phrase/Word	Phonetic Pronunciation
One	Uno	(*oo*-noh)
Two	Dos	(dohs)
Three	Tres	(trays)
Four	Cuatro	(*kwah*-troh)
Five	Cinco	(*sin*-koh)
Six	Seis	(says)
Seven	Siete	(see-*ay*-tay)
Eight	Ocho	(oh-choh)
The throat	La garganta	(lah gar-*gan*-tah)
Open your mouth.	Abra la boca.	(*Ah*-brah lah *boh*-kah)
Empty your bladder.	Orinar.	(Oh-ree-*narh*)
We need a urine specimen.	Es necesário una muestra de su orina.	(Ays nay-*say*-sar-ee-oh oo-nah moo*ay*-strah day oh-*ree*-nah)
You can only drink water.	Solo puede tomar agua.	(Soh-loh *pway*-day toh-mar *ah*-gwah)

Appendix D

Work Restrictions for Healthcare Employees

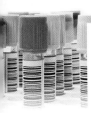

Table D-1: Conditions Requiring Work Restrictions for Healthcare Employees

Condition	Work Restriction
Chickenpox (varicella)	Off work until 7 days after appearance of first eruption and lesions are dry and crusted.
Ebola exposure	Off work until symptom free 21 days after exposure. According to the CDC anyone exposed to EBV who is symptom free 21 days after exposure will not get EBV. Follow local, state, and Federal guidelines.
Hepatitis A	Off work until cleared by a physician.
Hepatitis B	Off work until cleared by a physician.
Herpes zoster	May work if no patient contact.
Influenza	Work status determined by employee health department depending on work area.
Impetigo	Off work or no patient contact until crusts are gone.
Measles	Off work until rash is gone (minimum 4 days).
Mononucleosis	Off work until cleared by a physician.
MRSA (methicillin-resistant *Staphylococcus aureus*)	May work but no patient care until treatment is successful.
Pink eye (acute conjunctivitis)	Off work until treatment is successful.
Positive PPD test	May work depending upon evaluation and follow-up by employee health department.
Pregnancy	May work, but avoid contact with patients with rickettsial or viral infections, patients in isolation, and patients being treated with radioactive isotopes. Avoid areas with radioactive hazard symbol.
Tuberculosis (active)	Off work until treated and AFB smears are negative for 2 weeks.
Rubella (German measles)	Off work until rash is gone (minimum 5 days).
Salmonella	Varies depending on symptoms, treatment results, and employee health department evaluation.
Scabies	Off work until treated.
Shigella	Varies depending on symptoms, treatment results, and employee health department evaluation.
Strep throat (group A)	Off work until 24 hours after antibiotic therapy is started and symptoms are gone.
URI (upper respiratory infection)	Work status determined by employee health department.

Appendix E

Answers to Study and Review Questions and Case Studies

Chapter 1

ANSWERS TO STUDY AND REVIEW QUESTIONS

1. b	6. c	11. b
2. b	7. d	12. b
3. d	8. a	13. b
4. a	9. d	14. a
5. b	10. c	15. d

ANSWERS TO CASE STUDIES

Case Study 1-1: Telephone Etiquette and Irate Caller

1. Sally let the phone ring too many times, lost the caller when transferring the call, and kept the line open, allowing her conversation to be heard.
2. Leaving the line open. This allows the caller to hear conversations, which could violate HIPAA regulations if they should involve protected health information.
3. Sally should have prepared herself ahead of time by having the receptionist show her how to put callers on hold and transfer calls.
4. It is the laboratory administrator's responsibility to offer employees training in telephone etiquette.

Case Study 1-2: Phlebotomy and Protected Health Information

1. The nurse indicated that Matt needed to be quiet because he was broadcasting the patient's personal information across the common area, allowing others to hear.
2. The phlebotomist had ignored the patient's right to privacy as stated in the policies of several different facilities (i.e., the American Medical Association's Patient Care Partnership document).
3. Not only are there policies provided to prevent wrongful disclosure, but protected health information (PHI) is closely regulated by HIPAA, a federal law whose primary purpose is to secure and regulate patient privacy.

4. Matt should have handled the conversation in private. He should have waited for the requisition from the nurse and gotten any needed information at that time.

Chapter 2

ANSWERS TO STUDY AND REVIEW QUESTIONS

1. d	6. d	11. d
2. c	7. b	12. b
3. b	8. c	13. c
4. a	9. d	14. c
5. d	10. c	15. a

ANSWERS TO CASE STUDIES

Case Study 2-1: Scope of Duty

1. Although on the surface it seems like the proper thing to do, helping an inpatient walk to the bathroom is not within the phlebotomist's scope of duties and opens the phlebotomist up to liability issues, as illustrated by this case. It would have been better to have nursing personnel, who are properly trained in this area, assist the patient.
2. The hospital may have liability for the injury because of the liquid spilled on the floor that caused the patient to slip.
3. Vicarious liability and respondeat superior could come into play if a lawsuit is filed on behalf of the patient. However, it is also possible for the phlebotomist to be seen as individually liable because helping the patient is not a normal duty of a phlebotomist.

Case Study 2-2: Quality Assurance in the ER

1. The phlebotomist did not involve the patient in the identification process. Since the patient could communicate, he should have been asked to verify his name.
2. The Joint Commission NPSGs' number one goal for the clinical laboratory in 2014 was to identify patients correctly.

3. The screening criteria for accreditation of a health-care facility by TJC involve looking at activities in the facility and judging them based on four scoring categories. One of those categories is "Immediate Threat to Health and Safety," and the phlebotomist's misidentification of the ER patient for a transfusion falls under this scoring category. This means the facility was not in compliance with the standards set by TJC. This error would cause the accrediting team to be issued a Preliminary Denial of Accreditation until corrective action is validated.

Chapter 3

ANSWERS TO STUDY AND REVIEW QUESTIONS

1. c	5. a	9. b	13. c
2. d	6. b	10. a	14. b
3. a	7. c	11. d	15. d
4. a	8. d	12. d	

ANSWERS TO CASE STUDIES

Case Study 3-1: An Accident Waiting to Happen

1. The first thing the phlebotomist should do is wash the blood off of her arm, washing the scratch site thoroughly with soap and water for a minimum of 30 seconds.
2. The phlebotomist's actions that contributed to the accident included wearing heels and being in a hurry. It would have been better to wear appropriate shoes and change into heels just before going to lunch.
3. The phlebotomist should have had the scratch covered with a waterproof bandage.
4. The type of exposure she received can be classified as a parenteral exposure.

Case Study 3-2: Hitch-Hiking Microbes

1. Daren most likely got ill because his mother brought the "bugs" home to him from the ER. Daren rested his head on his mother's shoes and pants leg that were dragging on the contaminated hospital floor all day.
2. The pant legs need to be shortened so that they do not drag on the floor, or (2) better yet, the scrubs need to be removed before leaving work. (3) Daren's mother should have changed clothes before interacting with him or sitting down in the chair because the chair could also become contaminated.
3. It is technically not an HAI because it was not *acquired* in a healthcare facility. Facility policies need to be put in place to eliminate transferring healthcare-acquired infection outside of the healthcare setting.

Chapter 4

ANSWERS TO STUDY AND REVIEW QUESTIONS

1. a	5. b	9. d
2. c	6. a	10. b
3. b	7. c	
4. d	8. d	

ANSWERS TO CASE STUDIES

Case Study 4-1: Lab Orders

1. The blood culture specimens should be collected as soon as possible (ASAP). ASAP test orders have priority over routine collections. Facility protocol must be followed for exact time limits for collection.
2. The patient is in the emergency room (ER, also called the emergency department, or ED).
3. FUO stands for "fever of unknown origin." FUO indicates that the patient may have septicemia (or microorganisms in the blood), which can be detected by blood cultures.

Case Study 4-2: Misinterpreted Instructions

1. The student apparently did not notice the decimal point in the written instructions and filled the syringe with 1 mL of antigen.
2. The amount of antigen should have been written as 0.1 mL
3. The phlebotomist should not have left the student alone. If she had watched her throughout the process, she would have caught the error.
4. The patient received approximately five times as much antigen as the standard dose. If the patient had been exposed to TB, he or she could have a severe reaction.

Chapter 5

ANSWERS TO STUDY AND REVIEW QUESTIONS

1. b	5. d	9. c
2. d	6. b	10. b
3. c	7. c	
4. c	8. a	

ANSWERS TO CASE STUDIES

Case Study 5-1: Body System Structures and Disorders

1. The term for muscle pain is *myalgia*. Soreness of the tendons is most likely due to tendonitis (tendon inflammation).
2. The fluid-filled sac in the area of the elbow is called a bursa. Bursae help ease movement over and around areas subject to friction, such as prominent

joint parts or where tendons pass over bone. Inflammation of the bursa is called bursitis.

3. The student's leg muscles and tendons are probably stressed from the long weekend runs. Bursitis of the elbow most likely resulted from the long periods of lying on the floor resting on her elbows.

Case Study 5-2: Body Systems, Disorders, Diagnostic Tests, and Directional Terms

1. Glucose and insulin levels evaluate the endocrine system and the function of the pancreas, which is also an accessory organ of the digestive system.
2. The patient may be a diabetic who is either in insulin shock or diabetic coma.
3. The specimen was collected from the left arm, below the IV.

Chapter 6

ANSWERS TO STUDY AND REVIEW QUESTIONS

1. a	6. a	11. a
2. c	7. c	12. a
3. c	8. b	13. c
4. a	9. b	14. d
5. c	10. d	15. c

ANSWERS TO CASE STUDIES

Case Study 6-1: M-shaped Antecubital Veins

1. The median vein is the first choice for venipuncture in the M-shaped pattern.
2. The median cephalic vein is the second choice for venipuncture in the M-shaped pattern.
3. The median basilic vein is the last choice for venipuncture in the M-shaped pattern.
4. It is the last choice because it lies near the anterior and posterior branches of the medial cutaneous nerve and the brachial artery.

Case Study 6-2: Blood Specimens

1. The specimen was whole blood.
2. The part of the specimen that will be used for testing is the clear liquid called plasma, which was obtained by centrifuging the specimen.
3. A whole-blood specimen is collected in an anticoagulant tube. Blood collected in anticoagulant can be centrifuged right away to obtain plasma. The specimen was most likely whole blood because the processor was able to spin it right away, even though it had been collected only 5 minutes before she received it. In addition, most stat chemistry tests are performed on heparinized plasma, so as to save the time it would take to obtain serum from a clotted specimen.

Chapter 7

ANSWERS TO STUDY AND REVIEW QUESTIONS

1. d	5. b	9. b	13. d
2. b	6. a	10. b	14. d
3. d	7. d	11. d	15. b
4. b	8. c	12. b	

ANSWERS TO CASE STUDIES

Case Study 7-1: Proper Handling of Anticoagulant Tubes

1. Clots in EDTA specimens can be caused by inadequate mixing, a delay in mixing, or a delay in transferring a specimen collected in a syringe.
2. The clot in the CBC specimen was most likely caused by the delay in mixing it.
3. Yes. The problem with the second lavender-top tube led to an even greater delay in mixing the specimen, which most likely contributed to the clotting problem.
4. No. If Chi had mixed the first lavender-top tube as soon as he removed it from the tube holder, before putting it down, the problem with the second tube would not have affected it.
5. Chi can prevent this from happening in the future by mixing all additive tubes as soon as they are removed from the tube holder.

Case Study 7-2: Order of Draw

1. The green-top tube for the stat electrolytes is compromised.
2. The specimen is compromised because it was drawn after the EDTA tube and may be contaminated by carryover of EDTA. Sodium or potassium levels (depending on the type of EDTA) may be increased by EDTA contamination.
3. If the situation were to arise in the future, Jake could draw a few milliliters of blood into a plain discard tube to flush possible contamination from the needle before collecting the green-top tube. If he did not have a discard tube, he could use an SST or another green-top tube as the discard tube. Placing and removing a discard tube also helps remove residue on the outside of the needle. Jake should still indicate how the specimen was collected in case interference is suspected by lab personnel.

Chapter 8

ANSWERS TO STUDY AND REVIEW QUESTIONS

1. c	6. b	11. d	16. d
2. d	7. a	12. c	17. d
3. b	8. a	13. a	18. a
4. b	9. d	14. b	19. b
5. b	10. c	15. b	20. d

ANSWERS TO CASE STUDIES

Case Study 8-1: Patient Identification

1. Jenny didn't ask the patient to verbally state her name and date of birth.
2. Jenny assumed that because the woman was the only one left in the waiting room, she was the correct patient.
3. The patient may have been someone with a standing order who forgot to check in with the receptionist.
4. Specimens from the real Jane Rogers can be drawn after a new requisition and labels have been created. The identity of the other patient may be discovered when a physician's office calls for results and there are none. The specimens of the unknown patient will have to be discarded, which is especially unfortunate because the patient was a difficult draw.

Case Study 8-2: Blood Draw Refusal

1. The phlebotomists did not obtain parental permission personally or check with the child's nurse to see if parental permission had been given for the blood draw.
2. The phlebotomists made the assumption that because permission to draw a specimen from the child had been given previously, that it was all right to do so again this time. They also made the assumption that the child was not telling the truth.
3. A lawsuit alleging assault and battery could be filed by the parents.

Chapter 9

ANSWERS TO STUDY AND REVIEW QUESTIONS

1. b	5. a	9. b	13. a
2. b	6. b	10. d	14. c
3. c	7. a	11. a	15. b
4. c	8. b	12. a	

ANSWERS TO CASE STUDIES

Case Study 9-1: Physiological Variables, Problem Sites, and Patient Complications

1. Physiological variables associated with this collection site include the following: the patient is ill and may be dehydrated from vomiting, she is overweight, she has had a mastectomy on the left side, and she is normally a difficult draw. Charles will be limited to drawing from the right arm. He will most likely need to draw the specimen using a butterfly and the smallest tubes available. He should check the cephalic vein if he does not find another suitable antecubital vein. He may have to draw from a vein in the right hand, and he may have to warm the site to enhance blood flow. Because it is a physician office laboratory,

he should check with the patient's physician to see if it is advisable to offer the patient water, because she is probably dehydrated. Dehydration would make it even more difficult to find a vein.
2. Because the patient appears ill, she should be asked to lie down to prevent her from fainting during specimen collection. An emesis basin or wastebasket should be close at hand in case she vomits.
3. Charles should check the antecubital area of the right arm first, paying particular attention to the area of the cephalic vein if the median cubital vein is not palpable. If no suitable vein is found, he should check for a hand vein on the right arm, followed by veins on the right dorsal wrist and forearm. He should never consider using veins on the underside (ventral or palmar area) of the wrist or forearm.
4. If Charles is unable to find a proper venipuncture site, he should consider capillary puncture. Both the CBC and glucose specimens can easily be collected by capillary puncture. The site will have to be warmed to enhance blood flow because the patient may be dehydrated.

Case Study 9-2: Troubleshooting Failed Venipuncture

1. Blood most likely spurted into the tube because although Sara thought the needle was in the vein, it may have been only partially in the vein, with a tiny portion of it sticking out of the skin. Therefore the tube quickly lost vacuum.
2. The hissing sound and the fact that the tube no longer filled with blood even after the needle was repositioned are clues that the tube has lost vacuum.
3. Sara must position the needle in the vein, making certain that no part of the needle is out of the skin; then she must replace the tube with a new one.

Chapter 10

ANSWERS TO STUDY AND REVIEW QUESTIONS

1. b	5. d	9. b	13. b
2. d	6. a	10. d	14. d
3. d	7. d	11. b	15. b
4. c	8. b	12. c	

ANSWERS TO CASE STUDIES

Case Study 10-1: Capillary Puncture Procedure

1. The phlebotomist tried to collect the specimen as it was running down the finger. A scooping or scraping motion during collection may have activated the platelets and caused them to clump. In addition, because the child was uncooperative, the specimen was not collected and mixed quickly, which may also have contributed to platelet clumping.

2. It appears that the phlebotomist started to collect the specimen without wiping away the first drop of blood. Consequently the hemolysis may have been caused by alcohol residue. Trying to collect the specimen as it ran down the finger may have resulted in scraping the blood from the skin, which can also cause hemolysis in the specimen.

3. Improper direction of puncture and the presence of alcohol residue may have contributed to the blood running down the finger instead of forming drops, making it hard to collect the specimen. The phlebotomist's inexperience with children may have contributed to the child being uncooperative. In addition, if the phlebotomist had been more experienced with capillary puncture in children, he may have held the child's hand differently and prevented the child from pulling away.

Case Study 10-2: Stat Draw Turns Micro

1. Casey forgot to write on the labels that the microtubes contain venous blood. That is a problem because without that information it will be assumed that the specimens were collected by capillary puncture.

2. The results could be interpreted incorrectly because the concentration of glucose and potassium are higher in capillary blood than venous blood.

3. The CBC is compromised because the tube was not filled to the required level. Excess anticoagulant in an underfilled microtube can negatively affect test results. The delay in filling and in mixing the EDTA tube could also lead to microclots that would make the specimen unsuitable for testing.

Chapter 11

ANSWERS TO STUDY AND REVIEW QUESTIONS

1. a	5. c	9. d
2. b	6. c	10. b
3. a	7. c	11. b
4. b	8. c	12. b

ANSWERS TO CASE STUDIES

Case Study 11-1: Performing a Glucose Tolerance Test

1. Mr. Smith should finish drinking the glucose drink within 5 minutes.

2. The timing for all of the GTT specimens begins when the patient finishes the glucose drink. The patient was given the drink at 08:25. If he finishes it on time at 08:30, the 1-hour specimen would be collected at 09:30.

3. No. A level of 300 mg/dL at 30 minutes is abnormal according to the graph in Figure 11-12.

4. Normally, if a patient vomits within the first 30 minutes of a GTT, the test is discontinued and rescheduled. If the patient vomits after 45 minutes, the patient's physician should be consulted to determine if the test should be continued or not.

Case Study 11-2: POCT in the ER

1. The four electrolyte tests that are normally ordered are potassium, sodium, chloride, and carbon dioxide.

2. Yes, 2 to 3 drops of either venous or arterial blood can be used.

3. When an elevated potassium, such as 6.7 mEq/L, is reported and not supported by other clinical findings, the physician suspects a preanalytical error.

4. In this case, the nurse who drew the specimen through the IV valve did affect the results. Studies have shown that drawing blood through the valve of an IV will hemolyze the specimen and result in a falsely elevated potassium level.

Chapter 12

ANSWERS TO STUDY AND REVIEW QUESTIONS

1. b	6. c	11. a	16. b
2. d	7. d	12. a	17. c
3. b	8. b	13. d	18. b
4. b	9. d	14. d	19. c
5. a	10. d	15. c	20. c

ANSWERS TO CASE STUDIES

Case Study 12-1: The Case of the Missing Results

1. Nurse Susan may have used the label for Betty Smith on the specimens she collected from Mr. Jones.

2. The lab reports results according to the identification on the specimen, with the assumption that it is correctly labeled.

3. Nurse Susan will have to follow hospital protocol, which typically involves reprinting a lab slip and recollecting the specimen.

4. The results on Mrs. Smith will have to be removed from all records and the reason why they are being removed must be documented according to laboratory protocol.

Case Study 12-2: A Cooled Specimen Gets a Chilly Reception

1. Yes. The three tubes drawn could have been sufficient for all three tests. Ammonia specimens are typically collected in EDTA tubes. (Some methods require a heparin tube.) CBCs are drawn in purple tops. Stat electrolytes are typically drawn in lithium heparin tubes.

2. The most likely reason the electrolyte specimen needed to be recollected is that the specimen was

rejected for testing by the specimen processing technician. The likely reason it was rejected was because the phlebotomist put both the green top and the purple top in ice slurry because he wasn't sure which tube to use for the ammonia. Potassium is one of the electrolytes measured when electrolytes are ordered. Potassium levels artificially increase if the specimen is chilled because cold inhibits the glycolysis that provides the energy to pump potassium into the cells. With glycolysis inhibited, potassium leaks from the cells, falsely elevating levels in the specimen. An electrolyte specimen transported in ice slurry is a cause for rejection of the specimen for testing.

3. The problem could have been prevented if the phlebotomist had verified what type of tube was needed before he collected the specimen.

Chapter 13

ANSWERS TO STUDY AND REVIEW QUESTIONS

1. d	5. c	9. b	13. a
2. c	6. c	10. b	14. a
3. d	7. d	11. b	15. d
4. d	8. a	12. c	

ANSWERS TO CASE STUDIES

Case Study 13-1: 24-Hour Urine Specimen Collection

1. No. The specimen is missing a critical portion of urine.
2. The phlebotomist should not accept the specimen without first consulting a supervisor. Whether or not the specimen will be accepted depends upon the type of test and individual lab policy and may require consultation with the patient's physician. If it is determined that the specimen will be accepted, the phlebotomist should note the discrepancy in collection time and identify the person who authorized acceptance on the requisition or by computer entry.
3. Patients should be given verbal and written instructions in 24-hour urine collection procedures and verbal feedback should be obtained to ensure that the patient has complete understanding of the procedure. Patients should be made aware of the importance of timing and reminded to set an alarm if necessary.

Case Study 13-2: DNA Specimen Collection

1. The phlebotomist relied on her memory and did not appreciate the fact that procedures can change

quickly in the laboratory. She neglected to check the test catalog to find out what specimen should have been collected. Because she was in a hurry, she did not read the requisition carefully enough to see the important note attached.

2. The sample tested can be from a blood draw, but the buccal smear is the preferred specimen especially in this case, when the doctor specifically ordered "no blood draw."
3. When the patient returned with blood on his clothes from the puncture site that was still bleeding, the phlebotomist should immediately care for the patient until the bleeding has stopped. It is the laboratory's responsibility to notify the patient's physician/healthcare provider as soon as possible concerning the incident and to reimburse the patient for any cleaning bill associated with the incident.

Chapter 14

ANSWERS TO STUDY AND REVIEW QUESTIONS

1. b	5. b	9. d
2. d	6. b	10. c
3. b	7. c	
4. d	8. d	

ANSWERS TO CASE STUDIES

Case Study 14-1: Complications of ABG Collection

1. The phlebotomist should alert the patient's nurse to the problem.
2. A thrombus may be blocking blood flow and affecting the pulse.
3. The patient moving his arm very likely resulted in the phlebotomist missing the artery. In addition, the restless and agitated state of the patient may have contributed to an arteriospasm, which would have made it harder to hit the artery.
4. The phlebotomist should have made an attempt to calm the patient. In addition, he should have been prepared for movement by the patient, or he could have asked the patient's nurse to help steady the arm, since the patient was restless and agitated.
5. Although the specimen appears dark in color, the phlebotomist can be fairly certain that the specimen is arterial because it pulsed into the tube. It is probably dark in color because the patient has breathing difficulties.

Appendix F

Tube Guides

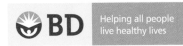

BD Vacutainer® Venous Blood Collection
Tube Guide

For the full array of BD Vacutainer® Blood Collection Tubes, visit www.bd.com/vacutainer.
Many are available in a variety of sizes and draw volumes (for pediatric applications). Refer to our website for full descriptions.

BD Vacutainer® Tubes with BD Hemogard™ Closure	BD Vacutainer® Tubes with Conventional Stopper	Additive	Inversions at Blood Collection*	Laboratory Use	Your Lab's Draw Volume/Remarks
Gold	Red/Gray	• Clot activator and gel for serum separation	5	For serum determinations in chemistry. May be used for routine blood donor screening and diagnostic testing of serum for infectious disease.** Tube inversions ensure mixing of clot activator with blood. Blood clotting time: 30 minutes.	
Light Green	Green/Gray	• Lithium heparin and gel for plasma separation	8	For plasma determinations in chemistry. Tube inversions ensure mixing of anticoagulant (heparin) with blood to prevent clotting.	
Red	Red	• Silicone coated (glass) • Clot activator, Silicone coated (plastic)	0 / 5	For serum determinations in chemistry. May be used for routine blood donor screening and diagnostic testing of serum for infectious disease.** Tube inversions ensure mixing of clot activator with blood. Blood clotting time: 60 minutes.	
Orange		• Thrombin-based clot activator with gel for serum separation	5 to 6	For stat serum determinations in chemistry. Tube inversions ensure mixing of clot activator with blood. Blood clotting time: 5 minutes.	
Orange		• Thrombin-based clot activator	8	For stat serum determinations in chemistry. Tube inversions ensure mixing of clot activator with blood. Blood clotting time: 5 minutes.	
Royal Blue		• Clot activator (plastic serum) • K₂EDTA (plastic)	8 / 8	For trace-element, toxicology, and nutritional-chemistry determinations. Special stopper formulation provides low levels of trace elements (see package insert). Tube inversions ensure mixing of either clot activator or anticoagulant (EDTA) with blood.	
Green	Green	• Sodium heparin • Lithium heparin	8 / 8	For plasma determinations in chemistry. Tube inversions ensure mixing of anticoagulant (heparin) with blood to prevent clotting.	
Gray	Gray	• Potassium oxalate/sodium fluoride • Sodium fluoride/Na₂ EDTA • Sodium fluoride (serum tube)	8 / 8 / 8	For glucose determinations. Oxalate and EDTA anticoagulants will give plasma samples. Sodium fluoride is the antiglycolytic agent. Tube inversions ensure proper mixing of additive with blood.	
Tan		• K₂EDTA (plastic)	8	For lead determinations. This tube is certified to contain less than .01 µg/mL(ppm) lead. Tube inversions prevent clotting.	
	Yellow	• Sodium polyanethol sulfonate (SPS) • Acid citrate dextrose additives (ACD): **Solution A -** 22.0 g/L trisodium citrate, 8.0 g/L citric acid, 24.5 g/L dextrose **Solution B -** 13.2 g/L trisodium citrate, 4.8 g/L citric acid, 14.7 g/L dextrose	8 / 8 / 8	SPS for blood culture specimen collections in microbiology. ACD for use in blood bank studies, HLA phenotyping, and DNA and paternity testing. Tube inversions ensure mixing of anticoagulant with blood to prevent clotting.	

(continued)

BD Vacutainer® Tubes with BD Hemogard™ Closure	BD Vacutainer® Tubes with Conventional Stopper	Additive	Inversions at Blood Collection*	Laboratory Use	Your Lab's Draw Volume/Remarks
Lavender	Lavender	• Liquid K_3EDTA (glass) • Spray-coated K_2EDTA (plastic)	8 8	K_2EDTA and K_3EDTA for whole blood hematology determinations. K_2EDTA may be used for routine immunohematology testing, and blood donor screening.*** Tube inversions ensure mixing of anticoagulant (EDTA) with blood to prevent clotting.	
White		• K_2EDTA and gel for plasma separation	8	For use in molecular diagnostic test methods (such as, but not limited to, polymerase chain reaction [PCR] and/or branched DNA [bDNA] amplification techniques.) Tube inversions ensure mixing of anticoagulant (EDTA) with blood to prevent clotting.	
Pink	Pink	• Spray-coated K_2EDTA (plastic)	8	For whole blood hematology determinations. May be used for routine immunohematology testing and blood donor screening.*** Designed with special cross-match label for patient information required by the AABB. Tube inversions prevent clotting.	
Light Blue / Clear	Light Blue	• Buffered sodium citrate 0.105 M (≈3.2%) glass 0.109 M (3.2%) plastic • Citrate, theophylline, adenosine, dipyridamole (CTAD)	3-4 3-4	For coagulation determinations. CTAD for selected platelet function assays and routine coagulation determination. Tube inversions ensure mixing of anticoagulant (citrate) to prevent clotting.	
Clear	New Red/ Light Gray	• None (plastic)	0	For use as a discard tube or secondary specimen tube.	

Note: BD Vacutainer® Tubes for pediatric and partial draw applications can be found on our website.

BD Diagnostics
Preanalytical Systems
1 Becton Drive
Franklin Lakes, NJ 07417 USA

BD Global Technical Services: 1.800.631.0174
BD Customer Service: 1.888.237.2762
www.bd.com/vacutainer

* Invert gently, do not shake
** The performance characteristics of these tubes have not been established for infectious disease testing in general; therefore, users must validate the use of these tubes for their specific assay-instrument/reagent system combinations and specimen storage conditions.
*** The performance characteristics of these tubes have not been established for immunohematology testing in general; therefore, users must validate the use of these tubes for their specific assay-instrument/reagent system combinations and specimen storage conditions.

Printed in USA   07/10   VS5229-13

Reprinted with permission from Becton Dickinson.

VACUETTE® Tube Guide
Venous Blood Collection Tubes

greiner bio-one

Cap Color	Additive	Number of Inversions	Testing Disciplines	Comments
	No Additive	5-10	Discard tube Transport/Storage Immunohematology Viral Markers	
	Sodium Citrate 3.2% (0.109 M) 3.8% (0.129 M)	4	Coagulation	If a winged blood collection set is used AND the coagulation specimen is drawn first, a discard tube is recommended to be drawn prior to this tube to ensure the proper anticoagulant-to-blood ratio.
	Clot Activator	5-10	Chemistry Immunochemistry Immunohematology Viral Markers	For complete clotting, 30 minutes minimum clotting time is required. Incomplete or delayed mixing may result in delayed clotting.
	Clot Activator w/Gel	5-10	Chemistry Immunochemistry TDMs	For complete clotting, 30 minutes minimum clotting time is required. Incomplete or delayed mixing may result in delayed clotting.
	Lithium Heparin Lithium Heparin w/Gel Sodium Heparin	5-10	Chemistry Immunochemistry	
	K_3 EDTA K_2 EDTA	8-10	Hematology Immunohematology Molecular Diagnostics Viral Markers	
	K_2 EDTA Gel	8-10	Molecular Diagnostics	
	Potassium Oxalate/ Sodium Fluoride	5-10	Glycolytic Inhibitor Glucose and Lactate	
	Sodium Heparin	5-10	Trace Elements	

Ring Indicator

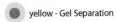 yellow - Gel Separation   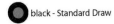 black - Standard Draw   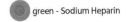 green - Sodium Heparin   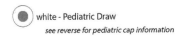 white - Pediatric Draw

see reverse for pediatric cap information

VACUETTE® Tube Guide

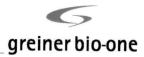

greiner bio-one

Pediatric or Small Volume Draw Tubes (2 ml or Less)

Cap Color	Additive	Number of Inversions	Testing Disciplines	Comments
	Clot Activator	5-10	Chemistry Immunochemistry Immunohematology Viral Markers	For complete clotting, 30 minutes minimum clotting time is required. Incomplete or delayed mixing may result in delayed clotting.
	Lithium Heparin Sodium Heparin	5-10	Chemistry Immunochemistry	
	Sodium Citrate 3.2% (0.109M) 3.8% (0.129M)	4	Coagulation	If a winged blood collection set is used AND the coagulation specimen is drawn first, a discard tube is recommended to be drawn prior to this tube to ensure the proper anticoagulant-to-blood ratio.
	Potassium Oxalate/ Sodium Fluoride	5-10	Glycolytic Inhibitor Glucose and Lactate	
	K_3 EDTA K_2 EDTA	8-10	Hematology Immunohematology Molecular Diagnostics Viral Markers	

Ring Indicator

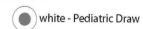 white - Pediatric Draw

Reprinted with permission from Greiner Bio-One.

Glossary

AABB: American Association of Blood Banks.

abdominal cavity: Body space between the diaphragm and the pelvis, which houses abdominal organs such as the stomach, liver, pancreas, gallbladder, spleen, and kidneys.

abducted: Away from the body; the position of the patient's arm for arterial blood gas collection.

ABGs: Arterial blood gases.

ABO blood group system: Four blood types, A, B, AB, and O, based on the presence or absence of two antigens identified as A and B.

ACA: Affordable Care Act.

accession: The process of recording in the order received.

accession number: A number generated by the laboratory information system (LIS) when the specimen request is entered into the computer.

acid citrate dextrose (ACD): An anticoagulant solution available in two formulations (solution A and solution B) for immunohematology tests such as DNA testing and human leukocyte antigen (HLA) phenotyping, which is used in paternity evaluation and to determine transplant compatibility.

acidosis: A dangerous condition in which the pH of the blood is abnormally low (acidic).

ACO: Accountable Care Organization.

ACT: Activated clotting time.

activated partial thromboplastin time (aPTT or PTT): Test used to evaluate the function of the intrinsic coagulation pathway and monitor heparin therapy.

additive: A substance (other than the tube stopper or coating) such as an anticoagulant, antiglycolytic agent, separator gel, preservative, or clot activator placed within a tube or collection container. An additive can be a liquid, powder, or spray-dried coating.

adipose: Denoting fat.

aerobic: With air.

aerosol: A fine mist of the specimen.

AFP: Alpha-fetoprotein.

agglutinate: To clump together; as in the antigen–antibody reaction between red blood cells of two different blood types.

agranulocytes: White blood cells (WBCs) that lack granules or have extremely fine granules that are not easy to see.

AHCCCS: Arizona Healthcare Cost Containment System.

AIIR: Airborne Infection Isolation Room.

airborne precautions: Precautions used in addition to standard precautions for patients known or suspected of being infected with microorganisms transmitted by airborne droplet nuclei.

airborne transmission: Transmission of disease by dispersal of evaporated droplet nuclei containing an infectious agent.

aliquot: A portion of a specimen used for testing.

alkalosis: A dangerous condition in which the pH of the blood is abnormally high (alkaline).

Allen test: A simple noninvasive test to assess collateral circulation before collecting a blood specimen from the radial artery.

alpha-fetoprotein (AFP): An antigen normally present in the human fetus that is also found in amniotic fluid and maternal serum. It is also present in certain pathological conditions in males and nonpregnant females.

alveoli: Tiny air sacs in the lungs where the exchange of oxygen and carbon dioxide takes place.

amniotic fluid: Clear, almost colorless to pale-yellow fluid that fills the membrane (amnion or amniotic sac) surrounding and cushioning a fetus in the uterus.

AMT: American Medical Technologists.

anabolism: A constructive process by which the body converts simple compounds into complex substances needed to carry out the cellular activities of the body.

anaerobic: Without air.

analyte: A general term for a substance undergoing analysis or being measured.

anatomic position: The position of standing erect, arms at the side, with eyes and palms facing forward. In describing the direction or the location of a given point of the body, medical personnel normally refer to the body as if the patient were in the anatomic position, regardless of actual body position.

anatomy: The structure of an organism, or the science of the structural composition of living organisms. In humans, the structural composition of the body.

anchor: To secure firmly, as in holding a vein in place by pulling the skin taut with the thumb.

anemia: An abnormal reduction in the number of red blood cells (RBCs) in the circulating blood.

antecubital fossa: The area of the arm that is anterior to (in front of) and below the bend of the elbow, where the major veins for venipuncture are located.

antecubital veins: Major superficial veins located in the antecubital fossa.

anterior: Pertaining to or referring to the front of the body; also called ventral.

antibody: Protein substance manufactured by the body in response to a foreign protein or antigen and directed against it.

anticoagulant: A substance that prevents blood from clotting.

antigen: A substance that causes the formation of antibodies directed against it.

antiglycolytic agent: A substance that prevents glycolysis, the breakdown or metabolism of glucose (blood sugar) by blood cells—e.g., sodium fluoride.

antimicrobial removal device (ARD): Blood culture bottle containing a resin that removes antimicrobials (antibiotics) from a blood specimen.

antimicrobial therapy: Use of antibiotics to kill or inhibit the growth of microorganisms.

antiseptic: A substance that inhibits the growth of bacteria and is used to clean the skin.

aorta: The largest artery in the body, arising from the left ventricle of the heart; it is approximately 1 inch (2.5 cm) in diameter.

APC: Ambulatory patient classification.

ARD: Antimicrobial removal device.

armband/wristband: Two other names for an identification band or bracelet.

arrhythmia: Irregularity in the heart rate, rhythm, or beat.

arterial line (A-line or Art-line): A catheter that is placed in an artery. It is most commonly placed in a radial artery and is typically used to provide accurate and continuous measurement of a patient's blood pressure, to collect blood gas specimens and other blood specimens, and for the administration of drugs such as dopamine.

arterialized: Arterial composition of capillary blood has been increased by warming the site to increase blood flow.

arteries: Blood vessels that carry blood away from the heart.

arterioles: The smallest branches of arteries, which join with the capillaries.

arteriospasm: A reflex (involuntary) contraction of the artery that can be caused by pain or irritation during needle penetration of the artery muscle or that may result from a patient's anxiety during arterial puncture.

arteriovenous (AV) shunt: Surgical fusion or artificial connection of an artery and a vein. It is typically created to provide access for dialysis; includes AV fistula and graft.

ASAP: As soon as possible.

ASCLS: American Society for Clinical Laboratory Sciences.

ASCP: American Society for Clinical Pathology.

aseptic: Sterile or pathogen free.

assault: An act or threat causing another to be in fear of immediate battery.

atria (singular, atrium): The upper receiving chambers on each side of the heart.

atrioventricular (AV) valves: The valves at the entrances to the ventricles.

autologous donation: Blood that is donated for one's own use.

avascular: Without blood or lymph vessels.

AV fistula: Permanent surgical fusion of an artery and vein that is typically created to provide access for dialysis.

AV graft: Surgical connection of an artery and vein using a piece of vein or artificial tubing.

AV shunt/fistula/graft: Permanent surgical fusion or artificial connection of an artery and vein that is typically created to provide access for dialysis.

avulsion: A tearing away or amputation of a body part.

axons: Threadlike fibers that carry messages away from the nerve cell body.

BAC: Blood alcohol concentration.

bacteremia: Bacteria in the blood.

bar code: A series of black stripes and white spaces of varying widths that correspond to letters and numbers.

bariatric: Pertaining to the treatment of obesity.

barrel: A term for the cylindrical body of a syringe, which has graduated markings in either milliliters (mL) or cubic centimeters (cc).

basal state: The resting metabolic state of the body early in the morning after fasting for a minimum of 12 hours.

basilic vein: Large vein on the inner side of the antecubital area that is the last choice vein for venipuncture.

basophils (basos): Normally the least numerous WBCs, they release histamine and heparin, which enhance the inflammatory response; identified by their large dark blue–staining granules, which often obscure a typically S-shaped nucleus.

battery: Intentional harmful or offensive touching or use of force on a person without that person's consent or legal justification.

BBP: Bloodborne pathogen.

bedside manner: The behavior of a healthcare provider toward or as perceived by a patient.

bevel: The point of a needle that is cut on a slant for ease of skin entry.

bicarbonate ion (HCO$_3^-$): An ion that plays a role in transporting carbon dioxide (CO_2) in the blood to the lungs and in regulating blood pH. HCO_3^- is formed in the red blood cells and plasma from CO_2.

bilirubin: A product of the breakdown of red blood cells.

biobank: A type of repository or bank where human biological samples such as, blood, saliva, plasma, skin cells, and organ tissues can be stored and used in research.

biohazard: Short for biological hazard; anything potentially harmful to health.

biosafety: Term used to describe the safe handling of biologic substances that pose a risk to health.

bleeding time (BT): Test that measures the time required for blood to stop flowing from a standardized puncture on the inner surface of the forearm.

blood alcohol concentration (BAC): Concentration of alcohol in a person's blood used as a measurement of intoxication for legal or medical purposes.

blood film/smear: A drop of blood spread thinly on a microscope slide.

blood pressure: A measure of the force (pressure) exerted by the blood on the walls of blood vessels.

bloodborne pathogen (BBP): Term applied to infectious microorganisms in blood or other body fluids.

Bloodborne Pathogens (BBP) Standard: OSHA regulations designed to protect employees with potential occupational exposure to pathogens found in blood or other body fluids or substances.

BNP: B-type natriuretic peptide.

body cavities: Large, hollow spaces in the body that house the various organs.

body plane: A flat surface resulting from a real or imaginary cut through a body in the normal anatomic position.

body substance isolation (BSI): Infection control precautions that preceded standard precautions and differed from universal precautions by requiring glove use when contacting any moist body substance.

brachial artery: Artery located in the medial anterior aspect of the antecubital fossa near the insertion of the biceps muscle; the second choice for arterial puncture.

bradycardia: Slow heart rate; less than 60 beats per minute.

breach of confidentiality: Failure to keep privileged medical information private.

bronchi (singular, bronchus): Two airways that branch off of the lower end of the trachea and lead into the lungs; one branch into the left and another into the right lung.

BT: Bleeding time test.

B-type natriuretic peptide (BNP): Cardiac hormone produced by the heart in response to ventricular volume expansion and pressure overload.

buccal swabs: Swabs of material collected from the inside of the cheek.

buffy coat: The layer of WBCs and platelets that forms between the RBCs and plasma when anticoagulated blood settles or is centrifuged.

bursae (singular, bursa): Small synovial fluid-filled sacs in the vicinity of joints; they ease friction between joint parts or tendons and bone.

butterfly needle: Another term for a winged infusion set.

C&S: Culture and sensitivity.

calcaneus: Medical term for heel bone.

calcium (Ca): A mineral that is essential to the clotting process and also needed for proper bone and tooth formation, nerve conduction, and muscle contraction.

CAP: College of American Pathologists.

capillaries: Microscopic one-cell-thick vessels that connect the arterioles and venules, forming a bridge between the arterial and venous circulations.

carbaminohemoglobin: Carbon dioxide combined with hemoglobin.

cardiac cycle: One complete contraction and subsequent relaxation of the heart.

cardiac output: Volume of blood pumped by the heart in 1 minute, averaging 5 L per minute.

cardiac troponin I (TnI): A protein specific to heart muscle.

cardiac troponin T (TnT): Heart muscle–specific protein; elevated longer than TnI.

carryover: Cross-contamination or transfer of additive from one tube to the next.

cartilage: A type of hard, nonvascular connective tissue.

case manager: The person who coordinates medical services on behalf of a patient.

catabolism: The process by which complex substances are broken down into simple ones, including the digestion of food.

catheterized: Term describing a urine specimen collected from a sterile catheter inserted through the urethra into the bladder.

causative agent: The pathogen responsible for causing an infection; also called the infectious agent.

CBGs: Capillary blood gases (CBGs); blood gas determinations performed on arterialized capillary specimens.

celite: An inert clay that enhances the coagulation process.

Celsius: A temperature scale on which the melting point is 0 degree and the boiling point is 100 degrees. Normal body temperature expressed in Celsius is 37 degrees; also known as the Centigrade scale.

Centers for Disease Control and Prevention (CDC): The division of the U.S. Public Health Service charged with the investigation and control of disease with epidemic potential.

Centigrade: *see* Celsius.

central nervous system (CNS): The brain and spinal cord.

central processing: Screening and prioritizing area where specimens are received and prepared for testing.

central vascular access device (CVAD): Indwelling line; tubing inserted into a main vein or artery used primarily for administering fluids and medications, monitoring pressures, and drawing blood.

central venous catheter (CVC): A line inserted into a large vein such as the subclavian and advanced into the superior vena cava, proximal to the right atrium. The exit end is surgically tunneled under the skin to a site several inches away in the chest; also called central venous line.

centrifuge: A machine that spins the blood tubes at a high number of revolutions per minute.

cephalic vein: The second-choice antecubital vein for venipuncture, located in the lateral aspect of the antecubital fossa.

cerebrospinal fluid (CSF): Clear, colorless liquid that circulates within the cavities surrounding the brain and spinal cord; it has many of the same components as plasma.

certification: Evidence that an individual has mastered fundamental competencies in a particular technical area.

CEUs: Continuing education units.

CF: Cystic fibrosis.

chain of custody: Special strict protocol for forensic specimens that requires detailed documentation tracking the specimen from the time it is collected until the results are reported.

chain of infection: A number of components or events that, when present in a series, lead to an infection.

chloride (Cl⁻): Electrolyte responsible for maintaining cellular integrity by influencing osmotic pressure and acid–base and water balance.

chordae tendineae: Thin threads of tissue that attach the atrioventricular valves to the walls of the ventricles to help keep them from flipping back into the atria.

circadian: Biologic rhythms or variations having a 24-hour cycle.

circulatory system: System that consists of the cardiovascular system (heart, blood, and blood vessels) and the lymphatic system (lymph, lymph vessels, and nodes) and is the means by which oxygen and nutrients are carried to the cells and carbon dioxide and other wastes are carried away from them.

civil action: Legal actions in which the alleged injured party sues for monetary damages.

Cl⁻: Chloride.

clay sealant: A type of sealer used for closing the end of a microhematocrit tube.

clean catch: Method of obtaining a urine sample so that it is free of contamination from the external genital area.

CLIA '88: Clinical Laboratory Improvement Amendments of 1988.

Clinical and Laboratory Standards Institute (CLSI): A global, nonprofit, standards-developing organization comprising representatives from the profession, industry, and government.

clot activator: A substance that enhances the coagulation process.

CLSI: Clinical and Laboratory Standards Institute.

CMS: Center for Medicare and Medicaid Services.

coagulation: The blood-clotting process.

coagulation cascade: Sequential activation of the coagulation factors.

collateral circulation: An area supplied with blood from more than one artery so that circulation can be maintained if one vessel is obstructed.

combining form: A word root combined with a vowel.

combining vowel: A vowel (frequently an "o") that is added between two word roots or a word root and a suffix to make pronunciation easier.

common pathway: Coagulation pathway involving the conversion of prothrombin to thrombin, which splits fibrinogen into the fibrin that entraps blood cells and creates the fibrin clot.

communicable: Able to spread from person to person, as a disease.

communication barriers: Biases or personalized filters that are major obstructions to verbal communication.

compatibility: Ability to be mixed together with favorable results, as in blood transfusions.

competencies: Educational standards for phlebotomy programs.

concentric circles: Circles with a common center; starting from the center and moving outward in ever-widening arcs.

confidentiality: The ethical cornerstone of professional behavior; the practice of regarding information concerning a patient as privileged and not to be disclosed to anyone without the patient's authorization.

contact precautions: Precautions used in addition to standard precautions when a patient is known or suspected of being infected or colonized with epidemiologically important microorganisms that can be transmitted by direct contact with the patient or indirect contact with surfaces or patient-care items.

contact transmission: Transfer of an infectious agent to a susceptible host through direct or indirect contact. *See* direct and indirect contact transmission.

continuous quality improvement (CQI): An ongoing effort to improve the quality of service.

continuum of care: A holistic, coordinated system for healthcare services.

coronary arteries: Arteries that branch off of the aorta just beyond the aortic semilunar valve that deliver blood to the heart muscle.

CPD: Citrate-phosphate-dextrose, an additive used in collecting units of blood for transfusion. Citrate prevents clotting by chelating calcium, phosphate stabilizes pH, and dextrose provides cells with energy and helps keep them alive.

CPT: Current procedural terminology.

CPU: Central processing unit.

CQI: Continuous Quality Improvement.

cranial cavity: Body space that houses the brain.

criminal action: Legal recourse for offenses committed against the law that can lead to imprisonment of the offender.

CRP: C-reactive protein.

C-reactive protein (CRP): A β-globulin found in the blood that responds to inflammation and therefore can be used as a sensitive though nonspecific marker of systemic inflammation.

crossmatch: A test to determine suitability of mixing donor and recipient blood.

CSF: Cerebrospinal fluid.

culture and sensitivity (C&S): Microbiology test that includes placing a specimen on special nutrient media which encourages the growth of microorganisms, identifying any that grow, and then performing sensitivity/antibiotic susceptibility testing to identify antibiotics that will be effective against them.

C-urea breath test: A test used to detect *Helicobacter pylori* bacteria based on the fact that the bacteria produce urease, an enzyme that breaks down urea and is not normally present in the stomach.

cursor: Flashing indicator on the computer screen.

CVAD: Central vascular access device.

CVC: Central venous catheter.

cyanotic: Marked by cyanosis or a bluish color from lack of oxygen.

cystic fibrosis: Disorder of the exocrine glands that affects many body systems but primarily the lungs, upper respiratory tract, liver, and pancreas resulting in abnormally high levels (two to five times normal) of chloride in the sweat.

data: Information collected for analysis or computation.

defendant: In a lawsuit, a person or persons against whom a complaint is filed.

delta check: Comparison of current results of a lab test with previous results for the same test on the same patient.

dendrites: Structures that carry messages to the nerve cell body.

deposition: A process in which one party questions another under oath while a court reporter records every word.

dermis: Corium or true skin; a layer composed of elastic and fibrous connective tissue.

diapedesis: Process by which WBCs slip through the walls of the capillaries into the tissues.

diaphragm: The dome-shaped muscle that separates the abdominal cavity from the thoracic cavity.

diastole: The relaxing phase of the cardiac cycle.

diastolic pressure: Pressure in the arteries during relaxation of the ventricles.

differential (diff): A test in which the number, type, and characteristics of blood cells are determined by examining a stained blood smear under a microscope.

direct contact transmission: Transfer of an infectious agent to a susceptible host through close or intimate contact, such as touching or kissing.

directional terms: Medical terms that describe the relationship of an area or part of the body with respect to the rest of the body or body part.

discard tube: Also called a clear tube; a tube used to collect and discard approximately 5 mL of blood to prevent IV or tissue fluid contamination of a specimen.

discovery: Formal process in litigation that involves taking depositions and interrogating the parties involved.

disinfectant: Substance or solution used to remove or kill microorganisms on surfaces and instruments.

distal: Farthest from the center of the body, origin, or point of attachment.

diurnal: Happening daily.

DNAR: Do not attempt resuscitation.

DNR: Do not resuscitate.

"Do Not Use" list: A list of confusing (or potentially dangerous) abbreviations, symbols, and acronyms that must be included on this list by every organization accredited by the Joint Commission.

dorsal: Posterior or pertaining to the back.

dorsal cavities: Internal spaces located in the back of the body.

DOT: Department of Transportation.

DRGs: Diagnosis-related groups.

droplet precautions: Precautions used in addition to standard precautions for patients known or suspected of being infected with microorganisms transmitted by droplets (particles larger than 5 µm) generated when a patient talks, coughs, or sneezes and during certain procedures such as suctioning.

droplet transmission: Transfer of an infectious agent to the mucous membranes of the mouth, nose, or conjunctiva of the eyes via infectious droplets (particles 5 µm in diameter or larger) generated by talking, coughing, sneezing, or during procedures such as suctioning.

drug screening: The practice of testing employees' or athletes' urine or blood to screen for illicit or illegal drugs.

due care: The level of care that a person of ordinary intelligence and good sense would exercise under the given circumstances.

edema: Swelling due to abnormal accumulation of fluid in the tissues.

EDTA: Ethylenediaminetetraacetic acid, an anticoagulant that prevents coagulation by binding or chelating calcium; it is used for hematology studies because it preserves cell morphology and inhibits platelet clumping.

electrocardiogram (ECG or EKG): An actual record of the electrical currents corresponding to each event in heart muscle contraction.

electrolytes: Substances such as potassium or sodium that conduct electricity when dissolved in water.

EMLA: A eutectic (easily melted) mixture of local anesthetics.

endocardium: The thin inner layer of the heart.

endocrine glands: Glands that secrete hormones directly into the bloodstream.

engineering controls: Devices such as sharps disposal containers and needles with safety features that isolate or remove a bloodborne pathogen hazard from the workplace.

"enter" key: Button on keyboard for data input.

Environmental Protection Agency (EPA): A federal agency that regulates the disposal of hazardous waste.

eosinophils (eos): WBCs that ingest and detoxify foreign protein, helping to turn off immune reactions; they increase with allergies and pinworm infestations and are identified by their beadlike, bright orange-red–staining granules.

EPA: Environmental Protection Agency.

epicardium: The thin outer layer of the heart.

epidermis: The outermost and thinnest layer of the skin.

epiglottis: A thin, leaf-shaped structure that covers the entrance of the larynx during swallowing.

epithelial: Consisting of epithelium.

epithelium: The avascular layer of cells that forms the epidermis and the surface layer of mucous and serous membranes.

EQC: Electronic quality control.

erythema: Redness.

erythrocytes: Red blood cells (RBCs); anuclear, disk-shaped blood cells whose main function is to carry oxygen from the lungs to the tissue cells and to transport carbon dioxide away from the cells to the lungs.

esophagus: The tube that carries food and liquid from the throat to the stomach.

ethanol: Ethyl or grain alcohol.

ETOH: Abbreviation for ethanol or blood alcohol.

evacuated tube: Type of tube used in blood collection that has a premeasured vacuum and is color coded to denote the additive inside.

evacuated tube system (ETS): A closed system in which the patient's blood flows directly into a collection tube through a needle inserted into a vein.

exocrine glands: Glands that secrete substances through ducts.

expectorate: Spit; the act of forcibly ejecting saliva or other substances from the mouth.

exsanguinate: To remove all blood.

exsanguination: Blood loss to a point where life cannot be sustained.

external: On or near the surface of the body; superficial.

external respiration: Exchange of respiratory gases in the lungs.

extrasystoles: Extra heartbeats before the normal beat.

extravascular: Outside the blood vessels.

extrinsic pathway: Coagulation pathway initiated by the release of thromboplastin from injured tissue.

FAA: Federal Aviation Administration.

fallopian tubes: Ducts that carry ova from the ovaries to the uterus.

FAN: Fastidious antimicrobial neutralization.

fastidious antimicrobial neutralization (FAN): Blood culture bottle that contains activated charcoal that neutralizes antibiotics in a blood specimen.

fasting: No food or drink except water for approximately 12 hours.

feather: Thinnest area of a properly made blood smear where a differential is performed.

fecal occult blood test: A test that detects hidden (occult) blood in stool (feces).

femoral artery: Large artery located superficially in the groin, lateral to the pubic bone; it is the largest artery used for arterial puncture.

fibrillations: Rapid, uncoordinated contractions.

fibrin degradation products (fibrin split products): Fragments remaining from the breakdown of fibrin.

fibrin: A filamentous protein formed by the action of thrombin on fibrinogen.

fibrinogen: Also called factor I; a protein found in plasma that is essential for the clotting of blood.

fibrinolysis: Stage 4 of hemostasis; a process that results in the removal or dissolution of a blood clot once healing has occurred.

FiO$_2$: Fraction of inspired oxygen, as in oxygen therapy.

fire tetrahedron: The latest way of looking at the chemistry of fire, in which the chemical reaction that produces fire is added as a fourth component to the traditional fire triangle components of fuel, heat, and oxygen.

fistula: A dialysis shunt created by direct permanent fusion of the artery and vein.

FIT: Fecal immunochemical test, also called immunochemical fecal occult blood test, iFOBT.

flanges: Extensions on the sides of an evacuated tube holder that aid in tube placement and removal.

flea: Small metal bar that is inserted into the tube after collection of a capillary blood gas specimen to aid in mixing the anticoagulant by means of a magnet.

FOBT: Fecal occult blood test.

fomites: Inanimate objects, such as countertops and computer keyboards, that can harbor material containing infectious agents.

forensic specimen: Specimen collected for legal reasons.

formed elements: Cellular portion of the blood.

fraud: Deceitful practice or false portrayal of facts by either words or conduct.

frontal plane: Divides the body vertically into front and back portions; also called coronal plane.

FUO: Fever of unknown origin.

galactosemia: Inherited disorder caused by lack of the enzyme needed to convert the milk sugar galactose into glucose, which is needed by the body to produce energy.

gallbladder: Accessory organ to the digestive system.

gametes: Sex cells.

gastric analysis: A test that examines stomach contents for abnormal substances and measures gastric acid concentration to evaluate stomach acid production.

gastrointestinal (GI) tract: The passageway that extends from the mouth to the anus through the pharynx, esophagus, stomach, and small and large intestines.

gatekeeper: Primary physician who serves as the patient's advocate and advises the patient on his or her healthcare needs.

gauge: A number that relates to the diameter of the lumen of a needle.

germ cells: Gametes or sex cells.

germicide: An agent that kills pathogenic microorganisms.

glomerulus: A tuft of capillaries that filter water and dissolved substances, including wastes, from the blood.

GLPs: Good laboratory practices.

glucose tolerance test (GTT): A test used to diagnose carbohydrate metabolism problems.

glycolysis: The breakdown or metabolism of glucose (blood sugar) by blood cells.

glycosylated hemoglobin: A substance that is increased in the RBCs of patients with diabetes mellitus and used as a retrospective index of glucose control over time.

gonads: Glands that manufacture and store gametes and produce hormones that regulate the reproductive process.

graft: A piece of a vein or tubing surgically made to form a loop from the artery to the vein that is just under the skin.

gram (g): The basic unit of weight in the metric system; approximately equal to a cubic centimeter or milliliter of water.

granulocytes: WBCs with easily visible granules.

great saphenous vein: The longest vein in the body, located in the leg.

GTT: Glucose tolerance test.

guaiac test: A test for hidden blood in feces; also called occult blood test.

HAI: Healthcare-associated infection.

hardware: Computer equipment used to process data.

Hazard Communication (HazCom) Standard: The OSHA Standard that requires employers to maintain documentation on all hazardous chemicals.

HazCom: Abbreviation for the OSHA Hazard Communication Standard.

HBV: Hepatitis B virus; the virus that cause hepatitis B.

hCG: Human chorionic gonadotropin.

HCO₃⁻: Bicarbonate ion.

HCS: Hazard Communication Standard (OSHA).

HCV: Hepatitis C virus; the virus that cause hepatitis C.

HDN: Hemolytic disease of the newborn.

healthcare-associated infection: Applies to infections associated with healthcare delivery in any healthcare setting, including home care.

Healthcare Infection Control Practices Advisory Committee: A federal organization established in 1991 that advises the CDC on updating guidelines regarding the prevention of nosocomial infection.

heart rate: Number of heartbeats per minute, which is normally around 72 beats per minute.

Helicobacter pylori (H. pylori): Bacterial species secreting substances that damage the lining of the stomach and cause chronic gastritis, which can lead to peptic ulcer disease.

hematocrit (Hct): Percentage by volume of red blood cells in whole blood.

hematoma: A swelling or mass of blood (often clotted) such as that caused by blood leaking from a blood vessel during or following venipuncture.

hematopoiesis: *see* hemopoiesis.

hemoconcentration: A decrease in the fluid content of the blood, with a subsequent increase in nonfilterable large molecule, or protein-based blood components such as red blood cells.

hemoglobin (Hgb or Hb): An iron-containing pigment in RBCs that enables them to transport oxygen and carbon dioxide and also gives them their red color.

hemolysis: Damage or destruction of RBCs and release of hemoglobin into the fluid portion of a specimen, causing the serum color to range from pink (slight hemolysis) to red (gross hemolysis).

hemolytic disease of the newborn (HDN): Destruction of RBCs of an Rh-positive fetus by Rh antibodies produced by an Rh-negative mother, which cross the placenta into the fetal circulation.

hemolyzed: The condition of serum or plasma that contains hemoglobin from broken RBCs.

hemopoiesis: Production and development of blood cells and other formed elements, normally in the bone marrow.

hemostasis: Process by which the body stops the leakage of blood from the vascular system after injury; also known as the coagulation process.

hemostatic plug: Blood clot formed from blood cells and platelets trapped in a network of fibrin strands.

heparin: Anticoagulant that prevents clotting by inhibiting thrombin formation.

heparin lock: A catheter or cannula with a stopcock or cap and a diaphragm to provide access for administering medication or drawing blood.

heparin management test (HMT): A test used in monitoring high-dose heparin, needed in catheterization laboratories and during surgery.

HICPAC: Healthcare Infection Control Practices Advisory Committee.

HIPAA: Health Insurance Portability and Accountability Act.

histologic/histological: Pertaining to the microscopic structure of tissue.

HIV: Human immunodeficiency virus.

HMOs: Health maintenance organizations.

HMT: Heparin management test.

homeostasis: The "steady state" (state of equilibrium or balance) of the internal environment of the body, which is maintained through feedback and regulation in response to internal and external changes.

hormones: Powerful chemical substances that affect many body processes.

hospice: A type of care for patients who are terminally ill.

HPC: Handheld PC.

H. pylori: *Helicobacter pylori.*

hub: The end of the needle that attaches to the blood collection device; also the threaded end of a tube holder where the needle attaches.

human chorionic gonadotropin (HCG or hCG): Hormone that appears in both urine and serum beginning approximately 10 days after conception. HCG is the substance detected in pregnancy tests.

human immunodeficiency virus (HIV): The virus that causes acquired immunodeficiency syndrome (AIDS).

hyperglycemia: A condition in which the level of sugar (glucose) in the blood is high, as in diabetes mellitus.

hyperkalemia: A high concentration of potassium in the blood.

hypernatremia: A high level of sodium in the blood.

hypersecretion: Secreting too much.

hypodermic needle: The type of needle used with the syringe system.

hypoglycemia: Condition in which the level of sugar (glucose) in the blood is low.

hypokalemia: A low concentration of potassium in the blood.

hyponatremia: A low level of sodium in the blood.

hyposecretion: Secreting too little.

hypothyroidism: A disorder characterized by insufficient levels of thyroid hormones.

hypoxemia: A low level of oxygen in the blood.

IACET: International Association for Continuing Education and Training.

IATA: International Air Transport Association.

iatrogenic: An adjective used to describe an adverse condition brought on by the effects of treatment.

iCa²⁺: Ionized calcium.

ICD-9-CM: International Classification of Diseases, Ninth Revision, Clinical Modification.

ICD-10-PCS: International Classification of Diseases, Tenth Revision, Procedural Coding System.

icons: Images used to request the appropriate programs or functions on a computer.

icteric: A term meaning "marked by jaundice"; used to describe serum, plasma, or urine specimens that have an abnormal deep-yellow to yellow-brown color due to high bilirubin levels.

icterus: Also called jaundice; a condition characterized by a high bilirubin (a product of the breakdown of red blood cells) level in the blood, leading to deposits of yellow bile pigment in the skin, mucous membranes, and sclerae (whites of the eyes), giving the patient a yellow appearance.

ID band/bracelet: Identification band/bracelet.

ID card: Clinic-issued patient identification document.

ID code: Unique identification for users.

IDS: Integrated healthcare delivery system.

immune: Protected from or resistant to a particular disease or infection because of the development of antibody through vaccination or recovery from the disease.

implanted port: A small chamber attached to an indwelling line that is surgically implanted under the skin in the upper chest or arm.

indirect contact transmission: Transmission of an infectious agent that occurs when a susceptible host touches contaminated objects such as patient bed linens, clothing, or wound dressings.

indwelling line: Another name for central venous catheter (CVC).

infant respiratory distress syndrome (IRDS): A respiratory condition in a premature infant caused by a deficiency of surfactant, which causes the alveoli to collapse.

infection: Invasion of the body by a pathogenic microorganism, resulting in injurious effects or disease.

infectious agent: The pathogen responsible for causing an infection; also called the causative agent.

inferior: Beneath, lower, or away from the head; also called caudal.

inflammation: Tissue reaction to injury, such as redness or swelling.

informed consent: Implies voluntary and competent permission for a medical procedure, test, or medication.

input: To enter data into a computer.

INR: International normalized ratio.

integrated: Connecting a network of computers with the appropriate "middleware" (software).

integument: Covering or skin.

integumentary system: The skin and its appendages, including the hair and nails; also referred to as the largest organ of the body.

interatrial septum: The partition that separates the right and left atria.

interface: Connect for the purpose of interaction.

internal respiration: Exchange of respiratory gases between the blood and cells in the tissues.

internal/deep: Within or near the center of the body.

interstitial fluid: Fluid in the tissue spaces between the cells.

interventricular septum: The partition that separates the right and left ventricles.

intracellular fluid: Fluid within the cells.

intravascular: Within the blood vessels.

intravenous (IV): Of, pertaining to, or within, a vein.

intravenous (IV) line: A catheter inserted in a vein to administer fluids and simply referred to as an IV.

intrinsic pathway: Coagulation pathway involving coagulation factors circulating within the bloodstream.

invasion of privacy: Violation of one's right to be left alone.

ionized calcium (iCa²⁺): Form of calcium used by the body for such critical functions as muscular contraction, cardiac function, transmission of nerve impulses, and blood clotting.

iontophoresis: Electrical stimulation from electrodes placed on the skin. Used in the production of sweat in the sweat chloride test.

IQCP: Individualized Quality Control Plan.

isolation procedures: Procedures intended to separate patients with certain transmissible infections from contact with others.

jaundice: Also called icterus; a condition characterized by increased bilirubin (a product of the breakdown of red blood cells) in the blood, leading to the deposition of yellow bile pigment in the skin, mucous membranes, and sclerae (whites of the eyes), giving the patient a yellow appearance.

Joint Commission on the Accreditation of Healthcare Organizations (JCAHO): A voluntary, nongovernmental agency, presently referred to as the Joint Commission, charged with (among other things) establishing standards for the operation of healthcare facilities and services.

K$^+$: Potassium.

keratinized: Having become hardened.

kidneys: Organs that form and excrete urine.

kinesics: The study of nonverbal communication.

kinesic slip: When the verbal and nonverbal messages do not match.

lactate: A form of lactic acid that is used as a marker of the severity of metabolic acidosis and a patient's stress response.

LAN: Local area network.

lancet: A sterile, disposable, sharp-pointed or bladed instrument that either punctures or makes an incision in the skin to obtain capillary blood specimens for testing.

large intestine: Part of the digestive system where undigested food is stored, formed into feces, and eliminated; also where normal intestinal bacteria act on food residue to produce vitamin K and some of the B-complex vitamins.

larynx: The enlarged upper end of the trachea that houses the vocal cords, the ends of which mark the division between the upper and lower respiratory tract.

lateral: Toward the side.

leukocytes: White blood cells (WBCs); nucleus-containing blood cells whose main function is to combat infection and remove disintegrated tissue.

leukopenia: An abnormal decrease of WBCs in the circulating blood.

lipase: Digestive enzyme secreted by the pancreas.

lipemia: Increased lipid content in the blood.

lipemic: Describing serum or plasma that appears milky (cloudy white) or turbid due to high lipid content.

LIS: Laboratory information system.

liter: The basic unit of volume in the metric system, which is equivalent to 1,000 mL.

liver: Accessory organ of the digestive system that stores glycogen, detoxifies harmful substances, secretes bile, and breaks down protein.

L/M: Liters per minute, as in oxygen therapy.

Lookback: Program that requires all components of a unit of blood to be traceable back to the donor and that also requires notification to all blood recipients when a donor for a blood product they have received has turned positive for a transmissible disease.

Luer adapter: In the Luer-Lok system, a device for connecting the syringe to the needle; when locked into place, it ensures a secure fit.

lumbar (spinal) puncture: Procedure in which a physician inserts a special needle into the spinal cavity to extract spinal fluid.

lumen: The inner space of a blood vessel or tube.

lungs: Organs that house the bronchial branches and the alveoli, where gas exchange takes place.

lymph: Lymphatic system fluid derived from excess tissue fluid; similar in composition to plasma. Also an abbreviation for lymphocyte.

lymph nodes: Structures of the lymphatic system that contain special tissue that traps and destroys both bacteria and foreign matter; lymph nodes also function in the production of lymphocytes.

lymphatic system: A system of vessels, nodes, and ducts that collect and filter excess tissue fluid, called lymph, and returns it to the venous system.

lymphocytes (lymphs): Normally the second most numerous WBCs and the most numerous agranulocytes. Two main types of lymphocytes are T lymphocytes and B lymphocytes.

lymphostasis: Obstruction or stoppage of normal lymph flow.

lyse: To kill or destroy, as in ruptured rbcs.

lysis: Rupturing, as in the bursting of red blood cells.

malpractice: A type of negligence committed by a professional.

mastectomy: Breast excision or removal.

material safety data sheet (MSDS): A written document containing general information as well as precautionary and emergency information for any product with a hazardous warning on the label.

MCOs: Managed care organizations.

measurand: The quantity or amount of a substance being measured.

medial: Toward the midline or middle.

median cubital vein: The preferred vein for venipuncture, located in the middle of the antecubital fossa.

median cutaneous nerve: A major motor and sensory nerve in the arm that lies along the path of the brachial artery and near the basilic vein.

Medicaid: A federal and state program that provides medical assistance for low-income Americans.

Medical Laboratory Scientist: A new ASCP designation for a person who generally has a bachelor's (BS)

degree plus additional studies and experience in the clinical laboratory setting. As of October 23, 2009, all CLS (NCA) certificants who had an active credential with NCA were transferred to the ASCP and the NCA merged Board of Certification as MLS (ASCP).

medical terminology: Special vocabulary of the health professions.

Medicare: Federally funded program that provides health care to people over the age of 65 and to the disabled.

megakaryocyte: Large bone marrow cell from which platelets are derived.

melanin: Dark pigment that colors the skin and protects it from the sun. Also found in the hair and eyes.

meninges: Three layers of connective tissue that enclose the spinal cavity.

menu: A list of options from which the user may choose.

metabolism: The sum of all the physical and chemical reactions necessary to sustain life.

meter: The basic unit of linear measurement in the metric system; equal to 39.37 inches.

microbe: Short for microorganism; a microscopic organism or one that is not visible to the naked eye.

microbiocidal: Destructive to microbes.

microclot: A tiny clot or thrombus that may not be visible to the naked eye.

microcollection containers: Small plastic tubes used to collect the tiny amounts of blood obtained from capillary punctures; also called capillary tubes and microtubes and sometimes referred to as "bullets" because of their size and shape.

microhematocrit tubes: Disposable, narrow-bore plastic or plastic-clad glass capillary tubes that fill by capillary action.

microtubes: Special small plastic tubes used to collect the tiny amounts of blood obtained from capillary punctures. Also called microcollection containers.

middleware: Term for any software that serves to "glue together" two separate, already existing programs.

midsagittal plane: Divides the body vertically into equal right and left portions.

midstream: Term applied to urine collection in which the specimen is collected in the middle of urination rather than at the beginning or end.

military time: Also called European time; based on a clock with 24 numbers instead of 12, eliminating the need to designate A.M. or P.M.

mitosis: A type of cell duplication that involves DNA doubling and cell division.

MLS: Medical Laboratory Scientist.

mnemonic: Memory-aiding code or abbreviation, as used in LIS, for example.

modem: Device that enables a computer to transmit data over telephone or cable lines, for example.

monocytes (monos): Normally the largest WBCs and 1% to 7% of total WBCs, they are mononuclear phagocytic cells and among the first lines of defense in the inflammatory process.

motor or efferent nerves: Nerves that carry impulses away from the CNS.

MR number: Medical record number used for patient ID.

multisample needle: A type of needle that allows multiple tubes to be collected with a single venipuncture.

murmurs: Abnormal heart sounds, often due to faulty valve action.

myocardial infarction (MI): Heart attack or necrosis (death) of heart muscle from lack of oxygen.

myocardial ischemia: Condition resulting from an insufficient supply of blood to meet the oxygen needs of the heart muscle.

myocardium: The middle muscle layer of the heart.

Na⁺: Sodium.

NAACLS: National Accrediting Agency for Clinical Laboratory Sciences.

NASH: The National Surveillance System for Healthcare Workers.

nasopharyngeal (NP): A term referring to the nasal cavity and pharynx.

National Fire Protection Association (NFPA): Federal agency that regulates disinfectant products and the disposal of hazardous waste, among other responsibilities associated with developing and enforcing regulations that implement environmental laws enacted by Congress.

NHSN: National Healthcare Safety Network.

National Institute for Occupational Safety and Health (NIOSH): The federal agency responsible for conducting research and making recommendations for the prevention of work-related injury and illness.

National Patient Safety Goals: Part of the Joint Commission's overall CQI requirements for accreditation.

needle phobia: Intense fear of needles.

needle sheath: Needle cap or cover.

Needlestick Safety and Prevention Act: Federal law that directed OSHA to revise the BBP standard in four key areas: the exposure control plan, selection of engineering and work practice controls with employee input, modification of engineering control definitions, and new record-keeping requirements.

negligence: Failure to exercise due care.

nephron: The microscopic functional unit of the kidneys.

network: A group of computers that are all linked for the purpose of sharing resources.

neuron: The fundamental working unit of the nervous system.

neutropenic: Pertaining to an abnormally small number of neutrophils in the blood.

neutrophils: Normally the most numerous WBC in adults, averaging 65% of the total WBC count, with granules that are fine in texture and stain lavender; also called polys, PMNs, or segs.

newborn/neonatal screening: The routine testing of newborns for the presence of certain metabolic and genetic (inherited) disorders, such as phenylketonuria.

NFPA: National Fire Protection Association.

NIDA: National Institute on Drug Abuse.

NIOSH: National Institute for Occupational Safety and Health.

noninvasive: Not penetrating the skin.

nosocomial infection: An infection acquired in a healthcare facility.

NP: Nasopharyngeal.

NPO: Nothing by mouth (from Latin, *nil per os*).

NSPGs: National Patient Safety Goals.

occlusion: Obstruction.

occult blood: Hidden blood. *See* guaiac test.

Occupational Safety and Health Administration (OSHA): U.S. government agency that mandates and enforces safe working conditions for employees.

O&P: Ova and parasites; a test to detect the presence of intestinal parasites and their eggs in feces.

order of draw: A special sequence in tube collection that is intended to minimize additive carryover or cross-contamination problems.

OSHA: Occupational Safety and Health Administration.

osteochondritis: Inflammation of the bone and cartilage.

osteomyelitis: Inflammation of the bone marrow and adjacent bone.

output: Return of processed information or data to the user or to someone in another location.

ovum: Female gamete or sex cell.

oxalates: Anticoagulants that prevent clotting by precipitating calcium.

oxyhemoglobin: Oxygen combined with hemoglobin.

pacemaker: In the heart, the structure that generates the electrical impulse that initiates heart contraction. *See* sinoatrial node.

palmar: Concerning the palm of the hand.

palpate: Examine by feel or touch.

pancreas: An accessory organ to the digestive system that secretes hormones and produces digestive enzymes.

papillae (singular, papilla): Small elevations of the dermis that indent the bottom of the epidermis and give rise to the ridges and grooves that form fingerprints.

papillary dermis: The dermal layer adjoining the epidermis.

parenteral administration: Administration by any route other than the digestive tract.

partial pressure (P): The pressure exerted by one gas in a mixture of gases.

partial pressure of carbon dioxide (pCO₂): A measure of the pressure exerted by dissolved CO_2 in the blood.

partial pressure of oxygen (pO₂): A measure of the pressure exerted by dissolved O_2 in the blood plasma.

password: A secret code that uniquely identifies a person and allows him or her to become a system user.

patency: State of being freely open, as in the normal condition of a vein.

pathogenic: Capable of causing disease.

pathogens: Microbes capable of causing disease.

patient ID: The process of verifying a patient's identity.

patient sample: A portion of a patient specimen used to obtain information by means of a specific laboratory test. *See* specimen.

pCO₂: Partial pressure of carbon dioxide.

PCP: Primary Care Physician.

PCR: Polymerase chain reaction.

PDA: Personal digital assistant.

peak level: Drug level collected when the highest serum concentration of the drug is anticipated.

pelvic cavity: Body space that houses the reproductive organs.

percutaneous: Through the skin.

pericardial fluid: Fluid aspirated from the pericardial cavity that surrounds the heart.

pericardium: A thin, fluid-filled sac surrounding the heart.

peripheral nervous system: All the nerves that connect the CNS to every part of the body.

peripherally inserted central catheter (PICC): A line inserted into the peripheral venous system (veins of the extremities) and threaded into the central venous system (main veins leading to the heart). It does not require surgical insertion and is typically placed in an antecubital vein just above or below the antecubital fossa.

peritoneal fluid: Fluid aspirated from the abdominal cavity.

permucosal: Through mucous membranes.

personal protective equipment (PPE): Protective clothing and other protective items worn by an individual.

petechiae: Tiny, nonraised red spots that appear on a patient's skin upon tourniquet application. They are minute drops of blood that escape the capillaries and come to the surface of the skin below the tourniquet, most commonly as a result of capillary wall defects or platelet abnormalities.

pH: Abbreviation for potential hydrogen, a scale representing the relative acidity or alkalinity of a solution in which 7 is neutral, below 7 is acid, and above 7 is alkaline.

phagocytosis: Process in which a WBC surrounds, engulfs, and destroys a pathogen or foreign matter.

phalanges (singular, phalanx): Bones of the fingers or toes.

pharynx: A funnel-shaped passageway that receives food from the mouth and delivers it to the esophagus; it also receives air from the nose and carries it into the larynx.

phenylketonuria: Disorder that results from a defect in the enzyme that breaks down the amino acid phenylalanine, converting it into the amino acid tyrosine.

PHI: Protected health information.

phlebotomy: Incision into the vein for the purpose of drawing blood.

PHS: Public Health Service.

physiology: The function of an organism or the science of the functions of living organisms.

PI: Process Improvement (tools).

PICC: Peripherally inserted central catheter.

Pictogram: An easily recognized and universally accepted symbol.

pilocarpine: A sweat-stimulating drug used in the sweat chloride test.

pituitary gland: Endocrine gland, under the control of the hypothalamus, which secretes hormones that control other glands; sometimes called the master gland.

PKU: Phenylketonuria.

plaintiff: Injured party in the litigation process.

plantar surface: The sole or bottom surface of the foot.

plasma: The top layer of clear liquid used for testing; also the fluid portion of the blood in the living body.

platelets: Cellular elements that play a role in blood clotting. *See* thrombocytes.

platelet adhesion: The adherence (or sticking) of platelets to an injured area.

platelet aggregation: The sticking of platelets to one another.

platelet plug formation: Stage 2 of hemostasis, in which platelets degranulate and stick to the site and each other, plugging the site of injury.

pleura (pleural, pleurae): Layer of thin membrane that encases the lungs.

pleural cavity/space: A small space between the layers of the pleurae of the lungs.

pleural fluid: Fluid aspirated from the pleural cavity surrounding the lungs.

plunger: A rodlike device that fits tightly into the barrel of a syringe and creates a vacuum when pulled back in the process of filling the syringe.

PMN: Polymorphonuclear.

PNS: Peripheral nervous system.

pO$_2$: Partial pressure of oxygen.

POCT: Point-of-care testing.

point-of-care testing: Alternate site testing (AST) or ancillary, bedside, or near-patient testing, often performed using portable or handheld instruments.

polycythemia: A disorder involving overproduction of red blood cells.

polymorphonuclear: Term used to describe a neutrophil whose nucleus is segmented (has multiple lobes).

posterior curvature: Medical term for the back of the heel.

posterior/dorsal: A term referring to the back.

postprandial: After a meal.

postural pseudoanemia: A condition that is the response to a change in position from standing to lying down.

potassium (K$^+$): A mineral that is essential for normal muscle activity and the conduction of nerve impulses.

potassium oxalate: An anticoagulant commonly used with the antiglycolytic agent sodium fluoride.

PP: Postprandial.

PPD: Purified protein derivative. *See* tuberculin test.

PPE: Personal protective clothing.

PPOs: Preferred provider organizations.

PPS: Prospective payment system.

PPTs: Plasma preparation tubes.

preanalytical: Prior to analysis.

pre-examination: Prior to analysis; a term the International organization for Standardization (ISO) uses in place of preanalytical.

prefix: A word element that precedes a word root and modifies its meaning by adding information, such as presence or absence, location, number, or size.

preop/postop: Before an operation or surgery (preoperative)/after an operation or surgery (postoperative).

primary care: Care by general physician who assumes ongoing responsibility for maintaining his or her patients' health.

primary hemostasis: The first two stages of the coagulation process, involving vasoconstriction and the formation of a platelet plug.

pronation: The condition of being prone, or the act of turning the body or body part face down.

prone: Lying face down.

protective isolation: Type of isolation in which protective measures are taken to keep healthcare workers and others from transmitting infection to a patient who is highly susceptible to infection.

prothrombin test (PT): A test used to evaluate the function of the extrinsic pathway and monitor coumarin therapy.

proxemics: The study of an individual's concept and use of space.

proximal: Nearest to the center of the body or point of attachment.

PSC: Patient Service Centers.

PSTs: Plasma separator tubes.

PTS: Pneumatic tube system.

Public Health Service: One of the principal units under the Department of Health and Human Services, whose mission is to promote the protection and advancement of the nation's physical and mental health.

pulmonary circulation: The vascular pathway that carries blood from the heart to the lungs, where carbon dioxide is removed, and then returns oxygenated blood to the heart.

pulse: Rhythmic throbbing caused by the alternating contraction and expansion of an artery as a wave of blood passes through it.

pulse rate: Same as heart rate.

QA: Quality assurance.

QC: Quality control.

QI: Quality improvement.

QNS: Quantity not sufficient.

QSE: Quality system essentials.

quality assurance: Refers to processes used to create standardization for quality service or product and prevention of problems.

quality control: Specific activities and techniques that are performed to fulfill the requirements for a quality service or product.

quality indicators: Guides used as monitors of all areas of patient care.

radial artery: The artery located at the thumb side of the wrist, which is the first choice and most common site used for arterial puncture.

Radio Frequency Identification (RFID): A form of wireless-based technology for identification; it uses both a tag or label that can be applied to a product or person and a wireless scanner that can track the items or identify persons beyond the line of sight of the reader.

RAM: Random-access memory.

random-access memory: Serves as temporary storage for data that will be lost when the computer is shut off.

RBC: Red blood cell.

read-only memory: Memory installed by the manufacturer that instructs the computer to carry out operations requested by the user and is permanently stored inside the computer.

reference laboratories: Large independent laboratories that receive and test specimens from many different facilities.

reference ranges: Normal laboratory test values for healthy individuals.

reflux: The backflow of blood into a patient's vein from the collection tube during venipuncture.

requisition: The form on which test orders are entered and sent to the laboratory.

res ipsa loquitur: A Latin phrase meaning "the thing speaks for itself."

reservoir: The source of an infectious microorganism.

resheathing devices: Equipment such as shields that cover a needle after use.

respondeat superior: A Latin phrase meaning "let the master respond." In other words, employers must answer for damages their employees cause within the scope of their practice.

reticulocytes (retics): Immature RBCs in the bloodstream that contain remnants of material from the nuclear phase.

reverse isolation: Same as protective isolation.

RFID: Radio Frequency Identification.

Rh blood group system: Blood group based on the presence or absence of an RBC antigen called the D antigen, also known as Rh factor.

Rh factor: Antigen called the D antigen, which is the basis for the Rh blood group system.

Rh negative (Rh–): Rh blood type of an individual whose RBCs lack the D antigen.

Rh positive (Rh+): Rh blood type of an individual whose RBCs have the D antigen.

risk management: An internal process focused on identifying and minimizing situations that pose risk to patients and employees.

ROM: Read-only memory.

router: A networking device that is customized to the tasks of routing and forwarding information through two or more network interfaces.

sagittal plane: The plane that divides the body vertically into right and left portions.

saline lock: A catheter or cannula that is often placed in a vein in the lower arm above the wrist to provide access for administering medication or drawing blood and that can be left in place for up to 48 hours. It is periodically flushed with saline or heparin to prevent clotting.

salivary glands: The glands that secrete saliva, which moistens food and contains enzymes that begin the digestion of starch.

sample: As defined by the CLSI, one or more parts taken from a system and intended to provide information on the system, often to serve as a basis for decision on the system or its production.

sclerosed: Hardened.

SDS: Safety Data Sheets.

sebaceous glands: Oil-secreting glands in the skin.

secondary care: Care by a physician (specialist) who can perform out-of-the-ordinary procedures in outpatient facilities.

secondary hemostasis: Stages 3 and 4 of the coagulation process, which involve fibrin clot formation and the ultimate dissolution of the clot after healing has occurred, respectively.

semilunar valves: Valves at the exits of the ventricles that are crescent shaped, like the moon (Latin, *luna*).

sensory or afferent nerves: Nerves that carry impulses to the CNS.

septa (singular, septum): Partitions consisting mostly of myocardium that separate the right and left chambers of the heart.

septicemia: Microorganisms or their toxins in the blood.

serous fluid: Pale-yellow, watery fluid found between the double-layered membranes that enclose the pleural, pericardial, and peritoneal cavities.

serum: Normally a clear pale-yellow fluid that can be separated from a clotted blood specimen and has the same composition as plasma except that it does not contain fibrinogen.

sex cells: Gametes.

shaft: The long cylindrical portion of a needle.

sharps container: A special puncture-resistant, leak-proof, disposable container used to dispose of used needles, lancets, and other sharp objects.

short draw: An underfilled or partially filled tube.

short-draw tubes: Tubes designed to be filled only partially without compromising test results.

shunt: A bypass of fluid to another fluid-containing system by forming a fistula, that is often done for dialysis.

silica: Glass particles used to enhance the coagulation process; a clot activator.

sinoatrial (SA) node: The structure that generates the electrical impulse that initiates heart contraction; also called the pacemaker.

skin antisepsis: Destruction of microorganisms on the skin.

small intestine: The longest part of the digestive tract where absorption of digested food, water, and minerals takes place.

sodium (Na$^+$): An extracellular ion in the blood plasma that helps maintain fluid balance.

sodium citrate: An anticoagulant that prevents clotting by binding calcium and is used for coagulation tests because it does the best job of preserving the coagulation factors.

sodium fluoride: An additive that preserves glucose and inhibits the growth of bacteria.

sodium polyanethol sulfonate (SPS): An anticoagulant used in blood culture collection that also reduces the action of a protein called complement, which destroys bacteria, slows down phagocytosis (ingestion of bacteria by leukocytes), and reduces the activity of certain antibiotics.

software: Programming or coded instruction required to control the hardware used in processing data.

solutes: Dissolved substances.

specimen (blood): As defined by the CLSI, the discrete portion of blood taken for examination, study, or analysis of one or more quantities or characteristics to determine the character of the whole. *See* patient sample.

spermatozoa: Male gametes or sex cells.

sphygmomanometer: Blood pressure cuff; a device used to measure blood pressure.

spinal cavity: Body space that houses the spinal cord.

sputum: Mucus or phlegm ejected from the trachea, bronchi, and lungs by deep coughing.

squamous: Scalelike.

SSTs: Serum separator tubes.

standard of care: The normal level of skill and care that a healthcare practitioner would be expected to practice to provide due care for patients.

standard precautions: Precautions intended to minimize the risk of infection transmission when caring for all patients regardless of their status. They apply to blood, *all* body fluids (including all secretions and excretions except sweat, whether or not they contain visible blood), nonintact skin, and mucous membranes.

stat: Immediately (from the Latin *statim*, meaning "immediately").

statute of limitations: A law setting the length of time after an alleged injury in which the injured person is permitted to file a lawsuit.

steady state: Stable condition required before obtaining blood gas specimens; that is, a condition in which there has been no exercise, suctioning, or respirator change for at least 20 to 30 minutes.

stomach: Organ of the digestive tract that mixes food with digestive juices and moves it into the small intestine.

storage: The preservation of data outside the CPU.

stratified: Arranged in layers.

stratum germinativum: Deepest layer of the epidermis; also called the stratum basale.

subcutaneous: Beneath the skin.

subcutaneous layer: A layer of connective and adipose (fat) tissue that connects the skin to the surface muscles.

sudoriferous glands: Sweat-secreting glands in the skin.

suffix: A word ending that comes after a word root and either changes or adds to the meaning of the word root.

superior: Higher, above, or toward the head; also called cranial.

supination: The condition of being supine or the act of turning the body or body part face up.

supine: Lying on the back with the face up.

Suprapubic aspiration: Term used to describe a way of obtaining a urine specimen by inserting a needle directly into the urinary bladder and aspirating (withdrawing by suction) the urine directly from the bladder into a sterile syringe.

surfactant: A substance that coats the walls of the alveoli, lowering the surface tension and helping to keep the alveoli inflated.

susceptible host: An individual who has little resistance to an infectious agent.

sweat chloride: A test that involves the stimulation of sweat production by electrical means and then collecting the sweat and measuring its chloride content to diagnose cystic fibrosis.

syncope (sin' ko-pe): Medical term for fainting—the loss of consciousness and postural tone that results from insufficient blood flow to the brain.

synovial fluid: Viscid (sticky), colorless fluid found in joint cavities.

syringe system: A sterile safety needle, a disposable plastic syringe, and a syringe transfer device.

syringe transfer device: A special piece of equipment used to safely transfer blood from a syringe into ETS tubes.

systemic circulation: The vascular pathway that carries oxygenated blood from the heart, along with nutrients, to all the cells of the body and then returns the blood to the heart, carrying carbon dioxide and other waste products of cellular metabolism.

systole: Contracting phase of the cardiac cycle.

systolic pressure: Pressure in the arteries during contraction of the ventricles.

tachycardia: Fast heart rate; over 100 beats per minute.

TAT: Turnaround time.

TDM: Therapeutic drug monitoring.

terminal: A computer screen and keyboard.

tertiary care: Highly complex care and therapy services from practitioners in a hospital or overnight facility.

TGC: Tight glycemic index.

therapeutic drug monitoring (TDM): Testing of drug levels at specific intervals to help establish a drug dosage, maintain the dosage at a therapeutic (beneficial) level, and avoid drug toxicity.

third-party payer: An insurance company or government program that pays for healthcare services on behalf of a patient.

thixotropic gel: An inert (nonreacting) synthetic gel substance in some ETS tubes (e.g., SSTs, PSTs, and PPTs) that forms a physical barrier between the cells and serum or plasma when the specimen is centrifuged.

TJC: The Joint Commission

thoracic cavity: Body space above the diaphragm that houses the heart and lungs.

threshold values: The level of acceptable practice beyond which quality patient care cannot be assured.

thrombin: An enzyme that converts fibrinogen into the fibrin necessary for clot formation.

thrombocytes: Medical term for platelets—cellular elements that play a role in the coagulation process and are the smallest of the formed elements.

thrombocytopenia: Decreased platelets.

thrombocytosis: Increased platelets.

thrombophlebitis: Inflammation of a vein, particularly in the lower extremities, along with thrombus formation.

thrombosed: Clotted—refers to a vessel that is affected by clotting.

tight glycemic index: Intensive insulin therapy that involves frequent monitoring of a patient's glucose level and administering insulin as required to keep glucose levels in a predetermined normal range and avoid hyperglycemia.

tissue thromboplastin: A substance present in tissue fluid that activates the extrinsic coagulation pathway and can interfere with coagulation tests when picked up by the needle during venipuncture.

TnI: Troponin I, a protein specific to heart muscle used in diagnosing an acute myocardial infarction (AMI) or heart attack.

TnT: Troponin T, a protein specific to heart muscle used in diagnosing a heart attack and also to monitor the effectivenesss of thrombolytic therapy.

tort: A wrongful act other than breach of contract committed against one's person, property, reputation, or other legally protected right.

tourniquet: A device (typically a flat strip of stretchable material) applied to a limb prior to venipuncture to restrict venous flow, which distends the veins and makes them easier to find and pierce with a needle.

trace element–free tubes: Tubes made of materials that are as free of trace-element contamination as possible.

trachea: A tube that extends from the larynx into the upper part of the chest and carries air to the lungs.

transfusion reaction: An adverse reaction between donor cells and the recipient.

transmission-based precautions: Precautions used in addition to standard precautions for patients known or suspected to be infected or colonized with highly transmissible or epidemiologically significant pathogens.

transverse plane: The plane that divides the body horizontally into equal upper and lower portions.

trough level: Drug level collected when the lowest serum concentration of the drug is expected, usually immediately prior to administration of the next scheduled dose.

trypsin: Digestive enzyme.

tube additive: Any substance placed within a tube other than the tube stopper or the coating of the tube.

tube holder: A clear plastic disposable cylinder with a small threaded opening at one end (the hub) where the needle is screwed into it and a large opening at the other end where an evacuated collection tube is placed.

tuberculin (TB) test: Tuberculosis test; also called PPD test. *See* PPD.

tunica adventitia: The outer layer of a blood vessel, made up of connective tissue and thicker in arteries than veins; also called the tunica externa.

tunica intima: The inner layer or lining of a blood vessel; made up of a single layer of endothelial cells, a basement membrane, a connective tissue layer, and an elastic internal membrane; also called the tunica interna.

tunica media: The middle layer of a blood vessel, made up of smooth muscle tissue and some elastic fibers and much thicker in arteries than in veins.

twenty-four–hour urine: Pooled urine specimen collected over a period of 24 hours, usually beginning in the morning.

UA: Urinalysis.

ulnar artery: Artery located on the medial aspect or little-finger side of the wrist.

unique plural endings: Plural forms of medical terms that follow the rules of the Greek or Latin languages from which they originated.

universal precautions (UP): Precautions established by the CDC and adopted by OSHA to prevent patient-to-personnel transmission of infection from bodily fluids. Under UP, blood and certain bodily fluids of *all* individuals are considered potentially infectious.

ureters: Ducts (tubes) that carry urine from the kidneys to the urinary bladder.

urethra: The duct (tube) through which urine is voided from the urinary bladder.

urinalysis (UA): A laboratory test that typically includes macroscopic, physical, chemical, and microscopic analysis of a urine specimen.

urinary bladder: A muscular sac that serves as a reservoir for urine.

urinary tract infection (UTI): Ailment caused by the presence of microorganisms in one or more structures of the urinary system.

USB drive: Universal Serial Bus; a device used for storing information.

uterus: Muscular organ in the female pelvis in which a fetus develops during pregnancy.

UTI: Urinary tract infection.

vacuum: Negative pressure, or artificially created absence of air.

VAD: Vascular-access device.

vasoconstriction: Stage 1 of hemostasis, in which a damaged vessel constricts (narrows) to decrease the flow of blood to an injured area.

vasopressin: Antidiuretic hormone (ADH).

vasovagal syncope: Sudden faintness or loss of consciousness due to a nervous system response to abrupt pain, stress, or trauma.

vector transmission: Transmission of an infectious agent by an insect, arthropod, or animal.

vehicle transmission: Transmission of an infectious agent through contaminated food, water, drugs, or the transfusion of blood.

veins: Blood vessels that return blood to the heart.

vena cava (plural, venae cavae): Either of two veins, the superior vena cava and inferior vena, that return blood to the heart and are the largest veins in the body.

venostasis: Trapping of blood in an extremity by the compression of veins.

venous stasis: Stagnation of normal blood flow.

ventral: To the front of the body.

ventral cavities: Internal spaces located in the front.

ventricles: The lower pumping or delivering chambers on each side of the heart.

venules: The smallest veins at the junction of the capillaries.

viability: Ability to stay alive.

vicarious liability: Liability imposed by law on one person for acts committed by another.

virulence: Degree to which a microbe is capable of causing disease.

WBC: White blood cell.

whole blood: Blood that is in the same form as when it circulated in the bloodstream.

whorls: Spiral pattern of the ridges and grooves that form a fingerprint.

winged infusion set: A ½- to ¾-inch stainless steel needle permanently connected to a 5- to 12-inch length of tubing with either a Luer attachment for syringe use or a multisample Luer adapter for use with the evacuated tube; also called a butterfly needle.

word root: The part of a medical term that establishes its basic meaning and the foundation upon which the true meaning is built.

work practice controls: Practices that alter the manner in which a task is performed so as to reduce the likelihood of bloodborne pathogen exposure.

Index

Note: Page numbers in *italics* denote figures; those followed by a "b" and "t" denote boxes and tables respectively.